The Hand: Diagnosis and Indications

Graham Lister

Clinical Professor of Surgery (Hand),
University of Louisville, Kentucky, USA.

SECOND EDITION

CHURCHILL LIVINGSTONE
EDINBURGH LONDON MELBOURNE AND NEW YORK 1984

CHURCHILL LIVINGSTONE
Medical Division of Longman Group UK Limited

Distributed in the United States of America by Churchill
Livingstone Inc., 1560 Broadway, New York, N.Y. 10036, and
by associated companies, branches and representatives
throughout the world.

First edition 1977
Second edition 1984
  Reprinted 1987

ISBN 0 443 02826 5

British Library Cataloguing in Publication Data
Lister, Graham
   The hand. —— 2nd ed.
   1. Hand —— Diseases —— Diagnosis
   2. Hand —— Surgery
   I. Title
   617'.575075   RC951

Library of Congress Cataloging in Publication Data
Lister, Graham.
   The hand : diagnosis and indications.
   Includes bibliographies and index.
   1. Hand —— Wounds and injuries —Diagnosis.
2. Hand —— Diseases —— Diagnosis. 3. Hand —— Surgery.
I. Title. [DNLM: 1. Hand. 2. Hand —— Surgery.
WE 830 L773h]
RD559.L57 1983   617'.575   82–23557

Printed and bound in Great Britain by
William Clowes Limited, Beccles and London

Preface to the Second Edition

Being a confessed cynic, I have always believed that second editions are inspired more by the publisher's avarice than by the author's greater enlightenment. It was therefore with the bitter satisfaction which comes with confirmation of a suspected fault in an otherwise perfect acquaintance that I received the request for this volume from Churchill Livingstone. I did not go beating on *their* door with ink-stained hands.

But I should have done. As I reluctantly reviewed the first edition, which with groundless conceit I had believed to be carved in stone, I found more than sufficient cause to kindle embarrassment—and enthusiasm. Certain omissions had been detected by reviewers, notably Barton[1]. Some were intentional, glibly rationalised at the time, but in retrospect clearly due to ignorance. Thus the second edition contains a chapter on congenital anomalies, that most complex of therapeutic decisions, and new or expanded sections on quadriplegia, cerebral palsy, compartment syndromes, fractures new and old, frostbite and other topics previously sidestepped or only lightly brushed. Other portions of the first edition were sufficiently unclear that even I found myself confused! These have been reorganised and include amongst others the texts on sensory examination and the selection of skin cover. Advances in knowledge have occurred in hand surgery during the past six years, both general and personal, and these have been incorporated throughout, but most notably in carpal injuries, in the detection of the malingerer and in those problems which cause almost daily encounters between the surgeon and the microscope. The courteous criticisms of Linscheid[2] and Albright[3] have been heeded, most obviously in the section on muscle testing, which has been clarified and enhanced, as has the entire volume, by the drawings of Grace vonDrasek Ascher, drawings which carry a unique blend of art and information. Furlow[4] politely hinted at a significant weakness of the first edition: references which are not annotated in the text are of much less value than those which are. This mistake has been corrected. In addition, classified references to the more esoteric infections, swellings and causes of nerve compression have been added to each chapter.

Giving thanks has similarities to throwing a party, one probably generates more resentment from those unintentionally omitted than appreciation from those justly included. Therefore, while recognising and being grateful for all the help given by the office staff of Hand Surgery Associates of Louisville, I will confine my acknowledgements to the following: Dr C. S. Wheeler who provided the arteriograms together with clear and often justifiably caustic elucidation; Drs Alain Carlier and John Stilwell and Ms Irene Ward who read and kindly criticised the text; Gloria Troutman and Cara Heybach who helped to type it. Most of all, my thanks are extended to Danny Smith and his Photographic Department, to the quality of whose work the following pages testify, and to my secretary Carol Smith, who under another name also converted the first edition from illegible manuscript to impeccable type.

Louisville, Kentucky, 1984   G.L.

REFERENCES

1. Barton N 1978 The Hand 10: 110–111
2. Linscheid R L 1977 Mayo Clinic Proceedings 52: 671–672
3. Albright J A 1977 Archives of Surgery 112: 1506–1507
4. Furlow L T 1978 Plastic and Reconstructive Surgery 62: 443

Preface to the First Edition

Most texts on hand surgery, while not ignoring diagnosis, concern themselves more with the technicalities of a surgical skill only now achieving recognition as a specialty in its own right.

By contrast, the purpose of this book is to describe in detail the techniques of diagnosis applicable in the various disorders of the hand and to indicate how different findings influence the choice of treatment.

Standard nomenclature has been adopted in the main. 'Medial' and 'lateral' lie uneasily on the hand, which is probably less used in the anatomical position than in any other. They have therefore been discarded in favour of 'ulnar' and 'radial'. 'Lateral', freed from the possibility of ambiguity, has been retained to refer to the side of the digit where *which* side is immaterial to the point under discussion. 'Middle' and 'small' have been used to refer to the third and fifth digits rather than 'long' or 'little', allowing initial letters to be used in clinical records as clearly understandable abbreviations for the fingers.

Fractures of the forearm and wrist are omitted for they clearly lie in the province of the orthopaedic surgeon and present no diagnostic problems to be considered in this text. By contrast, the chapter on compression wanders far from the hand for symptoms therein may have their origins as far proximal as the cervical spine and even beyond. Repetition is used throughout, I hope judiciously, and I make no apologies for its presence. It is valuable to the writer to aid in clarity and convenient to the reader as it eliminates irritating references to other parts of the book.

When first I heard of them, I searched unduly long for a description of the Allen or the Adson test, the Phalen or the Spurling. How to test for the superficialis of the index finger or the independent action of pronator quadratus; how did one reveal intrinsic tightness or distinguish a tendon adhesion from a joint contracture? These and many other questions fascinated and frustrated my study of the hand. If this book helps those like me, then it serves its purpose. If in the process it conveys my enthusiasm for the study then that would give me great personal satisfaction, for, as Ian Donald declared in the first sentence of his text on obstetrics: 'The art of teaching is the art of sharing enthusiasm'.

Louisville, Kentucky, 1976   G.L.

Contents

1

Injury

Like facial wounds, those of the hand are gory and obvious. This may mislead the harassed casualty officer into passing the patient on to a specialist surgeon without first excluding other hidden, more critical, damage. In turn, the specialist may assume that other injury has already been excluded and proceed with treatment, at worst under general anaesthesia where visceral or cranial complications may develop unheralded by symptoms. The first responsibility of any physician is that the patient should suffer no added harm through either his attention or neglect. It is therefore essential that every doctor who sees the patient should ensure that no other more urgent injury has been sustained than that to the hand. The patient with a hand injured beneath a car or through a windscreen may have sustained steering wheel injuries to thoracic and abdominal viscera. The patient with a gunshot wound of the hand may have sustained penetrating injuries to major vessels. The patient with a traction injury to the brachial plexus may have a middle meningeal haemorrhage. With one exception, hand injuries are never fatal and that fact should dictate their priority in management.

HISTORY

In assessing the injured hand, two matters concern the examiner. In being assessed, two matters concern the patient.

The examiner must establish, comprehensively and precisely, what structures have been injured. Secondly, he must decide what immediate steps he should take towards restoration of full function. Several factors play a part in making this latter decision. These are
the number and nature of structures damaged
the irreversible loss of viability of any tissues
the precision with which the extent of this loss
  of viability can be determined
the time between injury and repair
the surgeon's expertise.

By contrast, the patient has two different preoccupations. Firstly, what effect will his injury have on his everyday life,

both immediately and in the long term? Secondly, what is to be done to his hand and will it be done competently? In short, he requires information and assurance.

At this initial contact between surgeon and patient there are only a few highly significant facts which the examiner needs to know from the patient. A long and formal history is not required, for this makes only a minor contribution to resolving the prime concerns both of the examiner and of the patient. After preliminary introductions, the history, still systematic and exhaustive on significant points, should be taken while examining the injured hand.

Nature of injury
Assuming that the surgical care offered is of good quality, nothing influences the eventual recovery of hand function more than the mechanism and the force of the injury.

What happened to your hand?
This first question is likely to elicit a general statement of the incident and will usually indicate the region of the hand injured and the nature of the injuring force. This may well require to be clarified by supplementary questions before the mechanism of injury is fully understood. For example, factory workers will tend to use technical jargon in referring to machinery and the examiner must not let this pass if he is uncertain of the implications. As the answers are received, the surgeon mentally catalogues the probable damage he will encounter.

Does it have rollers?
What are they surfaced with?
What normally passes through them?
Do they have an automatic release mechanism?
How quickly were they stopped once your hand was caught?
Are they hot?
  Roller injuries[1,2] (Fig. 1.1) commonly produce avulsion flaps, usually distally based, and of questionable viability. The viability will be further compromised by burns, either from heat or from the friction of rollers with no automatic release or arrest (Fig. 1.2). Depending on the hardness of the rollers and on the size of the gap between them, transverse or comminuted fractures may or may not be

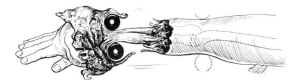

Fig. 1.1 Roller avulsion injury. The arm is drawn in by the rollers which, as the victim attempts to withdraw the limb, tear off distally based avulsion flaps.

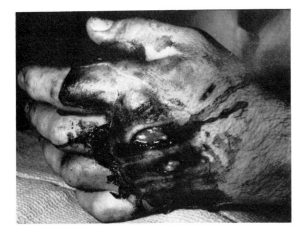

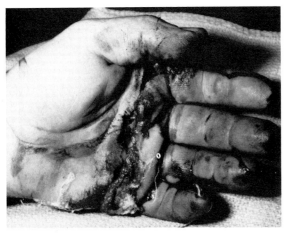

Figs. 1.2A & B Where the rollers come to rest and continue to rotate a full thickness burn is produced, the margins of which are undermined to a varying degree.

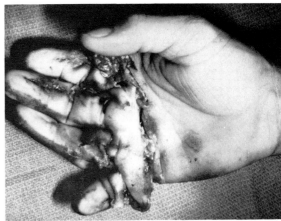

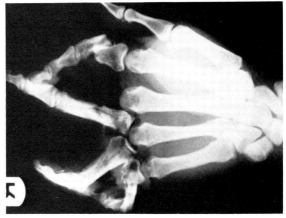

Figs. 1.3A & B The damage to the fingers distally may be so severe as to preclude revascularization.

present. Tendons and nerves may be intact and contused although either may be avulsed from proximal or distal. Vessels are likely to be disrupted or thrombosed, requiring interpositional grafts to restore flow. If the gap between the rollers is small, distal crush may be so severe as to preclude successful revascularisation (Fig. 1.3).

What roughly is the area and shape of the punch press?
What does it make?
How thick is that when it is complete?
  (i.e. *What is the space in which your hand was compressed?*)
Depending on what they produce, *punch presses* can inflict moderate to very severe injuries, more commonly the latter. Comminuted fractures, carpal disruption and soft tissue crush are the rule in the large area injuries (Fig. 1.4). In the smaller more defined injuries there is a greater likelihood of division of tendons and nerves than in roller injuries and this often at two levels, corresponding with either side of the recess.

What kind of saw?
What's the set on that blade?
  (set = amount of deflection in the saw's teeth from a straight line).
What were you cutting?
  Saw injuries resulting from a high-speed metal saw with a narrow set will approximate to a knife cut. By contrast,

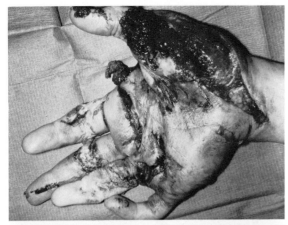
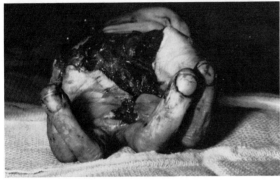

Figs. 1.4A & B Large area punch presses generate such great force as to totally disrupt the skeleton and all soft tissues.

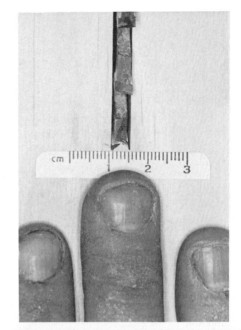
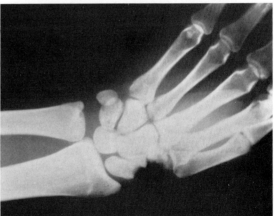

table rip saws and chain saws[3] used for heavy timber remove a swathe of all structures (Fig. 1.5), which precludes anatomical reduction of fractures and may dictate the use of grafts for all injured tissues. In addition, wide-set saws avulse as well as cut, producing damage distant from the skin wound which in particular makes revascularisation and replantation difficult (Fig. 1.6).

Does that have a sharp or a dull blade?
Did it come down squarely on your wrist or did it slice across it?
Show me the position of your hand when it slipped on the knife?

Lacerations of the hand may be produced by slicing with sharp instruments, little force being generated, or by the guillotine effect of heavy objects with a narrow edge. Lacerations both of the slicing and of the guillotine variety commonly divide tendons, which are usually under tension at the time of injury. Major nerves will be divided by a slicing wound but as they are not taut, may sustain no injury or only injury in continuity in guillotine lacerations, being pushed but not divided by the leading edge of the injuring agent.

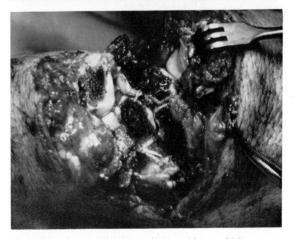

Fig. 1.5(A) Large table ripsaws have a wide set which removes a swathe of tissue (B & C).

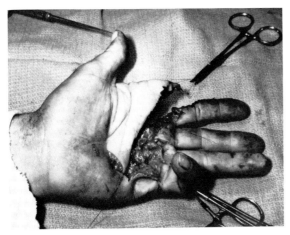

Fig. 1.6 Heavy tablesaw wounds produce devascularization which is difficult to overcome both because a segment of tissue has been removed, but also because the vessels are avulsed from proximal and distal.

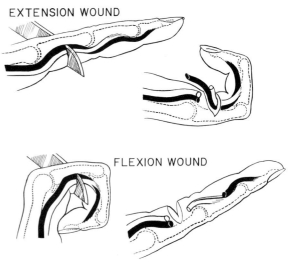

Fig. 1.7 Depending upon the posture of the hand at time of the injury, the distal tendon ends may be at the wound itself when the finger is extended on the operating table or alternatively if the finger was fully flexed then the distal tendon ends will be far removed from the skin laceration.

The relationship of the distal cut end of the long flexor tendons of the fingers to the skin wound varies according to the posture of the hand at the time of injury (Fig. 1.7). Where wrist and fingers were fully extended as in falling to the ground or warding off a stabbing attack, the free distal end will be level with the skin wound, even a little proximal to it. Where the fingers were firmly flexed as in holding a narrow-bladed knife which subsequently slipped the cut distal end will lie *distal* to the skin wound by a distance which may be as great as the maximum excursion of the tendon. Depending on age, sex, level of the wound and the finger involved, this excursion may be as much as 4 cm. In carrying out primary tendon repair, the cut distal end should be exposed and the proximal end retrieved to approximate to the distal end. The posture of the hand at the time of injury is therefore important in planning any incision to extend the skin wound.

What stuck into your hand?
What sort of an end does that have?
In what direction was it pointing?
Show me how it happened?

Penetrating injuries of the hand carry the same sinister implications of deep damage as do similar injuries to the abdomen or neck. An unimpressive skin wound may hide a remarkable amount of damage to deep structures[4]. Exploration in such situations is the absolute rule. What is to be found can often be predicted by knowing the site and direction of the injury and the nature of the wounding agent. Tapered, blunt-pointed objects may cause little damage to structures deep to the skin whereas the thin slivers of glass[5] which produce an unimpressive wound on the skin of the forearm commonly divide all flexor tendons and both major nerves (Fig. 1.8). The damage to deep

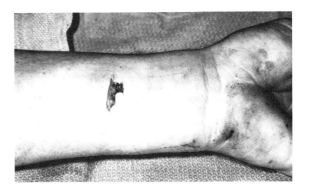

Fig. 1.8 This 2 cm wound on the anterior aspect of the forearm concealed a laceration of all eight flexor tendons of the fingers, of flexor carpi radialis and of the median nerve.

structures may be remote from the skin wound. Short, punctured lacerations over the knuckles should be the subject of deep suspicion. They are most likely to have been inflicted by a human tooth, but the victim may be unwilling to admit the fact. Such injuries are often the precursor of infection resistant to treatment (p. 231).

Pressure gun injuries (p. 73) should receive great respect. Depending upon the agent injected, they may or may not be painful immediately.[6] Whatever the patient's complaints, exploration should be undertaken and will often reveal a startlingly wide distribution of material (Fig. 1.9).

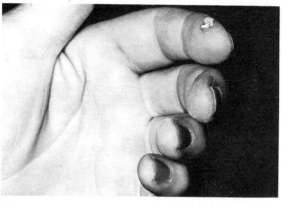

Fig. 1.9A This characteristically inconspicuous wound on the pulp of the left index finger was inflicted by a high pressure paint gun.

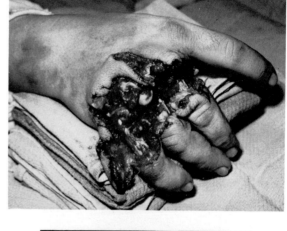

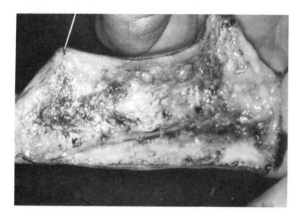

Fig. 1.9B Immediate exploration revealed that the paint had dissected along both neurovascular bundles of the index finger down as far as the distal palmar crease. Early debridement resulted in a vital digit with moderately good function.

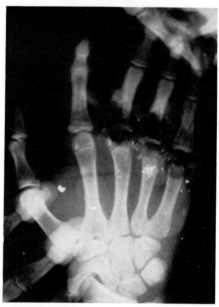

Figs. 1.10A & B This wound was inflicted by a large caliber revolver. It has removed a block of tissue from the region of the metacarpophalangeal joints.

Shotgun, revolver or rifle?
Range and calibre?

The damage caused by a *missile*[7-11] is related to the kinetic energy at the time of impact, which is equivalent to $MV^2/2$, where M = mass and V = velocity. Thus a high-velocity weapon will cause more damage than the low-velocity (a muzzle velocity of 2000 ft/sec being the dividing line), if range and caliber are equal (Fig. 1.10). Similarly, a large mass at a short range will cause a devastating injury even from a low-velocity weapon — the shot-gun is the prime example (Fig. 1.11). With a high-energy injury one should expect comminution and loss of bone, significant skin defects and a high incidence of vascular and nerve injury. Low-energy wounds, in contrast, often present as little more than a foreign body in the tissues (Fig. 1.12).

What height did you fall from?
Was there a lot of force behind it?
Did you realise you had broken something?

Very heavy falls on an outstretched hand are commonly associated with supracondylar fractures in children, carpal injuries in young and middle-aged adults and Colles fractures in older persons. Considerable direct force from a blunt object will produce a comminuted fracture, whereas mallet finger fractures and pathological fractures — most commonly through enchondromas in the hand — require very little force. The patient is often unaware in such circumstances that he has sustained an injury.

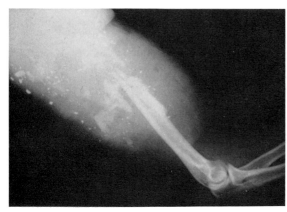

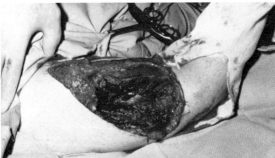

Fig. 1.11 (A) This exploded, comminuted fracture of the humerus was inflicted with a shotgun. (B) After debridement the resultant soft tissue defect extended from the shoulder nearly to the elbow.

Other mechanisms of injury have received individual study. A representative, but not exhaustive, list is shown below and the interested reader is referred to the appropriate paper.

Corn-picker[12, 13]	Woodworking tools[25]	Drug addiction[28-31]
Auger[14, 15] (Fig. 1.13)	X-radiation[26]	Snakebite[32-35]
Woodsplitter[16]	Electromagnetic	Spider bite[36]
Wool-carder[17]	radiation[27]	Karate[37, 38]
Snowblower[18] (Fig. 1.14)		Soccer[39]
Lawn mower[19]		
Sodium chlorate bomb[20] (Fig. 1.15)		
Escalator[21]		
Automobile roll-over[22-24] (Fig. 1.16)		

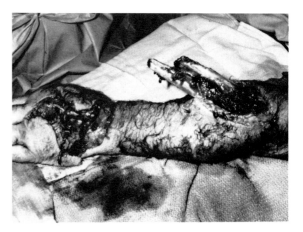

Fig. 1.13 Augers used for raising grain produce characteristic injuries which typically are multiple and separated by a distance which equals that between the spiral turns of the auger blade.

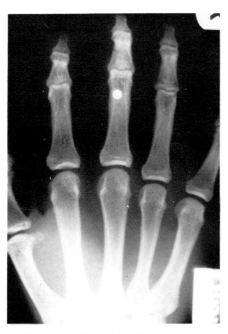

Fig. 1.12 By contrast with the high kinetic energy wounds of Figures 1.10 and 1.11, this patient who had sustained a gunshot injury presented with a small puncture wound, no loss of function and a pellet seen on X-ray.

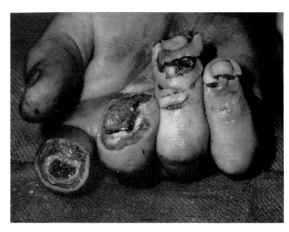

Fig. 1.14 Snow blowers and lawn mowers being of similar mechanism, produce similar injuries. The wounds are multiple, parallel, and separated by a distance which depends upon the speed both of the blade and with which the fingers were inadvertently put into the machine. Although they appear to be clean cut, there is an area of high pressure on either side of the blade which produces adjacent soft tissue damage.

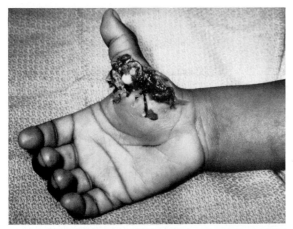

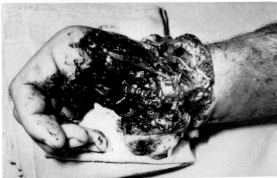

Fig. 1.15 Explosion of hand held devices, be they fireworks or bombs, produce a characteristic injury which is located primarily on the radial side of the hand. With smaller force the thumb is dislocated dorsally (A) whereas with more powerful explosives (B) the thumb is completely removed, and the radial and palmar aspect of the hand is severely mutiliated.

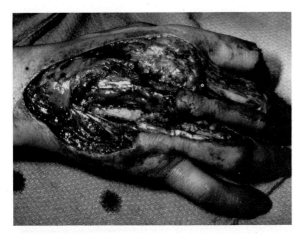

Fig. 1.16 Automobile roll-over injuries characteristically inflict deeply abrading wounds of the dorsum of the hand. The abrasion usually removes a large area of skin, underlying tendons, and the dorsal surface of the metacarpals and phalanges. This wound has been debrided, and repair of the extensor digitorum to the small finger already undertaken.

Time and injury

The time at which the patient was injured and at which the patient presented should be noted. Certain injuries require unusual expedition and should be treated as soon as they are recognised — *(in order of urgency)*

> vascular injuries producing significant haemorrhage
> hydrofluoric acid burns (p. 92)
> major vascular injury or compromise (due to fracture or dislocation) producing doubtful viability
> *macro-replantation* candidates, that is, where
> the amputated part contains significant muscle bulk
> pressure gun injuries (p. 73).

It is now recognised that there is no extreme urgency to replant parts containing little or no muscle. These have been designated *micro-replantations* and have been successfully performed in several replantation centers after more than 24 hours of *cold* ischaemia.

As emphasised earlier, hand injuries should take the place in operating room priority appropriate to their urgency. However, since there are 16 million hand injuries per year in the United States and 30% of the injuries seen in the emergency room are to the upper extremity[40], it makes good sense for management to keep at least one room staffed and free for hand surgery if the hospital has a significant emergency commitment.

If left untreated, the hand will undergo certain changes which may influence its eventual recovery of function:

1. Vessels occluded as a result of unstable fractures sustain permanent intimal damage at the site of occlusion and may require replacement; the ischaemia in the area they serve may become irreversible; if this includes muscle compartments, necrosis and contracture may result.
2. Contaminants become incorporated in the tissues.
3. Infection may become established.
4. Oedema in the hand increases, leading to
   (a) rise in intracompartmental pressures, with the consequences outlined in 1.
   (b) adoption of joint positions dictated by maximum laxity of the ligaments, namely wrist flexion, metacarpophalangeal joint extension, interphalangeal joint flexion and thumb adduction. If permitted to remain in this position, joint contractures will occur — an avoidable, and in truth iatrogenic, disaster.
   (c) friability of tissues, which will particularly hinder tendon, nerve and vessel repairs.
   (d) difficulty in skin closure, to the point of impairing skin circulation.

General health, current therapy, known allergies

Apart from scrupulously eliminating associated injuries, a brief general medical history should be obtained and examination performed, both aimed at discovering any cardiac or respiratory problems which may influence the choice of anaesthesia. Few, if any, medical conditions or drug therapies will interfere with adequate healing but uncontrolled *diabetes*, certain *skin conditions*, and *steroid intake* are associated with an increased sepsis rate, while psychiatric disorders or mental defect may severely limit postoperative cooperation. Known allergies should be recorded.

Social history

Much emphasis has been laid by some on the importance of occupation in choosing the operative procedure. This is true in reconstructive surgery of the hand and will be discussed more fully there. In the acute situation it is of lesser significance for the aim must always be to restore maximum function to the hand and to do that in the shortest time. However, with the great increase in digital replantation and revascularisation in the past ten years, the social history has assumed unaccustomed importance. The functional, economic and cosmetic factors involved in replantation must be discussed with the patient and his relatives and related to his or her individual situation. They must be told that

1. The average time off work is 7 months.
2. They have a 36% chance of having only protective sensation.
3. Motion in the joints of the replanted part will average 50% of normal.
4. Sixty per cent of patients require an average of 2.5 further operations.
5. The total cost of replantation exceeds that of revision of the amputation by a factor of 5 to 10 for a wrist amputation and 10 to 15 for a digital amputation. (These results averaged from personal unpublished data and from reports available 1/82)[41-45].

Armed with these facts a self-employed person, for example, or one with a non-compensation injury may well elect not to undergo replantation, while a child or a young woman may choose to do so.

To replant all amputated parts without concern for other factors than survival is a mechanical exercise, the work of a technician. To inform and discuss with the patient, covering all implications, even to the point of making the always arbitrary decision *not* to attempt replantation requires knowledge, time and tact. It is rightly the work of a physician.

Replantation referral

An increasing number of patients are referred for replantation over long distances involving expensive private air transport. The contraindications to replantation[46] should be carefully sought *before transfer* to ensure

that no patient, insurance carrier or Health Service incurs this expense in an ill-informed search for ill-advised treatment. The contraindications are detailed on page 00.

As the process of taking the history has been accompanied by the initial examination of the hand, a diagnosis accurate in general terms will have been made on conclusion of the dialogue with the patient. The nature of the injury should be explained in simple terms. By and large patients understand the words 'skin' and 'bones', but not 'joints', 'tendons', and 'nerves'. They do however generally understand hinges, ropes, and electrical cables and these can serve as useful analogies. Not only should the injury be described in outline but so also should the intended treatment, both immediate and secondary, and where it is to be employed, the technique of regional block. While any proposed line of treatment should be made clear to the patient, particular care should be taken to ensure that he fully understands the need for amputation, free skin grafts or distant flaps. The length of the patient's stay in hospital should be given, declared as an estimate assuming no complications. Possible complications and their management should be briefly touched upon, though not stressed unduly.

Where possible the time before he is able to return to full employment and recreation should be given in very approximate terms. The major difficulty in making such an estimate is doubtful viability. This is most likely where crush, electrical burning or pressure gun injury exists.

Where the injury is so severe that the patient is unlikely to be able to resume his former employment or recreations, this news should probably be withheld until that outcome is virtually certain and until the patient has adjusted to some extent to the fact that he has been injured.

This whole dialogue and the preliminary examination yet to be described usually takes no more than ten minutes. At the end of that time the diagnosis has been made, appropriate treatment chosen and in certain instances commenced, the patient has been informed and his anxieties allayed as far as possible.

SURFACE ANATOMY

At this juncture, when the hand is to be inspected and palpated, it is appropriate to consider where certain structures lie in relationship to surface marking and bony points. When the position of the skin wound is then considered in conjunction with the nature of the injury, suspicions will be aroused that specific deep structures may have been damaged.

The flexor surface of the wrist

There are two skin creases at the wrist. The distal crease overlies the proximal margin of the flexor retinaculum and the proximal carpal row (Fig. 1.17). The synovial sheath enveloping the flexors of the digits in the carpal tunnel extends to a point 2 to 3 cm proximal to this distal crease.

If the thumb is brought to touch the tip of the small finger and the wrist is then gently flexed, the tendon of palmaris longus stands out clearly (Fig. 1.18). This tendon lies superficial to the deep fascia of the forearm. It is absent in both hands in approximately 16% of subjects and present in only one or other hand in a further 14%. The median nerve lies beneath the fascia immediately deep to the tendon of palmaris longus, running parallel to it. The flexor carpi radialis lies deeply to the radial side of palmaris longus.

With the hand open, the proximal interphalangeal joint of each finger should be flexed in turn while observing the wrist (Fig. 1.19). It will be seen that the movement of all tendons of flexor digitorum superficialis occurs on the *ulnar* side of the palmaris longus and therefore of the

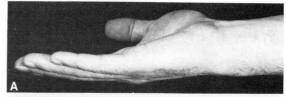
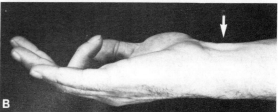

Figs. 1.19 A & B When the proximal interphalangeal joint of each finger is flexed in turn, it will be seen that all movement occurs on the ulnar side of the palmaris longus tendon producing a depression in that situation.

median nerve. The movement of flexor digitorum profundus tendons produced by flexing the distal interphalangeal joints is less easily observed but it can be palpated convincingly. Once again all movement is to the *ulnar* side of palmaris longus. Thus, *all flexor tendons to the fingers lie in the ulnar half of the wrist, together with the median and ulnar nerves and the ulnar artery.* Thus the majority of vital structures lie in the part of the wrist which is most vulnerable in falls on to sharp objects.

While attempting to flex the distal interphalangeal joints individually, a further fact will have been noted. It is not possible to flex the distal interphalangeal joints of the middle, ring and small fingers independently. This is

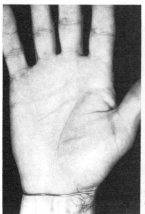
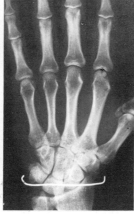

Fig. 1.17 A wire had been laid on the distal wrist crease. X–ray examination reveals the relationship of the crease to the carpus.

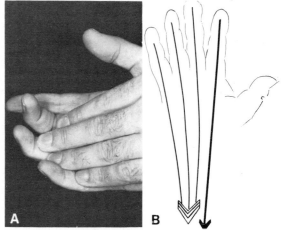

Fig. 1.20 (A) With the motion of the proximal interphalangeal joint blocked, flexion of the distal interphalangeal joint is produced by flexor digitorum profundus. This motion is invariably accompanied by involuntary flexion of the distal interphalangeal joints of the adjacent fingers. (B) This is due to the fact that the tendons of these three ulnar fingers all originate from a common muscle belly.

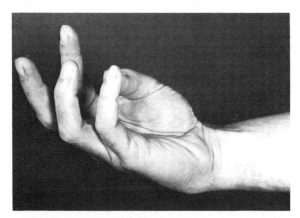

Fig. 1.18 If the wrist is gently flexed with the thumb in contact with the tip of the small finger, the tendon of palmaris longus, if present, will stand out clearly.

because the flexor digitorum profundus tendons which produce this movement have a common muscle belly (Fig. 1.20). If the fingers are now strongly *extended* and the wrist *flexed* against resistance, flexor carpi radialis and flexor carpi ulnaris together with palmaris longus can sometimes be seen and always palpated (Fig. 1.21). Flexor carpi ulnaris lies to the ulnar side of the finger flexor tendons and on its deep, somewhat radial, aspect lie the ulnar nerve and artery. The dorsal sensory branch of the ulnar nerve arises some 4-6 cm above the wrist and winding around the ulna deep to flexor carpi ulnaris it pierces the deep fascia to gain the subcutaneous tissue overlying the ulna head against which it can often be rolled beneath the finger. It proceeds distally to serve the dorsum of the hand and of the proximal phalanges of the small and ring fingers. It is at risk during excision of the ulna head.

ulnar side of the hook of the hamate lying between these bony prominences in a separate canal named after Guyon[48-51] (Fig. 1.22). The *floor* of the canal is formed by transverse carpal ligament (or flexor retinaculum, the *roof* of the carpal tunnel) and by the piso-hamate ligament. The *roof* consists of the volar carpal ligament and distally the aponeurotic origin of the hypothenar muscles, both covered by the palmaris brevis. Over this roof run the terminal branches of the palmar cutaneous branch of the ulnar nerve.[52] The divisions of the ulnar nerve finally separate in the canal and if palpation of the hook of the hamate is repeated using a firm rolling motion of the pulp of the examiner's thumb, the deep motor branch of the ulnar nerve can be felt moving from side to side over the hook. The ulnar artery leaves the nerve just beyond the hook of the hamate, turning radially just distal to the flexor

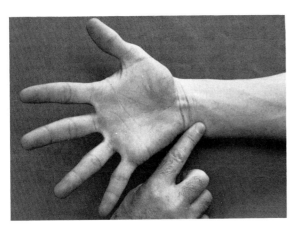

Fig. 1.21 Strong extension of the fingers produces powerful contraction of the flexor carpi ulnaris to stabilize the wrist. Since the long finger flexors are relaxed they do not obscure the wrist tendon.

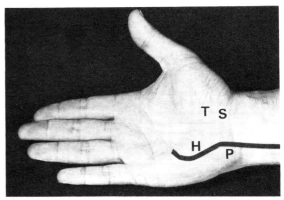

Fig. 1.22 The course of the ulnar artery and nerve can be deduced by palpating the pisiform P and the hook of the hamate H. The flexor retinaculum attaches at its ulnar end to these two bony prominences and at the radial margin to the tubercle of the scaphoid S and to the ridge on the trapezium T.

The tendon of flexor carpi ulnaris can be traced distally to its insertion into the pisiform bone which can be palpated at the extreme ulnar end of the distal wrist crease. Two centimetres distal to the pisiform and somewhat radially the hook of the hamate can be felt as a well-padded ridge proximal to the soft hollow of the palm. It lies beneath the broken crease line which runs from the junction of the palmaris longus with the wrist crease towards the small finger and which demarcates the hypothenar muscles. It lies at the bissection point of lines drawn along the ulnar side of the abducted ring finger and along the flexor surface of the radially abducted thumb — the cardinal line of Kaplan.[47] The ulnar attachment of the flexor retinaculum is to the pisiform and the hook of the hamate and therefore, all the flexor tendons lie on the radial side of these two landmarks. The ulnar nerve and artery in contrast, coming to lie on the radial side of the pisiform from their course beneath flexor carpi ulnaris, pass to the

retinaculum and superficial to the flexor tendons to form the superficial palmar arch. The vascular anatomy of the hand is subject to considerable variation.[53]

The tendon of flexor carpi radialis can be seen to the radial side of palmaris longus and traced out to the most obvious bony landmark on the flexor aspect of the wrist and hand, the tubercle of the scaphoid which marks the distal pole of that bone. The flexor carpi radialis tendon passes distal to the tubercle, immediately running to the ulnar side and beneath the overhang of the ridge of the trapezium to insert into the bases of the second and third metacarpals. This last stretch of tendon distal to the scaphoid Verdan has referred to as the 'forgotten tendon' and is the seat of inflammation in flexor carpi radialis tendinitis. It is to the scaphoid tubercle that all fingers point on flexion (Fig. 1.23). Immediately distal and somewhat radial to the tubercle lies the scaphotrapezial joint. The radial attachment of the flexor retinaculum is to the tubercle of

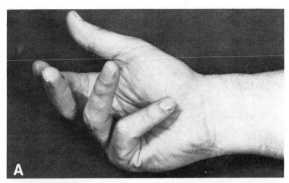

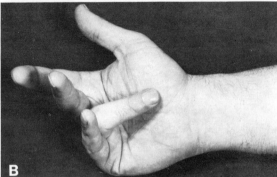

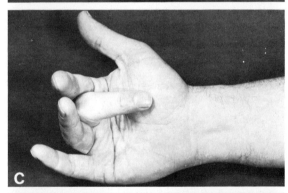

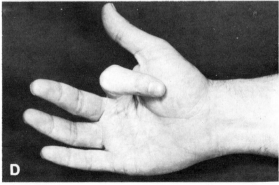

Figs. 1.23A–D All fingers on flexion at the metacarpophalangeal and proximal interphalangeal joints point to the tubercle of the scaphoid. This fact is of assistance in maintaining the correct rotation in fractures of the metacarpals and phalanges.

the scaphoid and the ridge on the trapezium. The motor branch of the median nerve, which is subject to many variations,[54,55], in most cases turns around the distal margin of the flexor retinaculum into the thenar mass. This it does at the point at which a line drawn distally from the scaphoid tubercle bissects Kaplan's cardinal line. The axis of the belly of the abductor pollicis brevis, the most important thenar muscle functionally and invariably median nerve innervated, runs from the tubercle on the trapezium to the metacarpophalangeal joint of the thumb. Between the tendons of palmaris longus and flexor carpi radialis the palmar cutaneous branch of the median nerve[56] emerges through the deep fascia some 5-6 cm proximal to the distal wrist crease to pass down superficial to the radial margin of the flexor retinaculum to serve the skin of the palm (Fig. 1.24) often as far distally as the proximal

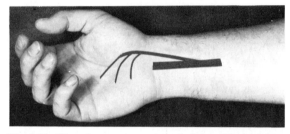

Fig. 1.24 The palmar cutaneous branch of the median nerve arises from its radial aspect some five to six centimetres proximal to the wrist, passes between the palmaris longus and flexor carpi radialis, crosses the base of the thenar eminence, and then gives numerous branches to serve the 'palmar triangle'.

phalanges. This nerve is commonly injured in release of the carpal tunnel. Beneath the flexor carpi radialis runs the tendon of flexor pollicis longus. It can be felt at this site if the wrist is relaxed in flexion and the thumb is actively flexed and extended. With this action, the muscle belly of flexor pollicis longus can be seen moving in the hollow to the radial side of flexor carpi radialis. On the belly the pulsations of the radial artery can be palpated. To the radial side of the artery the radius lies immediately beneath the skin. The insertion of brachioradialis can be felt to tighten along the border of the radius just above the styloid if the elbow is flexed against resistance in the neutral position between pronation and supination.

The extensor surface of the wrist
Distal to the insertion of the brachioradialis on the subcutaneous area of the radius a ridge can be palpated from which the extensor retinaculum passes around the dorsal aspect of the wrist to be attached on the ulnar border of the carpus to the pisiform and underlying triquetral, thus enclosing considerably more than half of the circumference of the wrist. The main bony landmark on the dorsum of the wrist is the ulnar head while on the dorsum of the radius midway between the ulnar head and

the ridge on the radial side of the wrist to which the extensor retinaculum gains attachment, a bony tubercle can be felt. Three centimetres distal to this radial tubercle in the adult hand a further bony prominence is evident. This is the base of the third metacarpal and between it and the dorsal tubercle lies the carpus. When the wrist is in the neutral position with respect to ulnar and radial deviation, the radial tubercle aligns with the scapholunate joint lying just distally.

Thirteen tendons pass beneath the extensor retinaculum in six synovial compartments. Their compartments and positions are detailed in Table 1.1.

The position of all these tendons can be confirmed by palpation during movement. It is especially difficult to distinguish the extensor pollicis brevis from the abductor pollicis longus. The former is a much narrower tendon than the latter and can be palpated on the first metacarpal just beyond its base to which abductor pollicis longus is inserted. The abductor pollicis longus invariably has several tendons. One or more of these, or the tendon of extensor pollicis brevis may lie in a separate unnamed compartment — 1A, perhaps? — which may be missed in releasing, and result in recurrence of, de Quervain's disease.

In the floor of the anatomical snuff box from proximal distally can be palpated the radial styloid, the scaphoid, the trapezium and the base of the first metacarpal. Palpation of the scaphoid should be practised by the examiner on himself for the act is mildly painful in the uninjured. If this is not realized an erroneous diagnosis of scaphoid fracture may be made on the evidence of normal tenderness. Across these structures the radial artery winds from the flexor aspect of the wrist beneath the tendons which define the snuff box to gain the space between first and second metacarpals. Overlying the artery lies the cephalic vein and bleeding from a wound in this region may be from this substantial channel rather than from the radial artery.

Running in the subcutaneous tissue overlying the snuff box and its tendons are the terminal branches of the superficial radial nerve of which there may be several, serving the dorsal surface of the thumb and to a varying degree the dorsum of the hand and of the proximal phalanges of the index and middle finger. One or more can commonly be palpated by rolling the finger over the radius proximal to the styloid process (Fig. 1.25). The radial nerve here is especially prone to injury during release of the first compartment for de Quervain's disease.

Table 1.1

Synovial compartment	Tendons	Situation
1st compartment	(1)st two tendons of 'anatomical snuff box', abductor pollicis longus and extensor pollicis	Palpable as the palmar boundary of the snuff box
2nd compartment	(2)radial wrist extensors, extensor carpi radialis longus and extensor carpi radialis brevis	These pass beneath extensor pollicis longus just distal to radius and can be palpated there with the wrist in resisted dorsi-flexion with the thumb flexed.
3rd compartment	(3)rd tendon of 'anatomical snuff box' extensor pollicis longus	Palpable as the dorsal boundary of snuff box; passes to ulnar side of the radial tubercle
4th compartment	(4)finger extensors, i.e. extensor indicis and 3(±1) tendons of extensor digitorum*	On the dorsum of the radius, between the radial tubercle and ulnar head
5th compartment	(5)th finger extensor, extensor digiti minimi, which usually has two tendons	In the groove between ulnar head and radius
6th compartment	Extensor carpi ulnaris	On ulnar aspect of the ulna, can be palpated just distal to the ulna head with the wrist in resisted ulnar deviation

*The tendon of extensor digitorum to the small finger is absent more often than not, arising as an intertendinous connection from the ring finger tendon on the dorsum on the hand.

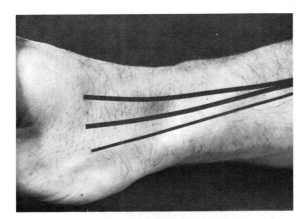

Fig. 1.25A The two or three branches of the superficial radial nerve can be rolled beneath the examiner's digit over the radial styloid beyond which the branches cross the snuff box to serve the skin of the dorsum of the first web space.

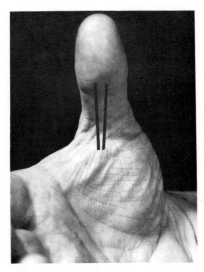

Fig. 1.26 The two digital nerves of the thumb can be palpated by the examiner in close proximity to one another on the palmar aspect of the matacarpophalangeal crease.

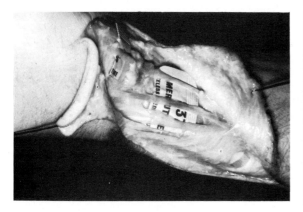

Fig. 1.25B These various branches of the radial nerve are seen together with the cephalic vein in the course of dissecting neuromata resulting from their division during release of a de Quervain's tenovaginitis.

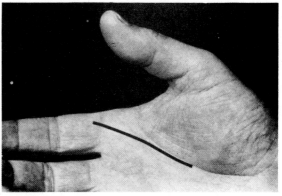

Fig. 1.27 The radial digital nerve to the index finger lies in a more ulnar position than might be supposed and can be palpated where it lies over the metacarpal head one centimetre from the radial end of the proximal palmar crease.

Palpable digital nerves

Both digital nerves to the thumb can be palpated at the metacarpo-phalangeal crease of the thumb — they lie close together over the sheath of flexor pollicis longus where they can be rolled beneath the examiner's thumb (Fig. 1.26).

The radial digital nerve to the index finger can be palpated where it lies over the metacarpal head at least one centimetre from the radial end of the proximal palmar crease (Fig. 1.27).

These three digital nerves are the most important in the hand. Ironically, they are also the most vulnerable, lying on unyielding structures and being devoid of the protection offered to the other digital nerves by the palmar aponeurosis. They are in addition those most at risk when sharp objects are grasped in the hand.

Skin creases and joints

Subcutaneous fat provides the padding on the palmar surface of the finger. It is however, absent beneath the skin creases, which are attached to the flexor sheath. This is significant in the spread of infection (Ch. 4).

The distal and middle digital creases approximate closely to the underlying interphalangeal joints, the distal tending to be just proximal to the distal interphalangeal joint, the middle just distal to the proximal interphalangeal joint (Fig. 1.28A,B). Knowing the attachments of the flexor tendons relative to the joints it is possible to deduce the likely damage to be found beneath skin lacerations in this region.

The flexor creases for the metacarpophalangeal joints are the proximal and distal palmar creases and the surface

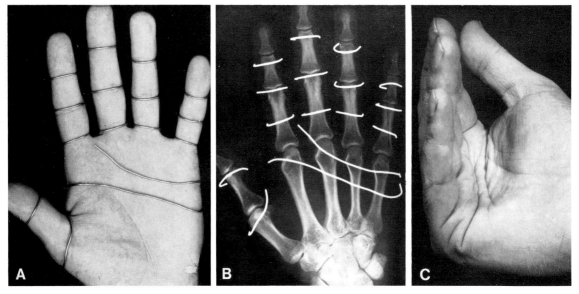

Figs. 1.28(A & B) Wires placed on the creases of a hand which was subsequently X-rayed reveals the relationship of those creases to the various joints. It will be noted in particular that the proximal digital creases do not correspond to any joint and that a line joining the ulnar end of the distal palmar crease to the radial end of the proximal palmar crease most closely approximates to the metacarpophalangeal joints. (C) Flexion of the metacarpophalangeal joints illustrates that their corresponding 'skin joints' are the proximal and distal palmar creases.

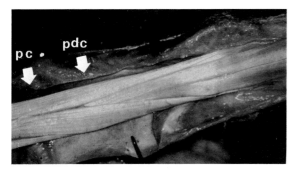

Fig. 1.29 The flexor digitorum superficialis divides beneath the distal palmar crease (PC) and the tendon of flexor digitorum profundus starts to become the more superficial of the two tendons at the level of the proximal digital crease (PDC). This relationship moves proximally when the fingers are strongly flexed. (Dissection by Dr D. C. Riordan.)

marking is a line joining the ulnar end of the distal crease to the radial end of the proximal palmar crease. This can be easily confirmed by flexing the metacarpophalangeal joints with the interphalangeal joints straight (Fig. 1.28C). The A$_1$ pulleys which constitute the proximal ends of the fibrous flexor sheaths arise from the palmar plates of the MP joints[57]. The flexor digitorum superficialis divides and starts to wind around the flexor digitorum profundus at the proximal end of the fibrous sheath, that is, deep to the palmar crease (Fig. 1.29). At the proximal digital crease,

level with the free margin of the finger webs, the flexor digitorum profundus is already becoming the more superficial of the tendons.

The long, curved thenar crease represents the skin joint which corresponds to the basal joint of the thumb and for that reason should be seen along its full length clear of the margin of any splint in which full movement of the thumb is intended.

INITIAL EXAMINATION (Fig. 1.30)

(Note that this is the first stage of examination, as performed in the emergency room or casualty department; the second is Exploration, done under aseptic conditions, see p. 59).

As already suggested examination should commence shortly after starting the dialogue with the patient. In children and in patients with more massive injuries, dressings may be left in place until after anaesthesia has been administered, for in such cases the initial examination yields no subtle information. In many other cases, where the patient, witnesses or the dressing testify to previous brisk haemorrhage which may recur, much information may be obtained by examination before removing that dressing. However, the dressings applied as a first aid measure should be gently removed at some stage in most cases, for knowledge can be gained from the site, configuration and appearance of the wound.

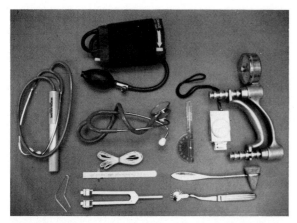

Fig. 1.30 The basic armamentarium for examination of the hand. All will be easily recognized with perhaps the exception of the instrument on the extreme left which is a Doppler flow meter and the instruments on the extreme right which are the grip and pinch dynamometer respectively.

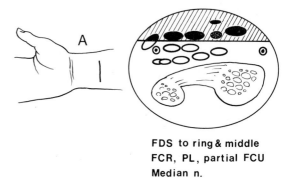

FDS to ring & middle
FCR, PL, partial FCU
Median n.

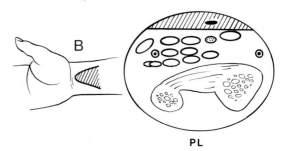

PL

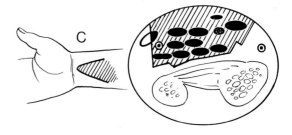

FDS to all
FDP to all
FCU, FCR, PL
Median n., Ulnar n.
Ulnar a.

The *site* leads the examiner with a good knowledge of surface anatomy to suspect which structures may be involved.

The *configuration* of lacerations can also give information (Fig. 1.31A and B). Where a slicing injury has been inflicted by a flat blade with a straight cutting edge, the wound will be more curved the more acute the angle of incidence of the blade to the skin. Thus a cut directly perpendicular to the skin will be straight and one virtually parallel to the skin will be almost a full circle, to the point of actually removing a piece of skin. Further, by mentally drawing a straight line joining the ends of the wound, the surgeon can deduce what deep structures are likely to be involved. With a straight blade, it can be generalised that the more curved the cut the longer the wound and the less deep the damage. He can also draw conclusions regarding the location of these structures relative to the wound since deep injury will always lie to the concave side of a curved wound.

After stabbing or laceration with an irregular flat instrument, such as a piece of glass, *no* prediction can be made regarding depth or extent of injury, but the direction is still indicated by the shape of the wound. This helps appreciably in planning extending incisions. The different potential of a slicing straight knife and a stabbing irregular piece of glass cannot be overemphasised and is well shown in Figure 1.31C.

The *appearance* of the wound may reveal damage to deep structures either by their presentation in the wound or, much more commonly, by the presence of dark red, gelatinous blood clot, *always* an indicator of injury to tendons, nerves, or vessels.

A point of management during examination arises. While it is probable that free arterial bleeding will not be evident

Fig. 1.31 Depending upon the nature of the cutting agent, that is, whether it has a straight or a ragged edge some conclusion can be drawn as to the nature of possible damage. (A) If it has a straight edge and the laceration is transverse, by mentally joining the two ends of the wound, the surgeon can deduce what structures will be lacerated. (B) If the edge is straight, but the wound V-shaped, then the laceration is likely to be fairly shallow. Once again, by joining the two ends some conclusion can be drawn as to the deep damage. (C) If the weapon has been ragged, such as a piece of glass or pointed, such as a knife blade, then no firm conclusion can be drawn since many structures can be damaged by the points of the instrument.

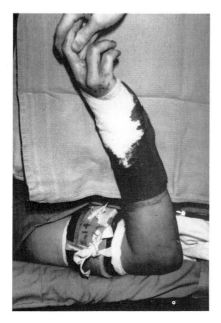

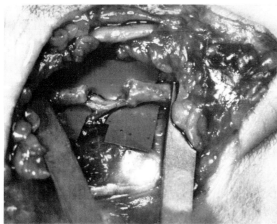

Fig. 1.32 Heavy bleeding through a compressive dressing suggests a partial laceration of a major vessel. Control of this wound required application of a tourniquet and immediate transportation to the operating room where indeed, (B) a partial injury of the ulnar artery was found.

on removing the dressing, the skin wound being filled with clot, it will occasionally be present. When free bleeding does occur it is probably due to a *partial* laceration of a major vessel (p. 37) and, as such, constitutes the only potentially fatal injury of the upper extremity (Fig. 1.32). The choice of action to control such haemorrhage which has been recommended variously is fourfold:

1. carefully ligate the very end of the vessel
2. apply an upper arm tourniquet
3. control the appropriate arterial pressure point
4. apply local pressure

Careful ligation of the very end of the vessel is a solution made attractive by its implied precision, but only to those who have never dealt with such a situation in the hand. Exposure of a bleeding vessel in the examination room sufficient to ligate it precisely requires quite unjustified exploration of the wound in conditions far from ideal and will probably result in excessive blood loss. Were it exposed, ligation could then only be achieved by the destruction of the distal portion of the proximal end of the artery. That portion may be essential for a straightforward tension-free anastomosis if vascular repair should subsequently be deemed necessary.

The application of an upper arm tourniquet in even the best ordered emergency room is fraught with the hazard of neglect and should for that reason be condemned. The tourniquet is acceptable only in that case where a collapsed patient is bleeding from a major vascular injury and is to be taken forthwith to the operating room.

To control bleeding by *digital pressure* on the appropriate pressure point — the brachial artery at mid-humerus — is acceptable and permits adequate examination preoperatively. It is not practicable or reliable during the time between examination and surgery.

Once the examination is completed using pressure point control, the bleeding should therefore be controlled by a *local pressure dressing* supplemented by *elevation of the arm*. This should be maintained under frequent supervision until the hand is being prepared in the operating room, when excessive blood loss can be prevented by the use of an upper arm tourniquet.

Description of the injury

The description of any injury usually states its *nature*, with or without qualification, its *site* and then details *deep structures* probably involved, for example, 'a punch-press injury of the left hand with multiple fractures' or 'a tidy, sliced laceration of the right middle, both flexors, radial digital nerve'.

Nature

This has largely been determined during the history and this is confirmed and refined during examination. A classification is helpful in separating those wounds and injuries likely to show healing by primary intention from those likely to pursue a more complicated course:

Tidy wounds
  incised
  sliced
    (a) with tissue loss
    (b) with flaps

  puncture

Untidy wounds
  crush ⎫
  avulsion ⎬ usually qualified by mechanism
  injection ⎭

Fractures

Finger tip
  (a) nail bed
  (b) pulp

Amputations
  (a) complete
  (b) incomplete — this implies an injury through bone and more than 50% of the skin circumference, viability doubtful or not

Tidy wounds are inflicted by sharp instruments and have well-defined edges. They are associated with little destruction of tissue and primary healing with minimal scarring results. Tendons, arteries, and nerves are commonly injured but cleanly, so that primary repair is easily achieved. Fractures are uncommon in such injuries. If they *are* present they tend to be transverse and not comminuted.

Multiple, parallel, tidy lacerations, especially on the wrist suggest a self-inflicted injury[58]. A number of small cuts beside one deep laceration suggests the same mechanism; such cuts are called 'hesitation marks' (Fig. 1.33). Indeed in any circumstance where the history does

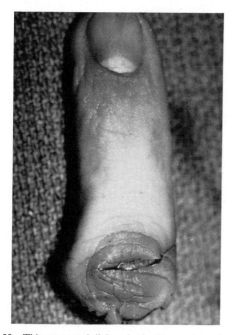

Fig. 1.33 This amputated digit arrived with a patient who it was stated had sustained an accidental amputation while alone chopping wood. Examination of the amputated part revealed a hesitation cut just distal to the point of amputation. Questioning revealed that this was a self-inflicted injury.

not fit the injury, the physician must pursue the truth. If he does not he may undertake inappropriate surgery and fail to offer appropriate ancillary treatment. Psychiatric consultation is required on all patients who injure themselves, for they need help. It may also be true that the more they object and protest, the more they need that help.

Untidy wounds result from tearing or bursting of the skin. They are caused by crush injuries, explosions and by such as rollers, power saws and farm machinery. The edges of the skin are irregular with many flaps of doubtful viability. Primary healing is less likely than in tidy wounds and extensive scarring tends to result. The full extent of injury to such patients may not be evident until days or even weeks after the accident. The nature of damage in untidy injuries is:

skin	indeterminable loss of viability
skeleton	fractures common, usually multiple and comminuted, with joint disruption
tendon	avulsion with or without loss of substance
	abrasion
nerve	avulsion
	crush ⎫
	traction ⎬ often in continuity
vessel	injury common, including avulsion
	partial tear in continuity
	thrombosis due to compression, torsion or traction

Viability

In *tidy lacerations* this is less likely to be in doubt than in injuries resulting from crush or avulsion. Depending upon the quality and integrity of collateral circulation division of the brachial artery or *both* radial and ulnar arteries may or may not result in insufficient perfusion of the distal limb. Where *either* radial *or* ulnar arteries have been divided at the wrist, the viability of the hand is not compromised. Lack of frank vascular inadequacy should by no means imply that the vessels should not be repaired, for otherwise late problems with hand function may arise from ischaemia.

In the finger, division of both digital arteries proximal to their dorsal branches will be evident from the greyish lividity of the pulp and even more of the nail bed. Vascular repair is necessary for survival of the digit. Since the digital artery lies dorsal to the nerve in the finger, division of the artery in palmar wounds is strong prima facie evidence that the nerve also has been divided.

In *untidy injuries* the paramount question, and often the one most difficult to answer is 'What tissues are viable?' No final decision regarding viability should be made until fractures are reduced and immobilized (Fig. 1.34). Torsion and compression of otherwise uninjured vessels may well arise through the instability of fractures and apparently nonviable digits may be amputated needlessly if this is not appreciated.

The *nonviable digit* is characteristically very white in colour with areas of pale violet. The pulp is collapsed and its temperature palpably lower than adjacent digits. With fingertip pressure it does not blanch and refill. Rotating the digit which is hanging loosely will not aid in determining whether or not vascular torsion or frank division is the cause of the pallor. Only exploration and fracture fixation can do so. In certain cases, however, flow *will* be improved by adjustment in the emergency room. This is especially true of the ring avulsion and the degloved skin should be repositioned pending formal exploration.

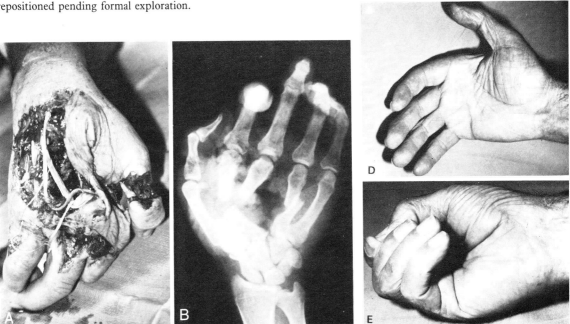

Fig. 1.34 (A) This patient sustained a massive crush injury beneath the platform of a tip-up, dumper truck which resulted in extensive metacarpal fractures and carpal-metacarpal dislocations. (B) On initial examination, all of the digits appeared to be nonviable. (C) After internal fixation of the fractures, however, flow returned to all digits without vascular repairs and two years later it can be seen (D) and (E) that the four digits survived with a reasonable return of function.

Replantation

Replantation of totally severed parts and *revascularisation* of incomplete amputations is becoming possible in an increasing number of centers.

In some the distinction is being made between two groups

Macro-replantation — the amputated part contains significant muscle bulk; speed is important; a high level of microsurgical skill and unlimited time are *not* necessary.

Micro-replantation — the amputated parts are usually digits; speed is of secondary significance; a high level of microsurgical skill and unlimited time are essential.

Certain factors have come to be recognized as *contraindications* to replantation:[59].

STRONG CONTRAINDICATIONS

1. Significant associated injuries — to torso and head; common in macro-replantation candidates (Fig. 1.35)
2. Extensive injury to the affected limb or to the amputated part — multiple level (Fig. 1.36); degloving; widespread crush
3. Severe chronic illness, such as to preclude transportation or prolonged surgery.

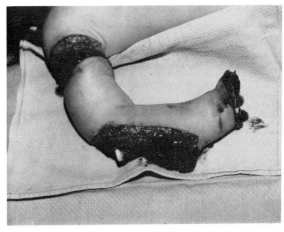

Fig. 1.36(A) This child sustained multiple level amputations and partial amputations when she fell beneath a lawn mower.

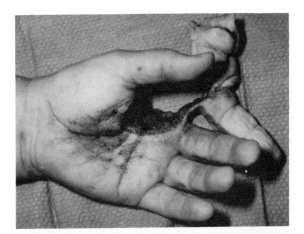

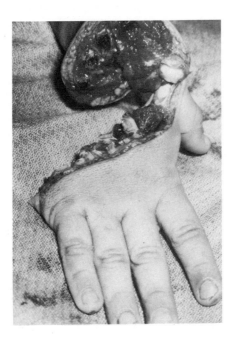

Fig. 1.35 The disc of a harrowing plow virtually amputated the right hand of this child. On arrival for replantation he was moribund, on account of an unsuspected fracture of the pelvis and retroperitoneal haematoma sustained when his body passed beneath the tractor wheel.

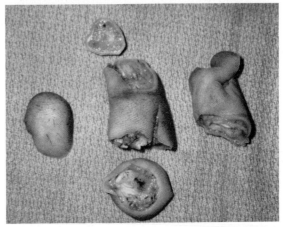

Fig. 1.36(B) Double level amputation of a single digit such as that shown here is a contraindication to replantation. (C) A common sight after lawn mower injury. These multiply amputated parts are none of them fit for replantation. When multiple parts present they should all be inspected carefully, because transplantation from one digit to another may provide function which could not be gained by any other means.

RELATIVE CONTRAINDICATIONS

These are often present in combination and therefore more discouraging.

1. Single digit amputation — especially proximal to the insertion of flexor digitorum superficialis (Fig. 1.37)
2. Avulsion injuries — as evidenced by
   (a) mechanism
   (b) structures dangling from part — usually nerves and tendons, this often indicates vessel avulsion *from* the part (Fig. 1.38 and Fig. 1.39)
   (c) 'red-streak' — bruising over the neurovascular pedicle indicating vessel disruption
3. Previous injury or surgery to the part
4. Extreme contamination
5. Lengthy warm ischemia — in practice only applicable to macro-replantation
6. Age — increased chance of vessel disease and systemic illness

SALVAGE REPLANTATION

Despite much of the above, replantation should be attempted in children or following amputation of the thumb or more than two fingers.

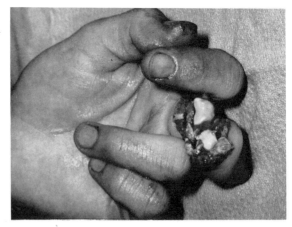

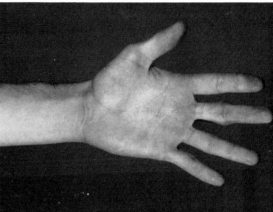

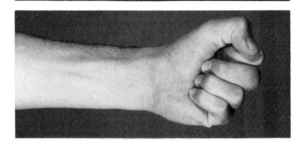

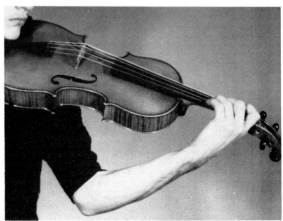

Fig. 1.37 Single digit amputation both complete and incomplete is usually a relative contraindication to replantation, however this teenager was not only skilful with a saw — as can be seen by the fact that he went through the proximal interphalangeal joint without damaging either articular surface — but was also a very competent violinist. His determination to recover resulted in perfect function. (B, C & D)

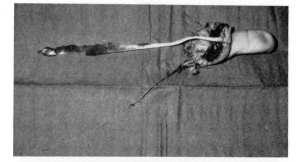

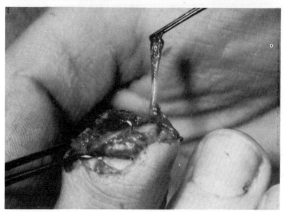

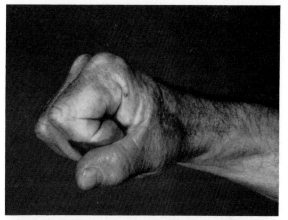

Fig. 1.38 (A) The presence of dangling nerves from these amputated parts suggests avulsion. This not only means that the eventual recovery of sensation would be unsatisfactory, but that it is probable that the digital arteries were avulsed from distally. (B) This was evident on exploration of the digit itself.

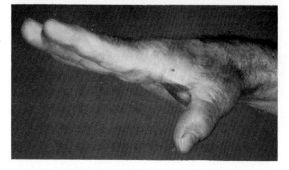

Fig. 1.39 (A) This thumb was avulsed by a zoo animal, and the long strands of digital nerve can be seen in the upper and lower parts of the photograph. (B & C) Because it was a thumb avulsion, it was nonetheless replanted employing long vein grafts. The patient at no time recovered normal sensation or motion, however the thumb functioned relatively satisfactorily.

RING AVULSION INJURIES

Other classifications of ring injuries are available[60], but that of Urbaniak et al[61] is best related to current microsurgical capabilities

Class I — circulation adequate (Fig. 1.40)

Class II — circulation inadequate: microvascular reconstruction will restore both circulation and function (Fig. 1.41)

Class III — complete degloving of skin or complete amputation of fingers (Fig. 1.42); microvascular reconstruction will restore circulation but only *poor* function; revision of the amputation is recommended, with or without a cross-finger flap to maintain competent length (Fig. 1.43).

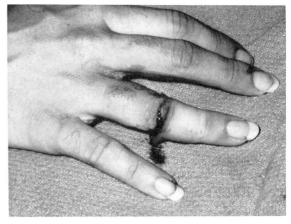

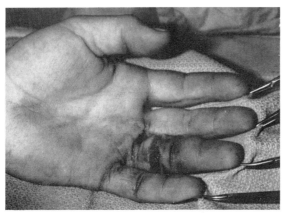

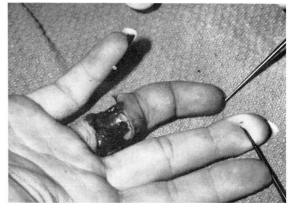

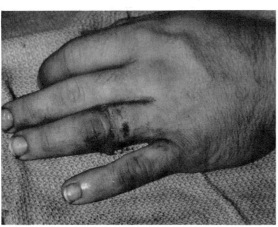

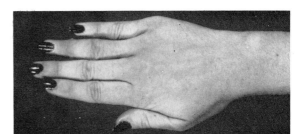

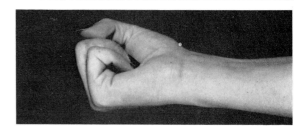

Fig. 1.40   *Class one ring avulsion.* Although the wound is circumferential, the circulation is identical to that in adjacent digits, and there was no damage to deep structures.

Fig. 1.41   (A & B) *Class two ring avulsion.* Here there was dislocation of the distal interphalangeal joint, and in addition the vascularization of the digit was compromised. (C & D) Very satisfactory function was achieved after revascularization.

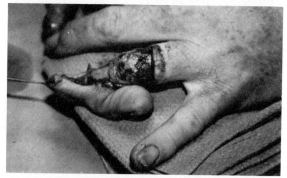

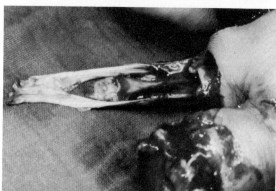

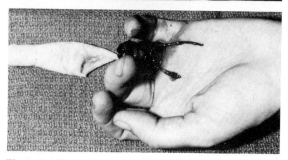

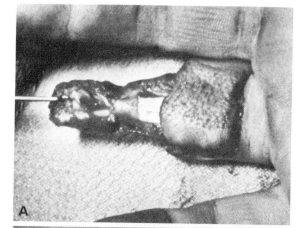

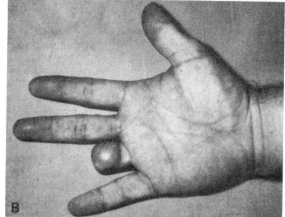

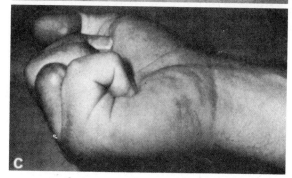

Fig. 1.42 *Class three ring avulsion.* (A & B) Although not completely removed, all of the skin of this digit has been avulsed, and there is a complex injury to the underlying skeleton. Largely due to devascularization of the underlying skeleton, the eventual functional result would be poor. (C) In this totally avulsed digit — one of two adjacent fingers damaged by rings — the entire extensor apparatus has been avulsed from the missing digit. (The incision in the upper right of the wound was for exploration of the proximal vessels which were damaged over a significant distance.) (D) Total avulsion — note long neurovascular structures.

Fig. 1.43 (A) A ring avulsion resulted in total loss of the skin of this construction worker's ring finger, the palmar defect being larger than the dorsal, as is commonly the case. A cross finger flap was raised from the dorsum of the adjacent finger and is seen here covering the proximal part of the palmar defect. Partial amputation was performed. This gave a competent hand which was functional and not unduly ugly (B & C).

Skin

Clean skin defects produced by tidy, slicing wounds can be evaluated in the emergency room and indications summarised as follows

		Defect	
		< 1 cm^2	> 1 cm^2
Bone	not exposed	NIL	free skin graft
	exposed	advance local skin	flap

The choice of skin graft and flap are considered in more detail in the section on exploration (p. 73).

Untidy wounds are much more difficult to evaluate since undermining both causes retraction of skin edges and impairs their blood supply. Thus the skin loss resulting from the injury and the skin excision necessary for adequate debridement must be finally assessed in the operating room (p. 73). Where the possibility exists the patient and family must be prepared for distant flap procedures.

Those wound margins and skin flaps which are of doubtful viability can be distinguished by:

1. *Colour.* The flap may be white or may show purplish lividity if there is an element of venous congestion. (In the congested dorsal flap, formerly doomed, a significant increase in survival has been achieved by microvascular venous repair).

2. *Design.* If the flap clearly has only a narrow pedicle it is unlikely to survive. Experience has shown that flaps raised on the limbs *surgically* have a precarious blood supply and certainly that proportions of length/breadth of 1/1 cannot be exceeded without risk of skin necrosis. Traumatically avulsed flaps have not been raised under such conditions and as a result those which exceed or even equal those proportions rarely survive. It is very important that the extent to which a flap is undermined is accurately assessed. This is especially true in roller and run over injuries where the flap may not be recognized as such, but where undermining may be very extensive and if left, much of the skin will die. The true state of affairs should be deduced from

history run-over
examination gaping wound, the edges of
which do not bleed
loss of skin sensation
exploration widespread undermining of skin edges

3. *Return of flow after exsanguination.* This is the most common clinical test of blood flow which is applied and involves observation of blood returning to the skin after its expression by the examiner's finger:

Slow return to an area of pallor suggests inadequate arterial supply;
Swift return to a purple, swollen area suggests inadequate venous drainage;
Swift return to a pink area indicates adequate blood flow.

Untidy hand injuries are often grossly contaminated, and because of this it may not be possible to assess the skin

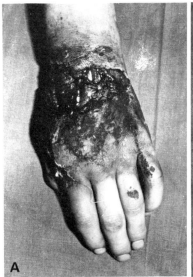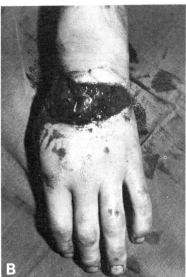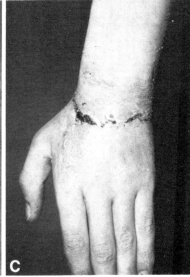

Fig. 1.44 (A) This twenty-one year old sustained a grossly contaminated injury to the dorsum of his hand when it was caught in a coal conveyer belt. It was not possible to assess the viability of the skin margins until after cleansing (B), when it became evident that skin viability was good. Suture resulted in primary healing (C).

viability with any accuracy. It may be necessary to wait until the limb has been anaesthetized and cleansed (Fig. 1.44).

In extensive injuries, especially if badly contaminated or if the treatment has been long delayed, the surgeon must be alert to the possibility of *gas gangrene*. Largely a clinical and radiological diagnosis, any evidence of gas in the tissues must be vigorously treated. Bessman and Wagner[62] drew attention to the high incidence of *non-clostridial gas gangrene*, especially in diabetics. It differs from the classical variety in that, while radical debridement is still required as an emergency measure, the extent of amputation necessary is somewhat less and cephalosporins and Kanamycin are more effective than the massive doses of penicillin required for clostridial gas gangrene. (for Skin exploration, see p. 73).

Tendon

HAND POSTURE

If the completely relaxed or anaesthetized normal hand is raised, with forearm supinated (Fig. 1.45), the weight of the hand causes the wrist to fall into some 30 degrees of dorsiflexion. The metacarpophalangeal joints lie in

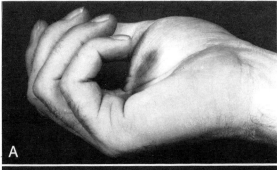

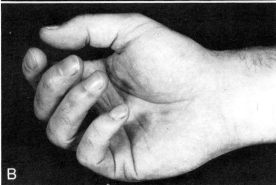

Fig. 1.45 (A) A completely relaxed hand in the fully supinated position lies with the wrist in some 30 degrees of dorsal flexion and with a 'cascade' of flexion in the fingers increasing from the index finger to a maximum at the joints of the small finger. (B) The thumb lies gently flexed so that its pulp comes to lie in close approximation to that of the index finger.

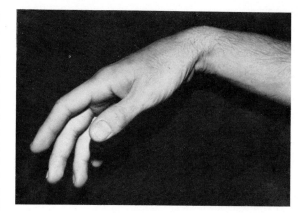

Fig. 1.46 With the arm in pronation, the wrist falls into palmar flexion and the fingers and thumb all extend.

increasing flexion from 40 degrees in the index finger to 50 degrees in the middle, 60 degrees in the ring and 70 degrees in the small and the proximal and distal interphalangeal joints adopt a similar posture. Thus, the distance from the digital pulp to the palmar crease decreases in smooth progression from the index to the small finger — the so-called 'cascade'. The metacarpophalangeal and interphalangeal joints of the thumb both lie in 30° flexion, the thumb abducted to the extent that the pulp lies closely adjacent to the pulp of the index finger.

When the unsupported, relaxed arm is then turned into pronation, the wrist falls into about 70° of palmar flexion and the fingers and thumb all extend, the thumb fully and the finger joints to within 20° of the neutral position (Fig. 1.46).

These postures in the relaxed hand are determined by the balance between the resting tone in the flexor and extensor tendons. Any change in the condition of the tendons will therefore appreciably alter the resting posture of the hand, assuming the absence of pre-existing pathology.

Complete division of all flexor tendons at the wrist (Fig. 1.47) results in full extension of all fingers in the supinated limb.

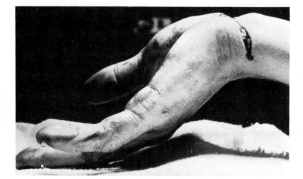

Fig. 1.47 Complete laceration of all flexor tendons at the wrist results in flaccid extension of all fingers in the supinated limb.

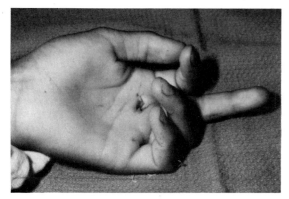

Fig. 1.48 The posture of the middle finger in this anaesthetized hand reveals division of both flexor tendons to that digit.

Complete division of both flexor tendons to one finger results in that finger lying in full extension, in marked contrast with the normal posture of those adjacent (Fig. 1.48). Division of the flexor digitorum profundus alone will result in loss of flexion at the distal interphalangeal joint. This will cause the finger tip to fall out of alignment with the others if it is an isolated injury. Lacerations of profundus do not produce hyperextension because the intact short vinculum prevents it. Such hyperextension of the distal interphalangeal joint suggests that the profundus tendon has been avulsed, a common injury sustained by players of rugby or American football, the ring finger being most often involved. This predilection has been shown to be due to a significantly weaker insertion of the profundus tendon there than in the middle finger[63]. Unfortunately, patients present late with this injury, on average over 2 months after the injury[64]. If the tendon has retracted into the palm, it should be repaired within the first week but if the end remains distal to the superficialis insertion, it can

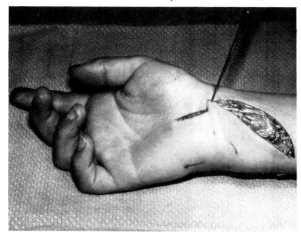

Fig. 1.49 No appreciable alteration in the posture of the finger occurs when all the superficialis tendons are divided at the wrist but the profundus tendons remain intact with the exception of that to the index.

be repaired successfully even after several months[65]. Later cases who have problems should have the distal interphalangeal joint fused.

It is important to appreciate, despite all that has been said about reaching a diagnosis on the basis of posture, that *division of superficialis tendons without injury to profundus* will result in *no* detectable change in posture (Fig. 1.49).

Division of flexor pollicis longus results in full extension of the interphalangeal joint of the thumb which, depending upon the normal range of the joint, may appear hyperextended (Fig. 1.50).

The extensor tendon division is less distinct in its effect on posture because the intrinsic muscles are responsible for much of the extensor contribution to the normal balance at the interphalangeal joints, and because of the inter-

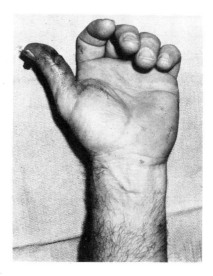

Fig. 1.50 Division of flexor pollicis longus as has occurred in this patient is evidenced by hyperextension of the interphalangeal joint.

tendinous connections of the long extensor tendons discussed more fully below. However, in an isolated injury on the dorsum of the hand the metacarpophalangeal joint may fall into more flexion than its neighbours.

Division of the long extensor tendon over the proximal phalanx will produce no postural change and little if any functional loss, as the long extensor will continue to extend the metacarpophalangeal joint acting through the transverse lamina while the lateral bands will extend the proximal interphalangeal joint. However, if the injury is not repaired, a traumatic boutonniere deformity will later result (Fig. 1.51). The presence of tendon injury will be suggested by pain on extension against resistance and confirmed by exploration.

Likewise where the extensor tendon has been divided or avulsed at its insertion into the terminal phalanx, the characteristic mallet finger deformity may not be obvious in the acute situation, developing some time later. (Fig. 1.52)

Postural changes in tendon injuries, though frequently diagnostic, are not always accurate for a variety of reasons:

1. Previous injury or disease.
2. Partial tendon division.

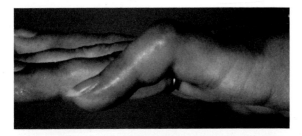

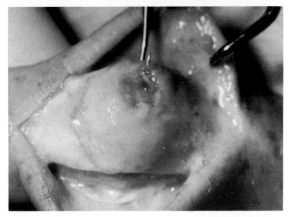

Fig. 1.51 This patient presented five weeks after a small laceration over the dorsum of the proximal interphalangeal joint. (A) represents maximum extension. Exploration of the finger (B) revealed an irregular injury to the central slip of the extensor apparatus.

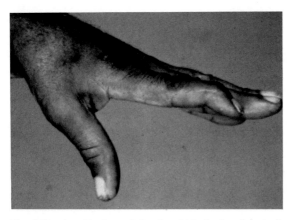

Fig. 1.52 A mallet finger deformity which developed gradually after a small laceration over the dorsum of the distal interphalangeal joint.

3. Tendon division proximal to a link with another intact tendon. This commonly occurs with
   (a) divisions of the extensors of the middle, ring, and small fingers proximal to their linking intertendinous connections;
   (b) isolated division at the wrist of flexor digitorum profundus to any of the middle, ring or small fingers, as these tendons are only independent from one another distal to the carpal tunnel.

TENDON TENSION

Gentle pressure exerted on each finger tip in turn is a surprisingly sensitive index of the integrity of the flexor tendons. Differences between the resistance encountered in adjacent fingers or between those in the injured and uninjured hands will certainly reveal complete division of either or both tendons and may also indicate when incomplete division is present. In the latter case, there is inhibition of normal muscle tone and the movement caused commonly proves painful.

Nerve injuries are *not* associated at the time of injury with an appreciable change in muscle tone. The tension in a tendon is therefore not altered by division of its nerve supply.

PASSIVE MOTION

Where doubt still exists regarding tendon injury, and the patient cannot cooperate in active motion it is possible to produce passive tendon movement in the flexor tendons. Especially useful in children, this is done by pressing firmly on the junction of middle and distal thirds of the ulnar half of the anterior aspect of the forearm. If the tendons are intact this results in flexion through 1 to 2 cm and is most marked in the ulnar three fingers (Fig. 1.53)[66]. If flexor pollicis longus is uninjured, when the pressure is exerted with one finger a little more distally over the anterior surface of the radius, the interphalangeal joint of the thumb will flex.

ACTIVE MOTION

Active motion can be assessed in any one of three ways: by asking the patient to perform the movement; by demonstrating what the examiner wishes him to do; by placing the appropriate joint in the position normally produced by the muscle being tested and asking the patient to maintain it. In all instances, resistance should then be offered to the motion since pain and even sudden release will clearly demonstrate the presence of a *partial tendon division*. 'Put your finger like that. Hold it there. Now, keep it there! Don't let me move it!'

Flexor digitorum profundus and flexor pollicis longus
The examiner should immobilize in turn the middle phalanx of each finger and the proximal phalanx of the thumb and ask the patient to flex the digit. Flexion at the

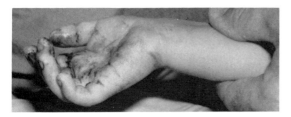

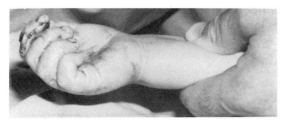

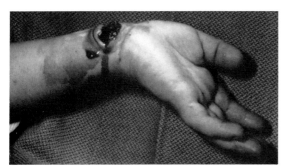

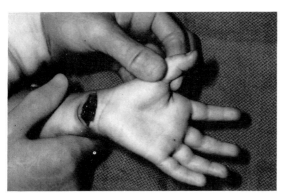

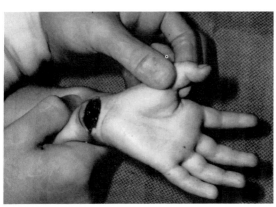

Fig. 1.53 (A & B) In this child with intact tendons, it can be seen that firm pressure exerted over the anterior aspect of the forearm with the examiner's thumb results in flexion of all the digits. (C) The posture following this wrist laceration suggests that all flexor tendons are divided with the exception, perhaps, of the thumb. When the thumb is supported (D) and then pressure exerted over the anterior aspect of the wrist (E) it can be seen that flexion occurs in the thumb suggesting the flexor pollicis longus is intact, but that none of the fingers move indicating that all long flexor tendons have been divided.

distal interphalangeal joint will confirm the integrity of the flexor digitorum profundus and, at the interphalangeal joint in the thumb, of the flexor pollicis longus (Fig. 1.54).

If the patient is unable to flex with tendons which have been shown to be intact by the passive flexion test described above, this is evidence of loss of innervation to the muscles in question. Such loss is probably due to nerve injury in the upper forearm, as follows:

Ulnar two fingers	Ulnar nerve *or* isolated injury to branch serving flexor digitorum profundus
Radial two fingers or the thumb	Median nerve above the antecubital fossa *or* anterior interosseous nerve in the forearm

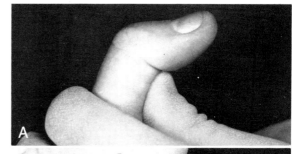

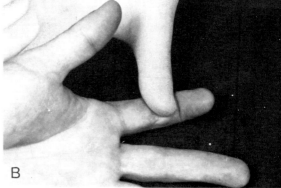

Fig. 1.54 Flexion of the distal joints of the thumb and finger respectively confirms the integrity of the flexor pollicis longus and flexor digitorum profundus.

Flexor digitorum superficialis[67]

As already discussed it is not possible to flex the ulnar three distal interphalangeal joints independently of one another on account of the common origin of the profundus tendons (p. 9). It follows that if two of the three are fixed in extension by the examiner and the patient asked to bend the third, this movement will be produced by the flexor digitorum superficialis and will occur at the proximal interphalangeal joint (Fig. 1.55). That flexor digitorum profundus is not responsible for any flexion during this test can be confirmed by passively moving the relaxed distal interphalangeal joint. The integrity or otherwise of flexor digitorum superficialis to the ulnar three fingers can thus be demonstrated. It should be noted that in one-third of normal patients the superficialis cannot achieve flexion of the small finger — in approximately half of those it will do so if the ring finger is permitted to flex simultaneously.[68] In others, more rare, there is no profundus to the small, the superficialis inserting to both middle and distal phalanges.[69,70] This test *cannot* be applied reliably to the index finger, the flexor digitorum profundus to it being independent (Fig. 1.56). The patient is asked to perform pulp to pulp pinch with the thumb and index finger as, for example, by gripping a piece of paper taken from the dressing pack. The more strongly this is performed the more it becomes an action of the flexor digitorum superficialis to the index finger with flexor digitorum profundus relaxed, as is shown by the hyperextension of

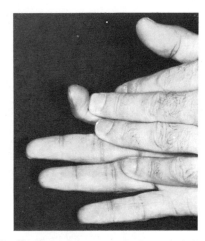

Fig. 1.56 The flexor digitorum profundus to the index finger having a separate muscle belly can act quite independently. The test previously described for superficialis of the ulnar three fingers cannot therefore be reliably applied to the index finger.

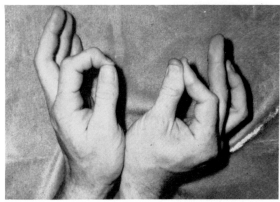

Fig. 1.57 The patient in this photograph is attempting to reproduce the posture achieved on his right hand with the one on the left. He fails to do this because of a previous division of his flexor digitorum superficialis which was subsequently demonstrated at exploration.

the distal interphalangeal joint. In contrast, if this test is performed in the presence of flexor digitorum superficialis division, the distal interphalangeal joint becomes progressively more flexed as flexor digitorum profundus substitutes for flexor digitorum superficialis (Fig. 1.57).

Flexor carpi radialis and flexor carpi ulnaris

With the fingers actively extended if possible, flexion of the wrist against gentle resistance will allow the examiner to palpate the tendons of the primary wrist flexors to ensure their integrity.

Extensors

The long and short extensor and long abductor of the thumb can be tested by asking the patient to extend his

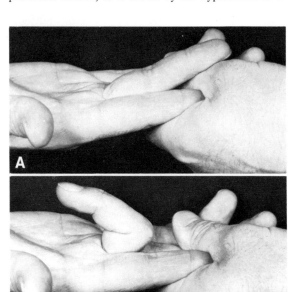

Fig. 1.55 (A) If two of the three ulnar digits are held firmly in extension, flexion of the remaining digit (B), can only be produced by action of the flexor digitorum superficialis. That this is the case can be confirmed by passive motion of the distal interphalangeal joint which will be found to be completely mobile.

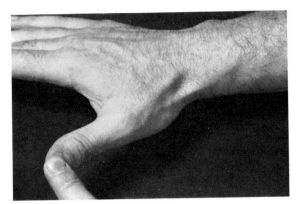

Fig. 1.58 The extensors of the thumb and the long abductor are tested by asking the patient to extend against resistance, when the tendons can be both seen and palpated.

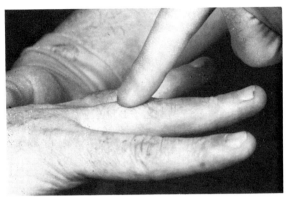

Fig. 1.59 The long extensor of the finger is tested by asking the patient to extend the metacarpophalangeal joint against resistance.

thumb against gentle resistance applied to the nail (Fig. 1.58), while the tendons are palpated. Unresisted extension alone may provide false reassurance regarding the integrity of extensor pollicis longus since the adductor pollicis and abductor pollicis brevis each contribute through the dorsal expansion to the power of extension of the interphalangeal joint.

Extensor pollicis longus rupture occurs as a result of
1. an extreme hyperextension injury in which it is crushed between the radial styloid and the base of the third metacarpal;[71]
2. a direct blow, with delayed rupture;[72]
3. chronic attrition through excessive use, or more commonly, over an old Colles fracture, which need not be displaced[73] (a similar mechanism of rupture of the extensor digitorum[74] and of the flexor tendons[75,76] has also been described);
4. attrition and synovitis in rheumatoid disease (Chapter 5);
5. secondary hyperparathyroidism, especially following chronic renal dialysis[77].

The long extensors of the fingers are similarly tested by asking the patient to extend against gentle resistance applied firstly to the dorsum of each proximal phalanx (Fig. 1.59) and secondly, with the middle phalanges supported on their palmar aspect, to the tips of the fingers (Fig. 1.60A). The second manoeuvre detects the presence of a *mallet finger* (Fig. 1.60B). With the use of gentle resistance to extension, division will be revealed by some lag in extension when compared with adjacent fingers and by pain over the site of division. This is particularly so if the test is conducted with the wrist and metacarpophalangeal joints in full flexion[78]. If the patient with division of a long extensor is asked to fully extend the metacarpophalangeal joint with the interphalangeal joints flexed a quite anomalous position will result in the affected finger, with the metacarpophalangeal joint flexed and the

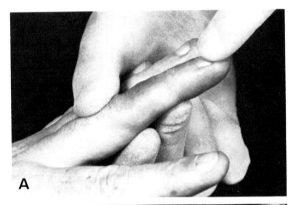

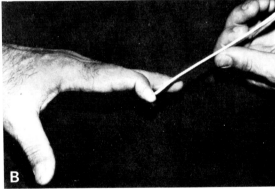

Fig. 1.60 (A) Supporting the middle phalanx, the ability of the patient to extend the distal interphalangeal joint against resistance will eliminate the presence of a mallet finger (B).

interphalangeal joints extended. When the extensor digitorum does not function but extensor indicis and digiti minimi are intact, the 'sign of the horns' will result[79] (Fig. 1.61). Other than direct laceration, this can also result from congenital absence of the muscle, selective injury or compression of the posterior interosseous nerve or its branches or from chronic lead poisoning.

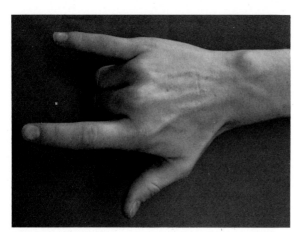

Fig. 1.61 The 'sign of the horns', evidence of intact extensor indicis and extensor digiti minimi.

Traumatic dislocation of a digital extensor, usually the long[80], results from a tear of the radial transverse fibres of the extensor hood over the metacarpophalangeal joint, permitting ulnar dislocation of the long extensor tendon. The occurrence is acute, associated with pain and a snapping sensation. The result is chronic dislocation with pain but normal extension. The treatment is repair.

Active extension of the wrist against gentle resistance will allow the tendons of intact primary wrist extensors to be palpated. The radial wrist extensors are subject to common variations[81].

The conclusions to be drawn from movement or lack of it in the untidy injury or that accompanied by a fracture must be much more guarded than in the uncomplicated tidy injury. Active movement may be inhibited or absent in the presence of intact tendons because of pain, oedema, joint injury, or fracture. Movement may, on the other hand, be produced by tendons which will not function in the long term for any of four reasons:

1. Partial division ───────────→ late rupture
2. Loss of blood supply
   (a) avulsion ⎫
   (b) crush   ⎬ ──────────→ necrosis
   (c) burn   ⎭
3. Abrasion   ──────────→ late rupture
   ──────────→ late adhesions
4. Severe peritendinous damage────→|late adhesions
   (for Tendon exploration, see p. 63)

Muscle
Lacerations of muscle are detected by the techniques described above for tendon injuries.

COMPARTMENT SYNDROMES
'A compartment(al) syndrome is a condition in which increased pressure within a limited space compromises the circulation (by lowering the arteriovenous gradient) and function of the tissues within that space.

Hypotension, haemorrhage, arterial occlusion, and limb elevation all appear to reduce the tolerance of limbs for increased tissue pressure'. Matsen, 1980[82]

All surgeons treating trauma would be well-advised to read Matsen's monograph, for all limbs subjected to trauma are susceptible to the development of a compartment syndrome. This is especially but not exclusively so where the injury is of a kind to produce increased compartment pressure, either by bleeding or by the accumulation of oedema fluid

vascular injury	burns
fracture	prolonged ischaemia
crush injury	

The physician may unwittingly compound the problem by the application of external splints, or worse casts[83], by elevation of a limb at risk and by failing to correct hypovolaemia[84].

Compartment syndrome in the upper extremity is most likely to afflict the flexor compartment of the forearm and the interosseous spaces, but can also occur in the dorsal compartment. The symptoms and signs are
1. *Pain* out of proportion to the injury
2. *Weakness* of the compartment muscles
3. *Increased tenseness* of the compartment envelope
4. *Hypesthesia* in the sensory distribution of nerves which pass through the compartment
5. *Pain on passive stretch* of the muscles of the compartment.

Flexor compartment in the forearm
Increasing pain and progressive weakness should alert the surgeon to the possibility of a compartment syndrome. Palpation of the forearm will reveal increased tension and will probably be very uncomfortable to the patient. Hypesthesia should be sought in all digits, although it will be most evident in the median nerve distribution.

Passive stretch test — with the fingers fully extended, if possible, the wrist should be gently and progressively extended also. Pain will result earlier in this sequence the more severe the condition. In fully established cases it is not possible to extend the fingers without pain, let alone the wrist. (Fig. 1.62).

Interosseous compartment[85]
This is more difficult to detect than forearm compartment syndrome, for several of the criteria do not apply: inappropriate pain may pass unheeded in the injured hand; hypesthesia does not occur; weakness of the muscles and raised compartment pressure are difficult to detect. Diagnosis therefore rests heavily on the

Passive stretch test[86] — the metacarpophalangeal joint of each finger in turn is held in hyperextension, the

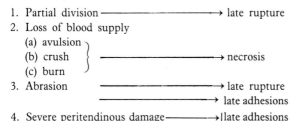

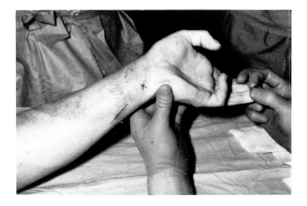

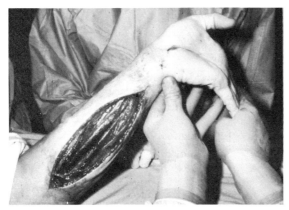

Fig. 1.62   (A) Even under anaesthesia it is not possible to fully extend the wrist and fingers in this patient who sustained a closed roller injury to his forearm. (B) After decompression of the forearm muscular compartment full extension was achieved with relative ease.

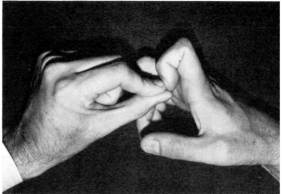

Fig. 1.63   Increase in the pressure within the intrinsic muscle compartments can be tested by placing each finger in turn in the intrinsic minus position as shown. If this manoeuvre cannot be undertaken without pain, it is an indication of a rise in intra-compartmental pressure.

interphalangeal joints are flexed and the finger is then deviated both radially and ulnarwards. (Fig. 1.63) If pain is elicited by the deviation or even more by the flexion, decompression is required. The interosseous compartments may be involved individually or in combination, thus

2nd compartment — 1st palmar and 2nd dorsal interosseous — stretch positive
3rd compartment — 2nd palmar and 3rd dorsal interosseous — stretch positive
4th compartment — 3rd palmar and 4th dorsal interosseous — stretch positive

It should be noted well that *the pulse is not lost* in either forearm or interosseous compartment syndrome since main arterial pressure is well above the critical closing pressure of vessels supplying the compartment tissues. If it is absent, that is probably evidence of major vascular impairment, which will coincidentally worsen the compartment syndrome by lowering the anteriovenous gradient. Both require urgent attention.

Angiography

In most circumstances where a probable compartment syndrome is accompanied by an absent pulse, exploration is urgently indicated and will reveal all pathology. Where, however, the patient's condition is critical for other reasons or vascular surgical capabilities are not available but angiography is — an unlikely circumstance — then angiography may be justified. The compartment syndrome which has advanced so far as to arrest flow will be revealed by a smooth tapering of the main vessels with absence of filling of small side branches as opposed to the sharp cut-off in the main vessel which is evidence of arterial injury.

Electrical stimulation[87]

Occasionally no active function is detected in the muscles of a compartment which may be due either to nerve injury more proximal or to raised compartment pressure. Electrical stimulation of the nerve close to the muscle will solve this dilemma

| Stimulation | CONTRACTION | proximal nerve injury |
| Stimulation | NO CONTRACTION | compartment syndrome |

Compartment pressure recording

When the signs are equivocal, the first requirement is for *frequent, regular, well-recorded reviews* of the patient. These will often reveal a deteriorating situation. When this is not so or when examination is complicated by other injuries, unconsciousness or age or when decompression is contraindicated unless absolutely necessary, then compartment pressure recording either with a wick catheter[88] or by the continuous infusion technique (Fig. 1.64) becomes valuable. If the clinical findings are confusing but the tissue pressure is above 40 mmHg, then decompression is indicated. The technique of pressure recording must be impeccable and should be perfected on

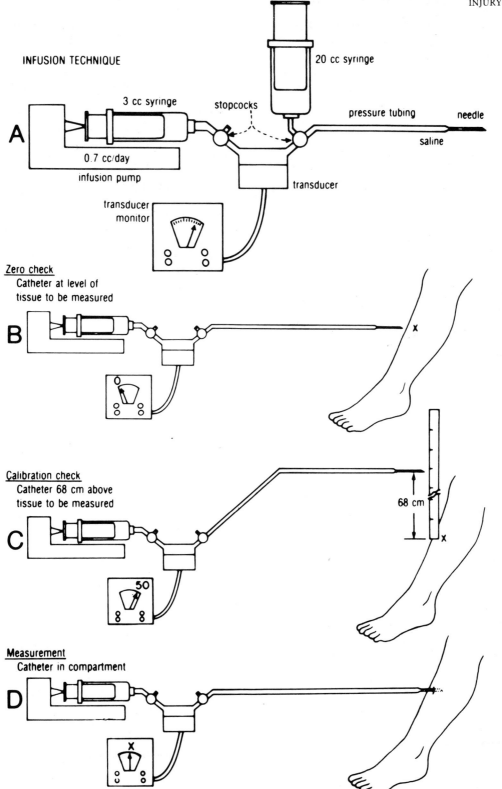

Fig. 1.64 Comparment pressure recording by the continuous infusion technique. (*From:* Matsen 1980 Compartmental syndromes. Grune and Stratton, New York, by courtesy of the author and publisher.)

normal volunteers. An erroneous reading is worse than no reading at all, since it will tend to supersede clinical signs.

Indications

Unequivocal cases and those confusing ones with tissue pressure over 40 mmHg should be submitted to effective release of dressings[89] and then to wide release of the tissue envelope — fasciotomy — of the forearm compartments or the interosseous spaces. (Fig. 1.62)[90] It must be remembered that significant post-ischaemic swelling may occur after release[91] and Matsen has drawn attention to the dangers of 'rebound' compartment syndrome. Vigilance must be maintained.

Three points concerning compartmental syndromes should be stressed:

1. The disappearance of pain after time may indicate necrosis, *not* recovery;
2. The syndrome may arise at any time during the first three days, and sometimes six, following an appropriate injury. The tests must therefore be repeated regularly until the surgeon is confident that danger has passed;
3. No surgeon or patient has ever regretted the performance of a fasciotomy, only the failure to do so. Therefore, if the surgeon feels that it *might* be necessary, it should be done. If decompression is not performed, muscle ischaemia will proceed to necrosis and in time to fibrosis — Volkmann's ischaemic contracture[92].

Nerve

SENSORY LOSS

Each side of each digital pulp and the dorsum of the metacarpal region of the thumb should be tested for *moving*[93] *two point discrimination*[94] (2PD) using a paper clip twisted to appropriate shape[95] (p. 156). This should be done in a definite sequence.

1. The ends are shown to the patient to reassure him that they are *not* sharp.
2. The ends should be set 5 to 8 mm apart for pulp testing and over 15 mm for dorsal testing.
3. The test should be performed holding the points in alignment along the axis of the digit and moving transversely across the axis. Pressure should be sufficiently light as to avoid blanching of a normal finger and thereby avoid overlap or recruitment.
4. The patient should be asked to observe the difference between one point and two points on the uninjured hand.
5. Each side of each digit should be tested until a clear difference is shown between different areas on the same hand or between the two hands. It is not necessary — nor probably would it be accurate — to

determine a precise figure for moving 2PD in the injured hand. It is sufficient to demonstrate a clear difference.

The nerves divided can then be deduced, knowing the site of the wound, and that usually the ulnar nerve serves the small finger and the ulnar half of the ring, the median nerve the remaining digits and the radial nerve the skin over the dorsum of the proximal phalanx and metacarpal of the thumb. Certain sources of difficulty may arise:

1. *Patient error.* This may be due to the patient being too young, too old, too confused, too inebriated or too disturbed by his injury to cooperate. If completely relaxed, children can cooperate from the age of three. If the patient is frightened, shocked or overawed, this age of cooperation may rise into the early teens. In any event, concentration swiftly flags and examination should be abbreviated accordingly by testing only appropriate areas of absolute sensory loss (see below). In patients such as those detailed above the *tactile adherence test* will frequently reveal the pattern of nerve loss (p. 154). A plastic pen is held lightly by the examiner. Its smooth surface is passed gently but firmly back and forward repeatedly through an amplitude of 1 to 2 cm across the pulp on each side of each finger. This should be tried first on the uninjured hand to determine how much pressure is necessary to demonstrate adhesion between the pen and the finger. Adhesion is shown by slight but definite movement of the finger and is due to the presence of sweat and will require somewhat firmer pressure in a cold than in a warm hand. Fortunately, young children and the inebriated all seem to perspire profusely! An insensate pulp will have no sweating and will therefore show no 'tactile adherence' and therefore no motion.

2. *Anomalous sensory loss*

   (a) ulnar and median nerves
   The number of fingers served by each nerve may vary. As an almost absolute rule, however, the palmar surface of the index and small fingers are served by the median and ulnar nerves respectively.

   (b) radial nerve
   Not infrequently the radial nerve distribution does not extend on to the thumb. On occasion the lateral cutaneous nerve of the forearm entirely replaces the radial nerve in carrying sensation from the hand[96].

Many other methods of sensory evaluation have been described and some are detailed in the next chapter (p. 154). All are either too painful, time-consuming or esoteric for routine use in the emergency room. The two described above are painless, swift, require no special equipment and give clear results in the great majority of patients. The remainder will be diagnosed by exploration.

POSTURE

The deformities associated with nerve injuries (p. 149), so characteristic particularly of ulnar nerve loss, are not seen in the acute situation.

PARALYSIS

The ulnar nerve in the hand usually serves the hypothenar muscles, all the interossei, the ulnar two lumbricals, the adductor pollicis and the deep head of flexor pollicis brevis. The median nerve in the hand serves the abductor pollicis brevis, the opponens pollicis, the radial two lumbricals and the superficial head of flexor pollicis brevis. This is a lengthy list for the trainee casualty surgeon to commit to memory and for the occasional examiner of the hand to recall. When this list is then qualified by the frequent variations which occur in the innervation of the lumbricals and of the thenar muscles, confusion arises or the attempt at recall is abandoned. For quick diagnosis of motor nerve injury at the wrist, *one muscle only* need be tested for each nerve:

Median — abductor pollicis brevis. With the hand flat and the palm up, the patient is asked to touch with his thumb the examiner's finger held directly over the thenar eminence and some 6 centimeters above it. If the patient is then asked to maintain this position against pressure from the examiner, the muscle belly can be seen and palpated between the scaphoid tubercle and the metacarpophalangeal joint of the thumb (Fig. 1.65).

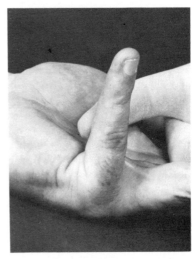

Fig. 1.66 The ulnar nerve invariably serves the flexor digiti minimi and this can be tested by asking the patient to flex the metacarpophalangeal joint to 90 degrees with the interphalangeal joints straight.

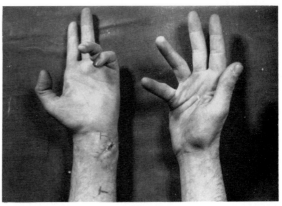

Fig. 1.67 This patient has sustained a division of the ulnar nerve at the left wrist. It can be seen that the action of his flexor digiti minimi in the normal hand produces the posture described in the previous figure, but that he cannot achieve this on the injured side.

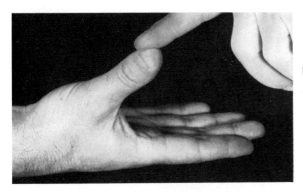

Fig. 1.65 The abductor pollicis brevis is innervated by the median nerve in the vast majority of cases. The integrity of the nerve therefore can be tested by asking the patient to reach up to meet the examiner's finger held over the hand in the line of the index finger.

Ulnar — flexor digiti minimi. In the same position, the patient is asked to raise the small finger vertically, that is, flex the metacarpophalangeal joint to 90° with the interphalangeal joints straight (Fig. 1.66). This posture cannot be achieved in ulnar nerve lesions. (Fig. 1.67)

When a patient is unable to cooperate with even these simple motor tests, some indication may be given by asking him

   (i)   to snap his fingers — abductor pollicis brevis — median

   (ii) to cross his fingers — 1st palmar and (middle over index)   2nd dorsal interosseous — ulnar[97].

This simplification of the examination of the hand for motor nerve loss does not release the surgeon from the responsibility of carrying out the full muscle test described in the Appendix (p. 351). This is especially necessary in multiple penetrating injuries, such as are sustained when the arm is put through a sheet of glass, since several injuries to both main nerve trunks and their branches are not uncommon. It is also desirable as a routine in all hand examinations as the surgeon thereby becomes more familiar with the full test. With practice, all muscles in the upper extremity can be tested in little over one minute. The routine also eliminates the presence of pre-existing muscle loss which might be the subject of later dispute. In high or proximal injuries the most significant sensory loss is still in the hand itself. By contrast, proximal motor loss must be detected for all the reasons listed above and also to determine the precise level of the nerve injury and to distinguish between complete and partial nerve lesions. This is particularly important in patients with fractures and gun shot wounds where neurapraxia is common. The preliminary examination draws the baseline from which future recovery is measured. If open reduction and internal fixation are performed, a complete record eliminates any embarrassing doubt as to whether a palsy arose after injury or after surgery.

The inability to initiate movement is not absolute evidence that the muscle or its nerve supply is divided. Pain in the hand or nervousness may well inhibit motion. It is better therefore to test the patient's ability to resist movement as described previously. This requires the examiner to place the limb in the position which the muscle being tested normally produces and then to instruct the patient to 'Keep it there! Don't let me move it!'

ACUTE CARPAL TUNNEL SYNDROME (p. 194)

This may arise either as a result of oedema or because dislocation or fracture has directed a bone fragment into the tunnel. The features characteristic of chronic median nerve compression are present but may be obscured by the symptoms and signs of the injury. The diagnosis is made on the basis of

an appropriate injury
a high level of suspicion
reduced sensation in median nerve distribution
a positive Tinel sign proximal to the wrist crease
weakness in abductor pollicis brevis

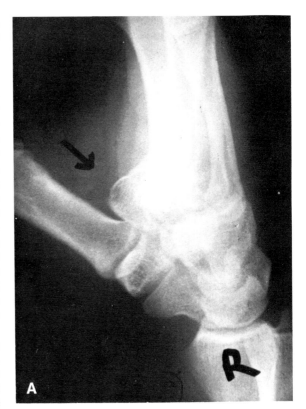

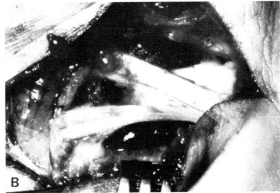

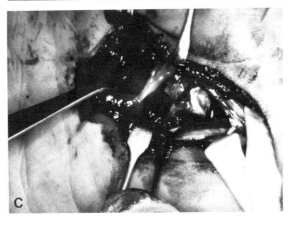

Fig. 1.68 A sixteen-year-old boy presented with numbness in his median nerve distribution which commenced shortly after a heavy fall onto his hand. (A) X-ray revealed an anterior carpal metacarpal dislocation and exploration of the carpal tunnel, (B) revealed the synovium to be grossly distended with blood. (C) Incision of the blood stained synovium revealed the base of the third metacarpal in the carpal tunnel. Reduction and internal fixation of the fracture dislocation resulted in a rapid return of normal median sensory function.

Phalen's test usually cannot be applied because of discomfort. If the injury is complex and the diagnostic signs confusing, *nerve conduction studies* will help, an increased distal motor latency in excess of 4.0 m secs. being diagnostic. Like other compartment syndromes, if the potential is there but the findings equivocal, then the patient should be re-examined regularly for 3 to 6 days after the injury or until conditions have improved.

Once diagnosed, acute carpal tunnel syndrome is treated by decompression (Fig. 1.68).

(For Nerve exploration, see p. 70.)

Vessel

OPEN INJURIES

Arterial lacerations which are *complete* are distinguished by a history of dramatic blood loss at the time of injury, sometimes described as pulsatile, which has ceased by the time of examination due to longitudinal and circumferential retraction of the arterial wall. The wound is filled with thick, shiny, gelatinous, dark red clot which may be oozing somewhat. Examination of the peripheral *pulses* is worthless[98] since retrograde flow may fill the lacerated vessel from distally. If the suspected laceration is in the radial or ulnar artery, obliteration of the other may eliminate the pulse spuriously present. In theory, the Allen test (p. 181) could reveal an injury of either forearm vessel. In practice, this manoeuvre is often too painful and may also provoke renewed bleeding, and exploration of all likely wounds becomes the rule.

Partial lacerations of a major vessel may be associated with continued arterial haemorrhage since the normally haemostatic retraction serves to *increase* blood loss (Fig. 1.69). Such lacerations are the only cause of death in the upper extremity and should be treated as such an emergency. They *may* present with no active bleeding, a large wound clot, and distal pulses present due to occlusion of the defect in the wall by the clot, thereby re-establishing the vascular conduit.

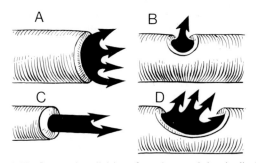

Fig. 1.69 In complete division of a major vessel, longitudinal and circumferential retraction results in dramatic reduction in blood loss. The same factors after partial injury tend to make the laceration in the wall of the artery wider, and therefore blood loss tends to be increased by the normally haemostatic mechanisms.

Lacerations in the correct site, of sufficient depth to have produced an arterial injury, require prompt exploration by a competent vascular surgeon.

CLOSED INJURIES (INCLUDING PENETRATING WOUNDS)
In open injuries, the surgeon need only speculate on what the necessary exploration will reveal. By contrast potential arterial injury in relatively closed spaces presents a much greater diagnostic challenge for here he must decide whether or not exploration is necessary.

Arterial compromise may result from several mechanisms

1. Gunshot wounds[99,100]
2. Fractures — humerus[101,102] and clavicle[103]
3. Dislocations — elbow[104] and shoulder[105]
   producing either
   (a) partial division —— false aneurysm
   or
   (b) extensive intimal disruption[106] —— thrombosis

The findings in the acute situation[107] in the upper extremity may be remarkably few. This is especially so and particularly hazardous in injuries to the subclavian and axillary arteries, where a neglected false aneurysm may result in later brachial palsy with less than 50% chance of recovery[108]. In order of appearance, the signs of major arterial trauma in the arm are:[109]

1. Diminution or absence of distal *pulses* — in the swollen limb or in the ischaemic digit the use of the Doppler flowmeter to check pulses is valuable[110,111].
2. *Pallor,* especially evident in the nailbeds which show very poor refill after blanching.
3. *Pain,* most evident on handling the limb.
4. *Paraesthesia,* hypaesthesia and anaesthesia.
5. *Paralysis* — when this degree of muscle ischaemia is present, compartment syndromes are inevitable; correction of the vascular interruption may increase the problem by inducing post-ischaemic oedema (p. 31) — it should be accompanied by fasciotomy.

It should be re-emphasised that few, if any, of those peripheral signs may be present. Delay may be disastrous, so if suspicions remain further steps must be taken, either by arteriography or exploration.

Arteriography is not indicated in open injuries since exploration can answer questions more directly with no loss of time. The value of arteriography in closed injuries has been questioned on similar grounds. However, exploration simply because major vessels may be injured is unnecessary surgery which may also be undesirable if other injuries or illnesses are present. Physical findings have been found to be unreliable, giving false negative indications in 20% and false positive in 42% of 86 patients subsequently evaluated by angiography[112].

Transfemoral subclavian arteriography is a swift, safe procedure. If it is undertaken to demonstrate the smaller, more distal vessels (p. 182) or prior to exploration to be done under axillary block, there is clear advantage and significant compassion in giving that block before the dye injection. The arteriogram may reveal

1. false aneurysm (Fig. 1.70)
2. thrombosis
3. intimal flap formation — seen either as a dissection of dye (Fig. 1.71) or suggested by an abrupt, sharp occlusion without haemorrhage (Fig. 1.72)

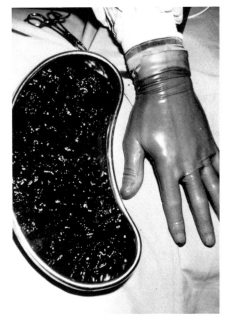

Fig. 1.70 (A) This patient presented with a massive swelling in his upper arm, but with good circulation to the hand and normal pulses. (B) Arteriography revealed a false aneurysm which (C) contained almost 3 units of blood.

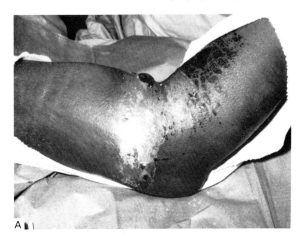

A

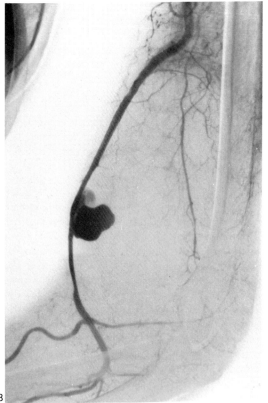

B

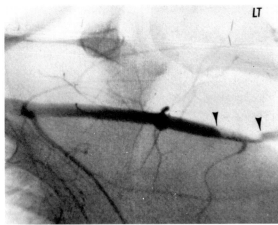

LT

Fig. 1.71 In this arteriogram the dissection of the intima is revealed by a sudden narrowing of the vessel indicated by the arrows.

4. extrinsic compression
5. acute arterio-venous fistula (Fig. 1.73)

Spasm[113] in terms of angiography is now a largely discredited word. It was used to imply a transitory constriction of a vessel following trauma, which may produce clinical signs and angiographic changes, but which would resolve spontaneously. All such cases should be explored — all will reveal vessel pathology.

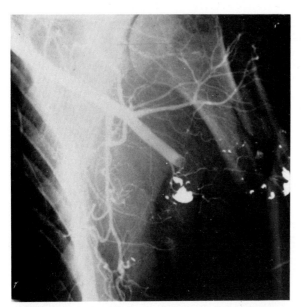

Fig. 1.72 An intimal flap is suggested by the sudden occlusion of the brachial artery following a gunshot wound without any evidence of haemorrhage.

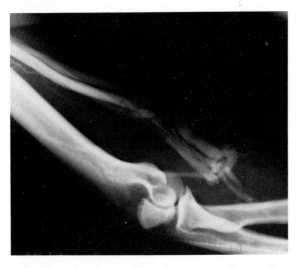

Fig. 1.73 An arteriovenous fistula is present here between the brachial artery and basilic vein.

Iatrogenic. A small but worrisome group of patients arise as a result of arterial puncture, intentional or otherwise. This may occur in the course of cardiac catheterisation (Fig. 1.74), radial cannulation for arterial blood gases — where the incidence of ischaemic complications in one series was 10%[114,115] — or misplaced intravenous lines[116]. The presentation may range from acute ischaemia as detailed above, to compartment syndromes, to intermittent claudication. Prevention requires avoidance of these techniques in anticoagulated patients[117] and careful evaluation of the arterial tree by Allen's test and Doppler studies before inserting radial lines. Treatment requires vein grafting, compartment decompression and, occasionally, fibrinolytic therapy[118].

NON-TRAUMATIC VASCULAR EMERGENCIES

A relatively small group of patients will present as emergencies due to vascular compromise of an acute nature not related to injury. Severe upper limb ischaemia may arise from a number of causes[119] including embolisation, thrombosis arising from atherosclerosis and small vessel occlusion resulting from Raynaud's phenomenon or disease (p. 184)[120]. Regardless of the site these patients present because of pain and changes in colour and temperature.

Examination reveals the classic features[121] detailed above

pulselessness
pallor and mottling of the skin
coolness of the part
paraesthesia, hypaesthesia and analgesia
paralysis, primarily in the intrinsic muscles and
    only if the occlusion is at or above the elbow
If the patient presents later,
ulceration will appear in digital occlusion
gangrene in forearm occlusions, with the addition of
compartment syndromes in more proximal blockage.

Emboli[122] usually arise from the heart, or more rarely from aneurysms, lodging either at the origin of the profunda brachii (Fig. 1.75) or at the bifurcation of the brachial artery into radial and ulnar. After full evaluation of the origin, brachial embolectomy is indicated[123]. The grave danger is that thrombus or additional emboli will have propagated distally, requiring lengthy, often fruitless, microsurgical exploration[124].

Thrombosis occurs on previously diseased vessels and is diagnosed partly by exclusion of a source of embolus and partly by evidence of peripheral vessel disease on examination, arteriography and exploration. Vein grafting is required, with or without resection.

Primary deep vein thrombosis (= effort thrombosis = Paget-Schroetter's syndrome)[125] arises as a result of a direct blow, prolonged pressure (as in sleep), adjacent major surgery or excessive stretch as in raking leaves, chopping wood or playing baseball, football or handball. It affects the subclavian or axillary veins and is characterised by swelling of the limb to a very variable degree, cyanotic discoloration and a feeling of discomfort and heaviness. A prominent venous pattern develops over the shoulder due to distension of collateral venous circulation. The limb may be anaesthetic and cooler than the contralateral one, but *all pulses are present.* The thrombosed vein may or may not be palpable on the inner aspect of the arm or in the axilla. Venography will reveal the venous thrombosis and the

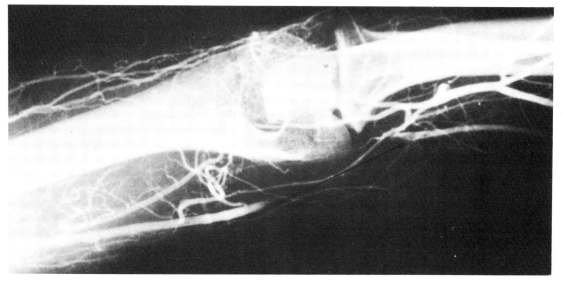

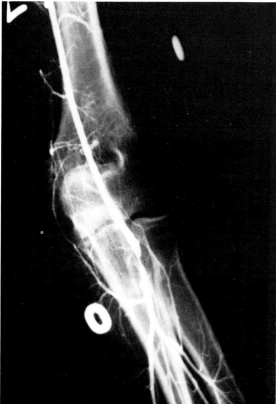

Figs. 1.74A & B These occlusions, complete and partial, both resulted from cardiac catheterization.

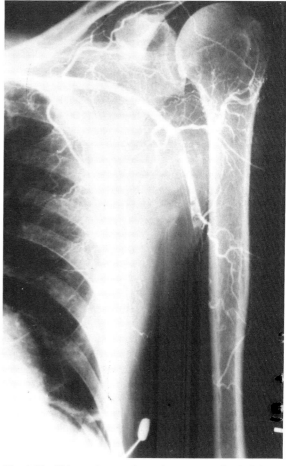

Fig. 1.75 This arteriogram shows the presence of emboli in brachial artery just proximal to the origin of the profunda brachii artery, in the brachial artery just distal to the circumflex humeral artery and also small emboli in the circumflex humeral artery itself.

marked collateral flow (Fig. 1.76). More severe cases may progress to venous gangrene[126] or be complicated by pulmonary embolism. Anticoagulation is required and venous thrombectomy or interpositional grafting is indicated in more severe cases.

(For Vessel exploration, see p. 72.)

Bone and joint

DEFORMITY

Significant swelling around a joint or bone is in itself sufficient to arouse suspicions of underlying skeletal injury. Any *bruising* beneath the skin, in the absence of any other cause, is pathognomonic of fracture or ligament tear. To state some general rules regarding angular deformity following fracture or dislocation in the hand

1. Deformity is more evident in the phalanges than in the carpus. This is partly because soft tissue coverage is less and partly because the force required to disrupt the skeleton is greater the more proximal the injury and there is therefore a greater accumulation of obscuring oedema.
2. *Fractures* angled in the line of digital motion that is, antero-posterior, are much less evident than those angled laterally or rotated.
3. *Joints* dislocated in the line of digital motion are more likely to remain so and are therefore more evident than those dislocated laterally or rotated which will often have reduced spontaneously.

A joint will only remain in the dislocated position if some element of the joint capsule either (i) remains intact and locks the bone ends in abnormal relationship or (ii) tears and becomes interposed between the bone ends. This is more likely to occur in antero-posterior dislocations than in lateral. In addition, the pull of the extrinsic tendons serves to tighten the locking in antero-posterior dislocations while tending to restore lateral dislocations to proper alignment.

These facts are important because they make more obscure some potentially more disabling injuries, for example, intercarpal dislocations and 'game-keeper's thumb' (p. 143).

The locking mechanism referred to in 3(ii) above is well illustrated by the comparison between the two types of dislocation most commonly seen in the index metacarpophalangeal joint:

Simple. Posterior dislocation which can be readily and effectively reduced in closed fashion; indeed, the majority of patients present with a history of angulation reduced spontaneously, personally or by someone present at the accident;

Complex[127,128]. Posterior dislocation in which the metacarpal head becomes trapped between the transverse metacarpal ligament on its palmar aspect and the displaced and

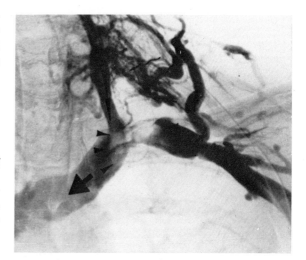

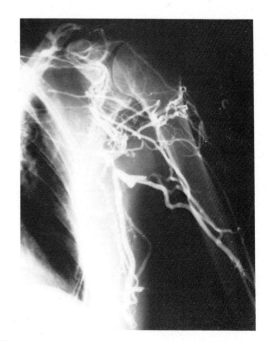

Figs. 1.76A & B Both these venograms show evidence of thrombosis in the main venous stream. This has completely occluded the axillary vein in (B) and in both there is evidence of unusual filling of the collateral venous system. (All angiograms courtesy of Dr C. S. Wheeler.)

ruptured palmar plate on its dorsal aspect; between the flexor tendons on its ulnar side and the lumbrical muscle on its radial side (Fig. 1.77). This usually requires open reduction, most effectively achieved through a *dorsal* approach, contrary to earlier teaching.

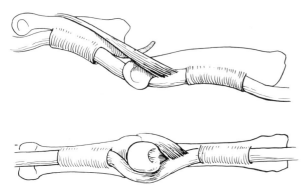

Fig. 1.77 This diagram illustrates the mechanism of a complex dislocation of the metacarpophalangeal joint. In the upper, lateral diagram it can be seen that the palmar plate is locked between the head of the metacarpal and the base of the proximal phalanx. In the lower diagram, an anterior view, the head of the metacarpal can be seen trapped between the flexor digitorum profundus on one aspect and the lumbrical on the other.

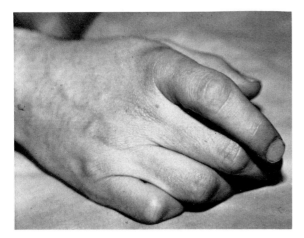

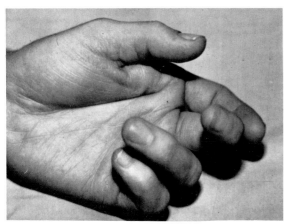

Fig. 1.78 (A) The typical posture of the complex dislocation is seen, the index finger being locked in some 30° of hyperextension. (B) The typical deep puckering at the palmar crease is evident, due to the traction on the palmar fascia and so through its skin attachment on the skin itself.

The posture of the dislocated finger is distinct for each type of dislocation. In the simple dislocation the proximal phalanx tends to lie in almost 90° of hyperextension while in the complex dislocation the angle of hyperextension is appreciably less. In the complex dislocation, the displaced metacarpal head forms a marked prominence in the palm, which also shows deep puckering of the proximal palmar crease due to traction on the skin attachments of the palmar fascia (Fig. 1.78). On radiological examination, an increased joint space results from the entrapped palmar plate while the presence of a sesamoid within the joint is diagnostic. In some cases of complex dislocation the circulation to the index finger may be embarrassed as the neurovascular bundles are stretched and trapped by the displaced metacarpal head. Complex dislocation may, more rarely, occur in the thumb and other fingers.

However tempting, no deformity should be corrected before thorough clinical and radiological evaluation. Nerve dysfunction, circulatory embarrassment and fractures should all be documented *before* any treatment is offered.

LIMITATION OF NORMAL MOTION
Active. The probable absence of injury to skeletal structures is most speedily checked by asking the patient to put each joint through a normal range of motion (p. 00). Apart from direct injury to the joint under examination or to the bones which form the joint, limitation or lack of active motion may be due to:

> tendon injury
> paralysis
> oedema
> pain
> significant injury proximally
> lack of patient co-operation — age, anxiety, intoxication.

Where *pain* limits active motion, note should be taken of its location and at what point in the joint range it occurs.

Passive. Where active motion is absent or limited, the examiner should attempt gentle passive motion both to detect any injury sustained and also to place on record any limitation of normal range present *before* the injury. Such limitation may influence treatment and postoperative care. The record also refutes any subsequent charge that the limitation arose as a result of the injury or treatment. Injury will become evident during passive motion by the presence of painful limitation of range.

In suspected carpal instability, the forearm should be carried through a full range of pronation and supination and the wrist then rotated — while applying axial compression — through a complete circle from radial deviation to extension to ulnar deviation to flexion. This may produce pain, often accompanied by a palpable 'popping' or 'clicking' in the carpus.

In recording joint range[129] the convention approved by all English-speaking Orthopaedic Associations, detailed later (p. 135), should be employed. Basically this dictates that all neutral joint positions, that is when the two bones coming together at the joint are in line, are recorded as 0°.

PRESENCE OF ABNORMAL MOTION

The most commonly injured joints in the hand are the ginglymus joints, probably because they are restricted to only one plane of movement. They are all of the interphalangeal joints and the metacarpophalangeal joint of the thumb. All have a similar structure[130]. The true and accessory collateral ligaments together form a fan of fibres which radiate out from a recess on the lateral aspect of the head of the proximal bone. These fibres insert, the true collateral into the bone of the base of the distal bone, the accessory into the lateral aspect of the palmar plate. The fibres are tight in all positions of the joint which shows no freedom for lateral motion. The palmar plate has two distinct portions[131,132]. The glenoid or fibrous part attaches to the palmar aspect of the base of the distal bone and by proximal lateral extensions to the margins of the anterior surface of the proximal bone. These extensions — called check-rein ligaments — when viewed anteriorly give the appearance of a swallow-tail. The fibrous palmar plate serves both to restrict hyperextension of the joint and as an extension of the articular surface of the base of the distal bone. It is through the fibrous part that tears of the palmar plate occur at its more distal portion. Such tears extend to a varying degree into the collateral ligament, splitting between the fibres of true and accessory parts (Fig. 1.79). The membranous part of the palmar plate lies between the check-rein ligaments and serves to transmit blood vessels to the vincular system. The extensor tendon closes the circle and in some joints is thickened to the extent that it has been referred to as a dorsal plate. If all the proximal attachments are cut, as in doing an arthrodesis, it can be seen that the base of the distal bone is indeed encircled by the attached structures with no bare areas (Fig. 1.80). The head of the proximal bone is enveloped by these structures through which it tears in dislocation.

True lateral dislocations of the hinge joints of necessity tear the true collateral ligament. Hyperextension injuries tear the palmar plate but need not tear all of either collateral ligament even when completely dislocated dorsally. Oblique dislocations tear *between* the fibres of the collateral ligament and through the palmar plate but often

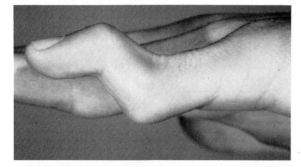

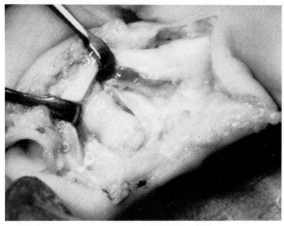

Fig. 1.79 (A) A typical hyperextension deformity resulting from tear of the fibrous part of the palmar plate to the proximal interphalangeal joint. (B) Exploration shows that the head of the proximal phalanx is protruding between the remnant of the fibrous portion distally and the major portion of the palmar plate proximally.

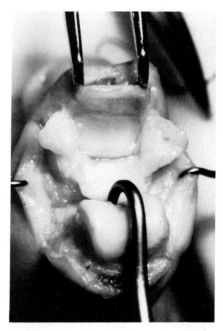

Fig. 1.80 Here in a patient undergoing distal interphalangeal joint arthrodesis for an old avulsion injury of the flexor digitorum profundus, the structure of the ginglymus joint is demonstrated. All margins of the base of the distal phalanx have attachments, the palmar plate below, the extensor tendon above, and the collateral ligaments on either side. In addition, the accessory collateral ligament can be seen attaching to the palmar plate forming 'a chair in which the head of the proximal bone will sit' (J. W. Littler).

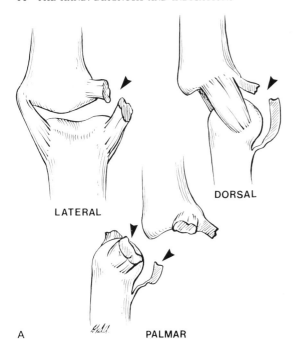

LATERAL

DORSAL

PALMAR

A

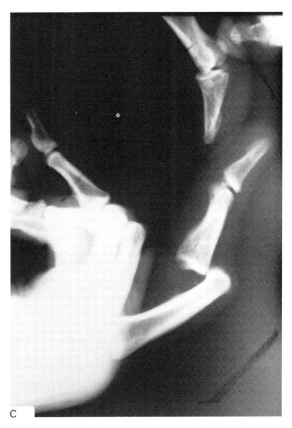

C

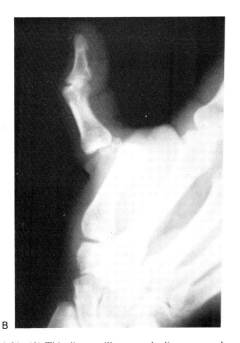

B

Fig. 1.81 (A) This diagram illustrates the ligamentous damage which results from dislocation of a hinge joint. (B) Although the bones in this dislocation appear to be widely separated, when the joint was explored it was found that both collateral ligaments were intact. (C) Although the bones are apparently much closer together than in (B) exploration of this anterior dislocation revealed a complete tear of the palmar plate and of one collateral ligament.

only partially. Anterior dislocations tear the palmar *and* one or other or both collateral ligaments (Fig. 1.81).

The palmar plates are tested by hyperextension. All collateral ligaments should be stressed by lateral angulation of the joint (Fig. 1.82). Those especially prone to injury are the collateral ligaments of the proximal inter-phalangeal joints and the ulnar collateral ligament of the metacarpophalangeal joint of the thumb, injured in forced abduction (gamekeeper's thumb)[133]. If a proximal inter-phalangeal joint cannot be fully extended, lateral stress may erroneously reveal apparent instability. This is due to normal *rotation* of the proximal phalanx permitted by laxity of the collateral ligament of the metacarpophalangeal joint. This spurious motion can be eliminated by firmly flexing the metacarpophalangeal joint. Similarly, injuries of the collateral ligaments of the metacarpophalangeal joints can only be tested by lateral stress on the proximal phalanx with the metacarpophalangeal joint in maximum *flexion*.

In many instances true lateral and true antero-posterior stress will show *painful stability*. In such cases, the joint should be stressed obliquely, placing tension on the accessory collateral ligament. Tears between the accessory and true collateral ligaments extending partially into the palmar plate are not uncommon and will be revealed by

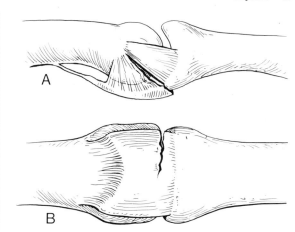

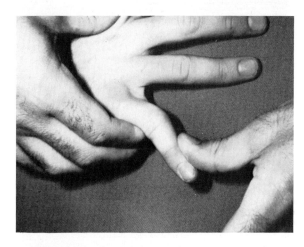

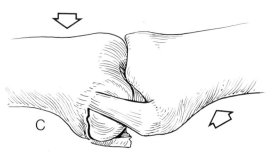

Fig. 1.83 Obliquely oriented injuries to a hinge joint tear between the fibres of the true and accessory collateral ligaments and part way across the palmar plate. Direct lateral and hyperextension stress fail to reveal instability. If, however, the stress is applied obliquely then the mechanism of injury is reproduced, and pain and instability are elicited.

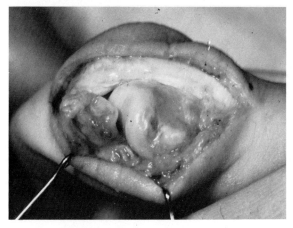

Fig. 1.82 (A) The collateral ligament of the proximal interphalangeal joint is stressed and in this case (B) reveals laxity to this true lateral stress which can only be due to a tear of the true collateral ligament. (C) Exploration revealed this to be true, the collateral ligament being torn from its attachment to the proximal phalanx. (Note the different mechanism from game-keeper's thumb in which the ulnar collateral ligament is torn from its distal attachment.)

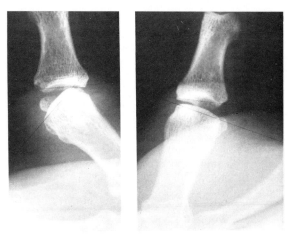

Fig. 1.84 Here the stress films of right and left thumb metacarpophalangeal joints are compared. That on the left opens to an angle of 45° compared with 10° on the right due to an ulnar collateral ligament tear — 'gamekeeper's thumb'.

severe pain and potential instability on such oblique stress (Fig. 1.83). All of these manoeuvres are painful in the presence of injury and should be done with this knowledge. If protective spasm or undue discomfort prevent a complete diagnosis, the test should be repeated under regional block, at which time stress X–rays should be obtained (Fig. 1.84).

The practice of moving broken bones to confirm the presence of fracture is painful, unnecessary and not without risk, for especially in the forearm major nerves and vessels lie close to the bones and can easily be damaged during such a manoeuvre. It should be condemned.

TENDERNESS

Tenderness elicited by the palpating finger can be a guide to the site and extent of injury. All such tenderness should be compared to the opposite, uninjured hand to ensure that it is different and therefore significant.

1. *Bone.* Fracture sites will be tender even on gentle pressure and in some sites, e.g. the scaphoid, this is diagnostic.
2. *Periarticular structures.* Where joint range is limited by pain, rupture of the capsule, collateral ligament or palmar plate is one cause. The precise location of the tear in more major injuries can be determined by careful pressure around the joint applied by the examiner's finger nail. With the wrist flexed each carpal bone and intercarpal joint should be palpated, the examiner mentally naming each in turn. Anteriorly the scaphoid tubercle should be palpated and the pisiform moved transversely on the triquetral. At any point, pain may reveal pathology.

RADIOLOGICAL EXAMINATION

All injured hands should be X–rayed, not only for reasons of litigation, but also because previous injury should be recorded and because the most confident clinical exclusion of fractures can be wrong. More than one view is always necessary and the surgeon and radiographer should ideally study the films together to determine whether further views will aid in diagnosis.

Special X–rays

Standard views of the hand are often inadequate and the hand surgeon should request any of the following which may seem necessary.

True lateral, anteroposterior and oblique of interphalangeal joints — to study articular alignment and detect small fragments attached to ligaments or tendons.

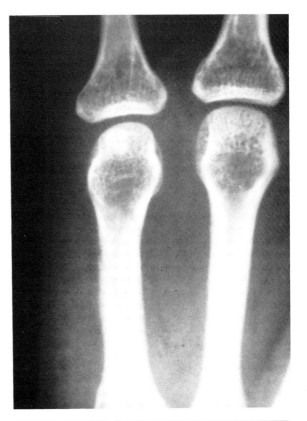

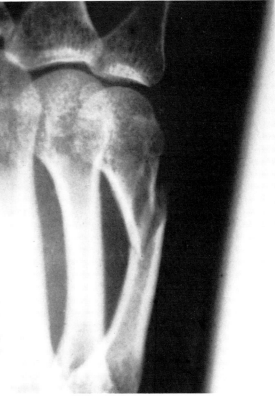

Fig. 1.85 (A) An anteroposterior X–ray yielded no clear evidence of a fracture of the fifth metacarpal. (B) In a lateral view supinated by 30° the fracture of the shaft was clearly evident.

Modified laterals of metacarpals are necessary since little can be seen on a true lateral of the hand. To study the index and middle the hand should be pronated 30° from lateral, for the ring and small supinated 30° (Fig. 1.85).

Scaphoid view — lateral and postero-anterior of the carpus, the latter in three positions: supinated by 45°, straight and pronated by 45° — while the majority of fractures show in the latter two views, some may show only in the others[134].

Carpal tunnel view[135] — may reveal fractures of the hook of the hamate and of the trapezial ridge[136] — the use of this view is sometimes eliminated by the need for extreme hyperextension of the wrist.

Hook of hamate view[137] — with the hand in mid-supination and the wrist dorsiflexed; it is often necessary to repeat this study, varying the position slightly to reveal the hamulus.

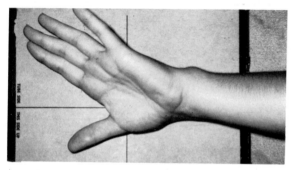

Fig. 1.86   The Robert view is taken with the forearm fully pronated, the shoulder internally rotated and the thumb abducted.

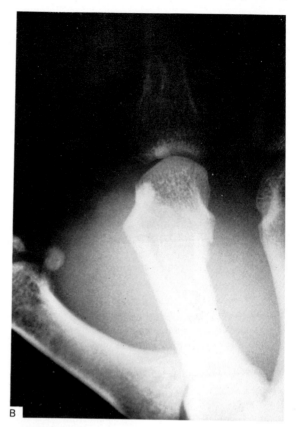

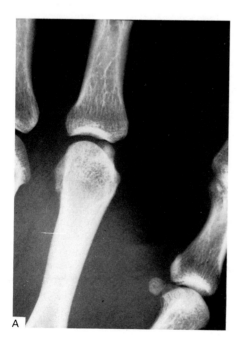

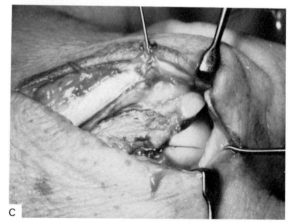

Fig. 1.87   (A) An anteroposterior view of this metacarpal head failed to reveal a fracture. (B) It was however evident on a Brewerton view. (C) Exploration revealed the degree of displacement in this comminuted fracture of the metacarpal head.

Six carpal views — true lateral, in which the metacarpal must be parallel to the radius, anteroposterior, clenched fist and postero-anterior views in three positions: neutral, and full radial and ulnar deviation — to study the carpal relationships (see below). The addition of a postero-anterior view in 20° of pronation has been suggested.[138]

Robert view[139] — taken with the arm fully pronated, the shoulder internally rotated and the thumb abducted — shows all articulations of the trapezium and first metacarpal (Fig. 1.86).

Brewerton view — taken with the fingers on the film and the metacarpophalangeal joints flexed to 65°, the tube at 15° ulnar to the vertical (p. 00) — may reveal fractures of the metacarpal head[140] (Fig. 1.87).

Stress films[141] under anaesthesia. Where instability of the basal joint of the thumb is suggested, the stress is achieved by pushing the tip of one abducted thumb against the other taking a simultaneous comparative view of both first carpometacarpal joints.

Arthrography[142].

While all bones should be scrutinised, particular attention should be paid to the following:

Points of insertion of ligaments and tendons (Fig. 1.88)
Even a small flake of bone at a point where it is known that a ligament or tendon is attached should command attention, otherwise an unstable joint or tendon imbalance may result. The mallet finger and post-traumatic boutonniere deformity may both result from such flake fragments. Splintage may suffice, but where the fragment is sufficiently separated from its origin, the tendon is also and open reduction is indicated (Fig. 1.89).

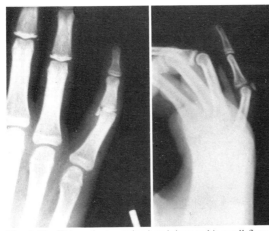

Fig. 1.88 This patient sustained an injury to his small finger while playing softball and presented with a swollen but clinically stable proximal interphalangeal joint. X-ray examination revealed, however, that the central slip of the extensor tendon had avulsed a small fragment of bone from the middle phalanx and likewise the collateral ligament a small fragment from the base on the radial aspect. Open reduction of these fragments ensured stability of the joint and prevented the development of a subsequent post-traumatic boutonniere deformity.

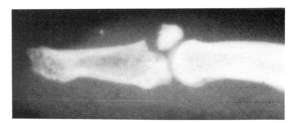

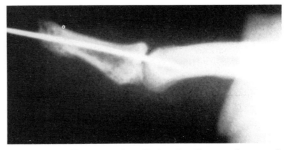

Fig. 1.89 (A) X–ray reveals a displaced mallet type fracture of the distal interphalangeal joint. (B) Open reduction and transfixation with a single Kirschner wire provides both reduction of the articular fragment and also the necessary splintage.

Alignment of articular surfaces
If intra-articular fragments are displaced even minimally, accurate reduction is imperative otherwise early osteoarthritis will be likely. Such reduction commonly requires operative intervention in a closed fracture. Many intra-articular fractures have ligaments or tendons attached to one or more of the fragments. This makes any reduction inherently unstable and internal fixation therefore necessary after reduction. In the fracture illustrated in Figure 1.90 the central slip of the extensor tendon is attached to the larger portion of the middle phalanx and only wiring prevented recurrent dorsal subluxation of the phalanx.

The mechanism is identical in the intra-articular fractures of the bases of the first and the fifth metacarpals. In the former, a Bennett's fracture[143], the abductor pollicis longus is attached to the larger metacarpal fragment, the ulnar collateral ligament to the smaller. In the latter, the extensor carpi ulnaris is similarly attached to the larger metacarpal fragment. Not only are these unstable, but even more, their displacement will become progressively worse through tendon traction if internal fixation is not employed.

The two other injuries at the basal joint of the thumb are simply variations on the Bennett's fracture —

Tear of the ulnar collateral ligament results in less pronounced but similar and equally disabling instability in the thumb skeleton. The reconstructive procedure of Eaton and Littler employing part of the flexor carpi radialis is indicated if stress films as described above or using a Robert view confirm this diagnosis.

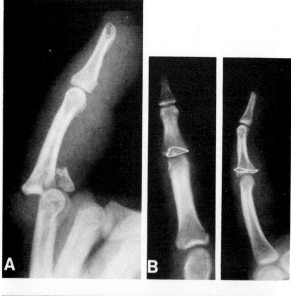

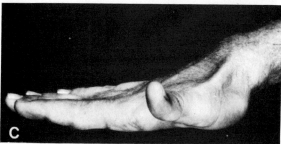

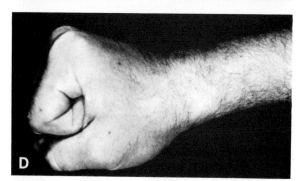

Fig. 1.90 (A) This X–ray shows a relatively common intra-articular fracture of the proximal interphalangeal joint. The small palmar fragment is still attached to the palmar plate and its relationship to the proximal phalanx is not markedly changed. The remainder of the middle phalanx is however dorsally dislocated. If this fracture is not accurately reduced, subsequent function in the joint will be compromised and early osteoarthritis assured. (B) Accurate reduction was obtained and maintained with intraosseous wiring through the triangular ligament region dorsally. This resulted in a full range of motion at eight weeks (C and D).

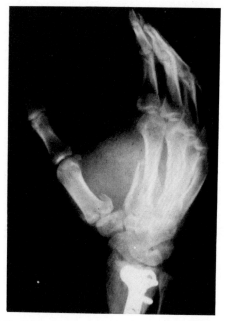

Fig. 1.91 This patient, who is clearly accident prone (evidence the plate on a Smith fracture of his radius), has sustained fractures of the metacarpal shafts and a Rolando fracture of the base of the thumb.

Rolando[144] *fracture* comes about when both abductor pollicis longus and the ulnar collateral ligament are attached to fragments broken from the main portion of the metacarpal (Fig. 1.91). Reduction and internal fixation in this less common fracture are much more difficult to achieve.

The alignment of articular surfaces in a different sense is important in avoiding minor degrees of lateral angulation in phalanges. On postero-anterior views of any phalanx the articular surfaces at either end should be parallel to one another. In the presence of swelling, some angulation may be obscured clinically but can be readily detected by drawing lines on the X-ray joining the condyles in each joint.

Fractures confined entirely to the cartilage can occur and of course do not show on any X-ray. If the injury is closed, such patients usually present late with persistent swelling and pain (p. 141).

Fractures of the metacarpal neck deserve special mention. Since the second and the third have virtually no motion at their carpo-metacarpal joint, no angulation can be accepted, otherwise the anterior displacement of the metacarpal head may produce a painful grasp. By contrast, since there is motion in the basal joint of the fourth and fifth metacarpals, some angulation can be accepted. In the common *boxer's fracture* of the fifth metacarpal neck, 40° of angulation is widely recommended as acceptable and by some as much as 70°. (Fig. 1.92.) Rather should hand

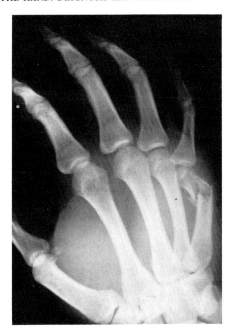

Fig. 1.92 Comminuted boxer's fracture of the head of the metacarpal.

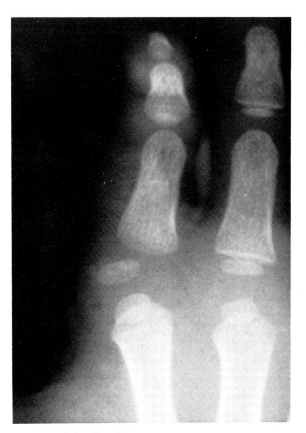

Fig. 1.94 *Salter Type I.*

function dictate management. If the patient can fully flex and fully extend his small finger, *without any tendency to claw* then the angulation should be corrected as best as possible closed and immobilised in a splint. If motion is abnormal, reduction and fixation will be necessary.

Epiphyseal fractures
Fractures which encroach on the epiphyseal plate deserve special study. They have been classified by Salter and Harris[145] into five categories (Fig. 1.93).

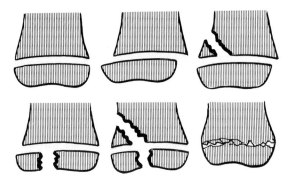

Fig. 1.93 The Salter classification of epiphyseal fractures (see text).

Type I — separation of the epiphysis from the metaphysis through the plate in a shearing manner (Fig. 1.94).

Type II — separation of the epiphysis, a small angle of metaphysis being broken off with it (Fig. 1.95).

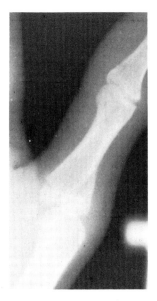
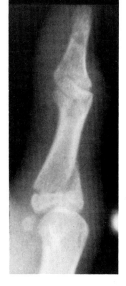

Fig. 1.95 *Salter Type II.*

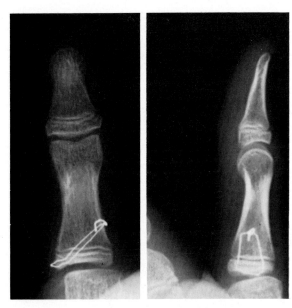

Fig. 1.96 *Salter Type III.* Here the fragment is held in place with an interosseous wire.

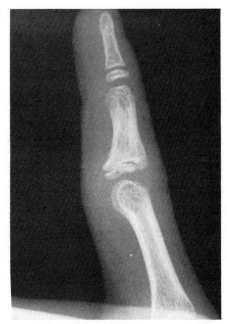

Fig. 1.97 Arrest of growth has occurred in the epiphysis of the middle phalanx consequent upon a Type V Salter fracture.

Type III — an intra-articular fracture of part of the epiphysis without interference with the epiphyseal plate (Fig. 1.96).

Type IV — a vertical, displaced fracture passing from the articular surface through epiphysis, plate and metaphysis.

Type V — a compression fracture of the cartilaginous plate with no evident injury of epiphysis or metaphysis. Type I injuries of the distal phalanx commonly produce a mallet finger appearance in the child, the extensor tendon being attached to the epiphysis, the flexor profundus to the metaphysis.

Provided they are accurately reduced Types I, II, and III carry a good prognosis as they do not interfere directly with the epiphyseal plate. Types IV and V, which do, may arrest growth of all or part of the bone with consequent shortening or angulation (Fig. 1.97). The surgeon should recognize this and warn the parents of the possibility.

Carpal-metacarpal relationship

Following heavy falls on the hand with consequent severe oedema, the junction of the carpus and the metacarpals should be scrutinized with care if no bony injury is apparent, for both dorsal (Fig. 1.98) and palmar (see Fig. 1.68) dislocation of the entire metacarpus may otherwise be overlooked.

Carpal bones

Scaphoid fractures, as is well known, may not be evident on early films. Such is the reputation of this bone for non-union, that despite lack of radiological evidence, all clinically probable cases should be treated by appropriate immobilization (Fig. 1.99).

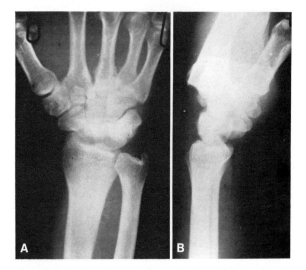

Fig. 1.98 (A) A standard anteroposterior view of the hand may not readily reveal any abnormality in the relationship between the carpus and the bases of the metacarpals, although comparison with a normal X–ray would show that there is some shortening and that no normal joint space is evident in any of these articulations. (B) A lateral view of the same patient reveals a dorsal dislocation of the metacarpals on the carpus.

Fracture of the hook of the hamate occurs after blows to the butt of the hand. It may easily be overlooked, going on to give persistent symptoms. If suspected, special radiological views should be obtained (Fig. 1.100). If detected, the fragment should be excised as non-union is common. The

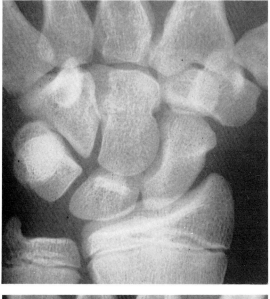

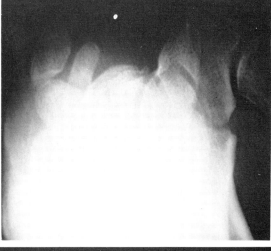

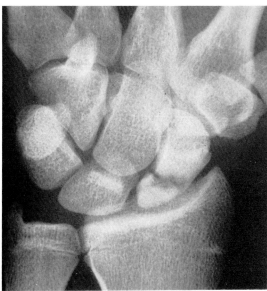

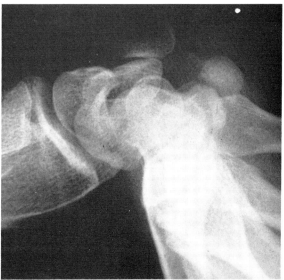

Fig. 1.99 This youth sustained a heavy fall but initial X–rays revealed no evidence of fracture. He presented some two years later complaining of wrist pain, and further X–ray (B) revealed a scaphoid fracture. It was at that time that the original films shown in (A) were reviewed.

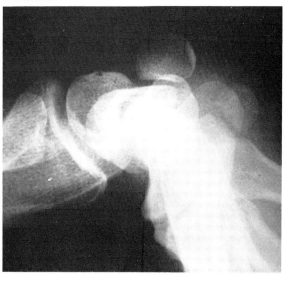

Fig. 1.100 (A) A carpal tunnel view in a suspected hamate fracture failed to reveal that fracture. The hamate view (B & C) showed the fracture at the base of the hook. Various slight adjustments should be made in this extended lateral view to be sure that the hook of the hamate is adequately visualized.

examiner must distinguish between a fracture and a persistent bipartite hamulus.

Carpal bone dislocation. Particular attention should be paid to the region of the lunate[146,147]. Dislocation of the lunate can be recognized in the antero-posterior view by its wedge-shaped appearance (Fig. 1.101) and in the lateral by the fact that the capitate does not articulate with the 'cup' of the lunate, which is rotated anteriorly out of place.

Transcaphoid-perilunate fracture-dislocation should be suspected whenever there is a palmar angulation of the hand at the carpal region, although this is often obscured by oedema, and where there is total loss of wrist extension. The radiological appearances show a widely separated fracture of the scaphoid and anterior displacement of the carpus, only the lunate and the proximal pole of the scaphoid maintaining their normal relationship to the radius (Fig. 1.102).

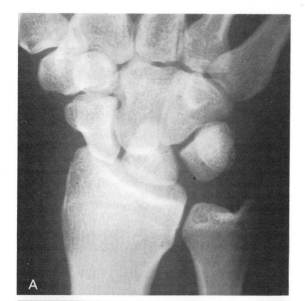

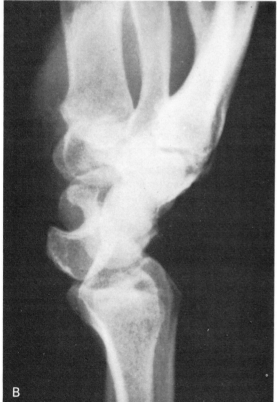

Fig. 1.101 Dislocation of the lunate is recognized on radiological examination by its wedge shaped appearance in the anteroposterior view (A) and in the lateral (B) by the fact that the capitate does not articulate with the 'cup' in the lunate.

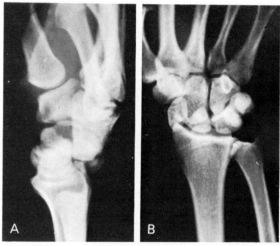

Fig. 1.102 This patient had sustained a trans-scaphoid perilunate dislocation eight weeks prior to presentation. (A) It can be seen that only the lunate and the proximal pole of the scaphoid maintain their normal relationship with the radius and that the remainder of the carpus lies dorsal to these portions of the carpus. (B) In the anteroposterior view there is wide separation of the two fragments of the scaphoid.

Traumatic carpal instability[148] has received intense attention during the past decade. While it has become evident that virtually any articulation may become unstable, it is also clear that the major group arises from heavy falls on the hand resulting in forced hyperextension, ulnar deviation and intercarpal supination. The extreme outcome is dislocation of the lunate (Stage IV), described above. Other stages[149] are recognized on X-ray as follows:

Stage I — scapho-lunate diastasis or instability

   AP view — widening of the scapho-lunate space beyond the accepted two millimetre upper limit of normal (the 'Terry-Thomas'[150] sign)

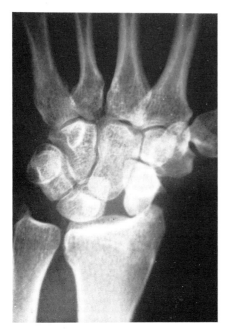

Fig. 1.103 Carpal instability. This X–ray shows considerable widening at the space between the scaphoid and the lunate. (The 'Terry Thomas' sign) In addition the scaphoid is foreshortened and superimposition of the distal pole on the body of the scaphoid results in the so-called 'signet ring' sign.

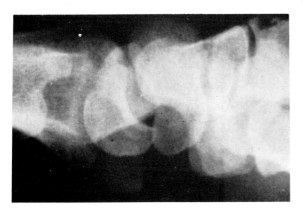

Fig. 1.104 Dorsal subluxation of the proximal scaphoid pole.

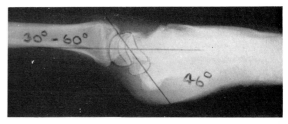

Fig. 1.105 The normal relationship has been drawn on this X–ray. The lunate is normally in neutral position relative to the radius and the metacarpal. The angle between the axis of the lunate and the scaphoid should be between 30° and 60° with an average of 46°. It should be noted that the interpretation of a true lateral can only be satisfactorily performed if the metacarpal is in direct line with the bones of the forearm.

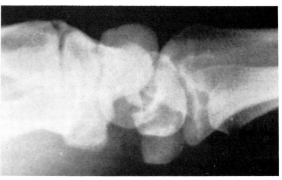

Fig. 1.106 A dorsal instability pattern of the lunate is demonstrated here, as well as in Figure 1.104. This is much more common than the palmar instability pattern.

1. *Lunate instability patterns*[152,153]: the axes of the radius, lunate, capitate and third metacarpal are usually aligned (Fig. 1.105). With carpal instability, the lunate may rotate posteriorly or anteriorly to create *palmar-flexed intercalated segment instability (PISI)* or, more commonly, *dorsi-flexed inter-calated segment instability (DISI)* (Fig. 1.106).
2. *Scapho-lunate angle:* formed by the longitudinal axes of these two bones, this averages 46° in the normal wrist with a range from 30° to 60°. Stage I instability results in a significant increase in this angle, which increases further in Stage II with the increase in dorsiflexion instability (DISI).

Radiological study of the severely disorganised carpus can often be aided by distracting the wrist. This is achieved under appropriate anaesthesia by suspending the hand using 'Chinese finger traps' and applying a weight over the distal end of the humerus.

Methods of surgical correction of carpal instability are still under evaluation and it would be wrong to express surgical indications which may well change before this volume is published! Suffice it to say that those carpal disruptions recognised early should be opened, reduced and fixed.

        — foreshortening of the scaphoid, with super-imposition of the distal pole on the proximal (the 'signet ring' sign) — rotatory subluxation[151] (Fig. 1.103).

lateral   — dorsal subluxation of the proximal scaphoid pole (Fig. 1.104).

Stage II — the same plus dorsal dislocation of the capitate

Stage III — triquetro-lunate diastasis with avulsion fracture of the triquetral.

Analysis of the true lateral view of the wrist should be performed.

In a few patients with carpal pain, even the most detailed evaluation by plain radiography will fail to reveal the cause. If a period of splintage fails to give relief, the following plan of investigation should be instituted.

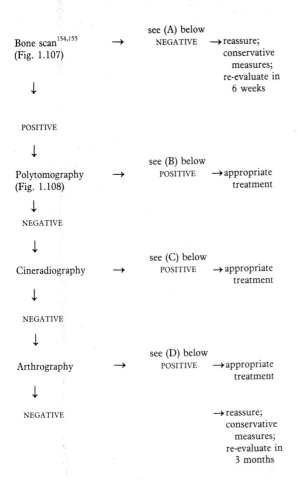

Bone scan[154,155]   →   see (A) below
(Fig. 1.107)   NEGATIVE → reassure;
                                            conservative
                                            measures;
                                            re-evaluate in
                                            6 weeks

↓

POSITIVE

↓

Polytomography   →   see (B) below
(Fig. 1.108)   POSITIVE → appropriate
                                             treatment

↓

NEGATIVE

↓

Cineradiography   →   see (C) below
                              POSITIVE → appropriate
                                               treatment

↓

NEGATIVE

↓

Arthrography   →   see (D) below
                              POSITIVE → appropriate
                                               treatment

↓

NEGATIVE   → reassure;
                                          conservative
                                          measures;
                                          re-evaluate in
                                            3 months

A = No significant pathology (while as a general rule this is true, ligamentous tears, *may* be 'cold'; if therefore problems persist at 6 weeks and the bone scan remains negative, one should re-enter the tree at 'cineradiography')

B = Occult fracture, bone cyst or tumour detected

C = Carpal instability: disruption of one or more ligaments

D = Partial ligamentous tear or loose body in joint

There appears to be almost no limit to the variety of dislocations which may appear in the hand. There is however a limit to the length of this manuscript and the reader is therefore referred to the literature in the following list of unusual injuries.

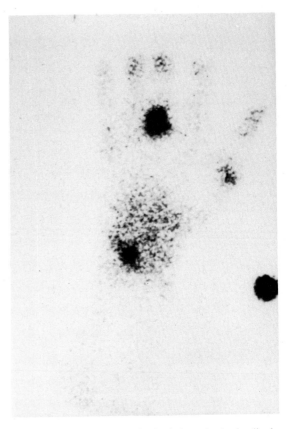

Fig. 1.107 A bone scan is of value in investigating localized carpal pain. This patient had a known injury to the region of the metacarpophalangeal joint of the middle finger, but in addition it can be seen on bone scan that he has an injury to the region of the lunatotriquetral articulation.

Dislocation of
   trapezoid[156,157]
   triquetral[158,159]
   trapezium[160,161]
   scaphoid and lunate[162,163]
   carpo-metacarpal[164-169]
   metacarpophalangeal[170-172]
   interphalangeal[173-177]
     (irreducible)
   simultaneous[178-183]

INDICATIONS in closed fractures of the metacarpus and phalanges

General comments
Once a fracture has been located and evaluated radiologically, the surgeon must decide on treatment. The aims should be those stated by the AO group
1. Accurate anatomical reduction
2. Rigid internal fixation
3. Early, active motion of the adjacent joints

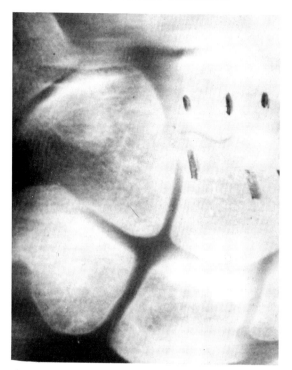

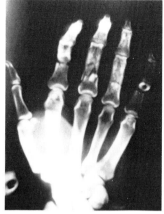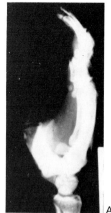

A

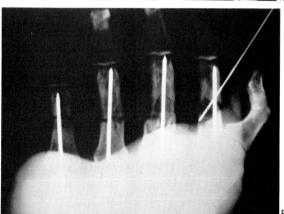

B

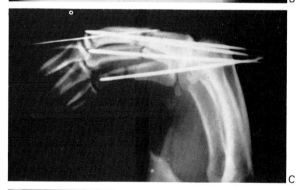

C

Fig. 1.108   Fractures of the capitate are relatively rare. *Polytomography* in this patient revealed a fracture of the waist of the capitate, thereby saving him from being labelled as a malingerer. The polytomography was only performed after bone scan had suggested the probable site of his difficulties.

In the hand, the most significant of these is the early institution of motion in the joints. With this in mind, the fracture should be studied in a set sequence:

Is the fracture reduced?
  if not, can it be reduced closed?
If it is reduced, or can be, is it then stable?
If it is not stable, can it be made so, closed?
If the fracture cannot be reduced or made stable without surgery, what will be necessary to make it so? Is that surgery justifiable?

Some closed fractures can be reduced and the reduction maintained by percutaneous pin fixation. This is particularly true of oblique fractures of the phalanges. Where previously the author opened many transverse fractures of the proximal phalanx, closed reduction and longitudinal fixation through the head of the metacarpal and the fully flexed metacarpophalangeal joint as recommended by Eaton has proved much more expeditious and at least equally successful (Fig. 1.109).

Certain closed fractures can only be reduced and made stable by complex surgery involving wide dissection, extensive use of fixation techniques and even requiring supplementary bone graft and transfixion of both adjacent

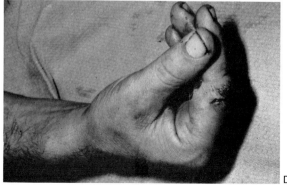

D

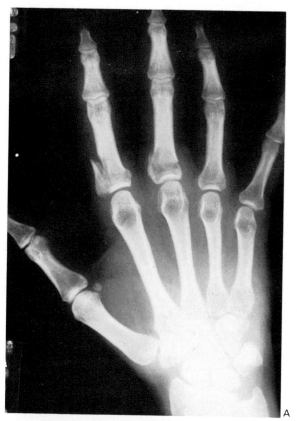

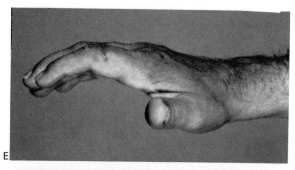

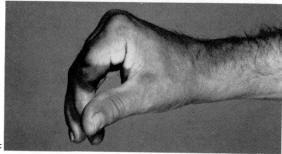

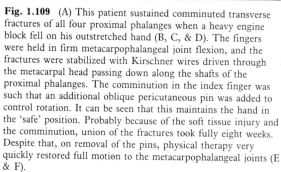

Fig. 1.109 (A) This patient sustained comminuted transverse fractures of all four proximal phalanges when a heavy engine block fell on his outstretched hand (B, C, & D). The fingers were held in firm metacarpophalangeal joint flexion, and the fractures were stabilized with Kirschner wires driven through the metacarpal head passing down along the shafts of the proximal phalanges. The comminution in the index finger was such that an additional oblique pericutaneous pin was added to control rotation. It can be seen that this maintains the hand in the 'safe' position. Probably because of the soft tissue injury and the comminution, union of the fractures took fully eight weeks. Despite that, on removal of the pins, physical therapy very quickly restored full motion to the metacarpophalangeal joints (E & F).

joints. In some cases this may be justifiable. In others, however, early active motion allied with the use of a splint for rest and protection may effect a better result. The hand surgeon must be aware of this and learn to decide which fractures require which approach (Fig. 1.110).

Fractures in children are often underestimated[184]. Remodelling can only occur in those fractures angulated in the line of pull of the tendons, that is antero-posterior, and then best at the metaphysis. Lateral angulation and rotational malalignment will *never* remodel and require accurate reduction (Fig. 1.111).

(For Bone and Joint exploration, see p. 59.)

Fig. 1.110 This patient sustained closed comminuted fractures of the bases of the proximal phalanges of the index and middle fingers. Scrutiny of the X–rays suggested that it would not be possible to reduce and fix all of the fragments were surgery to be undertaken. For this reason, the patient was commenced on early, active, protected motion. (B) This resulted in union of the phalangeal fractures with a full range of motion (C & D).

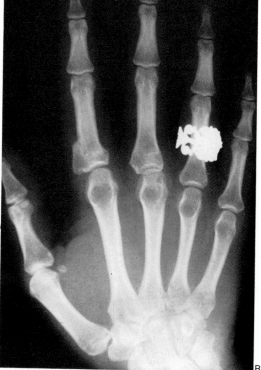

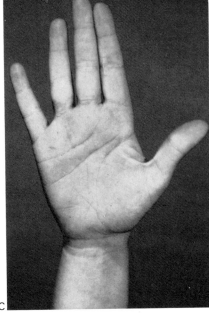

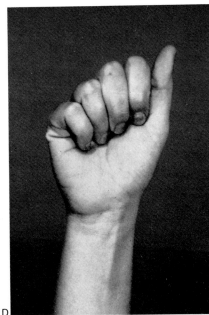

Fig. 1.110 C & D

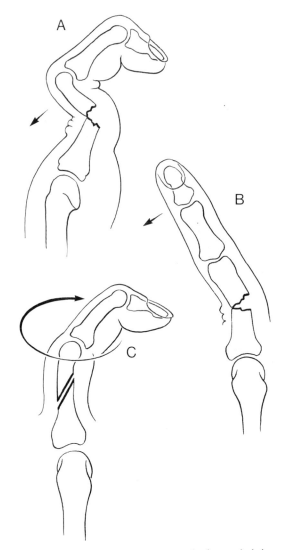

Fig. 1.111 Of the three malalignments of a fractured phalanx in a child only one will remodel, namely true palmar angulation (A). Lateral angulation (B) and rotatory malalignment (C) will not model with time and should therefore be corrected at the time of injury.

In concluding consideration of the initial emergency room examination, it is worth restating that in the crush injuries which form an increasing proportion of the hand injuries in an industrial society, examination (with the exception of radiological evaluation) plays a small role. The pain is so severe and the firm conclusions reached so limited that examination is often wisely postponed until formal exploration of the anaesthetised hand.

EXPLORATION

Although it has taken many pages to describe the history and initial examination, an experienced surgeon will complete the process in between five and fifteen minutes. As has become apparent, the examination can confirm only some of the suspicions aroused by the history. The final diagnosis is only made at exploration, the second examination.

This is always conducted under completely aseptic conditions in the operating room after thorough preparation and sterile draping of the limb. It may or may not be felt necessary by the surgeon to have tourniquet control during exploration but it does facilitate thorough cleansing of the wound and identification of structures.

The first step in exploration, often time consuming, is to thoroughly cleanse the wound. This should be carried out using some form of pulsatile flow of normal saline or Ringer's lactate achieved by the use of a large chip syringe or the 'water-pick'. The addition of local antibiotics to the irrigating fluid has been shown to significantly reduce the bacterial contamination[185] of the wound and a mixture of Polymyxin B 50 mg/ml and Bacitracin 50 u/s/ml[186] is a satisfactory choice. Cleansing of contaminated areas in the stream of saline is best done with the surgeon's glove finger. All interstices of the wounds must be sought out. The extent of a penetrating wound is often difficult to determine and partial division of tendons may be missed. In such a situation the presence of *blood staining of the tissue is a valuable guide* to the extent of the wound. Open joints should receive particularly careful scrutiny as foreign material may have been sucked into their far recesses.

The process should be continued patiently until all contamination has been cleaned out. The longer the delay between injury and surgery the more difficult this becomes. Where it proves impossible a choice must be made between

1. *sharp debridement of contaminated tissue.* This may be undesirable where it involves opening a joint, exposing bare bone or tendon or excising vital structures.
2. *leaving soiled tissue.* This will inevitably lead to inflammation and result in an increase in early oedema and late fibrosis. It will predispose to infection.

Widely scattered fragments of metal, which are relatively non-reactive, such as occur in shotgun injuries or explosions are commonly left but their pursuit may reveal unexpected injuries to deep structures. If difficulty is encountered in locating radiolucent foreign bodies, *xeroradiography* may be of assistance.[187,188].

Adequate exploration may require surgical extension of the skin wound. This practice has been criticised in the past but is completely justifiable provided cleansing as described has been meticulously performed. The line of the extending incision should be chosen with three factors in mind:

1. The viability of the skin flaps;
2. the avoidance of subsequent contracture by the careful choice of line. For example, on the flexor aspect of the digit, an appropriate modification of the mid-lateral or Bruner incisions should be used;
3. the history of injury, since the hand posture at that time indicates the probable site of tendon laceration in relation to the skin wound (p. 4).
4. the probable location of injured structures as suggested by the shape of the wound (p. 15).

In thoroughly cleansing all aspects of the wound the surgeon does more than that. He also compiles a list of injured structures, considers how they are to be repaired and establishes an order for the ensuing operation.

Bone and joint

In most compound injuries of the hand fractures can be palpated and visualized. Fragments entirely loose should be removed, those retaining periosteal attachments should be kept. Periosteum should be carefully preserved for its repair over a well reduced fracture will do much to prevent adhesion of overlying structures to the fracture site. Not uncommonly periosteal repair will be the only practical means of holding the reduction of some of the fragments in a badly comminuted fracture.

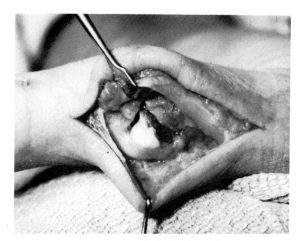

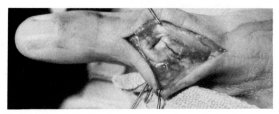

Figs. 1.112A & B Surgical exposure of an articular fracture permits accurate reduction and internal fixation to be performed.

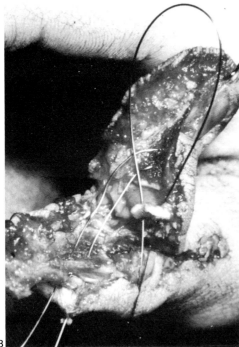
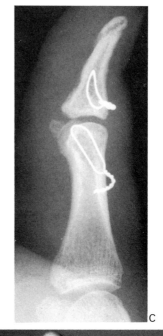
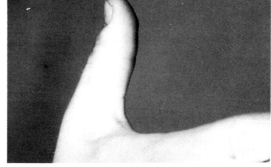
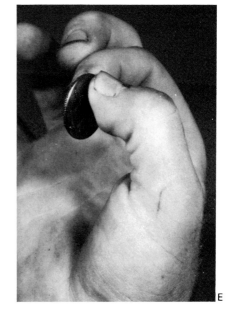

Fig. 1.113   (A) Saw injury of the distal phalanx passing through the distal interphalangeal joint requires careful interosseous fixation (B & C) of all fragments to preserve articular alignment. In this way restoration of function can be achieved (D & E).

All fractures should be reduced and immobilized as the first step for only then, in certain instances, can an accurate assessment be made of damage to other structures. Such instances include flow in vessels, viability of tissues and the presence and extent of defects in skin, vessel, tendon and nerve.

Particular attention should be given to obtaining an anatomically perfect reduction of fractures involving the articular surface[189] or, in children, the growing epiphysis (Fig. 1.112). In complex, open injuries this may require careful threading of various fragments on to interosseous wires in order to restore articular integrity (Fig. 1.113). In all fractures of the digits and metacarpal bones, rotational mal-alignments must be excluded or malfunction will result (Fig. 1.114). This is best achieved by visualization of the

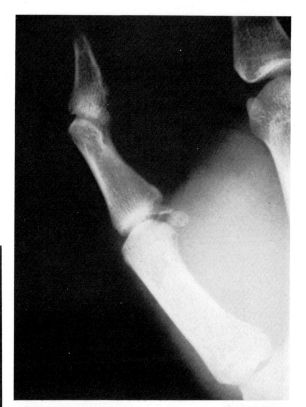

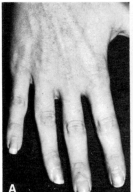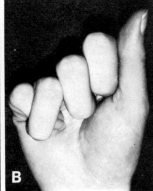

Fig. 1.114 This patient had sustained a fracture of the metacarpal of the right ring finger and insufficient attention was paid to obtaining the correct rotational alignment. This resulted in a deformity functionally and cosmetically unsatisfactory to the patient and embarrassing for the surgeon.

fracture during reduction and fixation. Where this is not possible or not applicable as in comminution with bone loss, the relationship of the planes of the finger nails with the interphalangeal joints flexed should be compared with that on the uninjured hand. A better known fact, but one it is not always possible to apply, is that all fingers when flexed at metacarpophalangeal and proximal interphalangeal joints point to the tubercle of scaphoid (Fig. 1.110). Repeated simultaneous flexion of injured and uninjured fingers to ensure that they are 'tracking' correctly is a further method of checking alignment. Appropriate fixation is selected.

The presence of dislocation should be confirmed and where reduction does not restore to the joint its original range and stability, the periarticular structures should be inspected. In the absence of juxta-articular fractures, instability will be due to disruption of the collateral ligament or plate. It is important to determine whether the disruption is in the substance of the ligament or is an

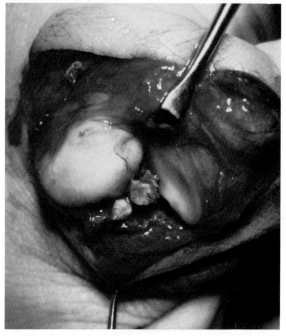

Fig. 1.115 (A) X-ray examination of this patient who sustained a game-keeper's thumb revealed a suspicious fragment on the palmar aspect of the joint. (B) Exploration of the joint revealed not only a fracture fragment from the anterior lip of the proximal phalanx, but also a depressed condylar fracture of the metacarpal head.

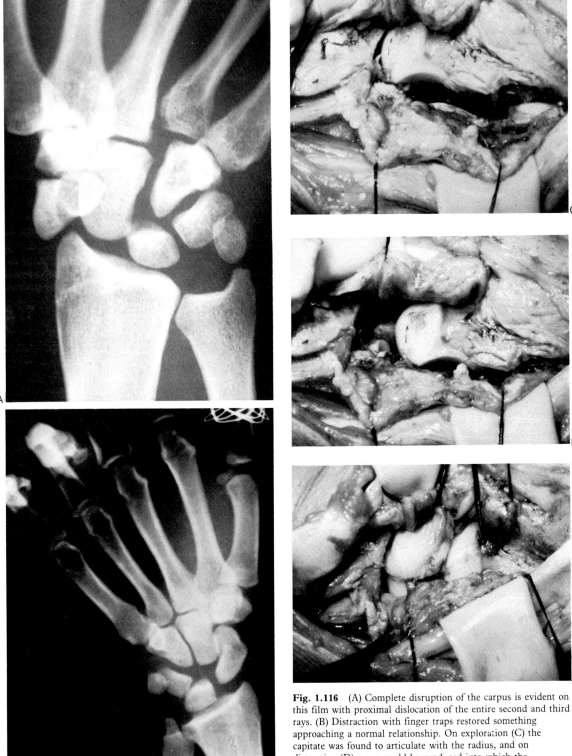

Fig. 1.116 (A) Complete disruption of the carpus is evident on this film with proximal dislocation of the entire second and third rays. (B) Distraction with finger traps restored something approaching a normal relationship. On exploration (C) the capitate was found to articulate with the radius, and on distraction (D) a gap could be produced into which the dislocated lunate could be replaced and fixed. (E) The ligaments were subsequently repaired, and the patient retrieved 70% of normal wrist motion.

avulsion of the ligament from the bone as the technique of repair may differ. Where the range of motion is decreased by reduction of the dislocation or where reduction cannot be achieved, it is probable that a portion of the periarticular structures is trapped in that joint space and this should be sought. Quite frequently, the entrapped tissue proves to be the palmar plate, torn in a hyperextension injury, as in complex dislocation of the index metacarpal already described. Alternatively, the trapped tissue may be unrelated to the joint — a so-called *complicated dislocation*[190]. This is especially common in the elbow joint where the brachial artery, median[191], ulnar and radial nerves can all become caught in an elbow dislocation and retained there after reduction.

If a joint is lying open or is surgically explored, the articular surface should be examined directly for fractures and also to determine that no flakes of cartilage are lying free in the joint (Fig. 1.115).

In *crush injuries of the carpus,* fractures and dislocations often coexist.[192] Displacement of the elements occurs either through the injuring force or because of the traction exerted by tendons at the time of the injury. Exploration should be aimed at determining the nature of any disorientation of these carpal bones and fragments. This is achieved by knowledge of the normal anatomy and by locating the articular facets and tendon insertions on each. Reduction is often facilitated by applying finger trap distraction and is further aided by repeated study of the X-rays (Fig. 1.116).

In *crush and friction injuries,* the viability of bone may be in question. This is most difficult to resolve at the time of primary exploration. Vessel refilling on release of the tourniquet, so helpful in assessing the skin, is of much less value in assessing blood supply to bone. In addition periosteal flow is not essential to survival of the cortex if medullary blood supply is good. Resection of bone, except where done as part of the process of resecting non-viable soft tissues, is therefore not performed as a primary procedure. The desirability of achieving primary skin cover in compound fractures whenever possible is a subject of debate. If one believes in its merits, as does the author, the need to cover exposed bone is heightened by absence of the periosteum or serious doubts concerning its viability.

Where there are significant defects in an exposed bone[193], correct alignment and rigid fixation of the remaining fragments is of equal, if not greater, importance. *Optimal skeletal length must be determined and maintained from the time of the initial surgery.* Once lost, wound contracture will prevent its recovery. Occasionally the object of alignment may be achieved by further bone resection to achieve good contact at the site of osteosynthesis but this has the distinct disadvantage of relatively lengthening the tendons (Fig. 1.117). This can be offset by equivalent shortening where they also are divided — this is common practice in the course of replantation and revascularisation where

shortening aids neurovascular repair. In those cases where shortening is inappropriate, fixation may be achieved internally or externally. Where internal, the fixation is most commonly achieved by Kirschner wires in the phalanges and by plates and screws[194] in the metacarpals. Clearly in the presence of a bone defect, compression techniques, such as interosseous wiring[195], are not applicable. Intramedullary fixation, using accurately cut selected Steinman pins, is an excellent method of managing a badly comminuted phalangeal fracture, especially in the elderly, for it best maintains the soft tissue attachments of the fragments[196] (Fig. 1.118). External fixation may employ a sophisticated device such as the mini-Hoffman[197] or may be constructed by Kirschner wires 'spot-welded' by methyl methacrylate[198] (Fig. 1.119). Wherever possible the fixation should be applied only to the bone which is fractured. This may however be inadequate and it proves necessary to go to the next bone. When this is done, the intervening joint must be transfixed or fracture fixation is not achieved and alignment will be lost.

Whenever, in applying either internal or external fixation, joints must be transgressed, then it is imperative to place them in the 'safe' position, that is, extension of the interphalangeal joints, flexion of the metacarpophalangeal.

The bone defect remains. If all tissues are clearly viable or can be made so, or if it is necessary to support a significant fragment such as an articular segment, then immediate cancellous bone grafting is indicated. In other circumstances, it can with benefit be left for 48 to 72 hours.

Where the skeletal defect is due to loss of a joint, length can be maintained by insertion either of a cortico cancellous bone graft to achieve fusion or of an immediate joint replacement. Although this sounds hazardous, the author has done it with success and with no complications in over ten cases (Fig. 1.120). The need for adequate debridement and good skin cover is heightened in all such procedures.

In the operative management of all fractures, from the most simple to the most complex, peroperative radiography plays an essential role.

Tendon and muscle

In the tidy hand injury, fairly firm conclusions will have been made about which tendons have been lacerated during the initial examination. These conclusions should be confirmed at exploration. The problems then remaining concern distinction of tendon and nerve, matching of tendon ends and exposure in the digit.

TENDON OR NERVE?

Locating the ends of divided structures for identification, matching and suture can be a frustrating exercise. Clearly flexing the wrist and fingers fully will help to bring the ends towards the wound but then, even with retraction, the ends may be obscured by blood clot. Herein lies the solution. By dissecting where the clot is most dense and

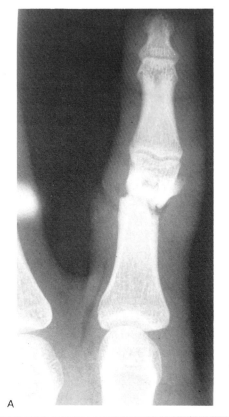

A

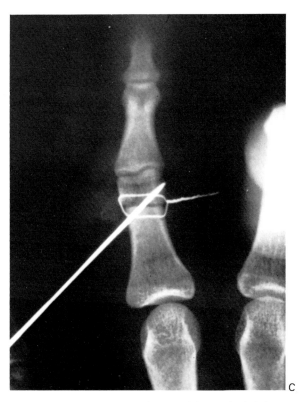

C

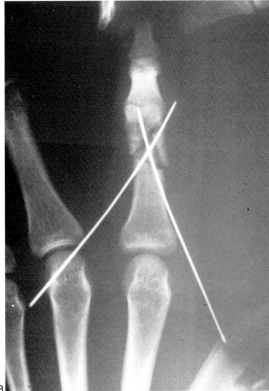

B

Fig. 1.117 (A) A comminuted fracture of the proximal phalanx proved impossible to internally fix with Kirschner wires. (B) Shortening of the two fragments with transverse osteotomies permitted rigid internal fixation (C) to be applied.

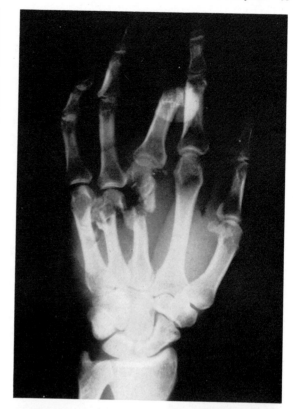

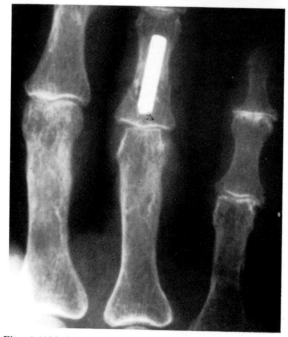

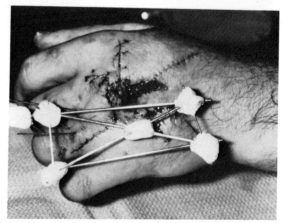

Fig. 1.119 (A) Following a gunshot wound this patient had a significant segmental loss of the third and fourth rays. (B) The length was maintained at the time of the initial debridement by the use of Kirschner wires 'spot welded' with methyl methacrylate.

Figs. 1.118A & B A comminuted fracture in a 93 year old lady with significant osteoporosis was effectively fixed using an intramedullary Steinmann pin. She proceeded to retrieve full motion in this digit.

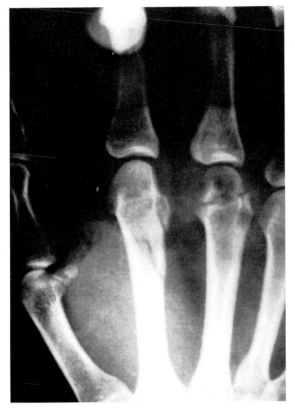

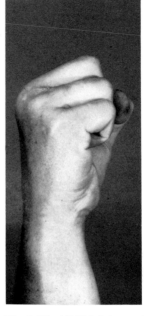
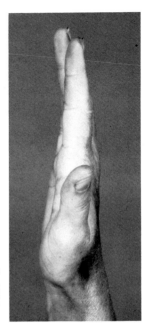

Fig. 1.120 (A) This lady sustained an open, untidy injury when her hand was caught in a cement mixer. Exploration revealed that the metacarpal head of the middle phalanx was loose, and that the fracture of the second metacarpal was stable. (B) Immediate joint replacement was undertaken, uneventful healing occurred, and she retreived full function as seen three years later (C & D).

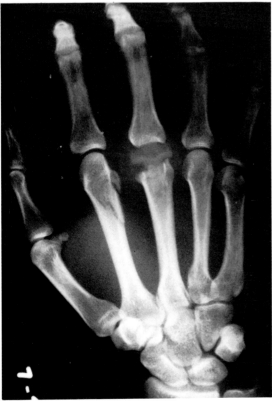

pure the ends will be revealed as white gleams through the gore (Fig. 1.121). Working in this bloodstained synovium is like wading through quicksand. Rather should it be excised sharply, revealing the contained structures, which can be identified by

Colour: Tendon — whitish yellow; nerve — whitish grey.

Texture of the surface: Tendon — smooth and firm; nerve — softer and somewhat more irregular due to the fascicular bundles appearing as longitudinal strands.

Median artery: If the structure believed to be the median nerve is inspected closely with magnification, an artery of differing diameter will almost always be found on its surface. Both nerve ends can be so identified. The artery also serves to ensure that the correct orientation of the nerve ends is selected.

Retraction: Nerve ends retract much less than do divided tendons.

Nerve fascicles: After irrigation, if the nerve end is turned end on and inspected with magnification, the fasicular bundles can be seen, shiny and hemispherical.

Passive movement: Selective flexion of the digital joints will identify individually the *distal* tendon ends. Once the *proximal* ends have been identified with a high degree of

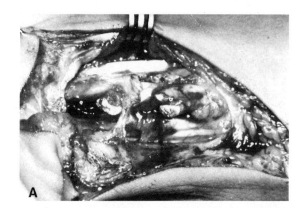

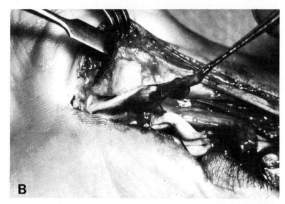

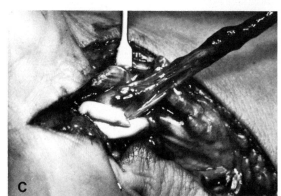

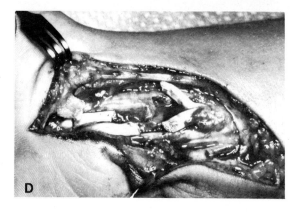

Fig. 1.121 (A) This patient had sustained a clean laceration of the palmar aspect of the wrist. The proximal tendon ends had been retrieved with little difficulty but even with full finger flexion the distal tendon ends were obscured in the dark blood clots seen at the proximal end of the carpal tunnel (on the left of the photograph). By dissecting where the blood clot was most dense (B and C), the distal tendon ends were revealed as a white gleam through the synovium. After transfixing the tendons with straight needles they were suitably approximated for subsequent primary tendon suture (D).

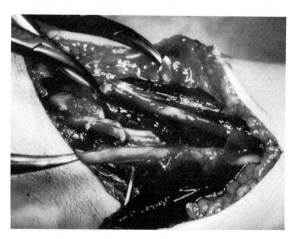

Fig. 1.122 Traction on the proximal ends of the probable tendons will reveal the presence of muscle bellies.

confidence, grasp then in turn by the cut end with fine toothed forceps and pull gently. Characteristic gliding motion will result and often the muscle belly will be revealed (Fig. 1.122).

TENDON IDENTIFICATION and PREPARATION

At the wrist: distal ends

In multiple flexor tendon injuries at the wrist, identification of the distal ends is straightforward after they have been located, profundus tendons flexing the distal interphalangeal joint, superficialis tendons the proximal interphalangeal joint. Traction on the distal end should be performed with the same care as on the proximal end by grasping the cut tendon end with fine toothed dissecting or mosquito forceps in order to avoid damage to the outer surface of the tendon (Fig. 1.123). Pulling on any finger flexor at the wrist, but especially a profundus tendon, will produce flexion to a varying degree in fingers adjacent to the finger to which the tendon goes, due to the interconnections between the tendons and due to the common synovial sheath. This spurious movement can be distinguished from that in the correct finger by gently resisting the pull with a finger on each digital pulp in turn.

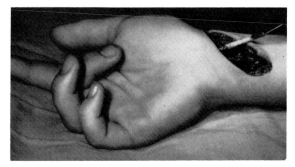

Fig. 1.123 Traction on the distal tendon end will effect flexion of either the proximal or the distal interphalangeal joint thereby revealing as here, a flexor digitorum superficialis.

In the correct finger there is a precise transmission of pull from tendon to finger tip compared with the 'dampened' pull in the adjacent finger.

Proximal ends

The correct matching of the proximal ends at the wrist is rather more taxing as all pass through the space which occupies only 3 cm to the ulnar side of the median nerve. Four features aid in identification:

Anatomy. The finger flexor tendons lie in three layers:
Superficial: Flexor digitorum superficialis to middle and ring (Fig. 1.124).
Middle: Flexor digitorum superficialis to index and small.
Deep: Flexor digitorum profundus to all fingers; those to middle, ring and small are conjoined; that to index is separate (Fig. 1.125).

Cross-section. No two tendons have identical cross-section either in diameter or shape.

Angle of cut. Despite the fact that all have been injured by the one blow it is surprising how the angle of the cut varies. This also affects the cross-sectional appearance.

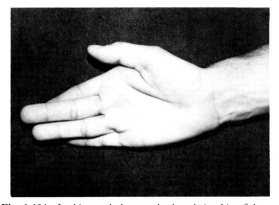

Fig. 1.124 In this posed photograph, the relationship of the superficialis tendons at the wrist is demonstrated. Those to the middle and ring fingers lie superficial to those to the small and index finger.

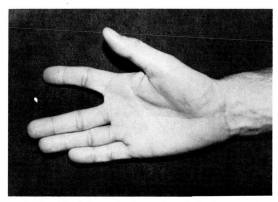

Fig. 1.125 All of the profundus tendons lie in the same plane. Those to the middle, ring and small fingers are, however, conjoined at the wrist, arising as they do from a common muscle belly while that to the index finger is quite separate.

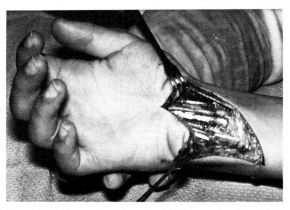

Fig. 1.126 The patient whose hand is illustrated in Fig. 1.121 had sustained an oblique laceration. After approximation and repair of the tendon ends it is evident that the correct proximal end was selected by the positioning of the fingers which lie in the normal cascade, the relationship of the fingers one to another being that which is seen in the uninjured hand.

Length. If the tendon ends are brought into exact apposition with no gap or overlap and held there, ready for suturing, by transfixion of the tendon ends with straight needles, the normal balanced posture of the finger should result (Fig. 1.126). Standard hypodermic needles should be used for this task, for they are sharp, inflict little damage and because of their hub they cannot stray or be forgotten.

While describing retrieval of proximal tendon ends, an anatomical point should be made with regard to the flexor carpi radialis. It lies neither above the fascia nor below it but rather within it, in its own separate tunnel. If the surgeon remembers this he will retrieve it either by looking for the tunnel end-on, where it will be marked by tell-tale blood clot or he will seek it from above or below the fascia where the tendon will shine through and can be released by incision.

In the digit

Having extended the incision as required to expose the distal end as dictated by the posture of the hand at the time of injury (p. 4) the flexor tendon sheath is exposed. Current theory and increasing practice dictate that the sheath should be preserved and repaired after flexor tendon repair.[199]. Sheath repair is relatively easy in its retinacular or cruciate portions and rather difficult in the annular pulleys. The latter should therefore be preserved intact whenever possible. With this in mind the cut end of the distal tendon should be located by looking through the sheath while flexing the finger. It will be seen as a moving junction of white tendon and dark red blood. The length of this tendon which can be seen in the retinacular portion of the sheath with full flexion is then measured (Fig. 1.127):

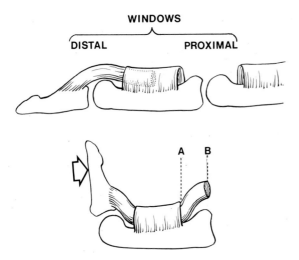

Fig. 1.127 Assessment for exposure during flexor tendon repair (see text).

AB	
1 cm or more	the entire tendon repair can be done by opening a 'window' in that retinacular portion of the sheath — a proximal window repair.[200]
0.5 to 1 cm:	the 'core' suture (Mason-Allen, modified Kessler etc.) cannot be placed in the distal tendon end through that window so both it and the next window distally must be opened — a combined window repair.
less than 0.5 cm:	even the peripheral running suture cannot be inserted through that window so that the major part of the work must be done in the next window — a distal window repair.

EXTENSOR TENDONS

The *distal ends* can be identified by the action produced on traction, bearing in mind the effect of the intertendinous connections.

The *proximal ends* can be classified into groups if they remain in their compartment beneath the extensor retinaculum or if they can be replaced there with confidence by tracing them into the sheath from which they have retracted. Which tendons come through which compartment can be recalled by using Table 1.1 (p. 12). Further identification depends, as with the flexor tendons, on studying

cross-section,

angle of cut,

length (Fig. 1.128)

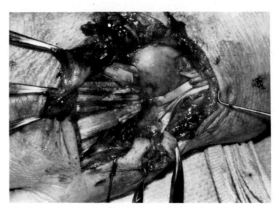

Fig. 1.128 In this clean cut laceration of all the extensor tendons at the wrist, the variation in cross-sectional dimension, in angle of cut and in the length of the various tendons can be seen.

PARTIAL DIVISION OF TENDONS

This may not have been revealed on examination but may subsequently result in tendon rupture if not repaired. Where some tendons have been totally divided this gives a strong clue as to the site of any partial divisions inflicted on others. In either case, partial divisions of tendons should be sought by inspecting each tendon in the vicinity of the skin wound along as much of its length as can be delivered into the wound by full flexion of all joints with traction alternatively proximally and distally directed. The traction should be exerted by gripping the tendon with a gauze swab moistened with saline or by the use of a smooth sharp tendon hook. This process should be repeated at all wounds for all tendons regardless of whether or not they have already been found to be divided in one wound. Injuries at multiple levels do occur and may be missed, especially if the division is only partial at one of them. It is worthy of re-emphasis that all blood clot and bloodstaining should be thoroughly pursued and explored for this frequently reveals partial injuries.

Although there is debate on the matter[201], partial tendon injuries should be repaired to avoid later triggering, entrapment or rupture[202] (Fig. 1.129).

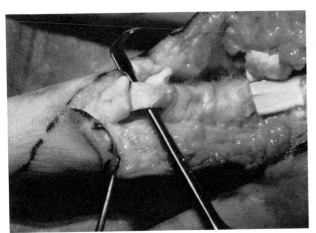

Fig. 1.129 This patient was explored secondarily because of lack of motion in a previously lacerated finger. He was found to have a partial laceration which was locking on the A² pulley, preventing motion.

ABRASION AND AVULSION OF TENDONS

Such injuries, especially of the extensors, are not uncommon in industrial and road traffic accidents. Much raw tendon is exposed to which adhesion can occur and the chance of successful function following primary repair is considerably less than in tidy lacerations.

Where the extensor tendon has only been partially abraded, the paratenon is lost and the blood supply of the tendon compromised. Gross contamination is the rule rather than the exception. These considerations apart, however, such unpromising material often does surprisingly well, although later tendolysis is very likely to be required. If satisfactory skin cover can be obtained, therefore, the tendon should be thoroughly cleansed, loose ends trimmed away and the tendon retained.

Tendons which have been avulsed are often found lying dangling from the wound in crush and roller injuries. However, their substance is often remarkably undamaged and if there is a chance that the part on which they act can be salvaged, they should be cleansed and sutured back in place, either from whence they came or to an adjacent motor better preserved, for they are difficult and in some instances impossible to replace.

MUSCLE

Muscle bellies are frequently injured in crush and avulsion injury. Dead muscle is an ideal medium for the growth of anaerobic organisms. At exploration the identification and excision of all non-viable muscle is therefore imperative. This is done using two criteria.

Appearance: Due to venous congestion and oedema the muscle which is probably non-viable bulges from its fascial covering and has a dark plum-red color contrasting with the brownish red of adjacent normal muscle.

Twitch: When normal muscle is grasped gently with toothed dissecting forceps, it twitches. Dead muscle does not. This test is valid regardless of the agents being used by the anaesthetist, but twitch decreases progressively with tourniquet ischaemia.

Perfusion: Especially in macroreplantation, it is important to know whether muscle in the amputated part will be perfused after vessel repair. Therefore perfusion through the major artery is undertaken before replantation with heparinised Ringer's lactate. Any muscle which does not ooze lactate is excised. This practice has markedly increased survival and decreased infection. It is equally applicable in revascularisation.

INDICATIONS

Opinions differ regarding primary repair of tendons. The author and his associates stand at one extreme end of the spectrum, believing that the primary repair of all injured tendons regardless of the site offers the best chance of speedy return of good function.[203] Contraindications are few. They include

loss of a segment of tendon — best judged by approximating the ends and assessing the resultant posture.

joint injuries of a nature sufficiently severe as to preclude early motion.

fractures which cannot be accurately reduced and securely fixed.

skin loss of a nature requiring distant flap coverage.

This is not the place to detail technique and postoperative management, only to stress that meticulous attention to these details is imperative if this philosophy is to prove successful.

Nerve

LACERATION

Where sensory and motor loss of characteristic distribution has been demonstrated on initial examination, exploration usually reveals a clear division of the nerve. Being softer and rather more adherent to adjacent soft tissue, nerve ends are somewhat less easy to locate than are the firmer tendon ends. The proximal end of the *ulnar nerve* divided at the wrist tends to adhere to the deep, radial surface of flexor carpi ulnaris and during exploration of the wound to be retracted with it. Likewise, the proximal end of the *median nerve* divided somewhat higher adheres to the deep surface of flexor digitorum superficialis. The ulnar nerve is further obscured by the more superficial and anterior ulnar artery with which it constitutes a neurovascular bundle invested by adipose tissue. Any difficulty encountered in locating nerve ends should be overcome by applying the rule which is absolute in secondary exploration — one must always dissect from normal tissue towards the injury. Thus in seeking out the end of a lacerated structure — and this is especially true in difficult exposures such as the upper forearm or the deep spaces of the hand — the incision should be extended adequately and the nerve, or vessel, displayed in uninjured tissue and traced from there. In applying this maxim to an injured nerve, there is clearly more hazard in dissecting the distal nerve end from distal proximally, for branches will be encountered and must be protected and incorporated in the nerve as the surgeon advances.

Once the ends have been located, correct orientation is essential in mixed nerves if the fullest recovery is to follow nerve suture. This is achieved using magnifying loupes, by
1. Matching blood vessels
2. Drawing a fascicular plan (Fig. 1.130): gripping the epineurium with very fine forceps, the nerve endings are rotated so that they can be examined either through strong loupes or the operating microscope. The fascicular bundles are of different size and, if the microscope is being used, can be seen to consist of differing number of fascicles. A plan should be drawn of each end in turn either mentally or using a sterile pen and paper and then the two ends matched.

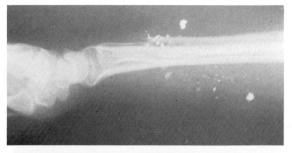

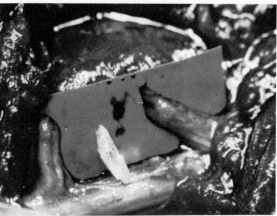

Fig. 1.131 A fracture of the ulna was inflicted on this child when she came between victim and assailant. The exploration revealed an injury of the ulnar nerve due to a bone fragment. The nerve damage was sufficiently well localized as to justify primary nerve graft.

PROXIMAL   DISTAL

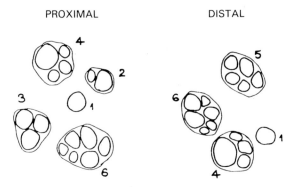

Fig. 1.130 This is a sketch of the fascicular bundles of the proximal and distal ends of a severed median nerve. It will be seen by comparing the size and number of fascicles contained in each bundle that accurate matching can be undertaken.

Primary or secondary repair of nerves has been the subject of some controversy. The ease of matching in the fresh injury, the impracticality of performing a delayed repair when tendons have been sutured primarily and the increased tension which results from the greater resection of nerve end necessary in secondary repair has made primary epineural suture supplemented by fascicular aligning sutures where necessary the method of choice for the author.

Where a defect exists in the nerve primary grafting should be performed only when the surgeon is confident that he is joining good nerve, that the skeleton is well stabilised, that the nerve graft has soft tissue cover which is well-vascularised and that healing will occur per primam (Fig. 1.131).

If *any* doubt exists as to the quality of nerve presenting for repair, it should be left and explored once the wounds are healed. An unsatisfactory suture does the patient a disservice because several months will pass before a decision will be taken to explore a nerve which is recorded as 'repaired' in the initial operation note. There is some merit in attaching the nerve ends one to the other to prevent retraction and thereby shorten the gap.

AVULSION

Where a nerve has been avulsed the injury is inflicted at differing levels in different fascicles and traction damage occurs both proximal and distal to the obvious division. This is revealed by several observations:
— the ends, both proximal and distal, are much thinner than expected or indeed than is the nerve itself when it is dissected out further away from the wound
— the ends frequently overlap
— when inspected with magnification the nerve can be seen to be the site of multiple sub-epineurial haemorrhages for some distance from its end.
Suture carries a greatly reduced hope of full function.

INJURIES IN CONTINUITY

When characteristic sensory and motor loss have been found on examination, but, despite exhaustive exploration of all wounds, the nerve in question is found to be intact an *axonotmesis* or *neurapraxia* (p. 166) has been sustained. In order to facilitate possible secondary neurolysis the exact site and extent of any bruising or swelling of the nerve should be recorded at exploration. If such swelling is significant primary epineurotomy *may* reduce nerve damage and speed recovery.

Traction injury

A long section of the nerve is damaged in traction injuries; it is swollen throughout to a varying degree and considerable quantities of extravasated blood may be visible through the epineurium. If this is creating tension evidenced by induration of the nerve on palpation, then it should be released by incising the epineurium.

Compression

Prolonged compression sufficient to produce lasting nerve disturbance is an unusual primary injury but may be found during exploration of an acute carpal tunnel or compartment syndrome. In the latter situation the nerve injury corresponds exactly to the extent of the forearm muscle bellies. The nerve is constricted, pale and avascular.

In all injuries in continuity, the significant point is whether or not the continuity of the axons themselves has been broken. The two possibilities have been given distinct names and the prognosis differs considerably.

Neurapraxia: axons intact — prognosis; early, full recovery;

Axonotmesis: axons divided — prognosis; late, possibly incomplete, recovery.

While it is not possible to distinguish between the two at the time of primary injury, neurapraxia is said to be associated in the majority of cases with retention of part or all of the sensory function of the nerve. Nerve conduction studies are of no value in making the distinction until some 48 hours to 8 days after injury, when conduction distal to the site of injury will remain only in the neurapraxia (the time until loss of distal conduction differs in various studies).

Vessel

Named arteries in the region of injury should be inspected, both under tourniquet control and after its release. Lacerations in large vessels should be occluded proximally and distally with bulldog clamps and in small with microvascular clamps. In the large vessel it is also prudent to dissect out the next most proximal branch and place a soft sling around the main vessel just above to afford immediate control should a clamp slip. The tourniquet should then be released and the speed of arterial inflow through other vessels to the region served by the lacerated one assessed before the choice between vascular repair and ligation is made.

Viability should not be the only criterion of the need to perform a vascular repair as relative ischaemia may produce later disability. Radial or ulnar arteries at the wrist should be repaired if the division is clean and the injury otherwise suitable. Most fingers have a dominant digital artery as evidenced by the calibre of the vessel. Where only one has been divided it should be repaired if experience is available both to judge that it is of significant calibre and to perform the microvascular repair. When neither carries flow, the finger is nonviable and vascular reconstruction is essential.

Partial lacerations are especially likely to produce considerable blood loss as haemostasis cannot be effected by the usual means of vessel retraction (p. 37).

Torsion and compression of vessels may result in marked spasm and this may persist despite removal of the cause. The vessel should be observed until the spasm settles. This may be encouraged by the application of a stream of warm lignocaine 1%. Where it does not resolve in vessels of consequence, flow should be restored by exploratory arteriotomy and replacement with a reversed vein graft where significant damage to the vessel is found.

Where vascular repair is to be performed, three major factors influence the outcome and these should be assessed during exploration.

1. *Proximal flow.* On release of the tourniquet it is probable that there will be no flow evident due to vasospasm and a small terminal thrombus. These problems should be overcome by dilatation of the vessel after resection of its cut end. This should result in brisk, pulsatile bleeding of considerable force which does not reduce provided the vessel is held out to length (Fig. 1.132). As a simple guide to desired force, blood from a digital artery should reach the end of the hand table, from the radial or ulnar the near side of the nurse's table and from the brachial artery the far side!

2. *Uninjured vessel ends.* These should be inspected under magnification appropriate to the vessel size, seeking any evidence of intimal damage or separation, of intramural or intraluminal thrombus or of vessel disease.

3. *Good run-off.* The amputated part or the limb distal to the vascular injury should be examined again for any evidence of injury likely to involve the distal vessel. The vessel distal to the injury should be exposed for a length which varies according to the degree of avulsion thought to be involved in the trauma. That vessel should be inspected for any evidence of damage, and in particular for
   (i) thrombus
   (ii) avulsed branches

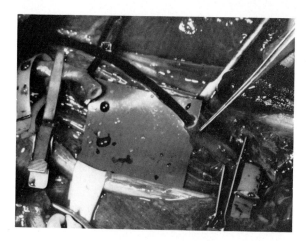

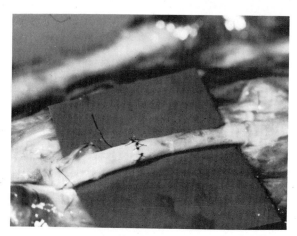

Fig. 1.132 (A) Exploration of this wound revealed a traumatic aneurysm due to a partial laceration in the ulnar artery. (B) After application of clamps and controlling slings, resection revealed good proximal flow. (C) Direct anastomosis proved possible.

(iii) intimal tears, which can be seen through the wall as transverse areas of discoloration and which can be felt as irregularities with micro-forceps moved gently along the vessel lightly gripped.

(iv) the 'ribbon sign'[204] — this is a series of curls in the course of a vessel normally straight, similar to those which can be produced in ribbons by pulling them firmly through a constriction. It is a sign of irreversible vessel damage.

Any damaged vessel must be resected and replaced by a suitable substitute, usually vein.

Skin

The possibility of deep damage underlying apparently innocuous puncture wounds has been emphasised. They must be explored to their full extent using a probe and the presence of blood staining as guides.

The urgency required in handling similar small wounds due to *high compression injection*[205-207] cannot be stressed too strongly. Such injuries may inject any number of substances — paint[208-210], grease[211], hydraulic fluid, molten plastic[212] are only the most common. The distance injected is a function of the pressure in the system — hydraulic fluid has been reported in the chest wall following a fingertip puncture. The damage done to the tissues is a function of the nature of the material enhanced by the passage of time. In those instances where the material is radio-opaque, X-ray will give some guidance as to the extent of spread and, after debridement, the adequacy of removal[213]. Regardless of the extent of the necessary incisions, the absolute responsibility of the surgeon is to remove all of the foreign material, no matter how many hours that may take (Fig. 1.133). If this is not done, the immediate result may be infection, gangrene and amputation and the longterm outcome, fibrosis and discharging sinuses from granulomas which cripple the hand[214,215] (Fig. 1.134). If the infected material is removed, the wounds sutured loosely and early motion begun, full function can be the reward (Fig. 1.135). The management of another potentially serious small wound — the human bite — is considered on page 231.

Total viable skin cover is of prime importance in the emergency management of hand injuries. Two facts have to be determined: skin viability and skin loss.

While viability has been assessed during examination on the basis of colour, design of flaps and return of flow after finger tip expression, the final decision is made at exploration

1. after all fractures have been reduced and immobilized;
2. after all vessels subjected to torsion or compression have been seen to be free of spasm;
3. after all appropriate vessels have been repaired and seen to transmit flow;
4. after the tourniquet has been applied for a period in excess of twenty minutes and then released;

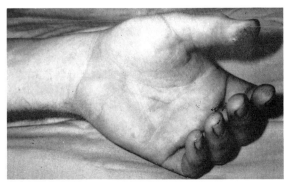

Fig. 1.133 (A) This patient sustained a high pressure injection injury with hydraulic fluid on the pulp of the left thumb. (B) The fluid was traced into all compartments of the hand, through the carpal tunnel and up above the wrist. After evacuation of all foreign fluid and thorough irrigation (C) the wounds were closed lightly and irrigating catheters inserted. The patient healed slowly but satisfactorily (D).

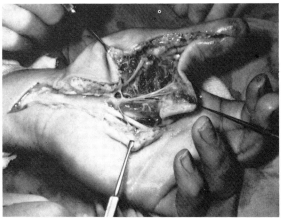

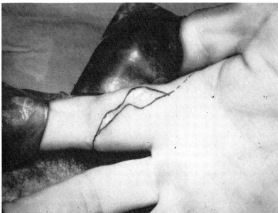

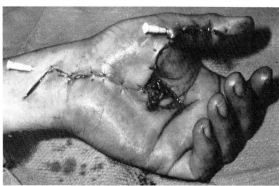

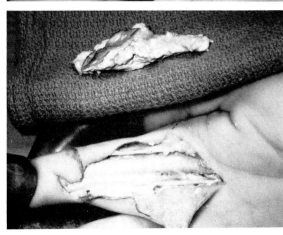

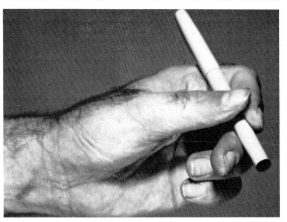

Fig. 1.134 (A) This patient had sustained a paint gun injection to the proximal phalanx of his index finger 18 months before presenting. Inadequate debridement had resulted in stiffness of the finger and persistent discharge from the sinuses. (B) Excision of all material, light closure of the wound, and subsequent irrigation restored satisfactory function.

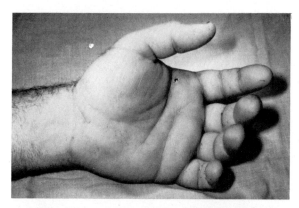

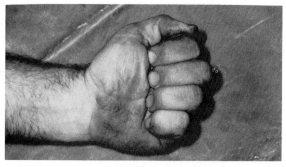

Fig. 1.135 (A) This patient presented 24 hours after injection of car undersealing with severe pain and oedema. (B) The material was followed throughout the hand and all removed. (C) Light suture and irrigation resulted in restoration of full function (D & E).

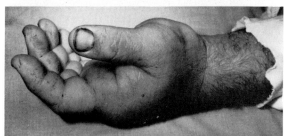

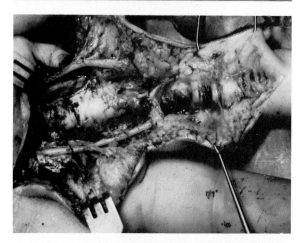

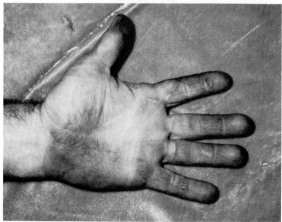

5. after ten minutes has been allowed to elapse following tourniquet release.

The release of the tourniquet will result in brisk oozing from the wounds in uncompromised cases. In more doubtful circumstances a very clear *line of demarcation* will appear between the region of *reactive hyperaemia* and the pallor of skin with no blood supply. This line should be marked with a skin pencil. If the decision were taken at this stage, however, too much would be sacrificed. Rather should the hand be elevated and compressed for a period related to the length of tourniquet application, then lowered, haemostasis achieved and the wounds washed free of blood. If the skin flaps are then re-examined, the line of demarcation will be less evident, for the hyperaemia will have settled, but in most instances circulation will be clearly seen beyond the mark made with the skin pencil. Provided no undue tension or distortion is subsequently applied to the flap, this second line can be selected for the excision. If, however, skin grafts or a flap are to be applied and wider excision does not expose an unsatisfactory bed for the former, then the excision can be more radical, approaching the first demarcation line. The most unequivocal evidence of acceptable skin blood flow, and that increasingly employed by the author, is brisk *dermal bleeding* on incision (Fig. 1.136). In extensive avulsion flaps these incisions are made parallel to the edge of the flap proceeding further and further from the edge until viability its unequivocally demonstrated.

Fluorescin[216] has been advocated by some to demonstrate flow. This it certainly will do, but it has been shown to be consistently pessimistic, resulting in unnecessary sacrifice of skin (Fig. 1.137). In extensive 'degloving' injuries of the limbs, immediate removal of the nonviable skin back to a bleeding margin is indicated, for valuable grafts can subsequently be cut from the less damaged portions of the excised tissue.

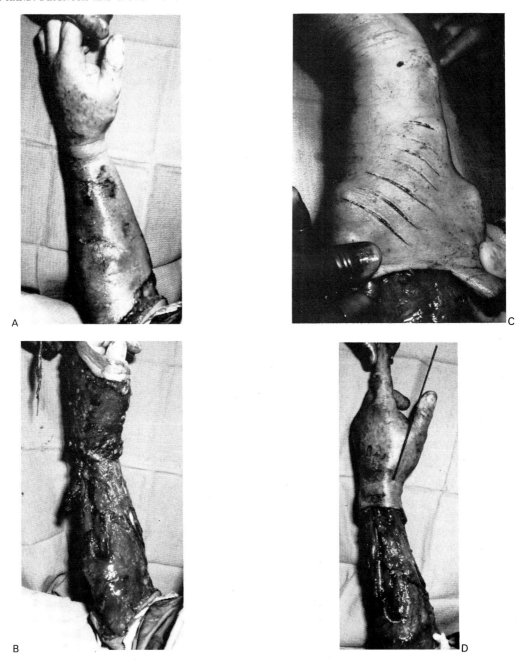

Fig. 1.136   (A & B) This patient had sustained a roller injury with degloving of the entire skin of the forearm. (C) Parallel incisions were made from the wound margin, and satisfactory dermal bleeding was not achieved until the level of the wrist had been reached. All this skin was therefore excised. (D) Drainage tubes were inserted between the muscle bellies, which were lightly sutured and skin grafted on the third day.

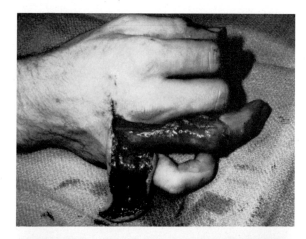

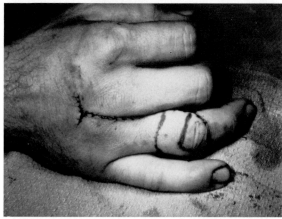

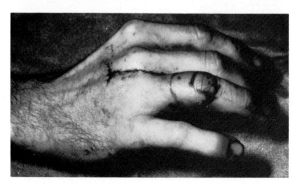

Fig. 1.137 (A) An avulsion flap of the proximal phalanx of the ring finger was evaluated using fluorescin. (B) The line of certain necrosis as predicted by fluorescin is the distal one and probable necrosis, the proximal line on the digit. (C) One week later, it can be seen that all skin had survived.

Some argue that flaps should be sutured back provided that all deep non-viable tissue has been removed, since survival cannot be predicted with absolute accuracy. While the premise is true, the conclusion is not acceptable since subsequent skin necrosis encourages sepsis and endangers repair performed deep to it. Marginally viable skin is probably worst of all because it multiplies the length of convalescence, delaying mobilization, promoting oedema and fibrosis in the hand and, if at length it survives, proving itself to be indurated and adherent (Fig. 1.138). If despite these considerations doubtfully viable flaps are placed into position this should be done without tension for they are more likely to survive than if they are stretched out to their original dimension[217].

SKIN LOSS AND REPLACEMENT

Especially in complex injuries, the wounds will gape apart and flaps of skin will retract markedly. *Landmarks* which correspond on either wound edge should sought. Those available in the hand are the many unique *skin creases,* the *nail folds* and the margins of *hair bearing skin* of the dorsum of forearm, hand, and fingers. Once these points have been matched the surgeon can decide whether or not skin has been lost.

Dorsal skin is more mobile than palmar, but it is so to accommodate finger flexion. Closure should not be achieved by 'pulling the wound edges together'.

Where the nail bed has been injured it is particularly important to locate all parts of this specialized structure. Not uncommonly portions are to be found on flaps of digital pulp which have carried the nail bed well away from its dorsal origin. These should be replaced accurately to avoid late deformity of the nail which can be functionally disabling. (Fingertip injuries are considered below, p. 85).

INDICATIONS

When skin has been lost, the replacement chosen should be the simplest compatible with the best and speediest functional recovery[218]. The simplest of skin cover is provided by the free skin graft. What is required by any skin graft is a bed which is vascular enough to produce capillary buds in sufficient quantity quickly enough to revitalize its dying cells (Fig. 1.139). The periosteum of bone paratenon and even cancellous bone are all capable of doing so, and therefore free split skin can be directly applied to them. Whether or not this is designed to produce the 'best and speediest *functional* recovery' is another matter entirely. For the very reason that they gain their blood supply by capillary budding from the bed, grafts in due course become firmly adherent to that bed. If movement of the bed is required through a greater range than that of the overlying skin — or vice versa, as in the movement of skin over bone — or if subsequent surgery such as tendon grafting will be required in the layer between skin and bed, then grafts are not suitable as a

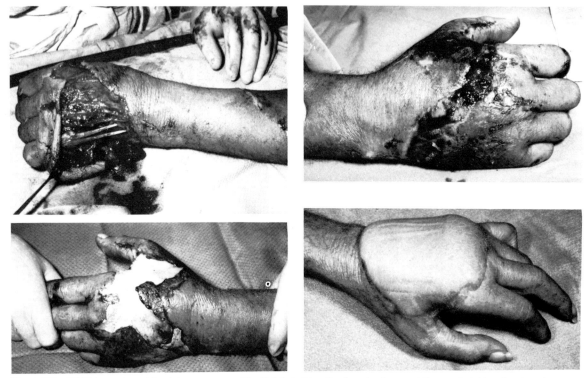

Fig. 1.138 (A) This crush avulsion injury was treated by lightly tacking the flaps in place, and then undertaking dressing changes on every second day. The necrosis proceeded in a rather scattered fashion. (C) Split thickness skin grafting after excision of necrotic tissue failed to take. (D) Distant flap cover was required by which time significant joint stiffness had ensued.

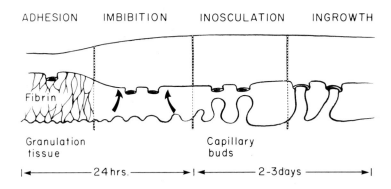

Fig. 1.139 A diagram of the normal process involved in skin graft take, proceeding from left to right (see text).

permanent cover. They may in complex injuries or in hands inexperienced in plastic surgical procedures be the correct *temporary* cover even in the situations described. If, however, the injury, the patient and the surgeon are fitted for immediate flap cover where it will eventually be undoubtedly required then an appreciable saving in time and money will be effected by the use of a primary flap.

Split skin is available in profusion and has the advantage that it takes readily. It can be meshed to cover large areas,

conform with contour defects or permit drainage of secretions (Fig. 1.140). The disadvantages of split skin are that it is associated with considerable contracture[219], which may produce joint deformities, and it is not as durable as full thickness skin. *Full thickness skin* is in relatively short supply, takes less well than split, but does not contract and is of course thicker and therefore more durable (Fig. 1.141). As will be evident from what is said above no skin graft takes on bare bone, tendon or ligament or over a cavity.

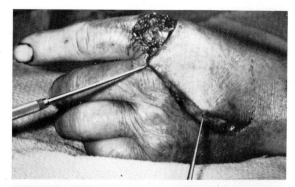

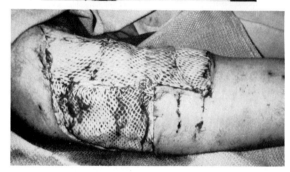

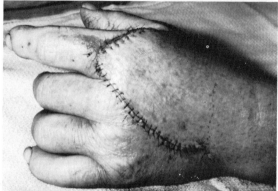

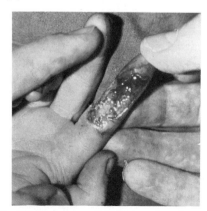

Fig. 1.140   Meshed skin grafts can be used to cover extensive areas as in this total degloving of the upper extremity (A) or to fit the contours of irregular defects and allow drainage of secretions (B).

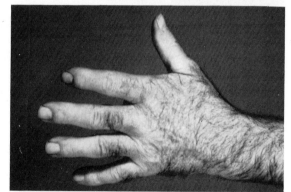

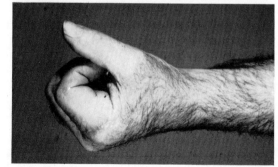

Fig. 1.141   This clean cut avulsion loss on the palmar aspect of the right index finger of a child exposed no significant deep structures. The bed showed a good blood supply and because of its extent, situation, and vascularity was ideal for the use of a primary full thickness graft.

Fig. 1.142   (A) An open saw injury of the metacarpophalangeal joint of the index finger has been repaired. The residual defect was triangulated during debridement and a transposition flap raised (B) to cover the defect with resultant good healing (C) and function (D).

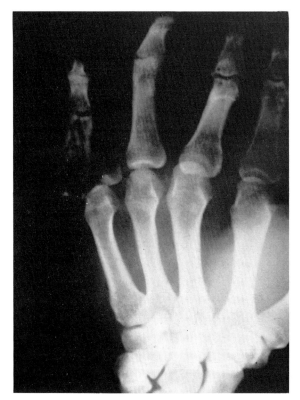

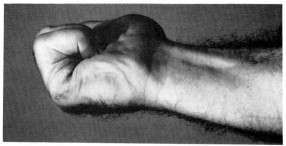

Fig. 1.143 *Palmar fillet flap.* (A) The small finger was irrevocably injured by crushing, but the skin remained viable. (B) A palmar fillet flap was therefore used to cover the reconstruction of the ring finger with resultant primary healing (C) and full range in the remaining digits (D).

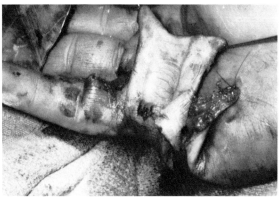

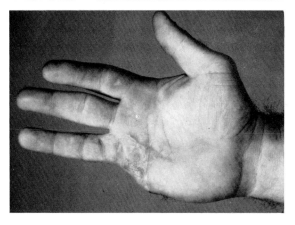

Bringing with it an intrinsic blood supply, a flap[220] is necessary in those circumstances. *Local skin flaps* are always preferred for several reasons — they are of the same texture, they can usually be transferred in one procedure and they bring with them some nerve supply. With this in mind the defect to be covered should be actually or conceptually triangulated — since this is the first step in local flap design — and then adjacent areas considered to determine whether or not they can, without detriment, provide a transposition or rotation flap (Fig. 1.142). While the planning of such flaps is outwith the scope of this text, suffice it to say that the larger the flap constructed, the more likely is it to achieve the objective. Occasionally the skeleton of a viable digit is irreparably damaged. This can then serve as an incomparable source of local skin as a filletted finger flap[221,222] (Fig. 1.143 and Fig. 1.144). If no local flap is available then other sources of hand skin should be considered for construction of a *regional flap*[223]. Such regional flaps include cross-finger, thenar, axial flag and neurovascular island — they are considered in somewhat greater detail under finger-tip injuries. If the defect is too large to be covered by a local or regional flap, then distant tissue must be used. *Distant flaps* may be of random blood supply, dependent upon the subdermal plexus, or axial[224] where a known vessel supplies the flap. *Random flaps* have the advantage of being thin and of potentially small dimension. Thus, *cross-arm flaps*[225-227] are ideal for resurfacing small, palmar defects and *tubed acromio-thoracic flaps* are ideal for cover of a thumb from which the skin has been avulsed (Fig. 1.145). Both have the disadvantage, especially in the female, of creating cosmetically unsatisfactory defects. *Axial flaps* may be of skin alone, or musculocutaneous (Fig. 1.146). They may be transferred on a pedicle or by microvascular techniques as a free flap. *The groin flap*[228-231] is the most widely used pedicle flap for the hand, almost to the exclusion of all others (Fig. 1.147). It provides predictably reliable skin cover of relatively good quality for large defects permitting

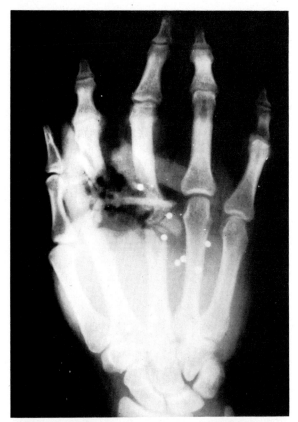

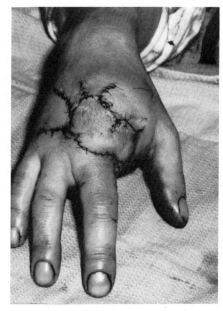

Fig. 1.144 *Dorsal fillet flap.* (A) A shotgun injury to the metacarpophalangeal joint region of the index and middle fingers resulted in extensive skeletal damage to the index, such that it was sacrificed to produce a long fillet flap (B) which could be employed to cover the immediate joint replacement in the metacarpophalangeal joint of the middle finger with undoubtedly viable skin (C).

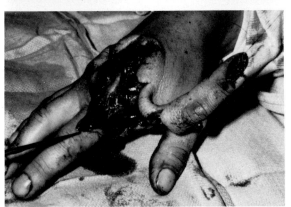

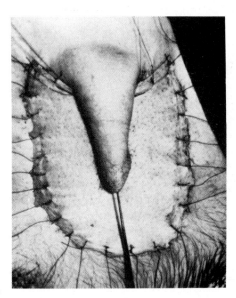

Fig. 1.145 A tube pedicle has been raised from the acromiothoracic region to provide immediate cover to a degloving of a thumb in which much of the skeleton was maintained but the skin removed by a water-ski tow-rope down to the level of the metacarpophalangeal joint.

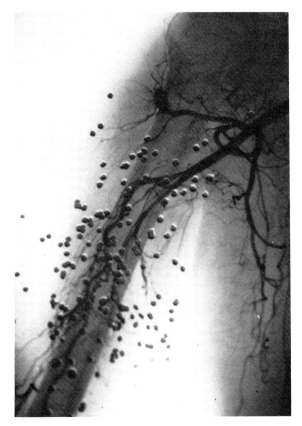

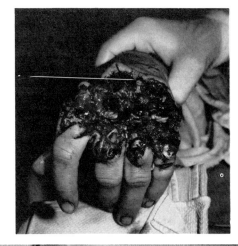

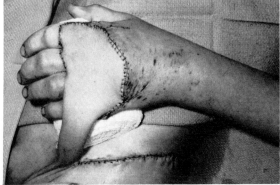

Fig. 1.147 (A) This high velocity gunshot wound of the metacarpophalangeal joint region required immedate bony stabilization and revascularization of one digit. (B) Immediate viable skin cover could be provided by a pedicle groin flap.

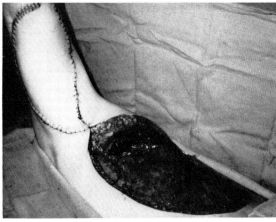

Fig. 1.146 (A) A shotgun blast to the upper arm resulted in loss of flow in the brachial artery. An immediate vein graft was performed, and (B) the resultant skin defect closed with a pedicle latissimus dorsi musculocutaneous flap.

immediate deep reconstruction where appropriate (Fig. 1.148). It can be split to a degree to cover two surfaces (Fig. 1.149) and on occasion has been used bilaterally to cover both hands simultaneously (Fig. 1.150). When even it cannot provide all the skin required it can be supplemented by free skin grafts (Fig. 1.151) or by the simultaneous use of a hypogastric[232,233] or tensor fascia lata[234] flap. Rarely, but increasingly, *emergency free flaps* are being used in departments with sufficient experience and adequate staff. The advantage of providing skin cover which has a permanent blood supply are clear, especially in injuries where the flow to the tissues of the hand is markedly improved, where circumferential flap cover is required, where the defect is too proximal for a groin flap, where external fixation of the forearm has been required, where major primary reconstruction of deep structures takes precedence in dictating the postoperative posture of the limb, where nerve supply is also required, as in restoring a thumb pulp (Fig. 1.152) or where illness, such as uncontrolled epilepsy, makes immobilisation a problem

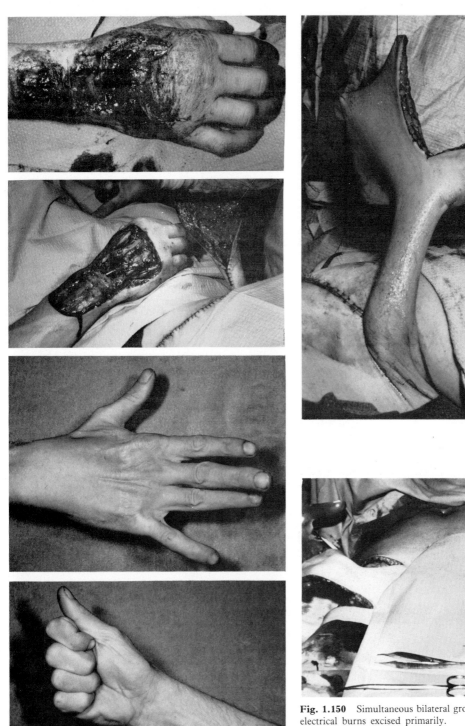

Fig. 1.150 Simultaneous bilateral groin flaps to cover bilateral electrical burns excised primarily.

Fig. 1.148 (A) This patient sustained a roll over injury in a truck which removed all extensor tendons plus the dorsal surface of the metacarpals. (B) Immediate groin flap cover permitted extensor tendon reconstruction and restoration of good function (C & D).

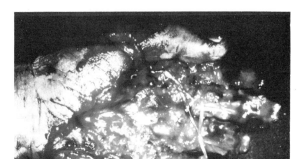

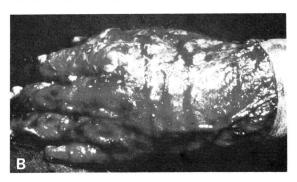

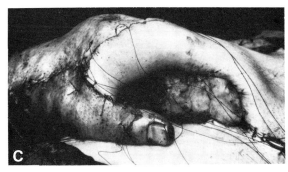

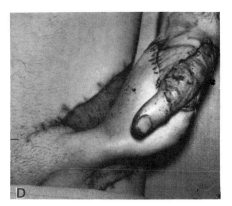

Fig. 1.151 (A, B) This patient suffered an avulsion injury while in his employment as a maintenance engineer, exposing both dorsal and palmar aspects of the hand. (C) A primary groin flap was applied to cover the digits and palmar surface of the hand, split thickness skin grafts being used on the dorsum. (D) On account of the tube pedicle, a primary groin flap allows adequate mobilization of the wrist and small joints of the hand while in place. (Further reconstruction on this patient is illustrated in Fig. 2.25).

(Fig. 1.153). Many free flaps carry with them an excessive amount of tissue and in circumstances requiring cover of a large area while avoiding bulk, the use of a *free muscle flap* with subsequent application of split skin grafts has decreased this problem. Summarizing the indications for different types of skin cover discussed above:

1. Areas with good blood supply, no exposed bone, tendon or ligament
   free skin graft
   (a) large areas on the dorsum or arm
   (b) non-contact side of the digit
       → split skin
           (i) irregular or discharging wounds
               → *meshed split skin*
   (c) small areas on flexion surface
   (d) contact side of digit
       → *full thickness skin*
2. Poor blood supply to bed, exposed structures, later surgery
   flap
   (a) small defects; skin available
       → local flap
   (b) small defects; no local skin available
       → *regional flap*
           (i) thumb pulp
           →*NVI flap*
   (c) small defects; no local or regional skin available
   (d) thumb skin avulsion
       → *distant random flap*
       infraclavicular
       cross-arm
   (e) large defects
       → *distant axial flap*
           (i) circumferential, forearm, external fixation
       or splint
       → *free flap*
           (ii) thumb pulp
               → *free NVI flap from great toe.*

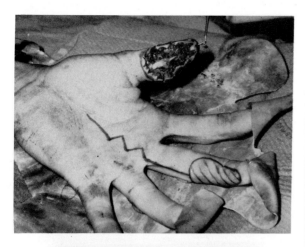

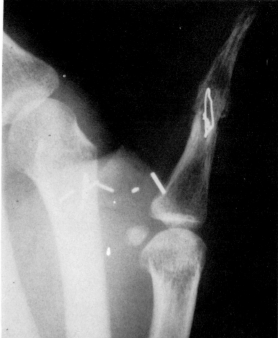

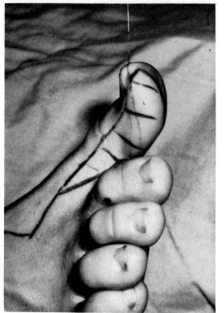

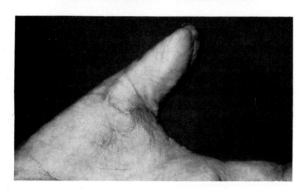

Fig. 1.152 A severe gouging injury of the pulp of the thumb required shortening of the skeleton with immediate arthrodesis of the distal interphalangeal joint. (A) The choice lay between a pedicle neurovascular island from the hand or (B) a free neurovascular island from the pulp of the toe. After discussion with the patient the latter was selected (C) Satisfactory healing and return of sensation resulted with good bony union of the osteosynthesis (D).

FINGER TIP INJURIES

The finger tip is an area in which examination of skin loss and the nature of the exposed tissue is unusually important in selecting the method of reconstruction and thereby influencing the outcome.

1. Pulp

Here sensation, adequate padding and total freedom from discomfort are essential. The points to be noted are:

a. *Whether or not bone is exposed.* If none is exposed and the defect is smaller than one square centimeter remarkable results have been reported from merely dressing the wound[235-237]. If the defect is larger than one square centimeter in an adult, a free skin graft is indicated. Split thickness skin is used for small defects particularly on the ulnar side of the digit, for contraction will draw in normally sensitive skin (Fig. 1.154). Full thickness grafts are employed on larger areas of well-vascularised soft tissue, especially on the radial, contact, aspect of the finger.

If bone is exposed, a graft may take but contraction would not occur and an adherent, tender scar would result. A flap is therefore required.

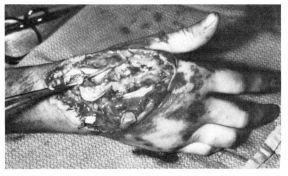

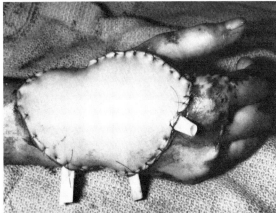

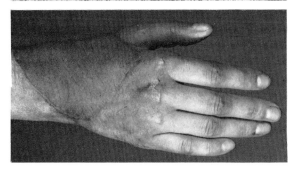

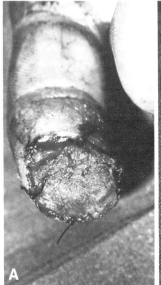

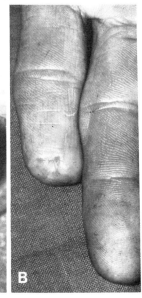

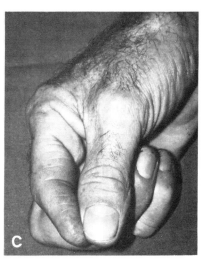

Fig. 1.153 This poorly-controlled epileptic sustained a deep road abrasion injury (A) which required stabilisation of the wrist, reconstruction of the capsule and immediate tendon transfer. Application of a free groin flap (B) as an emergency permitted appropriate splintage, avoided problems during two subsequent seizures and showed trouble-free healing (C). Her hospital stay was two days after injury.

Fig. 1.154 This amputation of an index finger just distal to the distal interphalangeal joint was covered with a split thickness skin graft in a casualty department. When seen for review, the skin graft appeared to be of good appearance and was left undisturbed. Subsequent contraction of the graft drew normal digital skin over the amputation stump and the patient made good use of this simple repair (B and C).

b. *The angle at which tissue loss has occurred.* If more tissue has been lost from the dorsal than from the palmar aspect, then if other factors make it appropriate, a local VY advancement flap is an excellent solution (Fig. 1.155)[240,241]. If the angulation is reversed, however, with more lost from the palmar than from the dorsal aspect, any attempt to use a local flap will be doomed to failure through undue tension, and another solution must be sought. In the thumb,

distal to the interphalangeal joint, a palmar angled defect, if not too great, may be closed by a Moberg advancement flap[242-243] (Fig. 1.156) or by a dorsal neurovascular island flap from the thumb itself[244].

Where bone is exposed and the angulation of the wound is unsuitable for local flap repair, the choice lies between:
Cross finger flap[245-247] — the most common solution, the main excluding factor is injury to the dorsum of the

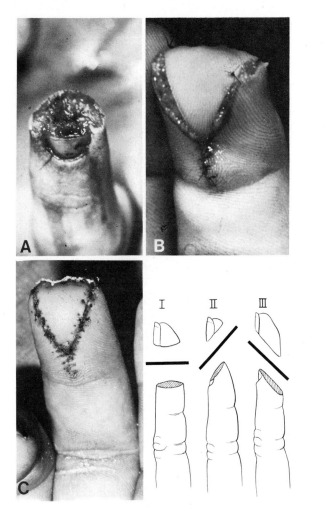

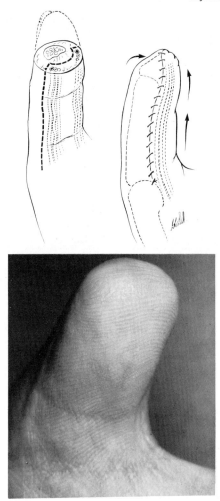

Fig. 1.155 The bone of the distal phalanx was exposed in this amputation of a middle finger and therefore flap cover was required. Since the angle of amputation was transverse a V–Y advancement, (B) was appropriate and this resulted in satisfactory healing (C). (D) The angle of amputation determines whether or not a local advancement flap can be used (not appropriate in Type III).

Fig. 1.156 (A) A Moberg advancement flap is possible on the thumb because the dorsal skin has a separate arterial supply. In addition, the interphalangeal joint is flexed down to enable the dorsal skin to meet the palmar advancement giving smooth, well-padded cover to the thumb (B).

adjacent donor finger. The cross finger flap to the thumb can be taken from the proximal phalanx of the index finger or from the middle phalanx of either the middle or ring fingers. When taken from the index finger, the radial nerve can be blocked at the wrist and the area of resultant anaesthesia mapped out. If it includes the proximal phalanx, the radial nerve branches can be preserved in raising the flap (Fig. 1.157). The proximal course of the nerve is then transferred to the thumb at the second stage. A nerve supply to the thumb tip is thereby preserved[248,249]. A word of caution should be offered on the radial-nerve innervated cross-finger flap. It may, at some point after the division, show gradually decreasing sensation. This

appears to be more common the longer the thumb and may be due to neurapraxia as the thumb is used in more and more abduction. It should probably therefore be reserved for thumbs amputated at the level of the interphalangeal joint. Where more mobility is required, especially in cross-finger flaps from the dorsum of the proximal phalanx, the axial flag flap can provide it[250], so covering difficult defects on adjacent digits (Fig. 1.158 and Fig. 1.159). Multiple cross-finger flaps are used for multiple fingertip amputations (Fig. 1.160).

Thenar flap[251] — where a cross finger flap cannot be employed, a flap from the metacarpophalangeal crease of the thumb is of use, but should be restricted to patients

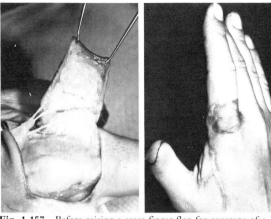

Fig. 1.157   Before raising a cross finger flap for coverage of a thumb defect the distribution of the radial nerve was mapped out by blocking it at the level of the wrist. It was found to include the donor area for the flap. In the process of raising the flap from the dorsum of the proximal phalanx of the index finger the terminal branches of the radial nerve were carefully dissected out and preserved (A). On division and inset of the flap, the radial nerve branch to the index finger was dissected back on the dorsum of the first web space and then transferred to the ulnar aspect of the thumb through another incision. With this innervated cross finger flap, the patient retained sensation on the tip of the amputated thumb (B).

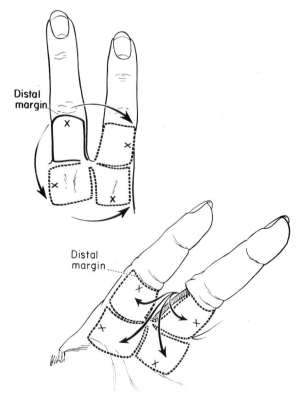

Fig. 1.158   (A) The axial flag flap taken from the dorsum of the proximal phalanx can be rotated to cover any area within reach through 360°. (B) A flap can also be brought through the web space to cover palmar defects.

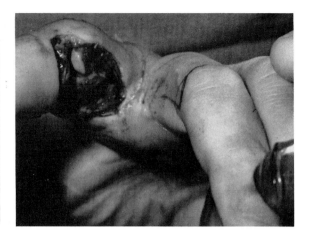

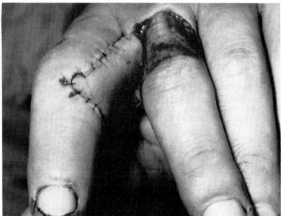

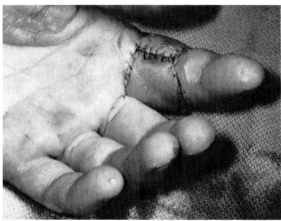

Fig. 1.159   (A) This defect revealing an open joint is on both the ulnar and palmar aspect of the index finger. Employing an axial flag flap with but a 2 mm pedicle, well vascularized cover was achieved for the lateral and (C) palmar aspect of the wound. (*From:* Lister G D 1981 The theory of the transposition flap and its practical application in the hand. Clinics in Plastic Surgery 8: 115.)

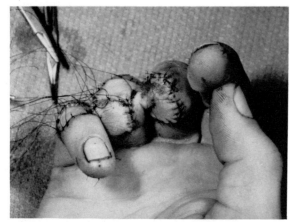

Fig. 1.160 Cross-finger flaps raised from adjacent fingers give very satisfactory cover for multiple fingertip amputations.

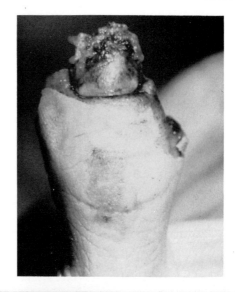

under 40 or unacceptable proximal interphalangeal joint contracture may result (Fig. 1.161). It is the flap of choice in younger women as it avoids an unsightly donor scar on the dorsum of a finger.

Immediate neurovascular island — only applicable where the pulp lost is that of the thumb, only where it is the major injury, only where the surgeon is experienced in the technique and only where the wound is sufficiently recent and clean as to mimic a surgical excision. Care must be taken to check that flow exists in all relevant vessels (p. 120). Some disrepute has fallen on this procedure on account of poor sensation in the transferred pulp[252]. This does not occur if care is taken to avoid all tension on the neurovascular pedicle, both during dissection, and even

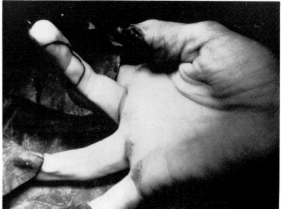

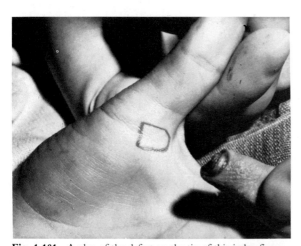

Fig. 1.161 A plan of the defect on the tip of this index finger of a twenty-two-year old girl has been marked out over the metacarpophalangeal crease of the thumb. A thenar flap was subsequently raised somewhat larger than the plan. The secondary defect was closed directly thereby eliminating the need for a skin graft.

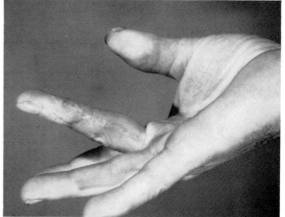

Fig. 1.162 This patient sustained a crush avulsion of the entire pad of the dominant right thumb. (A & B) Immediate neurovascular island flap was taken from the ulnar aspect of the middle finger with satisfactory restitution of the thumb pulp and good healing of the full thickness graft on the secondary defect (C).

more important after its application. At surgery, the pedicle must be seen to be loose with the flap in place on a fully abducted and extended thumb. Good results can then be expected[253-255] (Fig. 1.162).

Revision of amputation — sacrifice of length is always a disturbing procedure, but, where other solutions have been rejected, provides a sensitive well healed stump. It is appropriate in isolated loss of a finger tip in older patients where a cross finger flap is ruled out. It should not be employed on the thumb.

2. Nail bed

Here adequate support for the nail and avoidance of any significant nail distortion are necessary if the nail is not to be functionally a nuisance and cosmetically an embarrassment. The injured nail bed should be inspected with these points in mind and adequate inspection may dictate removal of part or all of the nail.

a. The distal half of the terminal phalanx should be present and if fractured, stably reduced usually with the help of a fine Kirschner wire. The more phalanx is missing the greater is the likelihood of a curved nail and ablation should be considered. A curved nail can only be avoided if the nail bed is *supported by bone throughout its length.* (Fig. 1.163).

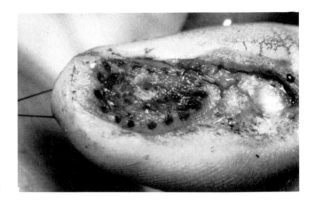

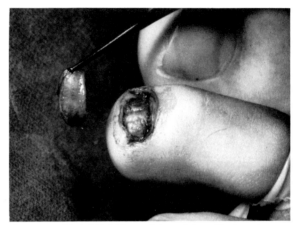

Fig. 1.164 (A) A full thickness defect of the nailbed can be reconstituted by a nailbed graft taken from the adjacent nailbed or, when insufficient is available, from the toe (B).

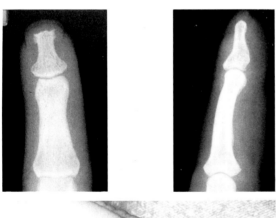

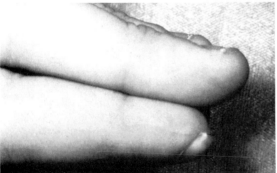

Fig. 1.163 (A) The tip of the distal phalanx has been trimmed back, as evidenced on this X-ray, to a point where it offers inadequate support to the nailbed. (B) This results in a curved nail, evident when it is compared with the normal finger on the opposite hand.

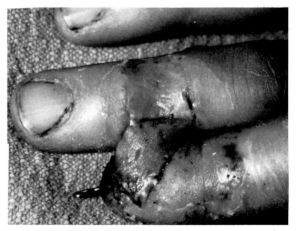

Fig. 1.165 Complete loss of all cover for the dorsal aspect of distal phalanx can be treated with a de-epithelialised inverted cross-finger flap, subsequently split skin grafted.

b. Accurate localization and matching of both germinal and sterile nail bed should be made prior to careful repair. Otherwise, deformity will result.

c. The eponychium should be similarly inspected. Any adhesion between it and nail bed will result in a grooved or split nail.

d. If any nail bed is missing, it is best replaced with a split thickness graft of nail bed, taken either from the injured finger or from a toe (Fig. 1.164).

e. When the nail is completely destroyed but distal phalanx remains, length can be maintained by covering the soft tissue defect with a reversed de-epithelialised cross-finger flap[223] (Fig. 1.165).

THERMAL INJURY

Burns

The basic question being asked when the burned hand is examined is 'What is the depth of the burn?' The answer to that question will determine

1. Whether or not skin cover will be required;
2. What type of skin cover will be appropriate and in due course functional;
3. What deep structures are likely to be damaged;
4. What steps should be taken primarily.

In all burns it has become the practice to classify the depth of skin destruction by degrees according to certain symptoms and signs. To some extent, this classification determines the line of treatment. These degrees are:

Degree	Appearance	Sensitivity	Graft
First-			
superficial	Erythema	Hyperaesthetic	No
Second-			
partial			Sometimes
thickness	Blistering	Hyperaesthetic	(see below)
Third-			
full	Hard, dry,		
thickness	waxy white	Anaesthetic	Yes

The vascularity or otherwise of the skin can be demonstrated by the speed of capillary refilling after finger tip pressure. In first and second degree burns, immediate refilling occurs whereas in third degree burns no change occurs either as a result of the pressure or of its release. Blood is present in the skin vessels of a third degree burn which might cause some confusion on cursory examination, but this blood, like all the tissues of the skin in full thickness burns, is coagulated and does not move with pressure. Nor does the finger bleed when stabbed with a needle (Fig. 1.166).

The classification laid out above is simple and fairly practical. However, like all simplifications it requires expansion.

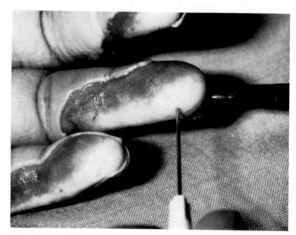

Fig. 1.166 A full thickness third degree burn does not bleed when stuck with a needle.

1. *Second degree burns.* It has become apparent that two distinct categories exist, having quite different implications as regards the eventual outcome (Fig. 1.167).

   (a) *Superficial partial thickness.* Characterized by blistering and erythema, this burn is very sensitive to touch. Without complications, it will heal of its own accord leaving stable, mobile, non-hypertrophic and uncontracted skin.

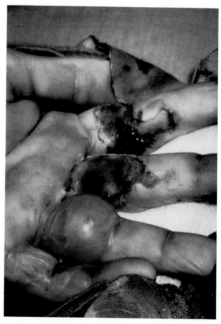

Fig. 1.167 This patient has sustained mixed superficial second, deep dermal, and full thickness burns. The blisters were debrided on the ring and small fingers and the burns on the index and middle excised and grafted.

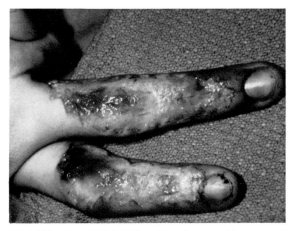

Fig. 1.168   An area of deep dermal burning treated by immediate excision and grafting.

(b) *Deep dermal.* Blistering is less marked and there may be some superficial coagulation and even loss of sensitivity (Fig. 1.168). Deep dermal burns are fairly pale. Pressure renders them even more pale over a wider area than in the superficial burn because of the tension already created by oedema. Sometimes a thin layer of redness persists due to very superficial intravascular coagulation. Although strictly partial thickness, this burn has destroyed the major part of the skin and only the deep dermis and appendages remain alive. Healing will slowly ensue from these structures only provided that infection does not destroy them. Even then the resulting skin will be alternately thin and hypertrophic, relatively immobile and liable to crack and ulcerate and contract. While healing does occur and therefore skin grafts are not essential, skin of such quality is quite unsuitable for satisfactory hand function. Early tangential excision and skin grafting are therefore desirable.

2. A category of *fourth degree* has much to commend it to the hand surgeon. Since the three standard degrees of burn indicate only the depth of skin loss and offer guidance only as to whether or not skin replacement will prove necessary, a fourth degree is helpful in distinguishing those cases in which structures of significance deep to the skin have been damaged by the burn injury.

History

CAUSE OF BURN[257]

Thermal

The temperature of the source has to be very high if third or fourth degree burns are to be inflicted before the hand is withdrawn. This is especially true of burns of the palm where the skin is thickest and sensitivity most acute. Thus scalds, kitchen accidents and coal fire contact will all tend to produce first or superficial second degree burns.

By contrast, where the temperature is indeed very high or where the hand cannot be quickly removed in response to pain, third and fourth degree burns are probable. These circumstances apply in contact with electric fires especially bar radiators, hot plates and in general body burns, as in nightdress accidents or when the patient is trapped in a house fire.

Electrical[258,259]

The electric fire burn[260,261] is usually a largely *thermal* injury unless the device is inadequately earthed or incorrectly wired or the conductive nature of the patient has been increased in some way, for example, by standing wet and barefoot on a stone floor.

True electrical injury is characterized by inability to release the live contact, sometimes by loss of consciousness, and less commonly by residual temporary paralysis and cardiac arrhythmias or arrest. The point of contact in the electrical burn almost invariably sustains a third or fourth degree injury (Fig. 1.169). The earth point, if sufficiently small in area, will also be the site of a burn and this should be sought.

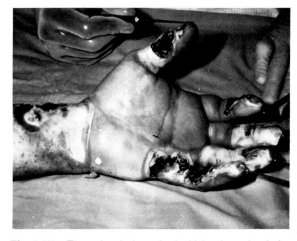

Fig. 1.169   The patient had sustained a high voltage electrical burn the point of entry being his non-dominant left hand. A fourth degree injury has been sustained, the full thickness loss evident at the wrist covering an area of destruction of superficial flexor tendons and the ulnar nerve and artery.

Chemical

The majority of chemicals which inflict burns will have done their worst by the time the patient arrives with the surgeon. One exception is *hydrofluoric acid.* This is widely used in industry in glass-etching and in the manufacture of germicides, dyes, plastics and rust-removing agents. It is characterized by progressive damage to the tissues caused by the fluoride ion. This can rapidly be neutralized by the infiltration of the tissues with 10% calcium gluconate until all pain is permanently relieved. This should be carried out urgently, and repeated if pain recurs.

Blast

Blast burns sustained in explosions commonly involve the face and hands. Although considerable oedema and crusting exudation ensue and can be alarming, these burns almost without exception are superficial second degree. The significant aspect of blast injuries is the damage caused to the airway both internally and through the later development of neck oedema.

Epilepsy, intoxication and unconsciousness

Where a localized burn has been sustained from a relatively low temperature, thermal source, the only common exception to the rule that full thickness burns do not result is in the patient where the response to pain has been dulled or totally eliminated. This occurs in grand mal seizures, usually in undiagnosed or uncontrolled epileptics and in gross intoxication with alcohol or drugs (Fig. 1.170). More

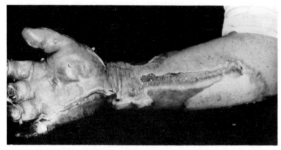

Fig. 1.170   This patient sustained a gross fourth degree burn to his right hand from an open coal fire. He had no other burns and he proved to be an untreated epileptic who at the time of injury was also heavily intoxicated.

rarely such burns may occur where unconsciousness has arisen through other causes; head injury, cerebrovascular accident or circulatory collapse. As these patients require help in ways other than in the management of their burn, localized full thickness thermal burns should always initiate more thorough investigation. If no systemic cause is present, then a local neurological deficit should be suspected and sought by examination.

Examination

Degree

The different areas of the burn should be classified (p. 91) as to the depth of the burn on the basis of inspection

(colour, blistering, coagulation, charring), palpation (expression and return of blood) and pinprick sensitivity.

By these criteria the distinction between superficial partial thickness, deep dermal and full thickness burns is more certainly made on the dorsum of the hand than it is on the palmar aspect. Splintage in correct posture (see below) and repeated examination are therefore more commonly employed than early surgery in burns of doubtful degree in the palm of the hand.

Extent

This should be carefully noted and can most efficiently be recorded on outline drawings of the hand. The area of burn should be broken up into the different regions with various degrees of probable skin loss and this is usually done by distinctive cross-hatching on the diagram.

Posture

Oedema, inevitable in the burned hand, will be most apparent on the dorsum but more significantly will also involve the periarticular structures. This results in the joints adopting the position in which the collateral ligaments are slack. Thus the metacarpophalangeal joints are straight and the interphalangeal joints flexed. Unless controlled by splintage and early motion, the ligaments will contract in this position causing fixed deformity.

In the fourth degree burn of the distal palm due to electric bar radiator injuries, the metacarpophalangeal and proximal interphalangeal joints of all fingers are in equal fixed flexion of about 80°.

Viability

The viability of digits distal to a burn should be checked by colour and circulatory return following expression. The significance and timing of vascular impairment differs with the site and degree of the burn.

1. *Palm or digit, fourth degree:* Immediate vascular embarrassment is not uncommon and indicates that both digital arteries have ceased to function. As the most *dorsal* of the vital structures on the *palmar* surface of the hand, this implies that both tendons and nerves have also been irrevocably destroyed. With this in mind and considering that vascular repair would require the use of a vein graft beneath a flap, salvage of the digit is an impractical proposition.

2. *Forearm, third degree:* Late vascular embarrassment in the hand may well occur, especially if the burn is circumferential. The mechanism and treatment is that of a compartment syndrome (p. 31). Oedema in the forearm beneath the unyielding eschar occludes the arterial inflow after a period of increasing venous congestion. The process can be arrested by slitting the eschar through its full thickness longitudinally until circulation is re-established. Every effort should be

made to avoid exposing vital structures in the escharotomy wound as they will be likely to become dessicated and die.

Conclusions

Will skin cover be required? If so, of what type?
This is desirable in all hand burns except first degree and superficial second degree, that is, the erythematous and the blistered burns. Split skin grafts will be totally adequate after early tangential excision of the deep dermal burn. In full thickness loss split skin will probably subsequently contract to an unacceptable degree (Fig. 1.171). Grafts will

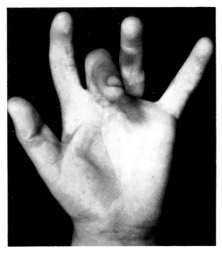

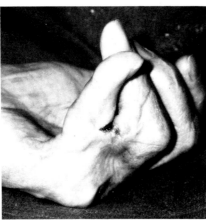

Fig. 1.171   (A) This child had suffered a full thickness burn of the palmar aspect of his middle finger which had been excised and covered with a split skin graft. At the time of examination, this was his maximum degree of extension.
(B) This patient sustained a full thickness burn to the fourth web space. Application of a split skin graft to the web space and the dorsal aspect of the metacarpophalangeal joint of the fifth finger resulted in flexion contractures of the metacarpophalangeal joint of the small finger, of the proximal interphalangeal joint of the ring finger and extension contractures of both interphalangeal joints of the small finger.

not take where bare tendons or bone are exposed by the burn. They are unsuitable as the final solution where tendon grafting will subsequently be required. Primary skin flaps are required where split skin grafts cannot provide the necessary cover.

What deep structures are damaged?
Electrical burns, the hook posture, skin charring, loss of digital viability, of sensation, and of movement all indicate injury to deep structures.

What immediate treatment is appropriate?
The best *posture* of the hand should be sought from the outset. That is, the wrist should be dorsiflexed, the metacarpophalangeal joints should be flexed as close to 90° as possible and the interphalangeal joints splinted in 20° of flexion. The collateral ligaments are so held taut and contraction is prevented. This position is very difficult to maintain in the burned hand. The use of Kirschner wires driven through the metacarpal head into the proximal phalanx has been found to hold the correct position most effectively without complication.

The alternative course, more applicable in more superficial and therefore less oedematous burns, is to commence immediate motion. This is facilitated by applying antibiotic cream and then covering the hands with only a loose plastic disposable glove[262] (Fig. 1.172).

Spontaneous separation of dead tissue may take several weeks and for this reason primary excision of hand burns has been recommended. This is certainly indicated as follows:

tangential excision of deep dermal burns of the dorsum with immediate grafting,[263-266] (Fig. 1.173).

full thickness excision of localized full thickness burns with immediate or delayed grafting or flap cover. (Fig. 1.174).

Electrical burns present similar problems to crush injuries, for tissues initially viable may subsequently die resulting in loss of grafts applied to an apparently satisfactory bed. By some, repeated excision with trial homografts or heterografts and by others, early flap cover have been recommended. The author has been impressed by the frustrations of the former and the relatively trouble-free healing obtained with early application of a flap.

In fourth degree burns, nerves and tendons in continuity and apparently involved by burn should not be excised as they often, surprisingly, show later function.

Escharotomy[267,268] should be considered in all third and fourth degree burns. The burn need *not* be circumferential for it to produce hazardous compression, since oedema in association with a significant burn can produce a tourniquet effect. Any distal circulatory or sensory changes or pain unrelieved by analgesics, should alert the surgeon to the need for decompression. As with fasciotomy —

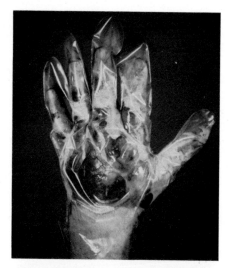

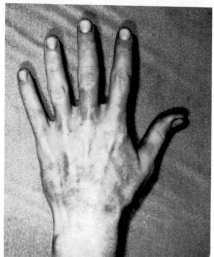

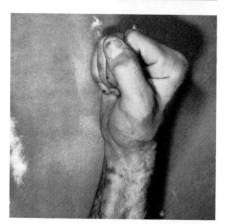

Fig. 1.172 (A) The application of antibiotic ointment such as silver sulphadiazine, covered with plastic dressing gloves which can be bandaged at the wrist, permits full function while treating superficial second-degree burns. This results in rapid healing (B) with maintenance of full function (C).

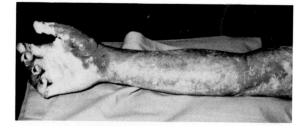

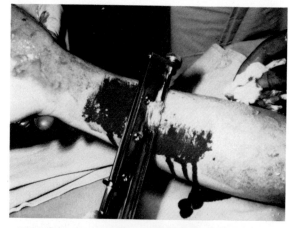

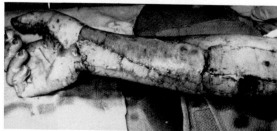

Fig. 1.173 Deep dermal burns (A) extending over a wide area should be tangentially excised (B) and immediately grafted with split thickness skin (C).

which should often be performed in conjunction with the escharotomy — if *any* indication exists, escharotomy should be undertaken.

Frostbite[269]

Frostbite results from exposure to cold. The rapidity of onset and severity of injury are influenced by the intensity of the cold, the duration of exposure, wetness of the part or immobility, which may result from sleep, inebriation or wounds. Any factors which reduce circulation will clearly increase the damage, including vascular disease or constrictive clothing.

The pathological process involves extreme vasoconstriction with a rapid drop in temperature of the part even to the point of tissue freezing. Rewarming results in hyperaemia due to increased blood flow but this is through

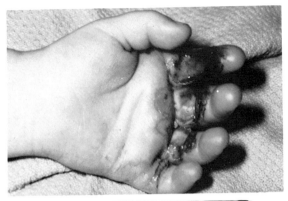

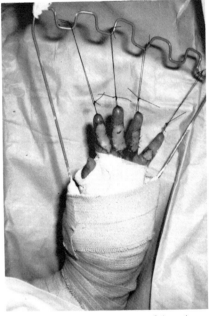

Fig. 1.174 Full thickness electrical burns of the palmar aspect of the fingers in a child (A) should be excised immediately and grafted with full thickness skin (B).

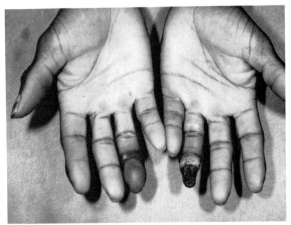

Fig. 1.175 Frostbite with some residual blister formation and frank necrosis.

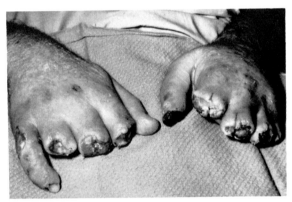

Fig. 1.176 Amputation some four weeks after frostbite injury to both upper extremities.

vessels damaged to a varied degree so that oedema and intravascular thrombosis may cause loss of a part apparently well-perfused.

Four degrees of frostbite have been described which correspond to the four degrees of burn

    1st — numbness, oedema, erythema

    2nd — blistering

    3rd — bluish-gray oedema (develops after hyperaemic phase)

    4th — cold, cyanotic, anaesthetic with *no* hyperaemic phase

One of the major problems in frostbite is presented by recognition of the various degrees but even more by the fact that several, or all, may be present simultaneously in the same digit, being worse peripherally, improving the more proximal the part. (Fig. 1.175). Loss of those portions of the digit with third and fourth degree changes is inevitable (Fig. 1.176). The late effects of frostbite may be due to sympathetic overactivity and are similar to established sympathetic dystrophy — pain, discoloration, oedema and sweating.

INDICATIONS

Rapid rewarming in a whirlpool at 42°C is required, with appropriate analgesia for the often severe pain which will accompany this process. If hyperaemia does not result, intra-arterial reserpine stellate ganglion block or immediate sympathectomy may reduce the area of tissue damage. Aspirin and low molecular weight dextran may reduce intra-vascular coagulation and improve flow. Control of treatment by use of the Doppler flowmeter and digital plethysmography (PVR)[270] and by analysis of blister fluid[271] may prove of value in the future. Conservation should be the theme with respect to the local injury which is too ill-defined for any other course. The late effects are greatly helped by sympathectomy.

REFERENCES

1. Sanguinetti M V 1977 Reconstructive surgery of roller injuries of the hand. Journal of Hand Surgery 2: 134–140
2. Strahan J, Crockett D J 1969 Wringer injury. Injury 1: 57
3. Haynes C D, Webb W A, Fenno C R 1980 Chain saw injuries: Review of 330 cases. Journal of Trauma 20: 772–776
4. Schwager R G, Smith J W, Goulian D 1975 Small, deep forearm lacerations. Plastic and Reconstructive Surgery 55: 190–194
5. Joseph K N, Kalus A M, Sutherland A B 1981 Glass injuries of the hand in children. The Hand 13: 113–119
6. Sharrard W J W 1968 Injection injuries. The Journal of Bone and Joint Surgery 50B: 1
7. Elstrom J A, Pankovich A M, Egwele R 1978 Extra-articular low-velocity gunshot fractures of the radius and ulna. Journal of Bone and Joint Surgery 60A: 335–341
8. Elton R C 1975 Gunshot and fragment wounds of the hand. Contemporary Surgery 7: 13–18
9. Luce E A, Griffen W 1978 Shotgun injuries of the upper extremity. Journal of Trauma 18: 487–492
10. Marcus N A, Blair W F, Shuck J M, Omer G E 1980 Low-velocity gun-shot wounds to extremities. Journal of Trauma 20: 1061–1064
11. Shepard G H 1980 High-energy, low-velocity close-range shotgun wounds. Journal of Trauma 20: 1065–1067
12. Robinson D W, Hardin C A 1955 Corn picker injuries. American Journal of Surgery 89: 780–783
13. Campbell D C, Bryan R S, Cooney W P, Ilstrup D 1979 Mechanical cornpicker hand injuries. Journal of Trauma 19: 678–681
14. Grogono B J S 1973 Auger injuries. Injury 4: 247–257
15. Beatty M E, Zook E G Russell R C, Kinkead L R 1982 Grain auger injuries: The replacement of the corn picker injury? Plastic and Reconstructive Surgery 69: 1 96–102
16. Jazheimer E C, Morain W D, Brown F E 1981 Woodsplitter injuries of the hand. Plastic and Reconstructive Surgery 68: 83–88
17. Smith J R, Asturias J 1968 Card injury of the hand: its characteristics and treatment. Journal of Bone and Joint Surgery 50A: 1161–1170
18. Barry T P, Linton P 1977 Biophysics of rotary mower and snowblower injuries of the hand: High vs. low velocity 'missile' injury. Journal of Trauma 17: 221–214
19. Ross P M Schwentker E P, Bryan H 1976 Mutilating lawnmower injuries in children. Journal of American Medical Association 236: 408
20. McGregor I A, Jackson I T 1969 Sodium chlorate bomb injuries of the hand. British Journal of Plastic Surgery 22: 16–29
21. Reid D A Campbell 1973 Escalator injuries of the hand. Injury 5: 47
22. Charters A C, Davis J W 1978 The roll-bar hand. Journal of Trauma 18:601–604
23. Harris C, Wood V 1978 Rollover injuries of the upper extremity. Journal of Trauma 18: 605–607
24. Mehrotra O N, Crabb D J M 1979 The pattern of hand injury sustained in the overturning motor vehicle. The Hand 11: 321–328
25. Heycock M H 1966 On the management of hand injuries caused by woodworking tools. British Journal of Plastic Surgery 19: 58
26. Caldwell E H, McCormack R M 1980 Acute radiation injury of the hands: Report on a case with a twenty-one year follow-up. Journal of Hand Surgery 5: 568–571
27. Ciano M, Burlin J R, Pardoe R, Mills R L, Hentz V R 1981 High-frequency electromagnetic radiation injury to the upper extremity: Local and systemic effects. Annals of Plastic Surgery 7: 128–135
28. McCabe W P, Ditmars D M 1973 Soft tissue changes in the hands of drug addicts. Plastic and Reconstructive Surgery 52: 538–540
29. McKay D, Pascarelli E F, Eaton R G 1973 Infections and sloughs in the hands in drug addicts. Journal of Bone and Joint Surgery 55A: 741–746
30. Neviaser R J, Butterfield W C, Wiechi D R 1972 The puffy hand of drug addiction. A study of the pathogenesis. Journal of Bone and Joint Surgery 54A: 629–633
31. Ryan J J Hoopes, J E Jabaley M E 1974 Drug injection injuries of the hands and forearms in addicts. Plastic and Reconstructive Surgery 53: 445–451
32. Snyder C C, Straight R, Glenn J 1972 The snakebitten hand. Plastic and Reconstructive Surgery 49: 275–282
33. Marten E 1979 Hand deformities in patients with snakebite. Plastic and Reconstructive Surgery 64: 554
34. Huang T T, Blackwell S J, Lewis S R 1978 Hand deformities in patients with snakebite. Plastic and Reconstructive Surgery 62: 32–36
35. Grace T G, Omer G E 1980 The management of upper extremity pit viper wounds. Journal of Hand Surgery 5: 168–177
36. Rees R, Shack R B, Withers E, Madden J, Franklin J, Lynch J B 1981 Management of the brown recluse spider bite. Plastic and Reconstructive Surgery 68: 768–773
37. Zeichner D M, Hoehn J G 1981 Karate-induced hand injuries. Orthopaedic Review 10: 127–131
38. McLatchie G R, Davies J E, Caulley J H 1980 Injuries in karate — a case for medical control. The Journal of Trauma 20: 956–958
39. Curtin J, Kay N R M 1976 Hand injuries due to soccer. The Hand 8: 93–95
40. Kelesy J L, Pastides H, Kreiger M, Harris C, Chernow R A 1980 Upper extremity disorders: a survey of their frequency and cost in the United States. C V Mosby, St Louis
41. Frey M, Mandl H, Holle J 1980 Secondary operations after replantations. Chirurgia Plastica 5: 235–241
42. Gelberman R, Urbaniak J, Bright D, Levin L S 1978 Digital sensibility following replantation. Journal of Hand Surgery 3: 313–319
43. Kleinert, H E, Jablon M, Tsai T 1980 An overview of replantation and results of 347 replants in 245 patients. Journal of Trauma 20: 390–398
44. Morrison W, O'Brien B, MacLeod A 1978 Digital replantation and revascularization. A long term review of one hundred cases. The Hand 10: 125–134
45. Scott F A, Howar J W, Boswick J A 1981 Recovery of function following replantation and revascularization of amputated hand parts. Journal of Trauma 21:3 204–214
46. Lister G D, Kleinert H E 1979 Replantation. In: Grabb, Smith (eds) Plastic Surgery, 3rd Edn. Little, Brown and Company, Boston
47. Kaplan E B 1965 Functional and Surgical Anatomy of the Hand. Lippincott, Philadelphia
48. Guyon F 1861 Note sur une disposition anatomique propre a la face anterieure de la region du poignet et non encore decrite. Bull Society Anat Paris 36: 184–186
49. Denman E E 1978 The anatomy of the space of Guyon. Hand 10: 69–76
50. McFarlane R M, Mayer J R, Hugill J V 1976 Further observations on the anatomy of the ulnar nerve at the wrist. Hand 8: 115–117

51. Lassa R, Shrewsbury M, 1975 A variation in the path of the deep motor branch of the ulnar nerve at the wrist. Journal of Bone and Joint Surgery 57A: 990–991

52. Engber W D, Gmeiner J G 1980 Palmar cutaneous branch of the ulnar nerve. Journal of Hand Surgery 5: 26–29

53. Coleman S S, Anson B J 1961 Arterial patterns in the hand based on a study of 650 specimens. Surgery Gynecology and Obstretrics 113: 409–424

54. Graham W P III 1973 Variations of the motor branch of the median nerve at the wrist. Plastic and Reconstructive Surgery: 51: 90—91

55. Lanz U 1977 Anatomical variations of the median nerve in the carpal tunnel. The Journal of Hand Surgery 2: 44–53

56. Taleisnik J 1973 The palmar cutaneous branch of the median nerve and the approach to the carpal tunnel. Journal of Bone and Joint Surgery 55A: 1212–1217

57. Brand P W, Cranor K C, Ellis J C 1975 Tendon and pulleys at the metacarpophalangeal joint of a finger. The Journal of Bone and Joint Surgery 57A: 779–783

58. Chuinard R G, Friermood T G, Lipscomb P R 1979 The 'suicide' wrist: Epidemiologic study of the injury. Orthopaedics 2: 499–502

59. Lister G D, Kleinert H E 1979 Replantation. In: Grabb, Smith, (eds) Platic Surgery, 3rd Edn. Little, Brown, and Co, Boston p 697

60. Carroll R 1974 Ring injuries in the hand. Clinical Orthopaedics 104: 175–182

61. Urbaniak J R, Evans J P, Bright D S 1981 Microvascular management of ring avulsion injuries. Journal of Hand Surgery 6:1 25–30

62. Bessman A N, Wagner W 1975 Nonclostridial gas gangrene. Report of 48 cases and review of the literature. Journal of American Medical Association 233: 958–964

63. Manske P R, Lesker P A 1978 Avulsion of the ring finger flexor digitorum profundus tendon. Hand 10: 52–55

64. Chang W H J, Thoms O J, White W L 1972 Avulsion injury of the long flexor tendons. Plastic and Reconstructive Surgery 50: 260–264

65. Leddy J P, Packer J W 1977 Avulsion of the profundus tendon insertion in athletes. The Journal of Hand Surgery 2: 66–69

66. Ferraiouli E B 1968 Repair of the disrupted flexor mechanism of the hand. Asoc Med Puerto Rico Bol 60: 11–16

67. Apley A G 1956 Test of the power of flexor digitorum sublimis British Medical Journal 1: 25–26

68. Baker D S, Gaul S, Williams V K, Graves M 1981 The little finger superficialis — Clinical investigation of its anatomic and functional shortcomings. Journal of Hand Surgery 6: 374–378

69. Kaplan E B 1969 Muscular and tendinous variations of the flexor superficialis of the fifth finger of the hand. Bulletin of Hospital Joint Disease 30: 59

70. Kisner W H 1980 Double sublimis tendon to fifth finger with absence of profundus. Plastic and Reconstructive Surgery 65: 229–230

71. Denman E 1979 Rupture of the extensor pollicis longus — a crush injury. The Hand 11: 295–298

72. Simpson R G 1977 Delayed rupture of extensor pollicis longus tendon following closed injury. The Hand 9: 160–161

73. Engkvist O Lundborg U & Lundborg G 1979 Rupture of the extensor pollicis longus tendon after fracture of the lower end of the radius. A clinical and microangiographic study. The Hand 11: 76–86

74. Mackay I, Simpson R G 1980 Closed rupture of extensor digitorum communis tendon following fracture of the radius. The Hand 12: 214–216

75. Southmayd W W, Millender L H, Nalebuff E A 1975 Rupture of the flexor tendons of the index finger after Colles' fracture. The Journal of Bone and Joint Surgery 57–A: 562–563

76. Younger C P, DeFiore J C 1977 Rupture of flexor tendons to the fingers after a Colles fracture. Case report. Journal of Bone and Joint Surgery 59–A: 828–829

77. Rosenfeld N, Rascoff J H 1980 Tendon ruptures of the hand associated with renal dialysis. Plastic and Reconstructive Surgery 65: 77–79

78. Carducci A T 1981 Potential boutonniere deformity — its recognition and treatment. Orthopaedic Review 10: 121–123

79. Furnas D, Spinner M 1978 The 'sign of horns' in the diagnosis of injury or disease of the extensor digitorum communis of the hand. British Journal of Plastic Surgery 31: 263–265

80. Kettelkamp D B, Flatt A E, Moulds R 1971 Traumatic dislocation of the long finger extensor tendon. A clinical anatomical and biomechanical study. Journal of Bone and Joint Surgery 53A: 229–240

81. Albright J A, Linburg R M 1978 Common variations of the radial wrist extensors. Journal of Hand Surgery 3: 134–138

82. Matsen F A 1980 Compartmental Syndromes. Grune and Stratton, New York

83. Garfin S R, Mubarak S J, Evans K L, Hargens A R, Akeson W H 1981 Quantification of intracompartmental pressure and volume under plaster casts. Journal of Bone and Joint Surgery 63A: 449–453

84. Zweifach S S, Hargens A R, Evans K L, Smith R K, Mubarak S J, Akeson W H 1980 Skeletal muscle necrosis in pressurized compartments associated with haemorrhagic hypotension. The Journal of Trauma 20: 941–947

85. Halpern A, Mochizuki R M 1980 Compartment syndrome of the interosseous muscles of hand. Orthopaedic Review 9: 121–127

86. Spinner M, Aiache A, Silver L, Barsky A S 1973 Impending ischemic contracture of the hand. Plastic and Reconstructive Surgery 50: 341–349

87. Matsen F A, Winquist R A, Krugmire R B 1980 Diagnosis and management of compartmental syndromes. Journal of Bone and Joint Surgery 62A: 286–291

88. Mubarak S J, Owen C A, Hargens A R, Garetto L P, Enneking W F 1978 Acute compartment syndromes. Diagnosis and treatment with the aid of the wick catheter. Journal of Bone and Joint Surgery 60A: 1091–1099

89. Bingold A C 1979 On splitting plasters. Journal of Bone and Joint Surgery 61B: 294–295

90. Wolfort F G, Cochran T C, Filtzer H 1973 Immediate interossei decompression following crush injury of the hand. Archives of Surgery 106: 826–828

91. Holden C E A 1979 The pathology and prevention of Volkmann's ischaemic contracture. Journal of Bone and Joint Surgery 61B: 296–300

92. Volkmann R 1967 Die ischaemischen muskellahmugen und-kontrakturen. Centrabl F Chir Translation by Edgar Bick. Clinical Orthopedics: 50: 5–6

93. Dellon A L 1978 The moving two-point discrimination test: Clinical evaluation of the quickly adapting fiber/receptor system. Journal of Hand Surgery 3: 474–481

94. Weber E H 1835 Ueber den Tastsinn. Archives Anat Physiol Wissenischs Med 152–160

95. Moberg E 1964 Evaluation and management of nerve injuries in the hand. Surgical Clinics of North America 44: 1019

96. Learmonth J R 1919 A variation in the distribution of the radial branch of the musculo-spiral nerve. Journal of Anatomy and Physiology 53: 371–372

97. Earle A S, Vlastou C 1980 Crossed fingers and other tests of ulnar nerve motor function. Journal of Hand Surgery 5: 560–565

98. Gelberman T H, Menon J, Fronek A 1980 The peripheral pulse following arterial injury. The Journal of Trauma 20: 948–950

99. Adar R, Schramek A, Khodadadi J, Zweig A, Golcman L, Romanoff H 1980 Arterial combat injuries of the upper extremity. Journal of Trauma 20: 297–302

100. Lord R S A, Irani C N 1974 Assessment of arterial injury in limb trauma. Journal of Trauma 14: 1042–1053

101. Linson M A 1980 Axillary artery thrombosis after fracture of the humerus. Journal of Bone and Joint Surgery 62A: 1214–1215

102. Broudy A S, Jupiter J, May J W 1979 Management of supracondylar fracture with brachial artery thrombosis in a child. The Journal of Trauma 19: 540–544

103. Tse D H W, Slabaugh P B, Carlson P A 1980 Injury to the axillary artery by a closed fracture of the clavicle. Journal of Bone and Joint Surgery 62A: 1372–1376

104. Sturn J T, Rothenberger D A, Strate R 1978 Brachial artery distruption following closed elbow dislocation. Journal of Trauma 18: 364–366

105. Lev-El A, Adar R, Rubinstein Z 1981 Axillary artery injury in erect dislocation of the shoulder. Journal of Trauma 21: 323–325

106. Shuck J M, Omer G E, Lewis C E 1972 Arterial obstruction due to intimal disruption in extremity fractures. Journal of Trauma 12: 481–489

107. Robbs J, Baker L 1978 Major arterial trauma: review of experience with 267 injuries. British Journal of Surgery 65: 532–538

108. Raju S, Carner D V 1981 Brachial plexus compression: Complication of delayed recognition of arterial injuries of the shoulder girdle. Archives of Surgery 116: 175–178

109. Ashbell T S, Kleinert H E, Kutz J E 1967 Vascular injuries about the elbow. Clinical Orthopaedics 50: 107–127

110. Scherr D D, Lichti E L, Lambert K L 1973 Tissue viability assessment with Doppler ultrasonic flowmeter in acute injuries of extremities. Journal of Bone and Joint Surgery 55A: 157–161

111. Yao S, Gourmos C, Papathanasiou K, Irvine W 1972 A method for assessing ischemia of the hand and fingers. Surgery, Obstetrics, and Gynecology 135: 373–378

112. McCormick T M, Burch B H 1979 Routine angiographic evaluation of neck and extremity injuries. Journal of Trauma 19: 384–387

113. Samson R, Pasternak B M 1980 Traumatic arterial spasm — rarity or nonentity. Journal of Trauma 20: 607–609

114. Grossland S G, Neviaser R 1977 Complications of radial artery catheterization. The Hand 9: 287–290

115. Mandel M, Dauchot P 1977 Radial artery cannulation in 1,000 patients: Precautions and complications. Journal of Hand Surgery 2: 482–485

116. Serafin D, Puckett C L, McCarty G 1976 Successful treatment of acute vascular insufficiency in a hand by intra-arterial fibrinolysin, heparin and reserpine. Plastic and Reconstructive Surgery 58: 506–509

117. Neviaser R J, Adams J, May G 1976 Complications of arterial puncture in anticoagulated patients. Journal of Bone and Joint Surgery 58A: 218–220

118. Kartchner M M, Wilcox W C 1976 Thrombolysis of palmar and digital arterial thrombosis by intra-arterial thrombolysin. The Journal of Hand Surgery 1: 67–74

119. Schmidt P E, Hewitt R L 1980 Severe upper limb ischemia Archives of Surgery 115: 1188–1191

120. Baur G, Porter J, Bardana E, Wesche D, Rosch J 1977 Rapid onset of hand ischemia of unknown etiology. Annals of Surgery 186: 184–189

121. Roberts B 1976 The acutely ischemic limb. Heart and Lung 5: 273–276

122. Saveyev V, Zarevakhin I, Stepanov N 1977 Artery embolism of the upper limbs. Surgery 81: 367–375

123. Sachagello C R, Ernst C B, Griffen W O 1974 The acutely ischemic upper extremity: selective management. Surgery 76: 1002–1009

124. Conklin W T, Dabb R W, Danyo J J 1981 Microvascular salvage of the embolized hand. Orthopaedic Review 10: 169–171

125. Adams J T, McEvoy R K, DeWeese J A 1965 Primary deep venous thrombosis of upper extremity. Archives of Surgery 91: 29–42

126. Paletta F X 1981 Venous gangrene of the hand. Plastic and Reconstructive Surgery 67: 67–69

127. Kaplan E B 1957 Dorsal dislocation of the metacarpophalangeal joint of the index finger. Journal of Bone and Joint Surgery 39A: 1081–1086

128. Green D P, Terry G C 1973 Complex dislocation of the metacarpophalangeal joint. Journal of Bone and Joint Surgery 55A: 1480–1486

129. Boyes J H 1980 The measuring of motions. Journal of Hand Surgery 5: 89–90

130. Eaton R G, Littler J W 1976 Joint injuries and their sequelae. Clinics in Plastic Surgery 3: 85–98

131. Bowers W H, Wolf J W, Nehil J L, Bittinger S 1980 The proximal interphalangeal joint volar plate. I. An anatomical and biomechanical study. Journal of Hand Surgery 5: 79–88

132. Bowers W H 1981 The proximal interphalangeal joint volar plate. II. A clinical study of hyperextension injury. Journal of Hand Surgery 6: 77–81

133. Smith R J 1977 Post-traumatic instability of the metacarpophalangeal joint of the thumb. Journal of Bone and Joint Surgery 59A: 14–21

134. Leslie I J, Dickson R A 1981 The fractured carpal scaphoid. Journal of Bone and Joint Surgery 63B: 225–230

135. Hart V L, Gaynor V 1941 Roentgenographic study of the carpal canal. Journal of Bone and Joint Surgery 23: 382–383

136. Palmer A K 1981 Trapezial ridge fractures. Journal of Hand Surgery 6: 561–564

137. Andress M R, Peckar V G 1970 Fracture of the hook of the hamate. British Journal of Radiology 93: 141–143

138. Moneim M S 1981 The tangential posteroanterior radiograph to demonstrate scapholunate dissociation. Journal of Bone and Joint Surgery 63A: 1324–1326

139. Robert P 1936 Bulletins et memories de la Societe de Radiologie medicale de France 24: 687–690

140. Lane C S 1977 Detecting occult fractures of the metacarpal head: the Brewerton view. Journal of Hand Surgery 2: 131–133

141. Bowers W H, Hurst L C 1977 Gamekeeper's thumb. Evaluation by arthrography and stress roentgenography. Journal of Bone and Joint Surgery 59A: 519–524

142. Engel J, Ganel A, Ditzian R, Militeanu J 1979 Arthrography as a method of diagnosing tear of the ulnar collateral ligament of the metacarpophalangeal joint of the thumb 'Gamekeeper's Thumb'. Journal of Trauma 19: 106–110

143. Bennett E H 1886 On fracture of the metacarpal bone of the thumb. British Medical Journal 2: 12–13

144. Rolando S 1910 Fracture de la base du premier metacarpien: et principalement sur une variete non encore decrite. Presse Medicale 33: 303

145. Salter R B, Harris W R 1963 Injuries involving the epiphyseal plate. Journal of Bone and Joint Surgery 45A: 587–622

146. Campbell R D, Lance E M, Chin Bor Yeoh 1964 Lunate and perilunar dislocations. Journal of Bone and Joint Surgery 46B: 55–72

147. Campbell R D, Thompson C, Lance E M, Adler J B 1965 Indications for open reduction of lunate and perilunate dislocations of the carpal bones. The Journal of Bone and Joint Surgery 47A: 915–937

148. Palmer A, Dobyns J, Linscheid R 1978 Management of post-traumatic instability of the wrist secondary to ligament rupture. Journal of Hand Surgery 3: 507–532

149. Mayfield J K., Johnson R P, Kilcoyne R K 1980 Carpal dislocations: Pathomechanics and progressive perilunar instability. Journal of Hand Surgery 5: 226–241

150. Frankel V H 1977 The Terry-Thomas sign. Clinical Orthopaedics 129: 321

151. Howard F, Thomas F, Wojeie E 1974 Rotatory subluxation of the navicular. Clinical Orthopaedics and Related Research 104: 134

152. Linscheid R L, Dobyns J H, Beabout J W, Bryan R S 1972 Traumatic instability of the wrist. The Journal of Bone and Joint Surgery 54A: 1612–1632

153. Sebald J R, Dobyns J H, Linscheid R L 1974 Natural history of collapse deformities of the wrist. Clinical Orthopaedics and Related Research 104: 140

154. Belsole R J, Eikman A, Muroff L R 1981 Bone scintigraphy in trauma of the hand and wrist. Journal of Trauma 21: 163–166

155. Batillas J, Vasilas A, Pizzi W, Gokcebay T 1981 Bone scanning in the detention of occult fractures. Journal of Trauma 21: 564–569

156. Meyn M A, Roth A M 1980 Isolated dislocation of the trapezoid bone. Journal of Hand Surgery 5: 602–604

157. Bendre D V, Baxi V K 1981 Dislocation of trapezoid. Journal of Trauma 21: 899–900

158. Frykman E 1980 Dislocation of the triquetrum. Scand. Journal of Plastic and Reconstructive Surgery 14: 205–207

159. Soucatos P N, Hartofilakidis-Garofalidis G C 1981 Dislocation of the triangular bone: Report of a case. Journal of Bone and Joint Surgery 63A: 1012–1014

160. Goldberg I, Amit S, Bahar A, Seelenfreund M 1981 Complete dislocation of the trapezium (multangulum majus). Journal of Hand Surgery 6: 193–195

161. Seimon L P 1972 Compound dislocation of the trapezium. Journal of Bone and Joint Surgery 54A: 1297–1300

162. Gordon S L 1972 Scaphoid and lunate dislocation. The Journal of Bone and Joint Surgery 54A: 1769–1772

163. Brown R H L, Muddu B N 1981 Scaphoid and lunate dislocation. The Hand 13: 303–307

164. Schutt R C, Boswick J A, Scott F A 1981 Volar fracture dislocation of the carpometacarpal joint of the index finger treated by delayed open reduction. Journal of Trauma 21: 986–987

165. Dennyson W G, Stother I G 1976 Carpometacarpal dislocation of the little finger. The Hand 8: 161–164

166. Lilling M, Weinberg H 1979 The mechanism of dorsal fracture dislocation of the fifth carpometacarpal joint. Journal of Hand Surgery 4: 340–342

167. Kleinman W, Grantham S A 1978 Multiple volar carpometacarpal joint dislocation. Case report of traumatic volar dislocation of the medial four carpometacarpal joints in a child and review of the literature Journal of Hand Surgery 3: 337–382

168. North E R, Eaton R G 1980 Volar dislocation of the fifth metacarpal. Journal of Bone and Joint Surgery 62A: 657–659

169. Weiland A J, Lister G D, Villarreal-Rios A 1976 Volar fracture dislocations of the second and third carpometacarpal joints associated with acute carpal tunnel syndrome. Journal of Trauma 16: 672–675

170. McCarthy L J 1980 Open metacarpophalangeal dislocations of the index, middle, ring and little fingers. Journal of Trauma 20: 183–185

171. Dray G, Millender L, Nalebuff E 1979 Rupture of the radial collateral ligament of a metacarpophalangeal joint to one of the ulnar three fingers. Journal of Hand Surgery 4: 346–350

172. Wood M B, Dobyns J H 1981 Chronic, complex volar dislocation of the metacarpophalangeal joint. Journal of Hand Surgery 6: 73–76

173. Posner M A, Wilenski M 1978 Irreducible volar dislocation of the proximal interphalangeal joint of a finger caused by interposition of an intact central slip. Journal of Bone and Joint Surgery 60: 133–134

174. Whipple T L, Evans J P, Urbaniak J R 1980 Irreducible dislocation of a finger joint in a child. Journal of Bone and Joint Surgery 62A: 832–833

175. Palmer A K, Linscheid R L 1977 Irreducible dorsal dislocation of the distal interphalangeal joint of the finger. Journal of Hand Surgery 2: 406–408

176. Paul A L 1976 Irreducible dislocation of a distal interphalangeal joint. British Journal of Plastic Surgery 29: 227–229

177. Salamon P B, Gelberman R H 1978 Irreducible dislocation of the interphalangeal joint of the thumb. Report of three cases. Journal of Bone and Joint Surgery 60A: 400–401

178. Levy I M, Liberty S 1979 Simultaneous dislocation of the interphalangeal and metacarpophalangeal joint of the thumb. A case report. Journal of Hand Surgery 4: 489–490

179. Cleak D K 1981 Simultaneous dislocation of the interphalangeal and metacarpophalangeal joints in a thumb. The Hand 13: 167–168

180. Weseley M S, Barenfeld P A, Eisenstein A L 1978 Simultaneous dorsal dislocation of both interphalangeal joints in a finger. Case report. Journal of Bone and Joint Surgery 60A: 1142–1143

181. Iftikhar T B, Kaminski R S 1981 Simultaneous dorsal dislocation of MP joints of long and ring fingers. Orthopaedic Review 10: 71–72

182. Adler G A, Light T R 1981 Simultaneous complex dislocation of the metacarpophalangeal joints of the long and index fingers. A case report. Journal of Bone and Joint Surgery 63A: 1007–1009

183. Espinosa R H, Renart I P 1980 Simultaneous dislocation of the interphalangeal joints in a finger. Case report . Journal of Hand Surgery 5: 617–618

184. Barton N J 1979 Fractures of the phalanges of the hand in children. The Hand 11: 134–143

185. Scherr D D, Dodd T A 1976 In vitro bacteriological evaluation of the effectiveness of antimicrobial irrigating solution. Journal of Bone and Joint Surgery 58A: 119–122

186. Scherr D D, Dodd T A, Buckingham W W 1972 Prophylactic use of topical antibiotic irrigation in uninfected surgical wounds. A microbiological evaluation. Journal of Bone and Joint Surgery 54A: 634–640

187. Carneiro R S, Okunski W J, Heffernan A H 1977 Detection of a relatively radiolucent foreign body in the hand by xerography. Plastic and Reconstructive Surgery 59: 862–863

188. Bowers D G, Lynch J B 1977 Xeroradiography for non-metallic foreign bodies. Plastic and Reconstructive Surgery 60: 470–471

189. Lee M H 1963 Intra-articular and peri-articular fractures of the phalanges. Journal of Bone and Joint Surgery 45B: 103–109

190. Fernandez D L 1981 Irreducible radiocarpal fracture-dislocation and radioulnar dissociation with entrapment of the ulnar nerve, artery and flexor profundus II–V — Case report. The Journal of Hand Surgery 6: 456–461

191. Matev I 1976 A radiological sign of entrapment of the median nerve in the elbow joint after posterior dislocation. Journal of Bone and Joint Surgery 58B 353–355

192. Green D P, O'Brien E T 1978 Open reduction of carpal dislocations: Indications and operative techniques. Journal of Hand Surgery 3: 250–265

193. Peimer C A, Smith R J, Leffert R D 1981 Distraction-fixation in the primary treatment of metacarpal bone loss. Journal of Hand Surgery 6: 111–124

194. Segmuller G 1973 Operative stabilisierung am handskelett. Hans Huber, Bern. 1977 Surgical stabilization of the skeleton of the hand. Williams and Wilkins, Baltimore.

195. Lister G 1978 Intraosseous wiring of the digital skeleton. Journal of Hand Surgery 3: 427–435

196. Grundberg A B 1981 Intramedullary fixation for fractures of the hand. Journal of Hand Surgery 6: 568–573

197. Bilos J, Eskestrand T 1979 External fixator use in comminuted gunshot fractures of the proximal phalanx. Journal of Hand Surgery 4: 357–359

198. Scott M M, Mulligan P J 1980 Stabilizing severe phalangeal fractures. The Hand 12: 44–50

199. Eiken O, Hagberg L, Lundborg G 1981 Evolving biologic concepts as applied to tendon surgery. Clinics in Plastic Surgery 8: 1–12

200. Lister G D 1983 Incision and closure of the flexor sheath during primary tendon repair. The Hand, in press

201. Weeks P M 1981 Invited comment on Three complications of untreated partial laceration of flexor tendons — Entrapment, rupture and triggering. Journal of Hand Surgery 6: 396–398

202. Schlenker J D, Lister G D, Kleinert H E 1981 Three complications of untreated partial laceration of flexor tendons — Entrapment, rupture and triggering. Journal of Hand Surgery 6: 392–396

203. Lister G D, Kleinert H E, Kutz J E, Atasoy E 1977 Primary flexor tendon repair followed by immediate controlled mobilization. Journal of Hand Surgery 2: 441–455

204. Van Beek A L, Kutz J E, Zook E 1978 Importance of the ribbon sign, indicating unsuitability of the vessel, in replanting a finger. Plastic and Reconstructive Surgery 61: 32–35

205. O'Reilly R J, Blatt G 1975 High-pressure injection injury. Journal of American Medical Association 233: 533–534

206. Gelberman R, Posch J L, Jurist J M 1975 High-pressure injection injuries of the hand. Journal of Bone and Joint Surgery 57A: 935–937

207. Schoo M J, Scott F A, Broswick J A 1980 High pressure injection injuries of the hand. Journal of Trauma 20: 229–238

208. Scher C, Schun F D, Harvin J S 1973 High pressure paint gun injuries of the hand. British Journal of Plastic Surgery 26: 167–171

209. Waters W R, Penn I, Ross H M 1967 Airless paint gun injuries of the hand 39: 613–618

210. Stark H H, Ashworth C R, Boyes J H 1967 Paint gun injuries of the hand. Journal of Bone and Joint Surgery 49A: 637–647

211. Stark H H, Ashworth C R, Boyes J H 1961 Grease gun injuries of the hand. Journal of Bone and Joint Surgery 43A: 485–491

212. Flint M H 1966 Plastic injection moulding injury. British Journal of Plastic Surgery 19: 70–78

213. Crabb D J M 1981 The value of plain radiographs in treating greasegun injuries. The Hand 13: 39–42

214. Ramos H, Posch J L, Lie K K 1970 High-pressure injection injuries of the hand. Plastic and Reconstructive Surgery 45: 221–226

215. Kaufman H D 1968 High-pressure injection injuries. British Journal of Surgery 55: 214–218

216. Dibbell D, Hedberg J, McGraw J, Rankin J, Souther S 1979 A quantitative examination of the use of fluorescein in predicting viability of skin flaps. Annals of Plastic Surgery 3: 101–105

217. Elliott R, Hoehn J, Stayman J W 1979 Management of the viable soft tissue cover in degloving injuries. The Hand 11: 69–71

218. London P S 1961 Simplicity of approach to treatment of the injured hand. Journal of Bone and Joint Surgery 43B: 454–464

219. Ross R 1979 Inhibition of myofibroblasts by skin grafts. Plastic and Reconstructive Surgery 63: 473–481

220. Horn 1951 The use of full thickness hand skin flaps in the reconstruction of injured fingers. Plastic and Reconstructive Surgery 7: 463–481

221. Lanier V C 1981 The fillet flap principle. Orthopaedic Review 10: 63–66

222. Chase R A 1968 The damaged index digit — a source of components to restore the crippled hand. Journal of Bone and Joint Surgery 50A: 1152–1160

223. Russell R C, Van Beek A L, Wavak P, Zook E G 1981 Alternative hand flaps for amputations and digital defects. Journal of Hand Surgery 6: 399–405

224. McGregor I A, Morgan G 1973 Axial and random pattern flaps. British Journal of Plastic Surgery 26: 202–213

225. Yeschua R, Wexler M R, Neuman Z 1977 Cross-arm triangular flaps for correction of adduction contracture of the web space in the hand. Plastic and Reconstructive Surgery 59: 859–861

226. Holevich J 1965 Early skin grafting in the treatment of traumatic avulsion injuries of the hand and fingers. Journal of Bone and Joint Surgery 47A: 944–957

227. Jarev A, Hirshowitz B 1978 A two stage cross arm flap for severe multiple degloving injury of the hand. The Hand 10: 276–278

228. Lister G D, McGregor I A, Jackson I T 1973 Groin flap in hand injuries. British Journal of Accident Surgery 4: 229–239

229. May J W, Bartlett S P 1981 Staged groin flap in reconstruction of the pediatric hand. Journal of Hand Surgery 6: 163–171

230. Schlenker J D, Averill R M 1980 The iliofemoral (groin) flap for hand and forearm coverage. Orthopaedic Review 9: 57–63

231. Schlenker J D 1980 Important considerations in the design and construction of groin flaps. Annals of Plastic Surgery 5: 353–357

232. Schlenker J D, Atasoy E, Lyon J 1980 The abdominohypogastric flap — axial pattern flap for forearm coverage. The Hand 12: 248–252

233. Shaw D T 1980 Tubed pedicle construction: The single pedicle abdominal tube and the acromiopectoral flap. Annals of Plastic Surgery 4: 219–223

234. Watson A C, McGregor J C 1981 The simultaneous use of a groin flap and a tensor fasciae latae myocutaneous flap to provide tissue cover for a completely degloved hand. British Journal of Plastic Surgery 34: 349—352

235. Louis D S, Palmer A K, Burney R E 1980 Open treatment of digital tip injuries. Journal of American Meidcal Association 244: 697–698

236. Allen M J 1980 Conservative management of fingertip injuries in adults. The Hand 12: 257–265

237. DeBoer P, Collinson P O 1981 The use of silver sulphadiazine occlusive dressings for fingertip injuries. Journal of Bone and Joint Surgery 4: 545–547

238. Illingworth C M 1974 Trapped fingers and amputated fingertips in children. Journal of Pediatric Surgery 9: 853–858

239. Das S K, Brown H G 1978 Management of lost fingertips in children. Hand 10: 16–27

240. Tranquilli-Leali E 1935 Ricostruzione dell'apice delle falangi ungueali mediante autoplastica volare peduncolata per scorrimento. Infort, Traum, Lavoro 1: 186–193

241. Atasoy E, Ioakimidis E, Kasdan M, Kutz J E, Kleinert H E 1970 Reconstruction of the amputated fingertip with a triangular volar flap. Journal of Bone and Joint Surgery 52A: 921–926

242. Macht S D, Watson H K 1980 The Moberg volar advancement flap for digital reconstruction. Journal of Hand Surgery 5: 372–376

243. Posner M A, Smith R J 1971 The advancement pedicle flap for thumb injuries. The Journal of Bone and Joint Surgery 53A: 1618–1621

244. Pho R W H 1979 Local composite neurovascular island flap for skin cover in pulp loss of the thumb. The Journal of Hand Surgery 4: 11–16

245. Cronin T D 1951 The cross-finger flap — a new method of repair. Annals of Surgery 17: 419–425

246. Curtis R M 1957 Cross-finger pedicle flap in hand surgery. Annals of Surgery 145: 650

247. Hoskin H D 1960 The versatile cross-finger flap. Journal of Bone and Joint Surgery 42A: 261–277

248. Adamson J E, Horton C E, Crawford H H 1967 Sensory rehabilitation of the injured thumb. Plastic and Reconstructive Surgery 40: 53–57

249. Gaul J S 1969 Radial innervated cross-finger flap from index to provide sensory pulp to injured thumbs. Journal of Bone and Joint Surgery 51A: 1257–1263

250. Lister G D 1981 The theory of the transposition flap and its practical application in the hand. Clinics in Plastic Surgery 8: 115–128

251. Flatt A E 1957 The thenar flap. Journal of Bone and Joint Surgery 39B: 80–85

252. Krag C, Rasmussen B 1975 The neurovascular island flap for defective sensibility of the thumb. The Journal of Bone and Joint Surgery 57B: 495–499

253. Henderson H P, Reid D A C 1980 Long term follow up of neurovascular island flaps. The Hand 12: 113–122

254. Markley J M 1977 The preservation of close two-point discrimination in the interdigital transfer of neurovascular island flaps. Plastic and Reconstructive Surgery 59: 812–816

255. Tubiana R, DuParc J 1961 Restoration of sensibility in the hand by neurovascular skin island transfer. Journal of Bone and Joint Surgery 43B: 474–480

256. Salisbury R E, Pruitt B A 1976 Burns of the upper extremity. Saunders W B, Philadelphia

257. Magierski M, Sakiel S, Buczak B, Koisar J, Kepny A, Ciembroniewicz W 1979 Analysis of reasons and locations of burns on hands. Scandinavian Journal of Plastic and Reconstructive Surgery 13: 141–142

258. Salisbury R E, Hunt J L, Warden G D, Pruitt B A 1973 Management of electrical burns of the upper extremity. Plastic and Reconstructive Surgery 51: 648–652

259. Sullivan W G, Scott F A, Boswick J A 1981 Rehabilitation following electrical injury to the upper extremity. Annals of Plastic Surgery 7: 347–353

260. Gunn A 1967 Electric fire burn. British Medical Journal 3: 764–766

261. Stone P A 1973 Hand burns caused by electric fires. Injury 4: 240–246

262. James J H, Morris A M 1977 The use of hand bags compared with a conventional dressing in the treatment of superficial burns of the hand. Chirurgia Plastica 4: 67–72

263. Chait L A 1975 The treatment of burns by early tangential excision and skin grafting. South African Medical Journal 49: 1375–1379

264. Wexler M R, Yeschua R, Neuman Z 1975 Early treatment of burns of the hand by tangential excision and grafting. Plastic and Reconstructive Surgery 54: 268–273

265. Levein B A. Sirinek K R, Peterson H D, Pruitt B A 1979 Efficacy of tangential excision and immediate autografting of deep second-degree burns of the hand. Journal of Trauma 19: 670–673

266. Malfeyt G A M 1976 Burns of the dorsum of the hand treated by tangential excision. British Journal of Plastic Surgery 29: 78–81

267. Salisbury R, McKeel D 1974 Ischemic necrosis of the intrinsic muscles of the hand after thermal injuries. Journal of Bone and Joint Surgery 56A: 1701–1707

268. Salisbury R E, Taylor J W, Levine N S 1976 Evaluation of digital escharotomy in burned hands. Plastic and Reconstructive Surgery 58: 440–443

269. Schumacker H B 1982 Frostbite In: Flynn J E (ed) Hand Surgery 3rd Edn, Williams and Wilkins, Baltimore p 591

270. Rakower S, Shahgoli S, Wong S 1978 Doppler ultrasound and digital plethysmography to determine the need for sympathetic blockage after frostbite. Journal of Trauma 18: 713–718

271. Robson M C, Heggers J P 1981 Evaluation of hand frostbite blister fluid as a clue to pathogenesis. Journal of Hand Surgery 6: 43–47

FURTHER READING

Books

Beasley R W 1981 Hand injuries. Saunders, Philadelphia
Eaton R G 1971 Joint injuries of the hand. Thomas, Springfield
Henry A K 1973 Extensile exposure. Churchill Livingstone, Edinburgh
Johnson M K, Cohen M J 1975 The hand atlas. Thomas, Springfield
Kaplan E B 1965 Functional and surgical anatomy of the hand. Lippincott, Philadelphia
Rockwood C A, Green D P 1975 Fractures. Lippincott, Philadelphia
Segmuller G 1977 Surgical stabilization of the skeleton of the hand. Williams and Wilkins, Baltimore

Journals

Adamson J E, Horton C E, Crawford H H 1967 Sensory rehabilitation of the injured thumb. Plastic and Reconstructive Surgery 40: 53–57
Alexander A H, Lichtman D M 1981 Irreducible distal radioulnar joint occurring in a Galeazzi fracture — Case report. Journal of Bone and Joint Surgery 63A: 258–261
Alpert B S, Buncke H J 1978 Mutilating multidigital injuries: Use of a free microvascular flap from a nonreplantable part. Journal of Hand Surgery 3: 196–198
Alpert B S, Buncke H J, Brownstein M 1978 Replacement of damaged arteries and veins with vein grafts when replanting crushed, amputated fingers. Plastic and Reconstructive Surgery 61: 17–22
Argamaso R V 1974 Rotation-transposition method for soft tissue replacement on the distal segment of the thumb. Plastic and Reconstructive Surgery 54: 366–368
Atasoy E 1980 The cross thumb to index finger pedicle. Journal of Hand Surgery 5: 572–574
Barton N 1977 Fractures of the phalanges of the hand. The Hand 9: 1–10
Barton N J 1979 Fractures of the shafts of the phalanges of the hand. The Hand 11: 119–133
Baruch A 1977 False aneurysm of the digital artery. The Hand 9: 195–197
Beasley R W 1967 Principles and techniques of resurfacing operations for hand surgery. Surgical Clinics of North America 47: 389–413
Biemer E 1980 Definitions and classifications in replantation surgery. British Journal of Plastic Surgery 33: 164–168
Bilos Z J, Hui P W T, Stamelso S 1977 Trigger finger following partial flexor tendon laceration. The Hand 9: 232–233
Burke F, Bondoc C C, Quinby W C, Remensnyder J 1976 Primary surgical management of the deeply burned hand. Journal of Trauma 16: 593–598
Burkhalter W E, Butler B, Metz W, Omer G 1968 Experiences with delayed primary closure of war wounds of the hand in Vietnam. Journal of Bone and Joint Surgery 50A: 945–954
Burkhardt B R 1972 Immediate or early excision and skin grafting of full thickness burns of the palm. Plastic and Reconstructive Surgery 49: 572–575
Caffee H H 1979 Anomalous thenar muscle and median nerve: A case report. Journal of Hand Surgery 4: 446–447
Cameron H U, Hastings D E, Fournasier V L 1975 Fracture of the hook of the hamate. Journal of Bone and Joint Surgery 57A: 276–277
Carter P R, Eaton R G, Littler J W 1977 Ununited fracture of the hook of the hamate. Journal of Bone and Joint Surgery 59A: 583–588

Chiu D T W 1981 Supernumerary extensor tendon to the thumb: A report on a rare anatomic variation. Plastic and Reconstructive Surgery 68: 937–939
Christensen S 1977 Anomalous muscle belly of the flexor digitorum superficialis in two generations. The Hand 9: 162–164
Cleveland J C, Ellis J, Dague J 1979 Complete disruption of axillary artery caused by severe atherosclerosis and trivial nonpenetrating trauma. Journal of Trauma 19: 635–636
Converse J M 1981 Alexis Carrel: The man, the unknown. Plastic and Reconstructive Surgery 68: 629–639
Conner A N 1971 Prolonged external pressure as a cause of ischaemic contracture. Journal of Bone and Joint Surgery 53B: 118–122
Crandall R C, Hamel A L 1979 Bipartite median nerve at the wrist. Report of a case. Journal of Bone and Joint Surgery 61A: 311–312
Culver J E 1980 Extensor pollicis and indicis communis tendon: A rare anatomic variation revisited. Journal of Hand Surgery 5: 548–549
Curtis R M 1957 Cross finger flaps in hand surgery. Annals of Surgery 145: 650–655
Dameron T B Jr 1975 Fractures and anatomical variations of the proximal portion of the fifth metacarpal. The Journal of Bone and Joint Surgery 57A: 788–792
DeLee J 1979 Avulsion fracture of the base of the second metacarpal by the extensor carpi radialis longus. A case report. Journal of Bone and Joint Surgery 61A: 445–446
Dell P C, Seaber A V, Urbaniak J R 1980 The effect of systemic acidosis on perfusion of replanted extremities. The Journal of Hand Surgery 5: 433–442
Demling R H, Buerstatte W R, Frentz G 1980 Management of hot tar burns. Journal of Trauma 20: 242
Denman E E 1977 An unusual branch of the ulnar nerve in the hand. The Hand 9: 92–93
Denman E E 1979 The volar carpal ligament. The Hand 11: 22–28
Diaz J E, Jones R S, Ciceric W F 1975 Perforation of the deep palmar arch produced by surgical wire after tenorrhaphy. A case report and review of the literature. The Journal of Bone and Joint Surgery 57A: 1150–1152
Dolich B, Olshansky K, Babar A 1978 Use of a cross-forearm neurocutaneous flap to provide sensation and coverage in hand reconstruction. Plastic and Reconstructive Surgery 62: 550–558
Edstrom L E, Robson M C, Macchiaverna J, Scala A 1979 Prospective randomized treatments for burned hands: Nonoperative vs. operative. Scandinavian Journal of Reconstruction Surgery 13: 131–135
Engber W, Clancy W 1978 Traumatic avulsion of the fingernail associated with injury to the phalangeal epiphyseal plate. Journal of Bone and Joint Surgery 60A: 713–714
Enna C D 1979 Isolated pathological fracture of the capitate bone. A case report. The Hand 11: 329–331
Fitzgerald M J T, Martin F, Paletta F X 1967 Innervation of skin grafts. Surgery, Gynecology, and Obstetrics 124: 808–812
Flatt A E, Wood R W 1970 Multiple dorsal rotation flaps from the hand for thumb web contractures. Plastic and Reconstructive Surgery 45: 258–262
Foucher G, Braun J B 1979 A new island flap transfer from the dorsum of the index to the thumb. Plastic and Reconstructive Surgery 63: 344–350
Fyfe I S, Mason S 1979 The mechanical stability of internal fixation of fractured phalanges. The Hand 11: 50–54
Gelberman R H, Blasingame J P, Fronck A, Dimick M P 1979 Forearm arterial injuries. The Journal of Hand Surgery 4: 401–408

Gibbs A N, Green A, Taylor J G 1979 Chip fractures of the Os triquetrum. Journal of Bone and Joint Surgery 61B: 355–357

Graham J M, Feliciano D V, Mattox K L 1980 Combined brachial, axillary, and subclavian artery injuries of the same extremity. Journal of Trauma 20: 899–901

Green D P 1973 True and false aneurysms in the hand. Report of two cases and review of the literature. Journal of Bone and Joint Surgery 55A: 120–128

Green D P, Anderson J R 1973 Closed reduction and percutaneous pin fixation of fractured phalanges. Journal of Bone and Joint Surgery 55A: 1651–1654

Halpern A A, Michizuki R, Long C E 1978 Compartment syndrome of the forearm following radial-artery puncture in a patient treated with anticoagulants. Journal of Bone and Joint Surgery 60A: 1136–1138

Harrison S H 1955 Unilateral digital-artery thrombosis: An industrial accident. The Lancet 486–487

Harvey F J, Bye W D 1976 Bennett's fracture. The Hand 8: 48–53

Henning K, Franke D 1980 Posterior displacement of brachial artery following closed elbow dislocation. Journal of Trauma 20: 96–98

Hentz V R, Pearl R M, Kaplan E N 1980 Use of the medial upper arm skin as an arterialised flap. The Hand 12: 241–247

Howard F M 1961 Ulnar nerve palsy in wrist fractures. Journal of Bone and Joint Surgery 43A: 197–201

Huffaker W H, Wray R C, Weeks P M 1979 Factors influencing final range of motion in the fingers after fractures of the hand. Plastic and Reconstructive Surgery 63: 82–88

Hunt J, Lewis S, Parkey R, Baxter C 1979 The use of technetium[99m] stannous pyrophosphate scintigraphy to identify muscle damage in acute electrical burns. Journal of Trauma 19: 409–413

Hurwitz P J 1980 The many-tailed flap for multiple finger injuries. British Journal of Plastic Surgery 33: 230–232

Iselin F 1973 The flag flap. Plastic and Reconstructive Surgery 52: 374–377

Jabaley M E, Wallace W H, Heckler F R 1980 Internal topography of major nerves of the forearm and hand: A current view. Journal of Hand Surgery 5: 1–18

Johnson R K, Iverson R E 1971 Cross-finger pedicle flaps in the hand. Journal of Bone and Joint Surgery 53A: 913–919

Joshi B B 1977 Neural repair for sensory restoration in a groin flap. The Hand 9: 221–225

Kaplan E B 1959 Anatomy, injuries and treatment of the extensor apparatus of the hand and digits. Clinical Orthopaedics 13: 24–41

Kaplan E N, Pearl R M 1980 An arterial medial arm flap — Vascular anatomy and clinical applications. Annals of Plastic Surgery 4: 205–213

Kiil J 1980 The need for replantation centers in view of the incidence of traumatic amputations. Scandinavian Journal of Plastic Surgery 14: 163–164

Kislov R, Kelly A P 1960 Cross-finger flaps in digital injuries, with notes on Kirschner wire fixation. Plastic and Reconstructive Surgery 25: 312–322

Kleinert H E, Kasdan M L 1963 Restoration of blood flow in upper extremity injuries. Journal of Trauma 3: 461–476

Kleinert H E, Kasdan M L, Romero J L 1963 Small blood-vessel anastomosis for salvage of severely injured upper extremity. Journal of Bone and Joint Surgery 45A: 788–796

Kleinert H E, Tsai T 1978 Microvascular repair in replantation. Clinical Orthopaedics and Related Research 133: 205–211

Kleinman W B, Dustman J A 1981 Preservation of function following complete degloving injuries to the hand: Use of simultaneous groin flap, random abdominal flap, and partial-thickness skin graft. Journal of Hand Surgery 6: 82–89

Komatsu S, Tamai S 1968 Successful replantation of a completely cut-off thumb. Plastic and Reconstructive Surgery 42: 374–377

Labandter H, Kaplan I, Shavitt C 1976 Burns of the dorsum of the hand: Conservative treatment with intensive physiotherapy versus tangential excision and grafting. British Journal of Plastic Surgery 29: 352–354

Lai M F, Krishna B V, Pelly A D 1981 The brachioradialis myocutaneous flap. British Journal of Plastic Surgery 34: 431–434

Lamberty B G H 1979 The supra-clavicular axial patterned flap. British Journal of Plastic Surgery 32: 207–212

Larson D L, Evans E B, Abston S, Lewis S R 1968 Skeletal suspension and traction in the treatment of burns. Annals of Surgery 168: 981–985

Lazar G, Schulter-Ellis F P 1980 Intramedullary structure of human metacarpals. Journal of Hand Surgery 5: 477–481

Leonard L G 1980 Adjunctive use of intravenous fluorescein in the tangential excision of burns of the hand. Plastic and Reconstructive Surgery 66: 30–33

Lichtman D M, Schneider J R, Swafford A R, Mack G 1981 Ulnar midcarpal instability — Clinical and laboratory analysis. Journal of Hand Surgery 6: 515–523

Linburg R M, Comstock B E 1979 Anomalous tendon slips from the flexor pollicis longus to the flexor digitorum profundus. The Journal of Hand Surgery 4: 79–84

Little J M, Zylstra J W, May J 1973 Circulatory patterns in the normal hand. British Journal of Surgery 60: 652–655

Lobay G W, Moysa G L 1981 Primary neurovascular bundle transfer in the management of avulsed thumbs. Journal of Hand Surgery 6: 31–34

Lokey H, Phelps D B, Boswick J A 1978 Traumatic false aneurysm of the hand in hemophilia. Journal of Trauma 18: 283–284

Lowrey, Chadwick R O, Waltman E N 1976 Digital vessel trauma from repetitive impact in baseball catchers. The Journal of Hand Surgery 1: 236–238

Lund F 1976 Fluorescein angiography especially of the upper extremity. Acta Clinical Scan Supplement 465: 60–70

Mack G R, Neviaser R J, Wilson J N 1981 Free palmar skin grafts for resurfacing digital defects. Journal of Hand Surgery 6: 565–567

MacLeod A M, O'Brien B M, Morrison W A 1978 Digital replantation. Clinical Orthopaedics and Related Research 133: 26–34

Malt R A, McKhann C F 1964 Replantation of severed arms. Journal of the American Medical Association 189: 716–722

Malt R A, Remensnyder J P, Harris W H 1972 Long-term utility of replanted arms. Annals of Surgery 176: 334–341

Mandal A C 1965 Thiersch grafts for lesions of the fingertip. Acta Chirurgica Scandinavica 129: 325–332

Maquiera N O 1974 An innervated full thickness skin graft to restore sensibility to fingertips and heels. Plastic and Reconstructive Surgery 53: 568–575

Martelo-Villar F J 1980 Bilateral anomalous flexor sublimis muscle to the index finger. British Journal of Plastic Surgery 33: 80–82

Mathison G W, MacDonald R I 1975 Irreducible transcapitate fracture and dislocation of the hamate. The Journal of Bone and Joint Surgery 57A: 1166–1167

McCarthy R E, Nalebuff E A 1980 Anomalous volar branch of the dorsal cutaneous ulnar nerve: A case report. The Journal of Hand Surgery 5: 19–20

McCraw J, Myers B, Shanklin K D 1977 The value of fluorescein in predicting the viability of arterialized flaps. Plastic and Reconstructive Surgery 60: 710–719

McCue F C, Honner R, Gieck J H, Andrews J, Hakala M 1975 A pseudo-boutonniere deformity. The Hand 7: 166–170

McFarlane R M, Hampole M K 1973 Treatment of extensor tendon injuries of the hand. Canadian Journal of Surgery 16: 366–375

McGrath M H, Adelberg D, Finseth F 1979 The intravenous fluorescein test: Use in timing of groin flap division. The Journal of Hand Surgery 4: 19–23

McGregor I M 1979 Flap reconstruction in hand surgery: The evolution of presently used methods. Journal of Hand Surgery 4: 1–11

McMurtry R, Youm Y, Flatt A, Gillespie T 1978 Kinematics of the wrist. II. Clinical applications. Journal of Bone and Joint Surgery 60A: 955–961

Meuli H, Meyer V, Segmuller G 1978 Stabilization of bone in replantation surgery of the upper limb. Clinical Orthopaedics and Related Research 133: 179–183

Meyers M H, Wells R, Harvey J P 1971 Naviculo-capitate fracture syndrome. Journal of Bone and Joint Surgery 53A: 1383–1386

Miller B J, Pers M, Schmidt A 1961 Fingertip injuries: Late results. Acta Chirurgia Scandinavica 122: 177–183

Milling M A P, Kinmonth M H 1977 False aneurysm of the ulnar artery. The Hand 9: 57–59

Milward T M, Stott W G, Kleinert H E 1977 The abductor digiti minimi muscle flap. The Hand 9: 82–85

Moberg E 1976 Reconstructive hand surgery in tetraplegia, stroke, and cerebral palsy: Some basic concepts in physiology and neurology 1: 29–34

Monawan P R W, Galaski C S B 1972 The scapho-capitate fracture syndrome. Journal of Bone and Joint Surgery 54B: 122–124

Moneim M S 1982 Unusually high division of the median nerve. Journal of Hand Surgery 7: 13–14

Morris A H 1974 Irreducible Monteggia lesion with radial nerve entrapment. Journal of Bone and Joint Surgery 56A: 1744–1746

Mosher J F 1977 Split thickness hypothenar grafts for skin defects of the hand. The Hand 9: 45–48

Murakami Y 1977 Dislocation of the carpal scaphoid. The Hand 9: 79–81

Murakami Y, Todani K 1981 Traumatic entrapment of the extensor pollicis longus tendon in Smith's fracture of the radius — Case report. Journal of Hand Surgery 6: 238–240

Murray J F, Ord J V R, Gavelin G E 1967 The neurovascular island pedicle flap. Journal of Bone and Joint Surgery 49A: 1285–1297

Noble J, Lamb D W 1979 Translunate scapho-radial fracture — A case report. The Hand 11: 47–49

O'Brien B McC 1976 Replantation and reconstructive microvascular surgery. Part I. Annals of the Royal College of Surgeons of England 58: 87–103

O'Brien B McC 1976 Replantation and reconstructive microvascular surgery. Part II. Annals of the Royal College of Surgeons of England 58: 171–182

O'Brien B M, Franklin J D, Morrison W A, MacLeod A M 1980 Replantation and revascularisation surgery in children. The Hand 12: 12–24

Nieminen S, Murmi M, Isberg U 1981 Hand injuries in Finland. Scand. Journal of Reconstructive Surgery 15: 57–60

Ogden J A 1972 An unusual branch of the median nerve. The Journal of Bone and Joint Surgery 54A: 1779–1782

Page R E 1975 Hand injuries at work. The Hand 7: 51–55

Pakiam I 1978 The finger as a donor site for skin grafts. British Journal of Plastic Surgery 31: 32–33

Park C N, Spinner M 1976 Irreducible fractures of the distal phalanx of the hand. Bulletin of the Hospital for Joint Diseases 37: 24–29

Parkes A 1975 Examination of the hand. The Hand 7: 104–106

Parks B, Arbelaez J, Horner R (1978) Medical and surgical importance of the arterial blood supply of the thumb. Journal of Hand Surgery 3: 383–385

Patxakis M J, Dorr L D, Ivler D, Moore T M, Harvey P 1975 The early management of open joint injuries. A prospective study of one hundred and forty patients. The Journal of Bone and Joint Surgery 57A: 1065–1071

Peacock E E 1960 Reconstruction of the hand by the local transfer of composite tissue island flaps. Plastic and Reconstructive Surgery 25: 298–311

Pho R, Chacha P, Yeo K 1979 Rerouting vessels and nerves from other digits in replanting an avulsed and degloved thumb. Plastic and Reconstructive Surgery 64: 330–335

Rayan G M, Elias L S 1981 Irreducible dislocation of the distal interphalangeal joint caused by long flexor tendon entrapment. Orthopedics 4: 35–37

Razek M S A, Mnaymneh W, Yacoubian H D 1973 Acute injuries of peripheral arteries with associated bone and soft tissue injuries. Journal of Trauma 13: 907–910

Reid D A C 1966 The neurovascular island flap for thumb reconstruction. British Journal of Plastic Surgery 19: 234–244

Richardson J D, Fallat M, Nagaraj H S, Groff D B, Flint L M 1981 Arterial injuries in children. Archives of Surgery 116: 685–690

Robb J E 1979 The termination of flexor tendon sheaths. The Hand 11: 17–22

Ruggeri S, Osternam A L, Bora F W 1980 Stabilization of metacarpal and phalangeal fractures in the hand. Orthopaedic Review 9: 107–110

Sachatello C, Ernst C, Griffen W 1974 The acutely ischemic upper extremity: Selective management. Surgery 76: 1002–1009

Salisbury R E, Loveless S, Silverstein P, Wilmore D W, Moylan A Jr, Pruitt B A 1973 Postburn edema of the upper extremity: Evaluation of present treatment. Journal of Trauma 13: 857–862

Schenck R R 1964 Variations of the extensor tendons of the fingers. The Journal of Bone and Joint Surgery 46A: 103–110

Schlenker J D, Kleinert H E, Tsai T 1980 Methods and results of replantation following traumatic amputation of the thumb in sixty-four patients. Journal of Hand Surgery 5: 63–70

Schultz R J, Furlong J, Storace A 1981 Detailed anatomy of the extensor mechanism at the proximal aspect of the finger. Journal of Hand Surgery 6: 493–498

Segmuller G 1978 Diaphyseal, metaphyseal, and epiphyseal fractures of the skeleton of the hand in childhood. Handchirurgie 10: 167–177

Shafiroff B B, Palmer A K 1981 Simplified technique for replantation of the thumb. Journal of Hand Surgery 6: 623–624

Shrewsbury M M, Johnson R K, Ousterhout D K 1972 The palmaris brevis — a reconsideration of its anatomy and possible function. Journal of Bone and Joint Surgery 54A: 344–348

Simodynes E E, Cochran R M 1981 Anomalous muscles in the hand and wrist — Report of three cases. Journal of Hand Surgery 6: 553–554

Smith A R, van Der Meulen J C, Kort W 1981 Oxygen levels in claudicating fingers: a 3 year follow-up after replantation. British Journal of Plastic Surgery 34: 342–344

Solem L, Fischer R P, Strate R G 1977 The natural history of electrical injury. Journal of Trauma 17: 487–492

Stark H H, Jobe F W, Boyes J H, Ashworth C R 1977 Fracture of the hook of the hamate in athletes. Journal of Bone and Joint Surgery 59A: 575–582

Stark H H, Otter T A, Boyes J H, Rickard T A 1979 Atavistic contrahentes digitorum and associated muscle abnormalities of the hand: A cause of symptoms. Report of three cases. Journal of Bone and Joint Surgery 61A: 286–290

Stripling W D 1982 Displaced intra-articular osteochondral fracture — Cause for irreducible dislocation of the distal interphalangeal joint 7: 77–78

Sturm J T, Bodily K C, Rothenberger D A, Perry J F 1980 Arterial injuries of the extremities following blunt trauma. The Journal of Trauma 20: 933–936

Suzki K, Takahashi S, Nakagawa T 1980 False aneurysm in a digital artery. Journal of Hand Surgery 5: 402–403

Tachakra S S, Smith J E M 1981 Severed limbs: the reattachment of major segments 26: 157–169

Taleisnik J 1976 The ligaments of the wrist. The Journal of Hand Surgery 1: 110–118

Tajima T 1974 Treatment of open crushing type of industrial injuries of the hand and forearm: Degloving, open circumferential, heat-press and nail-bed injuries. Journal of Trauma 14: 995–1011

Tempest M N 1952 Cross-finger flaps in the treatment of injuries to the fingertip. Plastic and Reconstructive Surgery 9: 205–222

Thompson R V S 1977 Closure of skin defects near the proximal interphalangeal joint — with special reference to the patterns of finger circulation. Plastic and Reconstructive Surgery 59: 77–81

Tubiana R 1968 Surgical repair of the extensor apparatus of the fingers. Surgical Clinics of North America 48: 1015–1031

Vance R M, Gelberman R H, Evans E F 1980 Scaphocapitate fractures. Patterns of dislocation, mechanisms of injury, and preliminary results of treatment. Journal of Bone and Joint Surgery 62A: 271–276

Verdan C E 1972 Half a century of flexor tendon surgery. Current status and changing philosophies. Journal of Bone and Joint Surgery 54A: 472–491

Vichare N A 1970 Anomalous muscle belly of the flexor digitorum superficialis. Journal of Bone and Joint Surgery 52B: 757–759

Vilain R 1973 Use of the flag flap for coverage of a small area on a finger or the palm. Plastic and Reconstructive Surgery 51: 397–401

Weber E R, Chao E Y 1978 An experimental approach to the mechanism of scaphoid waist fractures. Journal of Hand Surgery 3: 142–148

Weiland A, Villarreal-Rios A, Kleinert H, Kutz J, Atasoy E, Lister G 1978 Replantation of digits and hands: Analysis of surgical techniques and functional results in 71 patients with 86 replantations. Clinical Orthopaedics and Related Research 133: 195–204

Wenger D R, Boyer D W, Sandzen S C 1980 Traumatic aneurysm of the radial artery in the anatomical snuff box — A report of two cases. The Hand 12: 266–270

White J C 1969 Nerve regeneration after replantation of severed arms. Annals of Surgery 170: 715–719

Winkelman N Z 1980 Aberrant sensory branch of the median nerve to the third web space — Case report. The Journal of Hand Surgery 5: 566–567

Winspur I 1981 Single-stage reconstruction of the subtotally amputated thumb: A synchronous neurovascular flap and Z-plasty. Journal of Hand Surgery 6: 70–72

Wood R W 1968 Multiple cross finger flaps — 'Piggy-back' technique. Plastic and Reconstructive Surgery 41: 54–57

Wood V E, Frykman G K 1978 Unusual branching of the median nerve at the wrist. Journal of Bone and Joint Surgery 60A: 267–268

Worthen E F 1973 The palmar split skin graft. British Journal of Plastic Surgery 26: 408–411

Yoshizu T, Katsumi M, Tajima T 1978 Replantation of untidily amputated finger, hand, and arm: Experience of 99 replantations in 66 cases. Journal of Trauma 18: 194–200

Younger C P, DeFiore J C 1977 Rupture of flexor tendons to the fingers after a Colles fracture. Case report. Journal of Bone and Joint Surgery 59A: 828–829

Zook E G, VanBeek A L, Russell R C, Beatty M E 1980 Anatomy and physiology of the perionychium: A review of the literature and anatomic study. Journal of Hand Surgery 5: 528–536

Zweig J, Posch J, Larsen R 1969 Thrombosis of the ulnar artery following blunt trauma to the hand. Journal of Bone and Joint Surgery 51A: 1191–1197

2

Reconstruction

Before considering reconstruction of the previously injured hand the surgeon must not only possess a thorough knowledge of the deficiencies in structure and function in the affected limb. He must also understand the demands that the patient places on that limb both in his occupation and in his recreation. Knowing that nothing he does will prove successful without the active participation of the patient after surgery, he must in addition assess the patient's attitude and motivation.

Time may be on the patient's side, or against him. While nerve function is slow to return and time should be allowed for it to do so, joint contracture for whatever reason will become fixed and the joint itself increasingly damaged if intervention is unduly delayed. To choose the stage at which to operate is therefore a subtle art. One rule which proves helpful is never to operate while the patient shows steady improvement. This can be called 'plateau surgery' since it is undertaken when the patient ceases to progress in the climb to recovery. This necessitates regular repeated examination. Such repeated assessment is the key to management of patients likely to require reconstructive surgery of the hand. It not only permits close observation of slowly recovering function, but also gives the opportunity to adjust or change splints or physical therapy, to get to know the patient and his problems and to encourage him to take a positive, aggressive attitude, which will prove invaluable when operation is thought appropriate.

HISTORY

Original injury

Nature of injury — injuring agent, especially the presence of crush, heat or electrical damage.

Closed injuries in particular present problems. It is important to obtain details of the occurrence in order to clarify the mechanism, which may help in deducing the anatomical location and pathology. Whether or not the patient was able to continue work is some guide to the severity of the injury.

Date and time of injury. The circumstances under which an accident occurred may be of relevance. Whether or not it

happened at work is of great moment in some societies. The work, or compensation, injury offers the patient a cushion, in that he receives disability payment while off work, his medical bills are settled and he may receive lump-sum compensation for any permanent partial disability. This cushion is good in that it reduces the financial concerns of the injured. It may also have bad effects, leading to erroneous statements regarding the original circumstances, lack of effort in rehabilitation, reluctance to return to work and exaggeration of residual complaints.

Primary treatment. Details of primary treatment are often best obtained from the primary treating physician. In this time of litigation, questions regarding the original care may easily be misinterpreted as criticism. One must even be careful of emphasis and inflection in asking the simple question, 'Who was your original doctor?' The way in which the answer is phrased can also be enlightening with regard to the patient's attitude, which may strongly influence the outcome of the later treatment.

Subsequent progress and therapy.

Previous injury to the part. Previous injuries may materially influence both the presenting injury and the required treatment. This often requires prompting from the examiner which may reveal forgotten childhood falls, automobile wrecks and several sports injuries! The surgeon is then left at first medically, and later legally, to untangle the knot.

Occupation

The mental and economic well-being of the patient depends largely on his ability to return to his original employment. Ideally the surgeon would observe the man at work but this is not practicable. The patient can observe himself, however, and demonstrate subsequently what manoeuvres he is unable to perform. This often requires the patient to return to his place of work for trial employment. Many patients and even more employers are reluctant to participate in such a trial and this is frequently made more difficult by the attitude of insurance companies or government departments. Wherever possible, it should be arranged, especially where doubt exists as to whether or not further treatment is required. If after return to work the patient volunteers that he is fully capable of carrying out his original employment, then no matter how much loss of function in individual structures the surgeon may elicit on subsequent examination, he must be very guarded in suggesting any further surgical treatment.

Where he cannot do his job, the patient's explanation and demonstration of his difficulty should be carefully observed and analysed. That difficulty may be compounded from several elements — pain, loss of power or of the ability to adopt certain postures, diminished sensation or, more rarely, the intrusion of unused parts.

PAIN

The nature and location of pain and of factors which initiate it should be determined.

Where is your pain?

Does it radiate elsewhere?

The patient should be encouraged to indicate the site and radiation with one finger. This should later be correlated with tenderness on palpation or pain on manipulation. As a general rule, the more diffuse the pain, the greater is the problem diagnostically for the surgeon and the longer and more taxing will be his relationship with the patient.

How bad is it?

It is impossible to quantify pain. Some estimate can be obtained by asking them to indicate a number on a scale from 0 to 10, where 0 represents no pain and 10 constant, unremitting pain preventing sleep despite narcotics and making the patient feel suicidal.

Is it there all the time?

Does it keep you awake at night?

Constant pain which keeps the patient awake at night is more commonly of a neurological origin, with or without some psychological overlay, than of a musculo-skeletal.

What makes it worse?

What makes it better?

Rest helps most musculo-skeletal pain, activity makes it worse. This question may well elicit the demonstration by the patient of particular movements or postures which elicit pain. Once again, these should be noted and correlated with later examination.

Pain secondary to injury is usually one of three types:

1. Musculo-skeletal — this is due to distortion and stretch of injured or inadequate structures and is usually associated with activity.
2. Neuro-cutaneous — this is due to contact with neuromata, either at the macroscopic level of a neuroma (p. 00) or at the nerve endings in hypersensitive or unsuitable skin (p. 00). This is usually associated with contact.
3. Post-traumatic sympathetic dystrophy (= reflex dystrophy)[1-3]
   This symptom complex may arise after injury or surgery.

It can be recognised at three stages:

1. Immediate: inappropriate pain after injury or surgery should alert the physician to the potential for dystrophy. All circumferential dressings should be widely and correctly split. Intensive physical therapy should be instituted. There appears to be a direct correlation between the practice of splitting dressings before administering *any* prescription pain medication and a very low incidence of dystrophy.
2. Early dystrophy: the patient avoids all contact with the hand, which shows all the signs of sympathetic overactivity — it is cold, swollen, stiff, sweating and shows increased hair growth and reddish-blue discoloration. Management requires physical therapy with the addition of sensory re-education and transcutaneous nerve stimulation where helpful. It is at this stage that stellate ganglion blocks and even sympathectomy are indicated.
3. Late dystrophy (*Sudeck's atrophy*)[4]: less swollen and discoloured, the hand is now stiff, painful and atrophic. X-ray taken on the same film as the normal hand shows significant loss of bone substance. This stage is often accompanied by severe limitation of shoulder motion — the *shoulder-hand syndrome*. Most often seen after manipulation and unrelenting cast immobilisation of a Colles[5] fracture, this condition is treated by a combination of honesty, cheerfulness, physical therapy and other supportive measures.

LOSS OF POSITION AND POWER

Eight basic positions of the hand make up most manoeuvres and the ability of the hand to adopt these positions and to exert force while in them should be determined.

1. *Precision pinch.* The tips of finger nails of the index finger and thumb are brought together as in lifting a pin from a flat surface (Fig. 2.1).
2. *Pulp pinch.* The pulps of index and thumb are opposed with the distal interphalangeal joints extended as in gripping a sheet of paper (Fig. 2.2). The resistance to the thumb flexor can be increased by placing the middle finger on top of the index. The power exerted can be measured with a pinch dynamometer. Normal 5–10 pounds.
3. *Key pinch.* The pulp of the thumb is opposed to the radial side of the middle phalanx of the index finger, as in turning a key. The resistance exerted against the thumb is increased by 'stacking up' the other fingers behind the index using the interossei. The power can be measured again with a pinch dynamometer. Normal 13–20 pounds (Fig. 2.3).
4. *Chuck grip.* The digital pulps of index and middle fingers are brought into contact with the pulp of the thumb as in exerting longitudinal traction on a pencil.

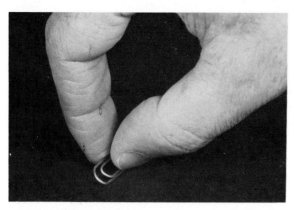

Fig. 2.1 Precision pinch.

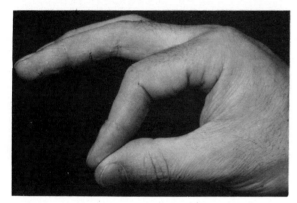

Fig. 2.2 Pulp pinch.

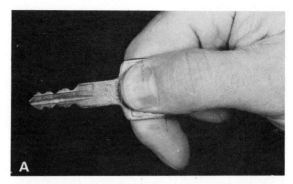

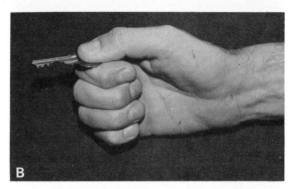

Fig. 2.3 (A) Key pinch. (B) The power exerted in key pinch can be increased by strong flexion of the thumb. The resistance offered by the index finger is supplemented by the 'stacking up' of the other fingers behind it.

The index finger pronates and the middle finger supinates so that the three digits come to resemble the chuck of a power drill (Fig. 2.4).

5. *Hook grip.* The fingers are all flexed at the interphalangeal joints and extended at the metacarpophalangeal joints as in carrying a suitcase (Fig. 2.5).

6. *Span grasp.* From the hook grip the interphalangeal joints are extended to approximately 30° and the thumb is abducted fully as in lifting a large glass or bottle (Fig. 2.6). Span is measured as the maximum distance attainable actively between the distal digital creases of thumb and index finger and of thumb and small finger. Alternatively, it can be assessed by the ability to lift cylinders of differing circumference.

7. *Power grasp.* The fingers are flexed fully and the opposed thumb is flexed over the fingers to increase the power as in using a hammer (Fig. 2.7). The force generated can be measured with a grip dynamometer[6] (normal 90–100 pounds). The grip is compared with that in the other hand. The normal variation between hands is some 10% but, rather surprisingly, the

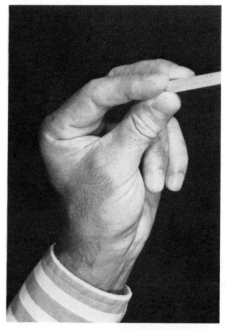

Fig. 2.4 Chuck grip, in which the thumb, index finger and middle finger come together round a narrow cylindrical object as does the chuck of a drill.

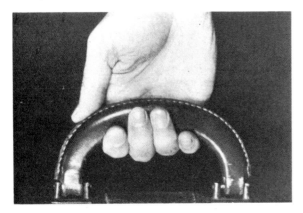

Fig. 2.5 Hook grip.

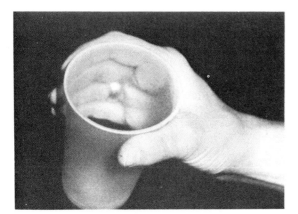

Fig. 2.6 Span grasp.

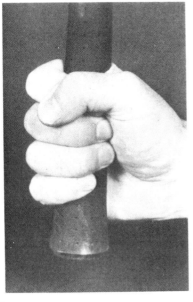

Fig. 2.7 Power grasp.

dominant is not always the stronger. When a grip dynamometer is not available a useful substitute is a pneumatic tourniquet cuff rolled up and bound with tape and inflated to 30 mm of mercury. The average male can grasp this with sufficient force to push the mercury off the usual scale, that is, 300 mm of mercury. Here comparison with the normal hand is even more important.

8. *Flat hand.* All fingers and the thumb are extended at all joints and the thumb is adducted to lie in the same plane as the hand, as in pushing against a flat surface, or inserting the hand between closely approximated surfaces (Fig. 2.8).

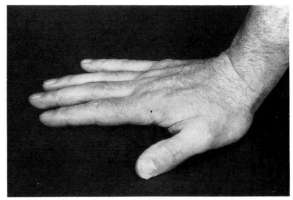

Fig. 2.8 The flat hand as used in pushing against a flat surface. It should be noted that in this posture the wrist requires to be in marked dorsal flexion.

It will be appreciated that the radial side of the hand plays the major role in fine movements and this is one reason why loss of median nerve sensation is much more significant than that of the ulnar nerve distribution. The ulnar side of the hand is more significant in powerful manipulations. The thumb is of prime importance in all except the hook grip and the flat hand and even the flat hand posture can be impeded by an immobile thumb fixed in palmar abduction.

The posture and movement of the wrist and forearm are very significant in most of these positions. Full dorsiflexion of the wrist is essential in pushing with either the flat hand or in applying full power grasp. Wrist flexion with power grasp is necessary in a pronated position in many reaching and lifting manoeuvres. Pronation and supination of the forearm are required in all powerful turning activities performed by the hand. Torque is applied to smaller objects by rolling movements of the digits engaged in a chuck grip — impossible without ulnar innervated intrinsics, difficult without median sensation.

Often a patient may lack several of the postures of the hand, but commonly one is of paramount significance in preventing him from resuming employment. This must be identified and then analysed during examination into specific structural and dynamic deficiencies. Thereafter, by correcting these deficiencies, treatment can be directly aimed at achieving occupational function.

Loss of sensation

The nature and distribution of sensory loss will be elicited during subsequent examination.

Unused parts

The presence of unused parts may inhibit the patient's ability to adopt one of the eight basic positions of the hand or to exert power in that position. This should be noted, for where the part cannot be rendered useful, judicious amputation may greatly enhance function. The stiff or painful index finger can often be disregarded, for all of the above positions can be assumed simply by using the middle and ring fingers as if they were index and middle (Fig. 2.9).

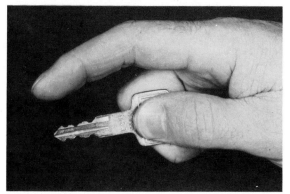

Fig. 2.9 The middle finger is substituted, often subconsciously, for the injured index.

The patient has in effect amputated his own index finger.

That a surgical program for the injured patient should be goal-oriented cannot be emphasised too strongly. To achieve this, an occupational therapist or rehabilitation counsellor should analyse both the patient and his job in terms of the functions detailed above. At his work place, the manipulations required are documented and the power in various postures are recorded. Much of this can be done swiftly and effectively by the use of a videotape which can subsequently be studied in detail by the counsellor. The limitations of the patient's hand are then charted alongside these occupational demands. By consulting this evaluation the surgeon can then focus on specific deficiencies, determine the anatomical cause and then prescribe surgery to correct it or declare that it cannot be corrected. In the latter instance, the patient learns at a much earlier stage than without analysis that he will be unable to return to his original employment. Negotiations can then proceed, contemporaneously with treatment, to rehabilitate and retrain the patient either with his original employer or with the relevant agency.

Personality, intelligence and reliability

It is not necessary to take a formal psychiatric history to gain an assessment of the patient's personality. Several simple guides can be offered in determining whether the patient is likely to respond well to further treatment, cooperate in rehabilitation and indeed whether or not he wishes to achieve full recovery.

Attendance

While most patients are genuinely unable to keep one appointment for unexpected reasons, the one whose record is repeatedly marked with failure to attend must be suspected of lacking interest.

Meeting the surgeon's gaze

A hypnotic stare lasting seconds is *not* implied, but even shy patients meet the surgeon's eye when he is explaining something or asking a question and failure to do so should raise fears of future problems. Failure of the surgeon to meet the patient's gaze is probably equally significant but is outwith the scope of this text.

Response to instructions

It is inevitable that some patients will be encountered who have insufficient intelligence to cooperate in their care. These should be recognized by their inability to perform with their normal hand simple movements carefully and repeatedly explained and demonstrated.

Honesty

Patients indicate to some degree their reliability in subsequent management by the honesty with which they answer questions. Some will, for example, claim to have used a splint continuously or left a dressing undisturbed when even cursory inspection shows this to be untrue.

Inappropriate affect

Patients who complain vehemently but with apparent relish of disability and especially pain, often ill-defined, but who show little other evidence of distress when the pain is elicited constitute a group little understood, difficult to manage and invariably unchanged by surgical intervention.

Liability

When a patient returns often to the matter of liability for his original injury, he must be suspected of wishing to extract maximum compensation. While such an attitude is understandable and often justified, it is not compatible with a single minded effort to achieve full recovery.

Malingering

A patient may malinger for financial gain, to avoid work, to inspire sympathy, possibly for other reasons. Whatever the cause, the surgeon must attempt to detect the fact for a number of reasons. Several manoeuvres are helpful.

The flat curve: Using the grip strength dynamometer, the patient's grip strength should be measured at all five settings from narrow to wide span grasp. However badly injured a hand may be the plot of the resulting strengths should always be a curve as in the normal hand (see below), skewed to right or left depending upon the injury. A flat curve, that is the same strength at every setting should raise suspicions. They can largely be confirmed by

Rapid exchange grip strength: When he has time to concentrate, the malingerer can produce less than maximal strength repeatedly. If he is encouraged to alternate rapidly from one hand to the other, strongly gripping the dynamometer, this control disappears. Normally with rapid exchange, grip strength falls slightly, but rises often dramatically in the patient who is malingering. Thus a suspicious recording might read as follows:

Hand	Dynamometer setting					Rapid exchange
	1	2	3	4	5	
Injured	20	20	20	25	20	90
Normal	85	100	110	140	120	120

Repeated 1, decreasing 2PD: If a patient claims total absence of sensation, it is relatively easy to disprove in that he shows a normal sweat or wrinkle pattern (p. 00) or occasionally he can be misled — 'Tell me each time you *do not* feel me touch you'. More subtle and difficult is the patient who attempts to deceive on testing of two point discrimination, knowing that to be some measure of sensory return. Initial testing may reveal a 2 PD of 15 mm in an area the examiner suspects to be normal. He should then apply a stream of 30 to 40 applications of 1 point alone, to the stage that the patient begins to doubt his own sensibility. This can be accompanied by occasional expressions of disbelief — 'Are you sure?' — and by the narrowing of the gap. The two points are at last applied, the patient in relief exclaims 'Two!' and the examiner has a 2 PD reading of 5 mm — and some information about the patient's veracity.

Breakaway: When testing muscle strength, if the examiner initially encounters resistance but, without his applying extra force, the offered resistance suddenly gives way and cannot be reproduced, this is evidence of an attempt to deceive.

Distracted function: The movement which the patient claims is impossible is reproduced passively by the examiner. While maintaining the position he then asks the patient to perform a new, and relatively complex, manoeuvre with his other hand. After the patient has attempted this for some moments, the examiner helps him, thereby releasing the passive hold on the limb in question. If the posture is maintained, active function exists and deception is proved.

Such deception may have complex causes, and the physician should remember that his first responsibility is to his patient, without ever being dishonest. As an example, take the high-achievement young violinist, an only child. Her expenses to audition for a prestigious school of music are being paid by a subscription raised by her township. Suddenly, without injury, she is unable to flex her small finger on her left hand. The *distracted function test* reveals her deception, but only to her physician. By informing her parents, he would disgrace and discredit her, when all she needs is some relief from the load of expectations and responsibility. Qualified reassurance is given, 'She will certainly recover, but may not be at her best for a while'. The load is removed, self-respect maintained, function returns, the audition is successful.

It may be seen from this example that the boundary between conscious malingering on the one hand and factitious injury and hysteria on the other is gray indeed.

From all or any of these criteria the surgeon must form an opinion of a patient's desire and ability to cooperate in any further surgery. While the benefits of any doubt should be given to the patient, where the surgeon has serious fears on this score, he should not undertake surgery. Much can often be gained by sharing these reservations with the patient. You may lose him, but this will only confirm your decision not to treat him.

Past medical history
Social history
Systematic enquiry
Quickly done, these questions frequently reveal fascinating and highly relevant information which the experienced examiner knows to pursue: the mastectomy five years previously in the patient with radiating pain; the 60 pack-years of smoking in the patient with a painful bony swelling; the polyuria and polydypsia in the patient whose wounds will not heal.

EXAMINATION AND INDICATIONS

Observation
Much can be learned by observing the hand at rest and in use before formal examination is begun.

Posture or balance
Any disturbance in the posture will quickly be detected. This may be due to disorders of bones, joints, tendons or nerves and will be discussed under each heading.

Protection
The posture adopted may not be due to joint or tendon problems but rather due to the desire to avoid pain. This is also a common cause of complete failure to use a hand which has sustained only a local injury. Examples of such protective postures include:

a. the flexed wrist held across the abdomen indicative of a median nerve neuroma at the wrist;

b. the finger excluded from pick-up movements due to digital nerve neuroma, a poorly healed nail bed or an adherent amputation stump;

c. the immobile hand cradled in the other arm, suggestive of early dystrophy. The hand at rest is never truly so, for the fit hand constantly moves in gesticulation, nervousness and personal mannerisms.

Cleanliness

That the hand which may be used in the consulting room is *not* used anywhere else is suggested by the extreme cleanliness of the palms, digital pulps and nails in contrast to the other hand. Cleanliness of one area of the hand may indicate lack of use. It may, however, be due to absence of sweating and because the skin ridges or 'finger-prints' are less pronounced, both a result of incomplete return of sensation.

The contrary is also true. Work staining on a hand or digit which is 'too painful to use' belies that claim.

Swelling

Oedema is always more evident on the dorsum of the hand. In the healed but little used hand it may not be striking but when that hand is compared with the dorsum of the other, swelling can be seen to have obliterated any intertendinous depression, making the extensor tendons more difficult to see. Variation in the amount of oedema can be recorded by volumetric displacement, immersing the hand to a precise landmark so that repeated tests may give comparable results. Oedema in the fingers can be most easily recorded by using a set of jeweller's sizing rings (Fig. 2.10).

Oedema from disuse arises in a somewhat passive fashion. More 'active' oedema results from infection, injury or venous or lymphatic obstruction and these are discussed elsewhere. Where the oedema is a major problem of obscure origin, the possibility of repeated infection, injury or obstruction inflicted by the patient must be considered.

Factitious lymphoedema[7]. Most factitious lymphoedema is caused by the surreptitious use of a tourniquet, the minority by repeated blows — often evidenced by recurrent bruising — or by self-injection[8] which may result in recurrent low-grade infection. The diagnosis is suggested by transverse marking at the proximal edge of the oedema (Fig. 2.11). It is often necessary to admit the patient to hospital where the diagnosis is confirmed by:

radiological exclusion of other causes; includes venography and lymphangiography
laboratory confirmation of normal chemistry
irregular nursing staff visits which may reveal the use of a tourniquet — it is usually obscured by clothing (Fig. 2.12)

bulky dressings; preventing access causes resolution.

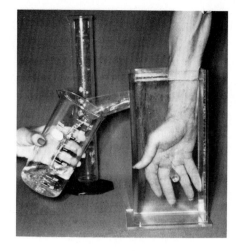

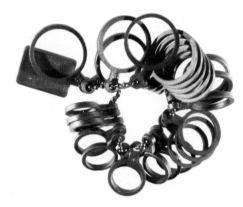

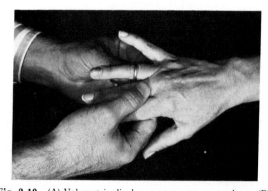

Fig. 2.10 (A) Volumetric displacement to measure oedema. (B) & (C) The progression of oedema of the fingers can be best and quickly recorded by the use of a set of jeweller's sizing rings.

Secretan's disease[9] is a hard oedema of the dorsum of the hand which results in peritendinous fibrosis. It is now believed by most[10] to be factitious in nature and surgery is no longer recommended[11].

Factitious ulceration[12] is another manifestation of self-inflicted injury (Fig. 2.13). It should be suspected if a wound fails to heal as expected, becomes virtually certain if

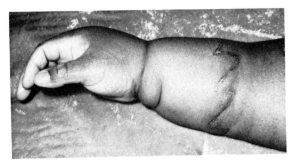

Fig. 2.11 This adult patient was referred after Z-plasty for an apparent constriction band had proved unsuccessful. The swelling in the hand in this somewhat obese patient is distal to circumferential markings which are evident just proximal to the Z-plasty — factitious lymphoedema.

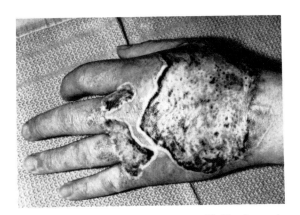

Fig. 2.12 Infrequently, a patient with a self-inflicted wound will present as an emergency. The full thickness burn shown here, the patients claimed, was caused by chemicals found in the toilet of a Greyhound bus. Histology showed it to be thermal in nature while enquiry revealed that the victim was known in psychiatric units throughout the state.

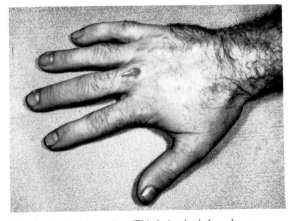

Fig. 2.13 Factitious ulcer. This lesion healed on three successive occasions when completely occluded in a cast only to recur on removal of that cast.

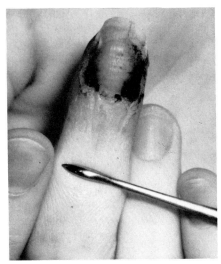

Fig. 2.14 This patient was treated for a variety of diagnoses for a painful finger. Only when fresh blood was seen around the base of the nail was the diagnosis made. On psychiatric consultation the patient admitted that her injury was self-inflicted.

evidence of interference appears such as fresh bleeding (Fig. 2.14) or excoriation, and can be confirmed by the application of tetracycline dressings beneath a removable window. Subsequent fluorescence of the opposite hand under ultra-violet light gives the confirmatory[13] evidence. Healing will result with application of an occlusive cast.

The diagnosis of factitious injury is made more difficult both by the fact that most cases commence with a definite, though minor, injury to the area and also by the friendly, relaxed, gentle, cooperative, but unconcerned, affect of the patient. This contrasts with the behaviour of patients with similar complaints

a. dystrophy — usually over-anxious
b. clenched-fist syndrome[14] — characterised by immovable digital flexion which is released by anaesthesia, these patients have poor defenses and may show great anger
c. SHAFT syndrome[15]. Sad, Hostile, Anxious, Frustrating, Tenacious.

'Malingering is feigning illness for secondary gain. Patients with factitious lymphedema are not *feigning* illness: they are *causing* illness' (Smith, 1975)[7]. All require psychotherapy.

Examination of the limb should first be directed at significant regions remote from the site of injury lest they be subsequently omitted.

Neck

The neck should be put through a full range of guided active motion — extension, flexion, lateral flexion and

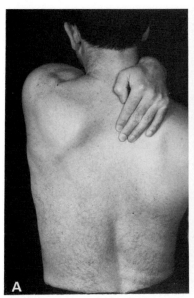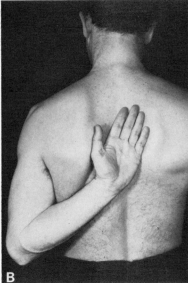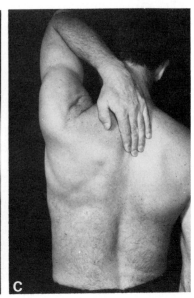

Fig. 2.15 The motion of the shoulder can be quickly checked by asking the patient to touch between the shoulder blades (A) over the contralateral shoulder which is performed by flexion and adduction, (B) under the homolateral axilla which demonstrates extension and internal rotation and (C) over the homolateral shoulder which demonstrates abduction and external rotation.

rotation. Any limitation or pain on these movements must be fully investigated for they may seriously affect function in the hand and may even be the origin of all residual symptoms. Investigations include:

> neurological examination of the trunk and lower limbs;
> X-ray of cervical spine: AP, lateral — in flexion and extension — oblique;
> myelogram where indicated.

Shoulder

The shoulder may have been injured in the same incident as was the hand, may be incapacitated by the same root injury or may be the seat of intrinsic derangement which contributes to the patient's disability. The joint should be put through a full range of guided active movement. This can quickly and reliably be effected by asking the patient to touch the interscapular region by three different routes:

1. Over the contralateral shoulder: *flexion, adduction* (Fig. 2.15A);
2. Under the ipsilateral axilla: *extension, internal rotation* (Fig. 2.15B);
3. Over the ipsilateral shoulder by carrying the arm directly out from the side: *abduction, external rotation* (Fig. 2.15C).

If difficulty is encountered in any of these actions then each component movement should be checked in turn and X-rays obtained.

More distal examination of the upper limb secondary to injury will be considered structure by structure.

Skin

Ideally the skin should provide an unbroken, mobile cover for the hand which can accommodate to any position adopted by the underlying joints, while being capable of withstanding certain forces, both direct and tangential. It must be fully sensible but not painful.

SCARS

These should be inspected for any evidence of incomplete healing, hypertrophy or contracture (Fig. 2.16). They should be palpated for adhesion to the underlying tissues, inelasticity or points of tenderness. When tenderness is located, the precise position and extent of the tenderness should be mapped out with a blunt-pointed instrument such as a probe and any area of associated numbness with a pin-wheel (p. 155). These should be marked with a skin pencil and photographed or drawn in the patient's record. In the case of burn scars, hypertrophy, inelasticity and fragility may follow on the spontaneous healing of a dermal burn.

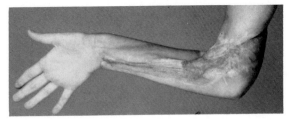

Fig. 2.16 Extensive scarring from the upper arm to the wrist has produced an immobile contracture of the elbow and less so of the wrist.

ULCERATION

Persistent or recurrent ulceration in the hand is caused by one of the following:

1. *loss of sensation* — discussed later; (p. 148).
2. *vascular insufficiency* — discussed later; (p. 179).
3. *unstable scars* — most commonly encountered following burns, they arise through repeated trauma to fragile or adherent skin or through the intermittent ischaemia produced by the raised tension created in extending or flexing a joint against a skin contracture;
4. *retained 'foreign body'* — this may be retained since the injury and may truly be a foreign body, including non-absorbable surgical material or may be necrotic tissue in the form of slough or sequestrated bone;
5. *factitious wounding* — suggested by the bizarre nature of the wound and the affect of the patients. (see p. 113)

SKIN GRAFTS

Not all grafts applied at the time of emergency surgery are employed because they provide the ideal solution. Frequently considerations of infection, coincident injuries, early mobilization or the experience of the surgeon may have dictated the use of the simplest and most sure means of achieving immediate skin cover. Grafts should be inspected as rather specialized scars, attention being paid to hypertrophy, contracture, adherence, inelasticity, fragility and ulceration, points of tenderness and differences in pigmentation. Plans to operate on structures beneath the graft (for example, the insertion of tendon grafts) should be considered, as should any likely increase in trauma to the area with return to work.

Revision, release or replacement of scars or grafts is one of the most rewarding forms of reconstruction. Particular attention should be paid to the *thumb-index web space*, where release of contracture in the adductor pollicis and first dorsal interosseous allied with introduction of better skin cover may convert a crippled to a functional hand (p. 145).

Several techniques of scar revision or replacement are available:

Full thickness grafts. These may be used after release of a scar contracture but they require a smooth, perfectly vascularized bed and therefore cannot be used where that is not available. They are therefore rarely applicable to the web spaces.

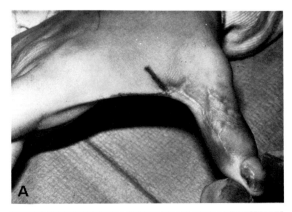
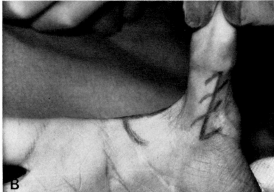
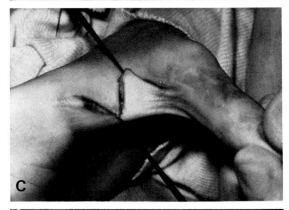
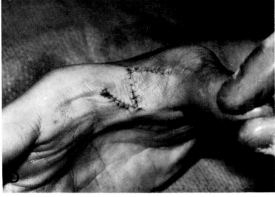

Fig. 2.17   As a result of a crush injury to the thumb, this patient had sustained a scar contracture on its ulnar aspect. This produced a limitation of span grasp by shortening of the web which was composed of good quality skin on both dorsal and palmar aspects. A Z-plasty was constructed, (A & B), and after exposure of the web space and release of some fascial contracture the flaps were transposed (C) and sutured into position, (D) providing increase in the depth of the first web space and also in the length of span grasp.

Z-plasty (Fig. 2.17). In this procedure the skin to release the contracture is gained from the transverse dimension, so the skin on either side of the scar should be inspected to see that it is of good quality and available in sufficient quantity. If it is constructed entirely within the scar the single contracture or bridle scar may become two, one to each side of the Z-plasty.

Local flaps. Transposition flaps, such as that from the dorsum of the index finger to the first web space described by Brand[16], are valuable in deepening a web space. The defect created when a flexion contracture of a digit is released can frequently be covered with a flap from the side of the same digit[17] — the flap where possible should include the dorsal digital arteries and nerves[18]. The planning and application of all such transposition flaps requires knowledge of the theory underlying their design[19].

Regional flaps, usually in the form of a cross-finger flap, provide appropriate cover when release of a contracture requires tendon and nerve surgery as well as scar excision (Fig. 2.18).

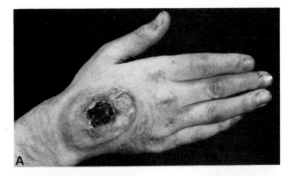

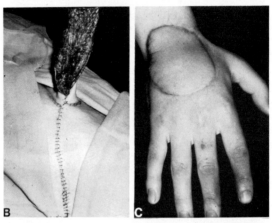

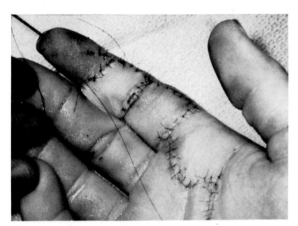

Fig. 2.18 The index finger was the seat of a severe contracture. Release required the insertion of a silastic rod and nerve graft, with excision of the scarred skin. Cover was achieved with a cross-finger flap.

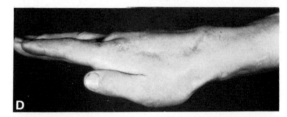

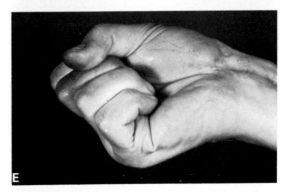

Distant flaps. These are necessary where inadequate local skin is available and full thickness grafts are not applicable or appropriate, for example prior to tendon grafting (Fig. 2.19). While on the dorsal aspect an axial groin flap can be used for scar replacement, in smaller defects or on the palm, thinner, random pattern flaps give superior results. These can come from the thorax (Fig. 2.20) or better still, from the other arm[20] (Fig. 2.21). Forearm defects require either a random pattern flap from the abdomen (Fig. 2.22) or a free flap (Fig. 2.23).

A note of caution should be sounded regarding scar or graft excision solely for treatment of points of tenderness. It is a procedure with a universally low success rate and should be so explained to the patient. Sensory re-education

Fig. 2.19 (A) This patient had sustained a full thickness fourth degree burn of the hand with destruction of the extensor tendons and contracture of the metacarpophalangeal joints in extension.

(B) A groin flap was raised and applied to the area following excision of the graft producing satisfactory cover, (C) through which extensor tendon grafting was performed after release of the metacarpophalangeal joints. The outcome was full extension, (D) and powerful flexion (E).

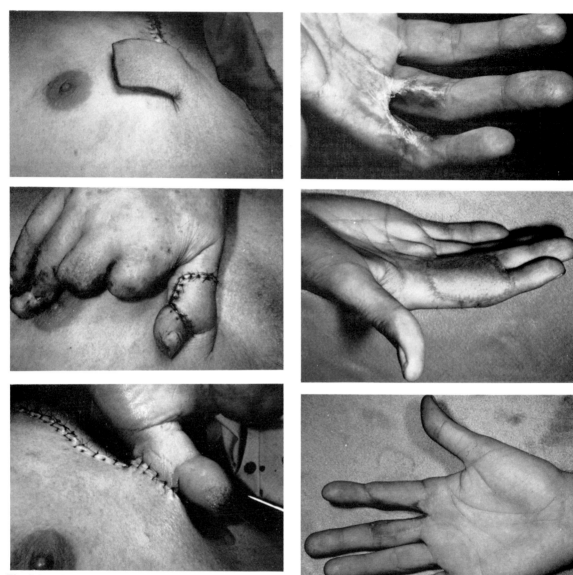

Fig. 2.20 (A) This small random infraclavicular flap provided a flap of suitable size and thickness to cover a bone graft in this mutilated hand (B). (C) The attachment is made secure by raising a small flap on the *recipient* site to suture to the free margin of the donor defect.

Fig. 2.21 (A) This small area of dense palmar scarring required excision both for comfort and also for access to the index finger for tendon and nerve grafting. This was achieved (B) with a cross arm flap which was subsequently divided (C) to provide good skin cover.

by exposure to a high frequency of different stimuli should be first employed. If surgery is later performed, such re-education should certainly be practised postoperatively at a very early stage.

FLAPS

Local flaps in the hand used at the time of injury, provided they were well-designed, are the least likely of all skin cover to require further attention. However, faults in design may result in any or even all of the problems referred to above in relation to scars in the hand.

Any secondary defects covered with skin grafts should be carefully examined for possible revision.

Distant flaps invariably present unsatisfactory features at secondary assessment:

Bulk. In the majority of distant flaps an excess of both skin and fat is introduced initially, mainly in the interest of preserving the blood supply of the flap. This bulk may limit motion purely by its presence (Fig. 2.24). Needless

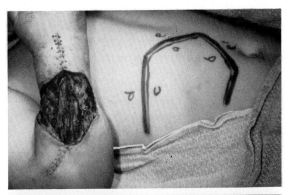

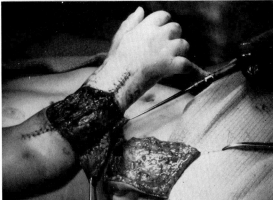

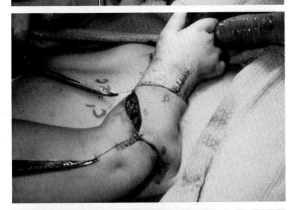

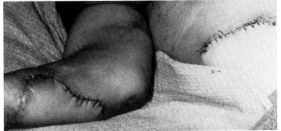

Fig. 2.22 (A) This congenital skin defect on the dorsal aspect of the forearm was too proximal for an axial groin flap. A random flap was therefore raised (B) and a secondary flap similar to that referred to in Figure 2.20 can be seen here raised from the forearm. The flap was applied (C) and divided three weeks later (D).

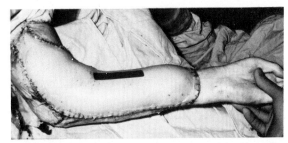

Fig. 2.23 After excision of extensive scarring of the arm and forearm, the only flap capable of providing sufficient cover was a latissimus dorsi musculocutaneous free flap. The contracted web space seen in the hand was subsequently released as shown in Figure 2.78.

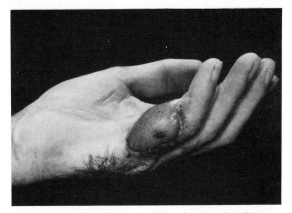

Fig. 2.24 A cross arm flap had been applied to the palmar aspect of the left small finger in this patient following an avulsion injury which exposed both tendons and neurovascular bundle. The bulk of this flap limited flexion of the small finger and revision was required before full function could be restored.

excision of skin should be avoided, however, for frequently none need be discarded. It should rather be redistributed by the use of Z-plasties in the marginal wound, which also serve to relieve any contracture in that wound.

Insensitivity. Sensation is always poor in distant flaps. This will improve with time and with thinning but rarely provides more than protective sensation. Usually little can be done to improve this situation but occasionally fine sensation may be imported to critical areas of a large flap, using a neurovascular island flap (Fig. 2.25).

PULP INJURIES and DIGITAL AMPUTATIONS

The digital pulp is a region where length should be preserved in the emergency situation and where split skin grafts are often employed both with this in mind and also in order to ensure primary healing. In other cases distant flaps may have been used ill-advisedly and will then require thinning, reduction and even replacement. The requirements in the digital pulp are freedom from pain, good sensation and stable padding which is adequate, but not excessive. Free graft reconstruction of the fingertip may

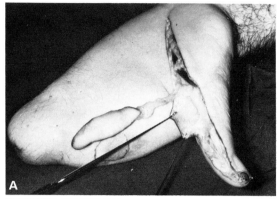

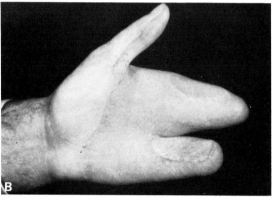

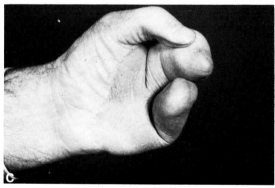

Fig. 2.25   (A) This patient who had sustained a gross avulsion injury of the left hand was treated primarily with a groin flap (Fig. 1.151, p. 84). Sensation was provided to the flap together with some augmentation of its blood supply by a neurovascular island taken from the non-contact, radial aspect of the thumb. The improved blood supply permitted a later conversion of the mitten hand to one of three digits, (B) with adequate flexion and key pinch between two areas with sensation. (C) The patient has since returned to his occupation as a maintenance engineer.

give an excellent result with good tactile gnosis[21]. As a general rule, it seems that the thicker the donor skin the better the functional result, the smaller the area the better the sensibility[22]. If the graft has retracted markedly, as it will do if not adherent to bone, sufficient pulp may have been drawn in to make the result satisfactory or alternatively to permit the use of a secondary local flap. The local flap employed may be of an advancement type, such as those described by Kutler[23], Moberg, and the V–Y advancement flap originally designed by Tranquilli-Leali (Fig. 2.26) and introduced into the English literature by Atasoy and others (p. 86). Joshi[24] has reported a transposition flap containing the dorsal digital nerve. All local flap procedures have the major merit of restoring sensation. If local flaps are not possible then the choice lies between reamputation more proximally, cross-finger flap, thenar flap, and neurovascular island flap.

The neurovascular island flap (p. 89) is justifiable only in the thumb and in a finger having unique occupational significance. Before undertaking a neurovascular island flap care should be taken to ensure that there is flow not only in the vessel which will supply the flap but also in the other digital artery of that finger and in the *contralateral*

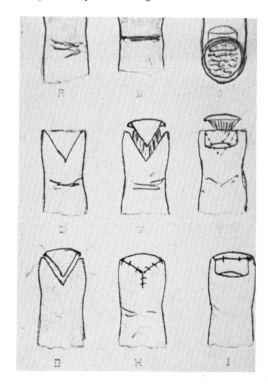

Fig. 2.26   This old illustration from the article of Tranquilli-Leali shows very clearly the steps in the production of a V–Y advancement flap.

vessel of the finger immediately adjacent (Fig. 2.27) — otherwise severe cold intolerance or even necrosis may result.

The choice between the remaining solutions should be made after explaining the time factor involved to the patient and discussing the choice with him in the light of his occupation.

Cross-finger and thenar flaps on the pulp have two major disadvantages:

insensitivity, which improves with time,[25,26]

stiffness in the involved digits, which is more common, more prolonged and therefore more significant in the older patient.

They do, however, provide satisfactory pain-free padding in the great majority of cases. If taken from the metacarpophalangeal crease of the thumb which can be closed directly, thenar flaps have the advantage that they create no cosmetically undesirable secondary defect, but the serious disadvantage of prolonged proximal interphalangeal joint flexion in the recipient finger[27]. They should therefore be reserved for young patients in whom the appearance of hand is unusually important. Even then, the need for vigorous physical therapy after division must be made clear to the patient before a thenar flap is used.

Reamputation more proximally is apparently a simple solution to the problem of tender pulp scars. It may have serious disadvantages of which the surgeon should be fully aware before embarking on this course:

1. The hazard of a tender scar remains, however careful the amputation technique, and to this must be added the possibility of the formation of a neuroma on either or both digital nerves. (p. 158)

2. A surprising amount of skeleton has to be resected if tension-free closure with good skin is to be achieved.

3. If the eventual amputation is through the middle phalanx, flexion of the proximal interphalangeal joint may be limited by the detached flexor digitorum profundus acting as an extensor via the lumbrical. This 'lumbrical plus' (p. 176) can be offset by suturing the tendon of profundus to the flexor sheath in the relaxed position.

4. *Quadriga syndrome.* The practice of suturing the flexor to the extensor tendon over the end of an amputation of middle, ring or small fingers seriously impairs the motion in the uninjured fingers due to the common origins of the flexors and of the extensors. This may even occur when the tendons have not been so tethered but due simply to scarring. This is predominantly of the flexor tendon and the patient complains of weakness of grip. Examination reveals a flexion deficit in the uninjured digits which have a normal passive range. It will be noted that the stump of the amputated digit is more strongly flexed than

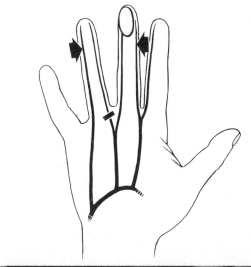

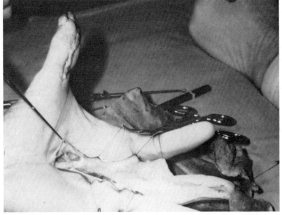

Fig. 2.27 (A) It is important in planning a neurovascular island flap that not only is flow in the vessel to the flap and in the remaining vessel to that digit confirmed, but also flow to the contralateral digital artery of the adjacent finger. This will provide the only flow to that digit, since its other side will be divided in the course of dissection. (B) The success of a neurovascular island transfer in restoring good sensation depends largely on insuring that the pedicle is not still under tension when the thumb is held in full palmar abduction and full extension as shown here.

the others. Verdan[28] termed this the quadriga syndrome after the Roman chariot in which the reins of all four horses were controlled in unison. Release of the flexor tendon remnant, done under local anesthesia to ensure effectiveness, restores full power (Fig. 2.28).

Ray amputation of a mutilated finger may prove beneficial. The disadvantage of the procedure is that, by removing one of the metacarpals, the leverage which the hand can apply is significantly reduced (Fig. 2.29). This adversely effects the use of a hammer, a spade, even a fishing rod.

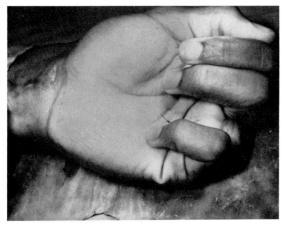

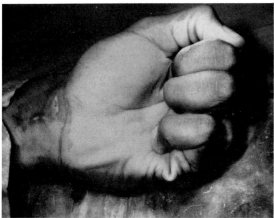

Fig. 2.28 Operative procedure under wrist block — *quadriga syndrome.*

(A) This patient is unable to fully flex his three remaining digits because the long flexor tendon is tethered out to length at the amputation stump.

(B) By division of the tendons to the ring finger in the palm, full flexion was achieved.

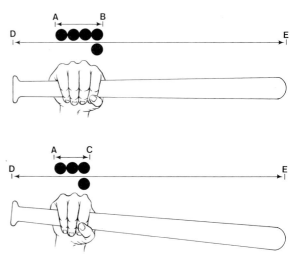

Fig. 2.29 This diagram illustrates how leverage is lost with removal of the index metacarpal ray. The length of the lever arm being reduced by one quarter has in fact been shown to reduce leverage by almost 50%.

It is therefore indicated for

stumps which impair function — for example the stiff flexed index stump which reduces thumb-finger span grasp or the painful small finger stump which is repeatedly struck

painful stumps — with the reservations expressed above

reasons of appearance — in salespersons, those engaged in communications and those concerned with cosmesis.

Ray amputation of the middle or ring should be accompanied by transposition of the index or small[29]. If not, 'scissoring' may occur (Fig. 2.30) or the remaining space will adversely affect the competence of the hand for containing liquids or small objects.

THUMB RECONSTRUCTION[30,31]

The best method of restoring the critical loss of a thumb is to undertake replantation. Where this has not proved possible or where the injury has been of a more complex nature than clean amputation, the requirements for a functional thumb must be understood during examination and reconstructive planning.

Position is the first requirement, for if the thumb cannot be opposed to the fingers it cannot serve its normal function. This can often be achieved by release of an adduction contracture and transfer of necessary motors.

Stability can be of two varieties, fixed and mobile. The latter is preferable and is fully achieved by restoring ligamentous integrity and by transfers appropriate to restore the movements normally produced by the nine muscles of the thumb. This may be impossible, in which case joints can be maintained in good position by tenodesis or arthrodesis. Wherever possible, the basal carpo-metacarpal joint is kept mobile.

Strength sufficient to resist the forces of the fingers is provided, as is stability, by judicious fusions, tendon grafts and transfers.

Motion for the thumb comes as a consequence of restoring mobile stability and strength. In order of importance, efforts should be directed at restoring opposition and abduction, adduction, and extension and flexion of the three joints in the sequence carpo-metacarpal, interphalangeal and finally metacarpophalangeal.

Sensation and vascularity of the terminal portion of the thumb are essential for its normal manipulative activity and are usually considered in conjunction with the final requirement, namely,

Length. The necessary length of a thumb depends upon the occupational and social demand the patient will place upon it. Some time must be spent, therefore, discussing this with each thumb amputee. Often the final decision

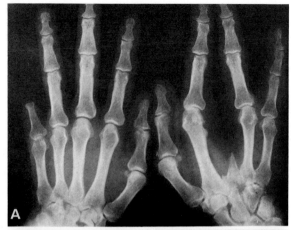

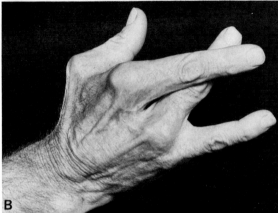

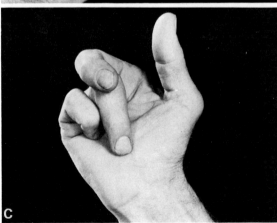

Fig. 2.30 This patient had sustained a mutilating injury to his middle finger which was treated by ray amputation. This resulted in severe functional incapacity as evidenced by scissoring in flexion and loss of the competence of the open hand. The situation was improved for the patient by transposition of the entire index finger on to the residual base of the middle finger metacarpal.

may be made after a period of trial, both of occupation and recreations. Fitting the available procedures to the needs of the patient is a complex and individual process and the following is intended to act only as a guide.

Acceptable length — poor covering

Better skin and sensation can be obtained from a *volar advancement* or *innervated cross-finger flap*[32,33] (p. 85). Where improved blood supply, sensation and a better pulp is required only a *neurovascular island flap*, pedicle or free transfer, can provide it.

Subtotal amputations

Subtotal amputations which have good skin cover and *nearly* acceptable length — which usually means an amputation at some point between the metacarpophalangeal and interphalangeal joints — can be restored either by *phalangisation*[34] (Fig. 2.31) or *metacarpal lengthening*[35] or *local flap and bone graft*[36].

Total amputations

Those in which there is no satisfactory function whatsoever, can be reconstructed by any one of three methods — *osteoplastic reconstruction*[37,38] (Fig. 2.32), *pollicisation*[39,40] (Fig. 2.33) or *toe-to-hand transfer*[41,42] (Fig. 2.34). In making the choice, the surgeon must pay heed to five factors:

1. *occupation* — manual workers may lose essential leverage across the palm of the hand by sacrificing the one metacarpal necessary in pollicisation[43]; athletes will be ill-advised to surrender a toe despite the fact that foot problems after toe-to-hand transfer have been shown to be few.
2. *sex* — women will be understandably dissatisfied by the cosmetic appearance of an osteoplastic thumb reconstruction and also with the donor scar of the tube pedicle.
3. *available digit* — if the patient is not prepared to surrender a toe and no finger can be sacrificed, — either because they are absent or essential — only one of the three options remains.
4. *basal joint* — of the three procedures only pollicisation adequately restores a basal joint to the thumb.
5. *palmar and digital vessels* — when injury or disease has damaged the neurovascular structures of the fingers, no pedicle is available for pollicisation or for conventional osteoplastic reconstruction, which requires a neurovascular island flap.

The influence of these five factors on the choice of procedure is shown in admittedly oversimplified form in Figure 2.35. It will be evident from the above that angiography (p. 182) plays an important role in selecting the procedure most likely to succeed.

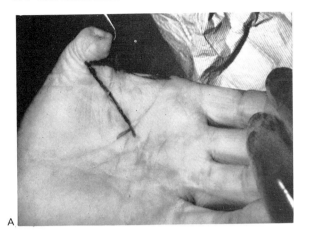

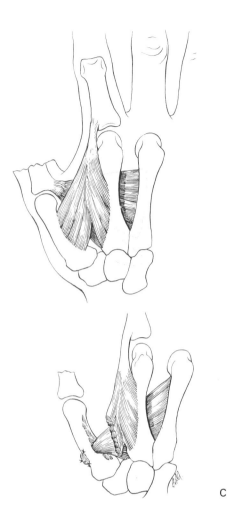

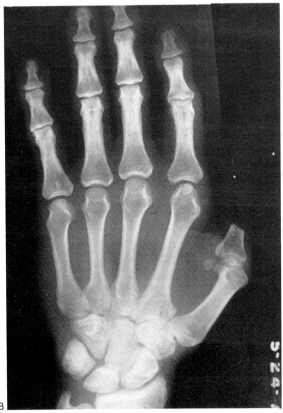

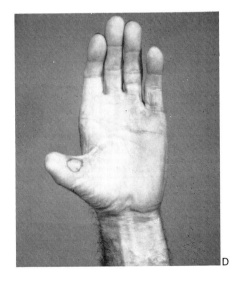

Fig. 2.31(A & B)   This patient had suffered a thumb
amputation at the midpoint of the proximal phalanx. As a result,
he had no first web space with which to effect span grasp. The
release of the muscles was performed as shown in (C), the first
dorsal interosseous being detached from the first metacarpal, and
the adductor pollicis being reinserted low on the metacarpal. A
Z-plasty was also performed resulting in the acceptable space
shown in (D).

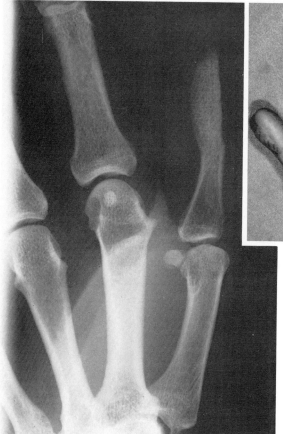
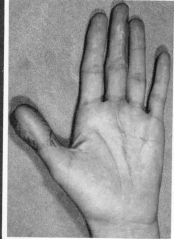
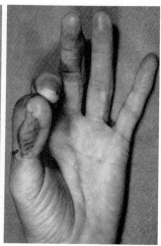

Fig. 2.32 Osteoplastic reconstruction. (A) This patient had sustained amputation at the mid-point of the proximal phalanx with degloving of soft tissue to a more proximal level while water skiing. An immediate bone graft was inserted, and subsequently incorporated satisfactorily. The bone graft was covered with a tube pedicle and a later neurovascular island was applied. In (B) and (C) it can be seen that the thumb is bulky and that the neurovascular island pedicle is somewhat unstable despite attempts to attach it to the bone graft. The markings on the thumb indicate the area in the skin remaining from the tube pedicle which receives innervation from the adjacent neurovascular island and from the thumb.

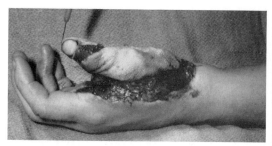

Fig. 2.33 (A) This patient sustained an extensive punch press injury to the radial aspect of the hand. It did not prove possible to revascularize the thumb. After provision of skin cover by a groin flap, the index finger was subsequently pollicized (B) providing good function, but (C) significantly narrowing the palm, as referred to in 2.29 above.

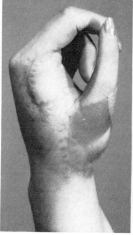
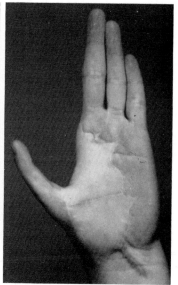

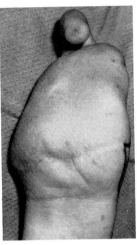
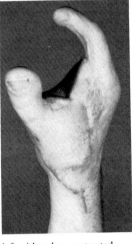
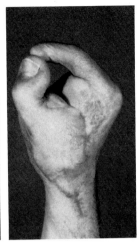

Fig. 2.34 (A) This patient was left with only a contracted middle finger after an industrial accident. The palmar defect had previously been covered with a groin flap. (B) By fusing the proximal interphalangeal joint of the middle at a satisfactory position and undertaking toe to hand transfer, a crude span grasp was achieved, and (C) some pinch was restored which gave him a good assist hand.

Fig. 2.35 This diagram summarizes the factors influencing the choice between pollicization, osteoplastic thumb reconstruction, and toe to hand transfer (see text).

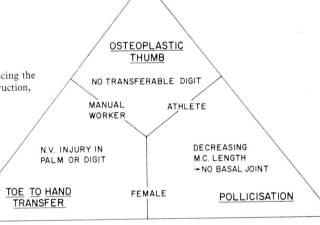

NAIL BED INJURIES[44]

Following nail bed injuries three distinct problems may be found all of which predispose to infection around the nail.

Remnants of nail

Where an unsuccessful attempt has been made to totally excise the germinal matrix small spicules of the nail persist, growing in irregular manner through the skin. These cause pain and annoyance. Formal ablation should be recommended.

Split nail

An injury of the nail bed in which the eponychium has been allowed to heal to the germinal matrix causes a longitudinal split in the nail (Fig. 2.36). This should be revised by excision and resuture under magnification.

Non-adherent nail

Where loss of sterile matrix has been replaced with a graft the nail which subsequently grows over it may not adhere resulting in painful packing of dirt under the nail. The area of nail bed which is failing in its function should be defined under magnification and shaved down to a bleeding bed to which a split thickness nail bed graft should be applied.

Before undertaking any revisionary surgery of the nail bed, the surgeon is well-advised to warn the patient of the unpredictability of the procedure.

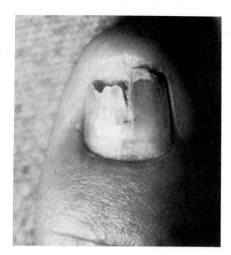

Fig. 2.36   The deformities arising from a nailbed injury are all shown in this nail which is split, nonadherent, and the source of recurrent discomfort and infection.

Bone

Three problems may arise following fractures of the hand: non-union, osteitis and malunion.

NON-UNION

Non-union comes about through *lack of adequate contact* between the bone ends or through *avascularity*. Lack of adequate contact may be due to

too large a gap — this may be due to appropriate debridement of damaged bone, say after a gunshot wound, but failure to insert a bone graft; to the interposition of soft parts such as a tendon or palmar plate (Fig. 2.37); to the presence between the viable ends of pieces of dead bone; to the interposition of tumor as in a pathological fracture; to excessive traction applied in attempting to immobilize the part.

excessive motion between the ends — this is more likely to occur in some situations than others — for example, diaphyseal fractures of phalanges move much more with flexion and extension than do the metaphyseal, where incidentally there is a better blood supply.

Avascularity notoriously occurs in the proximal pole of the scaphoid due to its unique pattern of blood supply, but may arise in the long bones of the hand as a consequence of crush injuries with resultant comminuted or segmental fractures, the fragments of which are deprived of their blood supply. Such injuries also cause scarring and poor perfusion of surrounding soft tissues. The effect, when established, is that the bone ends become sclerotic and the scar tissue forms a *fibrous union*, in which there may be motion — a *pseudarthrosis* (Fig. 2.38). On examination, the patient frequently has remarkably little pain and relatively good function. The presence of non-union may be detected

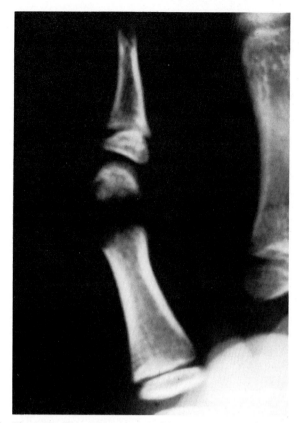

Fig. 2.37   This child presented with a persistently painful thumb after injury. X-ray revealed the presence of a wide gap, and exploration showed that this gap contained the long flexor tendon, preventing union.

by *tenderness on direct pressure* and by the presence of *motion*, either clinically or demonstrated on *stress x-ray* or *cineradiography* (Fig. 2.39). Treatment of non-union in the long bones requires removal of the cause, debridement of the bone ends, rigid fixation, cancellous bone grafting and provision of well-vascularised skin cover.

Non-union of the scaphoid: Patients with established non-union of the scaphoid may or may not know their diagnosis and may or may not have already received treatment. Knowing that a previously undiagnosed scaphoid fracture with no other pathology should be given a trial of proper scaphoid casting and assuming that the patient would not present if he had no pain and no loss of motion, a group of patients is left who can be managed according to the plan laid out in Figure 2.40. If the patient has been immobilised and presents with limited range of motion and pain, but no evidence of arthritis or aseptic necrosis, or of a definite gap between the fragments or of motion between the fragments on cineradiography, there is much to be gained and little to be lost by restoring to him the motion lost during many months of immobilisation. He may have a sound fibrous union. If retrieval of motion relieves his pain and gives him

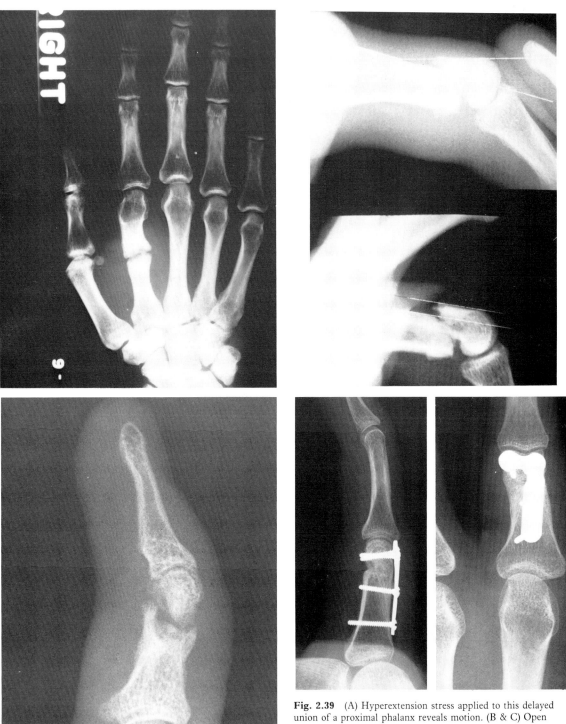

Fig. 2.39 (A) Hyperextension stress applied to this delayed union of a proximal phalanx reveals motion. (B & C) Open reduction and internal fixation with the minifragment set resulted in satisfactory union. (Osteosynthesis by Dr T. W. Wolff)

Fig. 2.38 The elements of pseudoarthrosis. (A) Sclerosis in the bone ends. (B) Ankylosis of an adjacent joint frequently plays a part in the development of motion at a nonunion.

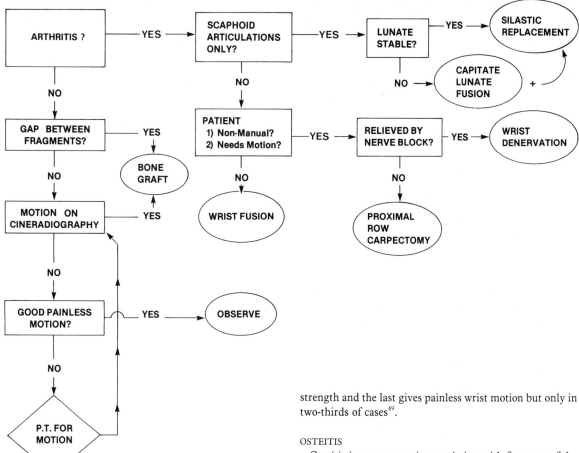

Fig. 2.40 Scaphoid nonunion. This flow chart outlines the decisions involved in choosing a line of treatment for scaphoid nonunion.

equal strength to the other hand, then he can be observed. If motion between the fragments exists or returns with no arthritis or necrosis, then bone graft is required (Fig. 2.41). If alternatively, there is evidence of arthritis, then the surgeon must look carefully for the distribution of those changes. If they are limited to the scaphoid and its articulations — the normal progression is scapho-radius, scapho-capitate, scapho-lunate and finally radio-lunate — then the lunate should be studied. If it is stable then a silastic scaphoid replacement will be stable also (Fig. 2.42). If it is not (Fig. 2.43), then the choice is the same as it is if there is radio-lunate arthritis, — that is, between limited[45,46] or complete wrist fusion, proximal row carpectomy[47] and wrist denervation. The first gives no motion but a strong, painless wrist, — although not without some complications[48], — while the second gives motion but loses

strength and the last gives painless wrist motion but only in two-thirds of cases[49].

OSTEITIS

Osteitis is uncommon in association with fractures of the upper extremity and is always due to *avascularity*, as outlined above. The findings are those of osteitis elsewhere: a chronically discharging wound surrounded by inflamed, indurated skin. X-ray will show a non-union, often with sequestration and sclerosis of bone fragments. Many organisms may be cultured, but they are merely opportunistic. They will disappear with adequate surgical treatment. That treatment is as for non-union — radical debridement of all avascular bone and soft tissue, adequate fixation, provision of well vascularised soft tissue cover and cancellous bone graft, either simultaneously or some six weeks later when it is seen that all infection has settled (Fig. 2.44).

MALUNION

Malunion is due to shortening or incorrect alignment at the time of the original fracture (p. 57). Malalignment may be *rotational* or *angulatory*, the angulation being antero-posterior or lateral. The direction in which the fragments point, or put another way, the convex side of the angle, is used to describe the angulation. The functional effects of malunion may be minor, as that following a boxer's fracture of the fifth metacarpal, or significant —

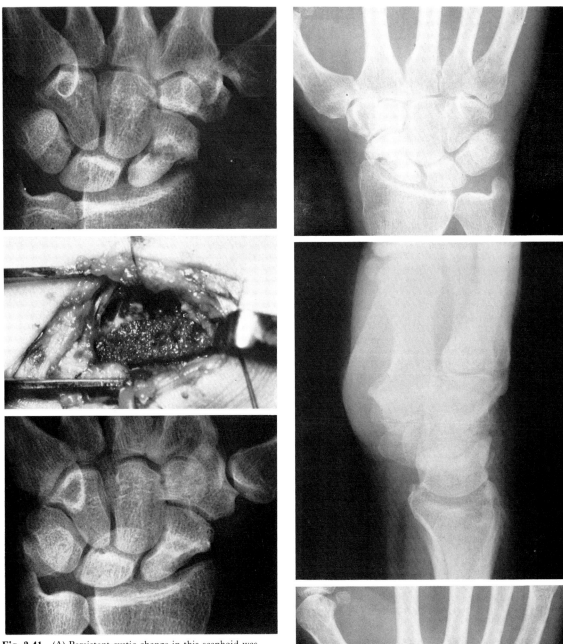

Fig. 2.41 (A) Persistent cystic change in this scaphoid was allied to motion evident on cineradiography but no clear evidence of aseptic necrosis or arthritis. (B) A cancellous bone graft was inserted resulting in (C) satisfactory late union.

Fig. 2.42 (A) Scaphoid replacement is required due to a failure of previous bone graft, extensive cyst formation, some evidence of aseptic necrosis, and also arthritis between the scaphoid and the capitate and radial styloid. The appearance of the lunate suggests that it is stable, and this is confirmed on lateral examination (B) where there is no evidence of any instability pattern. (C) Scaphoid replacement was therefore undertaken and proved stable and effective.

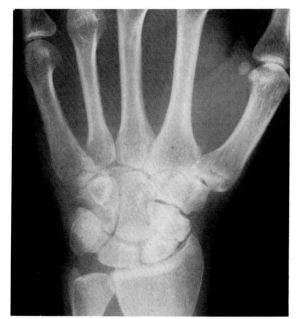

Fig. 2.43 Scaphoid replacement was indicated in this patient due to persistent nonunion of the scaphoid and evidence of arthritis changes between the scaphoid and the radial styloid. However, the configuration of the lunate indicates instability, and a scaphoid prosthesis would be difficult to maintain in position due to this instability pattern.

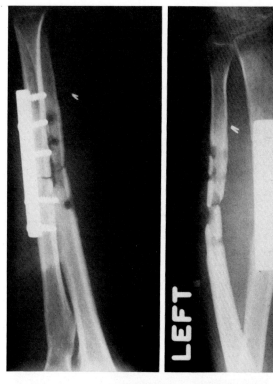

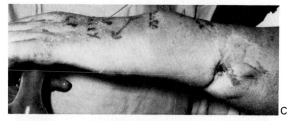

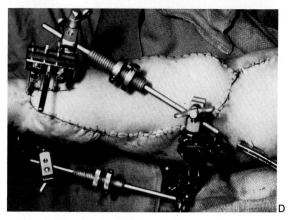

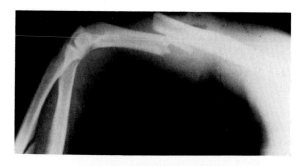

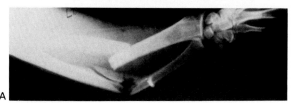

Fig. 2.44 Auger injury. (A) This inflicted incomplete amputations at two levels, the humerus and mid-forearm, requiring revascularization at both levels. This proceeded to infected nonunion of the forearm bones (B, C). (D) Rigid fixation was applied, and radical sequestrectomy was performed, the entire area being covered with a latissimus dorsi free flap. (Subsequent cancellous bone grafting and other procedures on the hand failed to restore satisfactory function to this extremity which was eventually amputated. However all bone infection was eliminated by this procedure.)

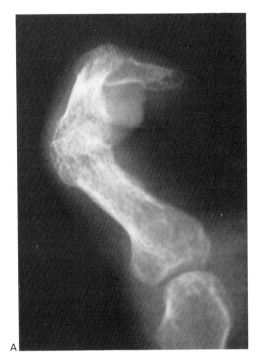

A

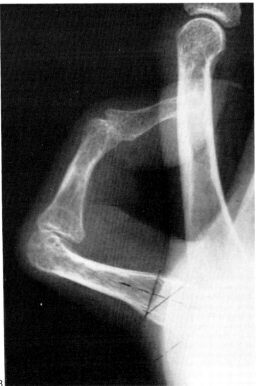

B

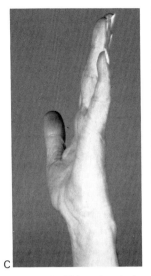

C

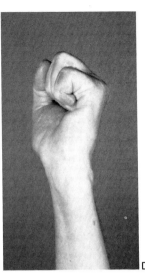

D

Fig. 2.45 This patient had gross malalignment of the proximal phalanx following a fracture at the junction of the proximal and middle thirds. In the anteroposterior view shown in (A) the malalignment can be partly appreciated. (B) In the lateral, as always, the metacarpophalangeal joint is obscured, but is indicated by the dotted line which bisects the line marking the axis of the proximal phalanx. The appropriate wedge for closing osteotomy is marked out on this X–ray. (C & D) With this correction of malalignment full range of motion was restored to the small finger.

scissoring, in which fingers do not run on parallel tracks, but cross one another or diverge, results most commonly from rotation, usually in an oblique or spiral fracture of the metacarpal, sometimes of a phalanx (Fig. 2.30, p. 123). It is corrected by rotational osteotomy.

reduced motion may be due to adhesions, or to relative lengthening of the tendons, as in the Z deformity (like that in rheumatoid, p. 254) seen after an anteriorly angulated transverse fracture of the diaphysis of the proximal phalanx. Passive motion of the proximal interphalangeal joint may remain, or a flexion contracture may have developed. In either event, motion will only be fully restored by correcting the malalignment (Fig. 2.45).

interference with normal function may arise as in lateral angulation of a border digit which may catch on sliding the hand into a narrow space (Fig. 2.46) or in posterior angulation of a second or third metacarpal which may produce a painful mass in the palm — the metacarpal head.

Cosmetic considerations may be significant and valid. The precise amount of lateral angulation in the phalanges can be deduced from study of true antero-posterior X-rays in which the articular surfaces should be parallel. On such X-rays the exact amount of bone to be removed in a closing wedge, or inserted in an opening wedge can be calculated (Fig. 2.47). Where corrective osteotomy[50] is not along the original fracture line, solid union of that fracture *must* be

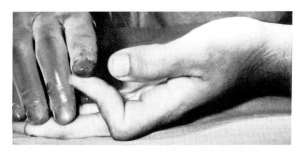

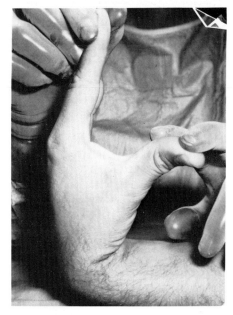

Fig. 2.58 (A) With the wrist fully extended the proximal interphalangeal joint here shows a 90° flexion contracture. (B) With full flexion of the wrist the index finger fully extends. From this it can be deduced that the long flexor tendon is adherent proximal to the wrist joint, and this proved to be the case on exploration.

In the great majority of cases flexion contractures are due to tightness of structures on the flexor aspect. Occasionally, however, the joint may be *prevented from extending* by incongruity of the articular surfaces, or adhesion of the dorsal capsule or of extensor tendon to the articular surface of the head of the proximal bone.

Where dorsal adhesions are the cause, not only will there be a flexion contracture but there will also be marked limitation of flexion.

Locking of a joint implies that it is *temporarily* fixed in a particular posture, but can be released by some manipulation of the joint, usually painful. This usually occurs in flexion and may, by progression of the process, result in a fixed flexion contracture. Trigger finger (p. 243) is by far the most common cause, but locking may also be due to loose bodies, osteophytes, capsular tears or distortion of the articular surfaces[56-57] (Fig. 2.59).

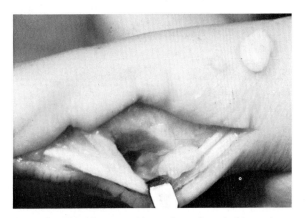

Fig. 2.59 This joint was subject to intermittent locking and periods of painful swelling. X-ray revealed nothing of note, but exploration of the proximal interphalangeal joint yielded the loose body shown in the photograph.

passive extension of the digital joints is limited in wrist extension, not so if the wrist is flexed (Fig. 2.58). Alternatively, if a flexor tendon functions on joints more proximal but not on the one being tested it may be assumed that one factor at least in the flexion contracture of that joint is adhesion of the tendon to the bone immediately proximal to the joint. In this circumstance, assuming the extensor tendon is healthy, passive flexion will exceed active flexion and may well be normal, while the extension deficit will be the same both actively and passively.

Capsular structures (collateral ligament, accessory collateral ligament, palmar plate). These may be the sole cause of limited extension, usually by shortening of the palmar plate or adhesions of the collateral ligament. Even where other structures are the primary cause of a flexion contracture in an *inter-phalangeal* joint the palmar plate becomes contracted at an early stage.

Dupuytren's[68] disease

Since micro-trauma[69,70] to the palmar fascia followed by myofibroblast contracture[71,72] is now blamed by many for the development of this disorder, the point may be stretched to include it at this juncture. A familial disorder, the patient when pressed can usually recall some member of his family, often distant, who has suffered from this complaint. It normally commences with the development of a nodule in the palm which is frequently painful. This may or may not proceed to the next stage, which is the development of bands of Dupuytren's contracture[73]. The bands develop in specific relationships to the flexor tendon sheath and neurovascular bundles of the finger[74] and affect, in order of frequency, the ring, small, middle, and rarely, the thumb and index fingers[75].

At examination the surgeon should determine whether or not the fascial bands are causing contracture. If they are not

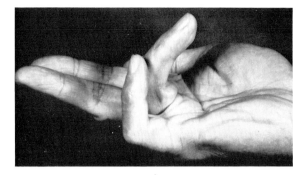

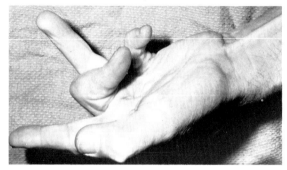

Fig. 2.60A & B   Dupuytren's contracture. Of the joints contracted, the metacarpophalangeal joint of the ring finger will be most readily released. The proximal interphalangeal joint contractures and the interphalangeal joint contracture of the thumb in (B) will prove most difficult to release.

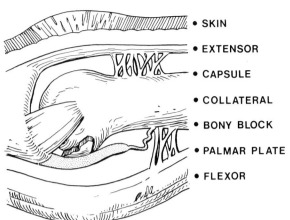

- SKIN
- EXTENSOR
- CAPSULE
- COLLATERAL
- BONY BLOCK
- PALMAR PLATE
- FLEXOR

Fig. 2.61   This diagram shows all of the factors which may be involved in loss of flexion (extension contracture).

then no surgery is required and the patient is advised to return when contracture commences. If contracture has occurred then fasciectomy should be scheduled. For the reasons outlined previously, full extension is more likely to be achieved after release of a metacarpophalangeal than of an interphalangeal contracture (Fig. 2.60). Other factors likely to have an adverse effect on the result are: early age of onset, the presence of Garrod's[76] knuckle pads[77], the number of rays involved[78] and the patient being an epileptic or an alcoholic — there is a higher incidence of coexistence with these conditions than would be expected randomly[79].

The examiner may attempt to predict the presence of a significant displacement of the neurovascular bundle by the method described by Watson[80] or by Doppler ultrasound examination[81]. Finally, he should ensure that no other areas are afflicted, for Dupuytren's-like fibromatosis can occur in the foot[82] and on the penis[83].

Limitation of flexion (Fig. 2.61)
This may be due to one or more of all the structures on the dorsal aspect of the joint.
  Skin — scar contracture.
  Long extensor. Again adjustment of the adjacent joints may yield a diagnosis of tendon shortening or of adhesion proximal to that adjusted joint. However, limited flexion caused by long extensor adhesion is most commonly seen in

the proximal interphalangeal joint, the adhesion being to the proximal phalanx consequent upon either a fracture or severe crush injury of the finger. Active extension of the joint will be severely limited or absent. Commonly it falls markedly short of passive extension.

  Intrinsics. Contracture of one or more intrinsics may follow ischaemia and muscle fibrosis (p. 31) or may occur for non-ischaemic reasons[84] (p. 275). If very marked this may be apparent from the 'intrinsic plus' posture of the hand in which the fingers are flexed at the metacarpophalangeal joints (Fig. 2.62). In less evident contracture, its presence is detected by attempting to flex the proximal interphalangeal joint while passively extending the corresponding metacarpophalangeal joint. In intrinsic tightness this movement is restricted (Fig. 2.63). The restriction can be differentiated from that caused by extensor muscle adhesion or capsular ligament disorder by thereafter allowing the metacarpophalangeal joint to flex. In other disorders the inability to fully flex the proximal

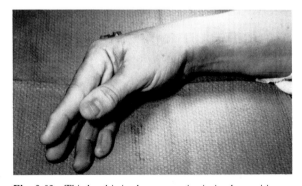

Fig. 2.62   This hand is in the extreme intrinsic plus position with metacarpophalangeal joint flexion and interphalangeal extension.

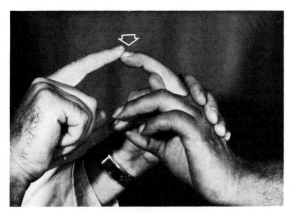

Fig. 2.63 With the metacarpophalangeal joint extended, attempts to flex the proximal interphalangeal joint in this patient with intrinsic tightness met with a rubbery resistance which limited flexion to a mere 20 degrees.

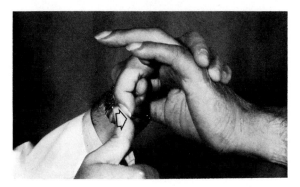

Fig. 2.64 When the metacarpophalangeal joint in the patient illustrated in Figure 2.63 was allowed to flex, significant increase in the flexion in the proximal interphalangeal joint resulted, demonstrating that the limitation of motion at that joint was due to intrinsic tightness.

interphalangeal joint will persist whereas in pure intrinsic tightness the proximal interphalangeal joint will increasingly flex as the metacarpophalangeal joint also flexes (Fig. 2.64). The intrinsic tightness present is recorded by noting the passive flexion which is possible at the proximal interphalangeal joint (a) when the metacarpophalangeal joint is extended and (b) when that joint is flexed. As an example, the record of the patient in Figures 2.63 and 2.64 read '0/20–60 (intrinsic tightness)'.

Capsular structures (dorsal capsule, collateral ligament, accessory collateral ligament, palmar plate). These structures alone may limit flexion by adhesion of any one of them to the head of the proximal bone of the joint. If other structures are primarily responsible, the capsular structures are likely to become involved in addition. In contrast with flexion contracture, which is more common in the interphalangeal joints and particularly the proximal, stiffness in extension due to collateral ligament shortening

is much more likely in the metacarpophalangeal joint. This is because that ligament is normally slack in extension and tight in flexion. Loss of flexion at the metacarpophalangeal joints can come about simply by immobilisation in the incorrect, extended position. In addition to a shortened collateral ligament, metacarpophalangeal flexion may be prevented by adhesion of the palmar plate to the palmar surface of the metacarpal head. It is possible to distinguish between palmar plate adhesion and collateral ligament tightness as the cause of metacarpophalangeal joint fixation in extension. If the collateral ligaments are the cause then abduction and adduction of the fingers, normally at least 45° combined in this extended position, will be virtually eliminated. In the less likely situation in which the palmar plate is the major or sole culprit, attempted passive flexion will produce an opening of the dorsal aspect of the joint. This comes about as the anterior lip of the base of the proximal phalanx jams against the adherent plate and the unaffected and therefore still loose collateral ligament permits the flexion force to rock the dorsal lip away from the metacarpal head. This is subtle, is felt as a recess dorsally between head and base and may be best appreciated under anaesthesia (Fig. 2.65).

Apart from factors on the extensor aspect and in the joint capsule limiting flexion, it may be blocked by palmar structures:

Flexor tendon: a flexor tendon adherent within the sheath may be sufficiently bulky to block full flexion of an interphalangeal joint;

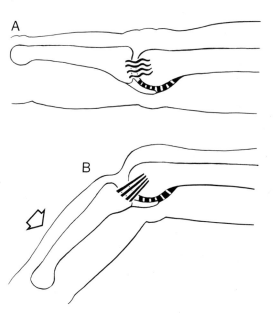

Fig. 2.65 Adhesion of the palmar plate to the head of the metacarpal with no involvement of the collateral ligament results in rubbery resistance to flexion and causes an opening of the dorsal aspect of the joint.

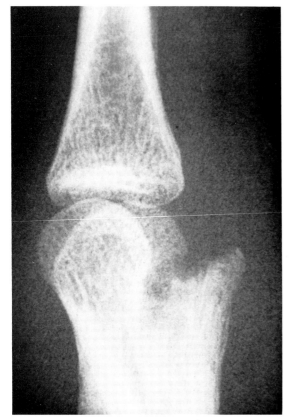

Fig. 2.66   A bony block clearly limiting flexion.

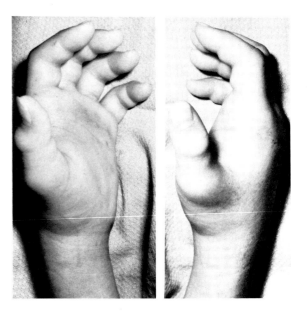

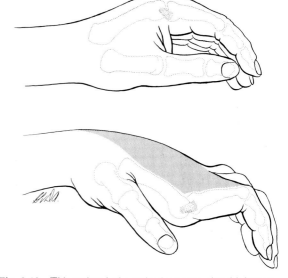

Fig. 2.68   This patient had sustained a severe, closed injury to the hand resulting in significant oedema. This is most evident on the dorsum (B), and the effect on the wrist, metacarpophalangeal and interphalangeal joints is diagramatically shown in (C). The resultant posture is undesirable for all three joints.

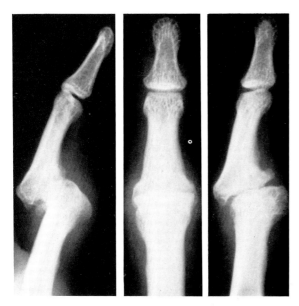

Fig. 2.67   This patient had previously sustained a fracture-dislocation of the proximal interphalangeal joint which was not adequately reduced. This has gone on to posttraumatic osteoarthritis.

Bone: this may take the form of a true block (Fig. 2.66) or may be the result of articular incongruity or destruction (Fig. 2.67).

Chondral fractures may present a diagnostic problem. The patient complains of a persistently painful joint which remains swollen, although the swelling tends to wax and wane, limiting flexion to a varying degree. X-ray reveals nothing. This condition most frequently affects the metacarpophalangeal joint and persistent questioning may cause the patient to recall an injury, usually minor, but which involved a direct blow to the metacarpal head or a twist which could have caused the proximal phalangeal base to impinge on the head. Exploration may reveal the fracture and often a consequent loose body in the joint cavity (Fig. 2.59).

The severely injured hand becomes very oedematous. Unless prevented from doing so the joints assume the posture in which their ligaments are most relaxed. Ligamentous contracture and fibrosis causes the joints to become virtually immobile in this position, which is characteristically

Wrist	— flexion
Thumb	— adduction
Metacarpophalangeal	— extension
Proximal interphalangeal	— flexion (Fig. 2.68)

The first procedure the surgeon may have to undertake in such a neglected or mismanaged hand is to release the contractures (Fig. 2.69).

Recording range of motion

As each joint is carried by the examiner to its full *passive* range and this is recorded the patient should be invited to 'keep it there'. The *active* range can then be recorded also. It is common practice to record active range only. This can be misleading as it is not a true reflection of the capabilities of that joint but rather of the limitations of the muscles acting upon it. Paralysis or tendon adhesions, for example, will cause the active range to fall far short of the passive and only the two can accurately pinpoint the problem (Fig. 2.70).

The active range should be recorded as recommended by Koch and Mason, adding the passive range in brackets

$$\frac{\text{maximum extension}}{\text{maximum flexion}} \quad \text{e.g.} \quad \frac{(10)\ 60}{90} \quad \begin{array}{l}\text{in the patient shown} \\ \text{in Figure 2.70}\end{array}$$

All recordings should be made with a goniometer applied to the dorsal aspect of the joint. Only in this way can accurate measure be taken, especially by different observers, of improvement or deterioration between visits.

Indications

If active range does not equal passive, there is no benefit whatsoever to be gained from operating on the joint alone. Rather should the cause of loss of active motion be located

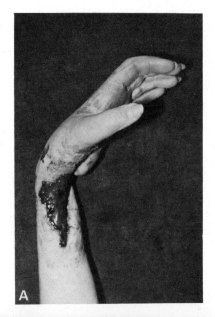

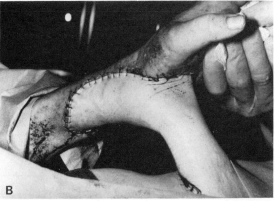

Fig. 2.69 This patient presented a history of having sustained a full thickness burn to the anterior aspect of the left wrist some six months previously during which time wet dressings had been applied. No splintage had been employed nor had skin cover been provided. As a result the wrist was in flexion, the thumb in adduction, the metacarpophalangeal joints in extension and the proximal interphalangeal joints in a degree of flexion. All these deformities were fixed. All could have been avoided by appropriate splintage.

(B) Treatment was commenced by application of a groin flap to the large skin defect on the wrist following release of the scar contracture present therein.

and remedied whereafter passive range may improve appreciably through exercise of the muscles which normally produce the full range. Conversely, no substitution surgery, either tendon graft or tendon transfer, will have sufficient power to improve the passive range of motion in a joint. Thus, for example, it is fruitless to recommend a flexor tendon graft to a patient with stiff digital joints or, as happens more commonly, to perform an

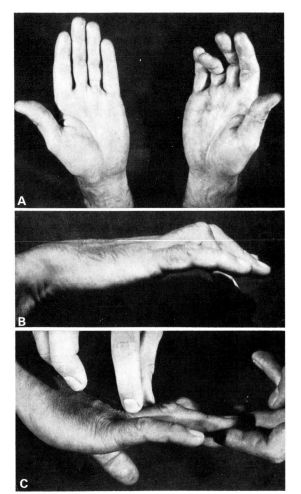

Fig. 2.70A & B This patient presented with an inability to extend the proximal interphalangeal joints of both ring and middle fingers. His active range of motion in the ring finger was recorded as 60 to 90 degrees.

(C) His passive range was however 10 to 90 degrees indicating that the cause of his loss of extension lay in the tendon and not in the proximal interphalangeal joint itself.

opponensplasty on a patient with limited passive abduction of the thumb.

Since active range cannot *exceed* passive range, there is no way in which the surgeon can determine at examination whether or not the tendon acting on a joint can take advantage of any improvement he may achieve by operating to relieve a limited passive range. Thus it is most important at surgery to check, for example, that the flexor tendon is capable of actively achieving the new found flexion attained passively, either by working under local anaesthetic and enlisting the patient's help or by exposing the tendon away from the joint and pulling on it. Otherwise a puzzling discrepancy will exist postoperatively between the active function present then and the passive range achieved at operation.

ABNORMAL MOTION

Having recorded the passive and active range of *normal* movement of the joints, the surgeon should test for the presence of *abnormal* movements. Chronic *hyperextension* or *recurrent dorsal dislocation*[85-87] may follow an untreated tear of the palmar plate or fracture-dislocation of the proximal, or more rarely distal, interphalangeal joint. This may present openly or masked as a swollen, 'weak' joint. Clinically it can be revealed by passive stress with or without anaesthesia. The collateral ligaments of each joint should be stressed by placing the examiner's thumb or index finger on the opposite side of the joint to act as a stable fulcrum while holding the joint in extension and stressing the collateral ligament using the distal part of the limb or digit as a lever arm to exert force. This may reveal frank laxity and sublux the joint. More commonly the patient withdraws his hand, complaining of pain over the collateral ligament under test. The precise point of tenderness on the collateral ligament should be sought by pressure with the digital pulp. Lateral stress X-ray films should be taken. If pain is severe, this should be performed under appropriate nerve block. Care should be taken to avoid rotation, and therefore spurious lateral movement, of the proximal interphalangeal joint which has a flexion contracture, by testing for lateral instability in the presence of such a contracture with the metacarpophalangeal joint locked in full flexion. That flexed posture is also the one in which lateral stability of the metacarpophalangeal joint should be tested since it tightens the collateral ligament.

Recording abnormal motion is done by placing skin marks over the mid-point of the lax joint and also of the joints immediately adjacent. The angle produced by stress between these joints can then be measured with varying degrees of difficulty and therefore inaccuracy (Fig. 2.71).

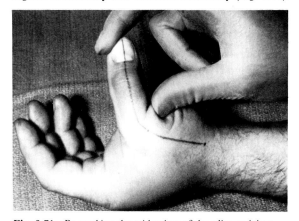

Fig. 2.71 By marking the mid-points of the adjacent joints angulation can be appreciated on stress, even when it is of a much less significant degree than in this tear of the ulnar collateral ligament.

Greater ease and accuracy can be achieved by measuring on stress X-rays.

Gamekeeper's thumb[88]. The joint most afflicted by laxity is the metacarpophalangeal joint of the thumb. Tears of the ulnar collateral ligament are common and disabling. The injury was said to be sustained by keepers while breaking the necks of small game — hence the name. Now the injury most commonly results from falling on the outstretched hand — a combined extension and radially deviating stress — often with some additional force applied by something wrapped around the thumb itself, as in skiing[89]. The injury involves avulsion of the collateral ligament from the base of the proximal phalanx with or without a fragment of bone[90] together with tearing of the palmar plate and accessory collateral ligament. This differs from the proximal interphalangeal joint where rupture is much more common proximally[91]. The torn ligament in the thumb may come to lie superficial to the adductor expansion, which normally overlies it, eliminating any chance of healing — the Stener lesion[92] (Fig. 2.72) (described also in the proximal interphalangeal joint[93]). Since a stable thumb is essential, these should be explored and repaired at the time of injury[94], the only necessary indication being laxity and bruising. However, they are frequently ignored by the

patient or splinted by his physician. When he presents later the patient will have painful weakness of his thumb and show radial instability and some palmar subluxation on examination. The palmar plate offers some stability with the joint in extension, so with lesser degrees of instability the stress should be applied with the joint in flexion[95]. As mentioned previously, care should be taken to prevent rotation of the proximal bone when applying lateral stress to a flexed joint, lest an incorrect diagnosis of instability be

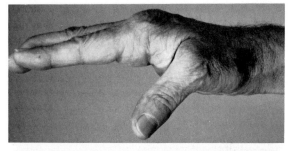

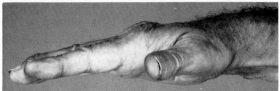

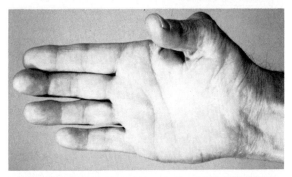

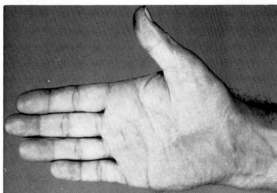

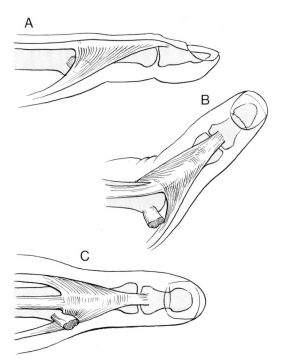

Fig. 2.72 *Stener lesion.* After a tear of the ulnar collateral ligament of the metacarpophalangeal joint of the thumb from its distal attachment, the ligament may come to lie outside the adductor contribution to the extensor expansion. Thus healing cannot occur.

Fig. 2.73 Restoration of function by arthrodesis for chronic instability of the metacarpophalangeal joint. (A & B) Restoration of alignment in extension. (C & D) Restoration of radial abduction.

made. In the future arthrography may become a routine part of the investigation, helping to predict the pathology more accurately[96]. Depending on the state of the joint surfaces the choice lies between reconstruction and arthrodesis (Fig. 2.73).

RADIOLOGICAL EXAMINATION

| Interphalangeal joints | — true anteroposterior, lateral and obliques |
| Metacarpophalangeal joints | — anteroposterior, Brewerton (p. 000) and two *angled laterals* — 30° pronation for index and middle — 30° supination for ring and small |

Study of these X-rays will reveal *incongruity* due to a healed intra-articular fracture, a bony block, or chronic dislocation, or evidence of *traumatic arthritis* in the form of loss of joint space, eburnation — sclerosis — of the bone ends, cyst formation and osteophytic spurs. The findings may dictate what line of treatment can be pursued.

INDICATIONS

Significant *abnormal* motion is a definite indication for exploration and reconstruction or stabilisation. Except where X-ray has shown definite incongruity or advanced degeneration, *limited motion in a stable joint* should always be treated initially by dynamic splintage, only to be abandoned when no further gain can be achieved as evidenced by unchanging measurement on successive visits.

If the articular surfaces are good, soft tissue release may well restore motion[97,98]. The procedure in most cases will involve a dorsal approach and exploration of all possible causes of contracture — extensor tendon, dorsal capsule, true collateral, accessory collateral, palmar plate[99], flexor sheath and flexor tendon in that sequence. After each is released, motion should be checked and for this and other reasons local anaesthesia is most helpful, for the patient can provide the power to move the joint (Fig. 2.74). In addition, his active function obviates the need, otherwise essential, to check through separate incisions that the motor tendons of the joint are free to function. Further, the range achieved can be demonstrated to the patient, potent reinforcement during immediate postoperative therapy. Hyperextension of the joint can be corrected by palmar plate repair, advancement or reconstruction[100].

If the articular surface is destroyed, soft tissue release will not suffice. Evaluation of perichondrial arthroplasty, by which it is hoped to restore cartilage cover to the bone ends, is still in progress[101-106]. Joint replacement in the young, post-traumatic hand is quite different from that in the crippled rheumatoid and should only be embarked upon

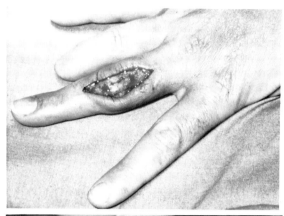

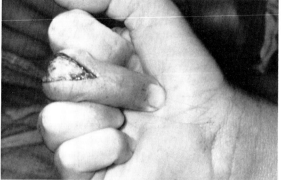

Fig. 2.74 Local anaesthesia in capsulectomy (see text).

after full discussion with the patient of the relatively limited experience available with respect to long-term results. If it is still requested, replacement arthroplasty is more likely to do well in the joints supported by adjacent normal joints in most activities, namely the carpometacarpal joint of the thumb all the metacarpophalangeal joints and the proximal inter-phalangeal joints of the middle and ring. In all other digital joints arthrodesis[107-109] should be strongly recommended. Selection of the angle of arthrodesis must be considered at the time of examination. The metacarpophalangeal joint and interphalangeal joint of the thumb should be fused in 20° of flexion, and the *distal* interphalangeal joints of the fingers at 10°, 20°, 30° and 40° of flexion, reading from index to small. These figures are adjusted to individual functional needs but less so than in the *proximal* interphalangeal joints where other considerations apply, as follows. In the index finger, the position should be such as brings the pulp of the finger in firm contact with that of the thumb (Fig. 2.75). In the ulnar three fingers, a position should be chosen which brings the finger down into power grasp, while avoiding undue malalignment of the pulp of the digit with the other fingers when the hand is extended. The latter depends entirely on the ability of the metacarpophalangeal joint to hyperextend (Fig. 2.76). Fortunately, this tends to increase from the radial to the ulnar side of the hand as does the need for proximal interphalangeal joint flexion to give powerful grasp. Thus, as a general rule, the angles chosen for arthrodesis are index 20°, middle 30°, ring 40°, and small 50°.

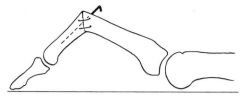

Fig. 2.76   The angle at which the proximal interphalangeal joint should be fused is determined by the available hyperextension of the metacarpophalangeal joint which permits the tip of the flexed digit to remain in the plane of the palm.

ADDUCTION DEFORMITY OR CONTRACTURE OF THE THUMB

This crippling loss of thumb function can come about as a result of one or any combination of a number of disorders:

  skin contracture
  adductor fibrosis
  basal joint disease (p. 234)
  loss of active opposition (Fig. 2.77)

It is imperative that all factors be dealt with in such a way

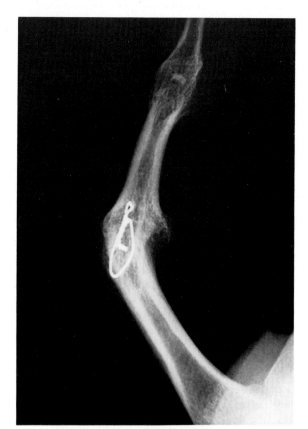

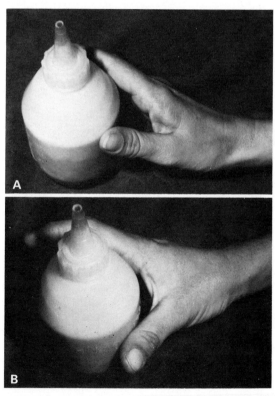

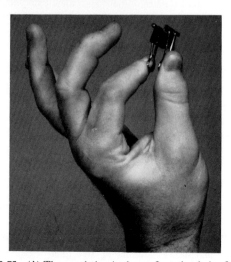

Fig. 2.75   (A) The angulation is chosen for arthrodesis of the proximal interphalangeal joint of the index finger that approximates the pulp of that digit to that of the thumb. (B) This is particularly important in this patient who has previously undergone fusion of the distal interphalangeal joint.

Fig. 2.77   This patient had sustained a high median nerve injury with resultant loss of opposition. Her attempts to grasp objects of large diameter are impeded by her inability to abduct the thumb. In this case, she has compensated to some extent by hyperextension of the metacarpophalangeal joint of the index finger. Span grasp in a hand with normal abduction is shown for comparison.

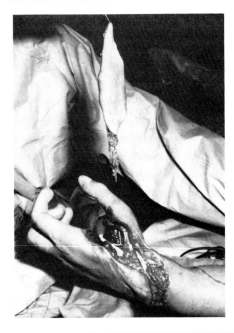

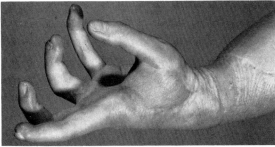

Fig. 2.78 Release of a severe first web space adduction contracture creates a large skin defect. This is best covered with pliable skin which does not fill the space gained with a bulky flap. Here a free dorsalis pedis flap is being applied. The patient is previously shown in Figure 2.23. (Case done in conjunction with Dr R. D. Acland).

as to avoid swift recurrence. For example, adductor release without provision of mobile adequate skin would be valueless (Fig. 2.78). Release with provision of skin will fail to give maximum benefit if the patient has no means to hold the thumb out in abduction, either static, in the form of a carpometacarpal arthrodesis or a temporary internal splint, or better dynamic, by provision of a strong opponensplasty at the time of release. In planning therefore, the surgeon should test all muscles commonly used for such a transfer. There are many satisfactory motors. One cautionary word may not be out of place. In considering and testing superficialis to the ring finger, the most popular tendon for opponens transfer, it is wise to carefully check the profundus to that finger, thus avoiding the embarrassing result of a powerful opponensplasty — and an immobile ring finger.

WRIST

Following injury to the wrist, problems present usually as a combination of pain and loss of motion and of grip strength. This pain is usually well-localized and characteristically is related to movement and is virtually, if not completely, relieved by immobilisation. This symptom-complex results in significant loss of grip strength. The presentation may be early, with a clear memory of the injury, or late with little or no recall. In the first case, the mechanism of injury should be elicited for it may offer guidance to the location and probable nature of the pathology. In particular, a history of a 'popping' or 'snapping' sound at the original incident suggests intercarpal ligamentous disruption. In the late case, it is possible that osteoarthritis or aseptic necrosis will be found.

Tenderness

Tenderness to palpation should be sought, first by gently flexing the wrist with the elbow resting on the examination table and palpating the radius, ulna, each carpal bone and intercarpal joint and finally each metacarpal base in turn; secondly, by extending the wrist and palpating the scaphoid and pisiform. Well-localized tenderness should be compared with the opposite hand and its position noted. This is an unusually important step since, in certain instances, it may prove to be the only guide to the pathology.

Pain on motion

The wrist is now carried passively into all positions — flexion and extension, supination and pronation, ulnar and radial deviation and finally rotated through the extremes of flexion, deviation and extension. Any limitation in *range of motion* should be noted but in particular, pain should be recorded, once again with particular reference to its site. The test should then be repeated while applying longitudinal compression, provided this does not cause excessive discomfort. During this manipulation 'popping'[110] may be felt and not infrequently subluxation of a carpal bone can be detected. Painful 'popping' may also be due to *recurrent subluxation of the extensor carpi ulnaris*[111] over the ulnar head. This is due to rupture of the restraining septum of the sixth dorsal compartment[112] and is reproduced by supination, flexion and ulnar deviation.

Recording range of motion

It is difficult to measure range of motion in the wrist joint in a consistent manner. Flexion and dorsiflexion can be recorded by marking the skin over four points — the head of the fifth metacarpal and the prominent styloid on its base to give a line for the hand; the ulnar head and its subcutaneous border for a line for the forearm. Still radial and ulnar deviation remain difficult to document. The whole process is made simple and accurate by making the measurements on X-rays taken in the extremes of motion.

Radiological examination

Radiological examination should now be undertaken employing any or all of the views detailed on p. 46. This may reveal

carpal instability p. 53
Kienbock's disease p. 238
Osteoarthritis — radiocarpal, intercarpal or carpo-metacarpal p. 233
Non-union of the scaphoid p. 127

The four conditions listed above will account for the great majority of patients with painful wrists of skeletal origin. A fifth, closely related to the wrist joint often proves difficult to treat, namely, disorders of the

Inferior radio-ulnar joint —

(a) *with Colles' fracture:* in many patients the ulna become relatively too long as a result of collapse of the radius causing *impingement* on the triquetral and lunate. If pain persists after wrist motion has reached a plateau and especially if supination causes added pain, ulnar head resection is usually efficacious.

(b) *subluxation:* traumatic subluxation is evidenced by undue prominence of the ulnar head and often painful dislocation and relocation of the ulna on pronation and supination. If seen immediately after it occurs, the torn triangular fibrocartilaginous complex (TFCC) *may* heal with immobilisation in full supination for six weeks,[114] or, despite persistent subluxation, pain may resolve.

(c) *perforated TFCC*[114]: This can be demonstrated by arthrography, and is associated with *positive ulnar variance* and also with symptomatic chondromalacia of the points of abnormal contact between ulna and lunate.

These latter two conditions may be treated by ulnar head resection if conservative measures fail but the results may be disappointing. This differs from the good results in troublesome Colles' fractures, probably because of the demands of a different age group and also because (b) and (c) above are isolated injuries, not masked by the problems of a concomitant radial fracture.

Those wrist disorders not revealed by simple X-ray will require additional investigation.

Local anaesthesia infiltrated into the previously identified tender area may prove both therapeutic and diagnostic. This should be done very precisely so the examiner is certain of the anatomical location of each serial injection. If all other studies are negative but symptoms persist, this may be the only evidence for exploration as in *chronic sprains of the carpometacarpal joints of the fingers*[115] for which arthrodesis is curative.

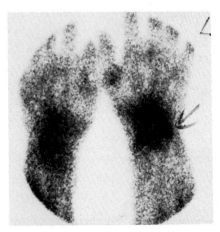

Fig. 2.79 Bone scan of this persistently troublesome carpus revealed increased uptake in the ulnar portion of the carpus.

Technetium bone scan (Fig. 2.79) if negative, will reassure and dictate conservative management; if positive, will help to localise the area for further study (see also diagnostic plan on page 55).

Polytomography (trispiral or ellipsoid) may highlight undetected fractures or small bone lesions.

Arthrography will reveal ligamentous lesions which are incomplete but may have been suspected by tenderness and by relief with local anaesthetic. If such a lesion is shown and does not settle with rest, limited carpal fusion will effect relief (Fig. 2.80).

If the more obvious skeletal causes have been eliminated by X-ray, the soft tissue causes of pain around the wrist — deQuervain's and other inflammatory disorders (p. 242) — should be pursued before the sophisticated tests listed above are embarked upon.

Nerves — peripheral

In assessing the effect of nerve injury, which may have been complete or partial, single or multiple, accurately repaired or not, after a period of recovery which may still be progressing the surgeon requires knowledge of the anatomy of the upper limb possibly more complete than in any other aspect of hand examination. Since recovery may be incomplete the assessment can be of value only if the same tests are repeated at regular intervals of six weeks, wherever possible by the same examiner. The tests selected should be as objective as can be devised.

In observing the hand of a patient known or believed to have a nerve injury, clues to the location of the injury may be seen.

SKIN CHANGES

a. *Site of scar.* The site of scars in the arm allied to a knowledge of the surface markings of the major structures at risk, leads the surgeon to suspect which nerves may be involved.

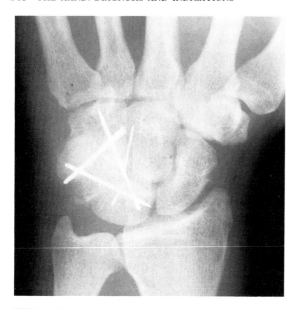

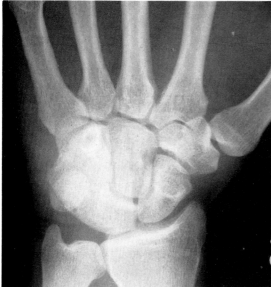

Fig. 2.80   The patient in Figure 2.79 was subjected to exploration and changes were found between the triquetral and the hamate and lunate. (A) Intercarpal fusion was undertaken. (B) The patient was subsequently free of all pain and achieved a grip strength equal to that of the opposite hand.

b. *Ulcers.* Areas with no protective sensation are injured inadvertently — these are most commonly on the finger tips.

c. *Smoothness, dryness and cleanliness of skin.* The skin ridges in areas of sensory loss become less pronounced. This smoothness and loss of sweating minimizes dirt retention. Allied to reduced use this results in the area being much cleaner than those adjacent.

d. *Absence of calluses.* The hands of workmen show thickening of the palmar skin. In areas of sensory loss the skin becomes softer and calluses disappear.

e. *Circulatory and colour changes.* Due to absence of sympathetic control the colour of adjacent innervated and denervated areas often differs markedly, the denervated area being most frequently red and shiny.

f. *Temperature changes.* For the first few weeks after nerve injury the denervated digits are warm, as their vessels have been freed from sympathetic control. Thereafter the fingers become cold to the touch when compared with adjacent, innervated areas.

ALTERATION OF CONTOUR

Muscle wasting
Paralysed muscles become increasingly atrophic. Those muscles in the hand which do so most markedly are
  abductor pollicis brevis — median nerve (Fig. 2.81)
  abductor digit minimi ⎫
  1st dorsal interosseous ⎭ ulnar nerve

The wasting is most easily appreciated if the injured is compared with the uninjured hand. The deformity has two components — depression due to loss of muscle bulk and prominence of bones normally masked by muscle. In more proximal injuries, the arm and forearm lose bulk and this should be recorded as a difference in circumference from the unaffected arm at a measured 10 cm distance above and below the olecranon.

Spindling of the fingers
The bulk of subcutaneous tissue becomes reduced in most fingers deprived of their sensory supply and this results in a

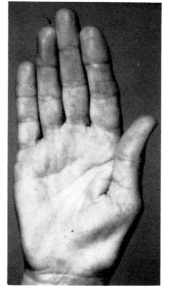
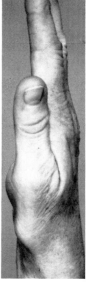

Fig. 2.81A & B   Atrophy of the abductor pollicis brevis in median nerve injury.

noticeable tapering of the distal portion of the affected digits.

PATHOGNOMONIC POSTURES

Changes in posture due to nerve injury may be very evident at rest or may only be observed or become more pronounced when the patient is asked to perform certain functions. As a general rule, the higher the lesion, the more likely is the postural change to be seen immediately. With the passage of time also, a postural *deformity*, which is passively correctable, becomes a *contracture*, which is not. This is due to joint changes and one of the major responsibilities of those following a patient with a nerve injury is to prevent contracture by correct splinting. Such splinting often serves to improve function also.

Cerebral palsy

This differs from all other nerve lesions commonly affecting the upper extremity — apart from a cerebrovascular accident, which resembles it in many ways — in that the lesion is of an upper motor neuron rather than a lower and there is therefore usually a marked degree of *spasticity*. There are two groups of disorder:

extrinsic —   flexion contracture of elbow, wrist and fingers
                 pronation contracture of the forearm
                 adduction ± flexion contracture of the thumb
intrinsic —   intrinsic-plus deformity of the fingers, that is, flexion of the metacarpophalangeal joints and extension, often swan-neck, of the interphalangeal joints.

(The further evaluation of cerebral palsy patients is on p. 170.)

Upper roots of the brachial plexus — 'Erb's palsy'[116] (Fig. 2.82)

Originally described in relation to birth injuries this injury may be produced by any powerful blow to the shoulder with associated contralateral flexion of the cervical spine. This is not uncommon in motorcyclists wearing a crash helmet, which skids on landing throwing the force on to the angle of the neck and shoulder. The roots are disrupted from above in turn.

C5 and C6. Due to loss of shoulder abduction (deltoid) and external rotation (spinati), of elbow flexion (biceps, brachialis, brachioradialis) and forearm supination (biceps, supinator) the arm hangs by the patient's side internally rotated, extended at the elbow and pronated.

C7. The additional loss of elbow extension (triceps) increase the limpness of the posture while the loss of wrist extension (extensor carpi radialis longus et brevis and ulnaris) results in some wrist flexion. In its full form this

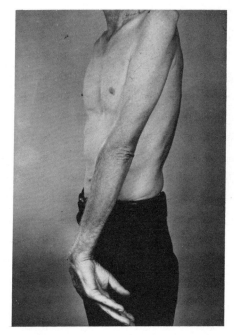

Fig. 2.82 *Erb's palsy.* The patient sustained a brachial plexus gunshot injury. He shows shoulder adduction, elbow extension, forearm pronation and wrist flexion — the 'porter's tip' position.

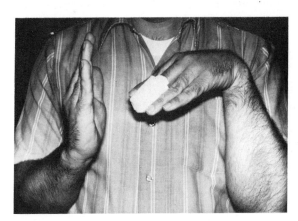

Fig. 2.83 This patient had sustained a spontaneous radial palsy and demonstrates the characteristic 'drop wrist' posture.

turns the palm of the hand upwards to the rear at the level of the mid-thigh, a posture adopted for the surreptitious receipt of money — 'porter's tip' position.

Radial nerve above the elbow

Due to loss of the wrist and finger extensors, a 'drop wrist' posture results (Fig. 2.83). The fingers may appear to extend remarkably well but this is due to (i) the tenodesis effect of wrist flexion in extending the metacarpophalangeal joints and (ii) active intrinsic extension of the interphalangeal joints.

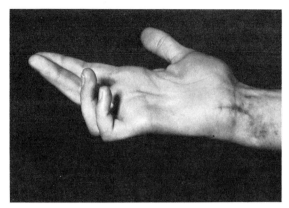

Fig. 2.84   An ulnar claw hand.

Ulnar nerve at the wrist — 'claw hand' (Fig. 2.84)[117]
The characteristic posture of hyperextension of the metacarpophalangeal joints and flexion of the interphalangeal joints is adopted by the ring and small fingers only in pure ulnar nerve loss at the wrist. Paralysis of the flexor digit minimi and the lumbrical muscles of these fingers disturbs the balance of the meta-carpophalangeal joints of which these muscles are the prime flexors. If the joints are sufficiently mobile, the long extensors hyperextend them and in young hands this it may do by as much as 60°. The long extensors thus lose and the long flexors gain mechanical advantage at the interphalangeal joints, which therefore adopt a flexed posture.

'Ulnar clawing' does not result in all ulnar nerve lesions. This can be for any one of the following reasons:
1. *The ulnar nerve does not serve the lumbricals.* The lumbricals exercise control over the metacarpophalangeal joints, as is evidenced by the absence of clawing in the middle and index fingers in ulnar nerve injuries, when all intrinsics to these fingers other than the lumbricals are paralysed. The innervation of the lumbricals varies and hence, so will the presence of clawing. High ulnar nerve injuries in the presence of a Martin-Gruber anastomosis (p. 00) will also show no clawing.
2. *The metacarpophalangeal joint is not hyperextensible, through age, disease, injury, or inherent stiffness.* This fact can be demonstrated in the recently acquired ulnar claw hand. By blocking the hyperextension of the metacarpophalangeal joint, clawing no longer occurs with extension. Prevention of metacarpophalangeal hyperextension is the basis of many operative procedures for ulnar claw hand.
3. *Either the long flexors or the long extensors are not functioning*
    (a)   If the ulnar nerve injury is above the motor branch to the flexor digitorum profundus of the

ring and small fingers, clawing does not occur. As the nerve recovers proximal to distal, the long flexors will recover first, and temporary clawing may then be seen.
    (b)   In the unusual event of an associated radial nerve injury above the branch to extensor digitorum or to the tendon itself.

Ulnar abducted finger[118] (Fig. 2.85)
If the metacarpophalangeal joint cannot hyperextend, the hand does not claw. In some of these patients, the loss of the third palmar interosseous causes the small finger to abduct markedly in extension. This is often an impediment when sliding the hand into narrow spaces, such as into a trouser pocket.

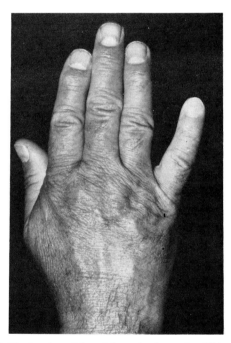

Fig. 2.85   An ulnar abducted finger in ulnar palsy. This occurs in patients in whom the metacarpophalangeal joint cannot hyperextend and thus the long extrinsic extensors abduct the finger, no resistance being offered by the paralysed third palmar interosseous.

Froment's sign[119] (Fig. 2.86)
The patient is asked to pull on a sheet of paper with index finger and thumb while the examiner withdraws it strongly. The normal patient maintains maximum contact of his digital pulp with the paper by extending the interphalangeal joint of the thumb. In ulnar palsy, for the reasons explained on page 30, the flexor pollicis longus is too powerful for the combined interphalangeal joint extensors weakened by the loss of the contribution from adductor pollicis. In addition, the control of the

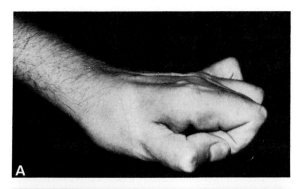

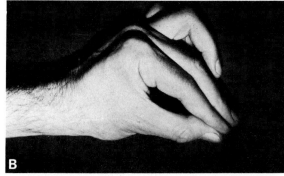

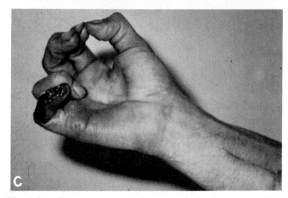

Fig. 2.86 *Froment's sign.* (A) In attempting to exert powerful key pinch in which the interphalangeal joint of the thumb is normally extended that joint flexes. Note the clawing of the small and ring fingers and also the wasting of the first dorsal interosseous.

(B) Froment's sign, wasting of the first dorsal interosseous and clawing, are again demonstrated in this patient with an ulnar nerve lesion.

(C) This patient shows all the deficits of an ulnar nerve injury — the Froment posture, clawing and sensory deficit as evidenced by the full thickness burn of the small finger which was sustained when it was inadvertently immersed in hot oil.

metacarpophalangeal joint is lost through the paralysis of adductor pollicis and the deep head of flexor pollicis brevis. It collapses into hyperextension, balance is lost and the interphalangeal joint flexes. Many other active postural tests have been described to confirm ulnar nerve paralysis[120].

Median nerve

The radial half of the hand becomes flattened. This is partly because of thenar muscle wasting but also because the loss of abductor pollicis brevis results in an adducted posture of the thumb. This is for two reasons:

a. adductor pollicis is unopposed;

b. extensor pollicis longus, always an adductor of the adducted thumb, becomes more strongly so due to shift of the dorsal expansion under the action of the unopposed adductor pollicis.

Combined median and ulnar nerve at the wrist[121] — 'simian hand'

A full claw hand *plus* thenar and hypothenar flattening *plus* thumb adduction and flexion results. This posture is very characteristic and has been called the 'simian hand' because of its similarity to the hand of the ape. Apart from combined ulnar and median nerve injuries, this posture is also seen in

Charcot-Marie-Tooth disease — an inherited disorder, this is characterised by palsy commencing peripherally, firstly in the lower limb. It affects primarily median and ulnar innervated intrinsics, sparing the radial nerve and usually leaving sensation intact (Fig. 2.87).

Lower roots of the brachial plexus: 'Klumpke paralysis'[122]: C8 and T1. This results from violent upward traction on the upper limb such as can occur obstetrically in management of breech or arm presentation. The roots are disrupted from below. Loss of all intrinsic muscles of the hand produces flattening and marked wasting but there may be no dramatic change in posture due to weakness or absence of function in the long flexors.

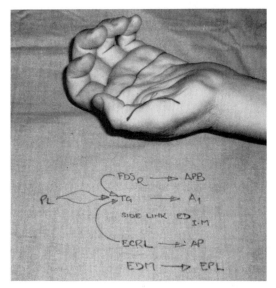

Fig. 2.87 The characteristic flat claw hand of median and ulnar nerve motor loss is seen here in a patient with Charcot-Marie-Tooth disease. The planned transfers and tenodeses are drawn out on the sterile sheet.

TINEL'S SIGN[123,124]

If the ends of growing axons are tapped, tingling paraesthesiae are felt in the area of sensory distribution of the nerve to which these axons belong. It should be clearly understood that the Tinel's sign gives no indication whatsoever of

1. *the quality of eventual recovery,* which may be anything from mere paraesthesiae to acceptable two point discrimination,

2. *the quantity of eventual recovery,* for the sign can be evoked from a very small percentage of the total nerve axon population.

The test is performed by lightly tapping as in percussing the chest commencing distally and proceeding proximally along the line of the nerve (Fig. 2.88). The Tinel's sign is elicited over a varying length of the nerve. The most

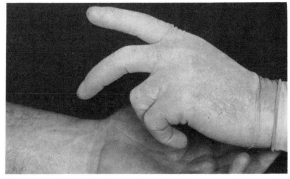

Fig. 2.88 A Tinel's sign can be elicited by percussing over the line of the involved nerve with the flexed middle finger as in percussing the chest.

proximal and distal points of the Tinel's sign are localised by measuring their distance from chosen fixed bony points.

Table 2.2   Dermatomes and cutaneous nerve distribution

Dermatomes (Figs. 2.89 and 2.90)

on top of the shoulder	C4	ulnar aspect forearm and hand	C8
outer aspect upper arm	C5	inner aspect elbow	T1
radial aspect forearm and hand	C6	inner aspect upper arm	T2
hand *(overlapped by adjacent dermatomes)*	C7		

Abbreviation in Figure	*Nerve*	*Cutaneous nerve distribution* (Figs. 2.89 and 2.90)
	supraclavicular nerves (C3, 4)	on top of shoulder
A	axillary nerve (C5, 6)	proximal lateral aspect of upper arm
LIC	lateral inferior cutaneous nerve of arm (C5, 6, a branch of the radial nerve)	distal lateral aspect of upper arm
LCF	lateral cutaneous nerve of the forearm (C5, 6, the termination the musculocutaneous nerve)	radial aspect of forearm
R	superficial radial nerve (C7, 8)	radial dorsum of the hand to the PIP joints[1]
M	median nerve (C6, 7, 8)	thumb, index, middle and radial side of ring finger
PCM	palmar cutaneous branch of the median nerve (C6, 7, 8)	palmar triangle[2]
U	ulnar nerve (C8, T1)	small and ulnar side of ring finger hypothenar eminence
DSU	dorsal sensory branch of the ulnar nerve (C8, T1)	ulnar dorsum of the hand to the PIP joints[3]
MCF	medial cutaneous nerve of the forearm (C8, T1, from the medial cord)	ulnar border of forearm
MCA	medial cutaneous nerve of the arm (C8, T1, from the medial cord)	inner aspect of the upper arm (distal)
ICB	intercostobrachial nerve (T2)	inner aspect of the upper arm (proximal)
PCF	posterior cutaneous nerve of the forearm (C5–8, from the radial nerve)	dorsum of forearm

1. The dorsal innervation of the fingers distal to the proximal interphalangeal joints is from the digital nerves via constant dorsal digital branches.
2. The 'palmar triangle' is that small area defined by the proximal palmar crease and the thenar and hypothenar creases. Sensory change there is significant since the palmar cutaneous nerve arises some centimetres above the wrist and does not pass through the carpal tunnel. The nerve may supply more distal palmar skin, as far as the PIP joints.
3. Sensory change in dorsal sensory territory has similar significance in ulnar nerve disorders as palmar cutaneous loss in median nerve problems — it localizes the lesion proximal to the wrist.

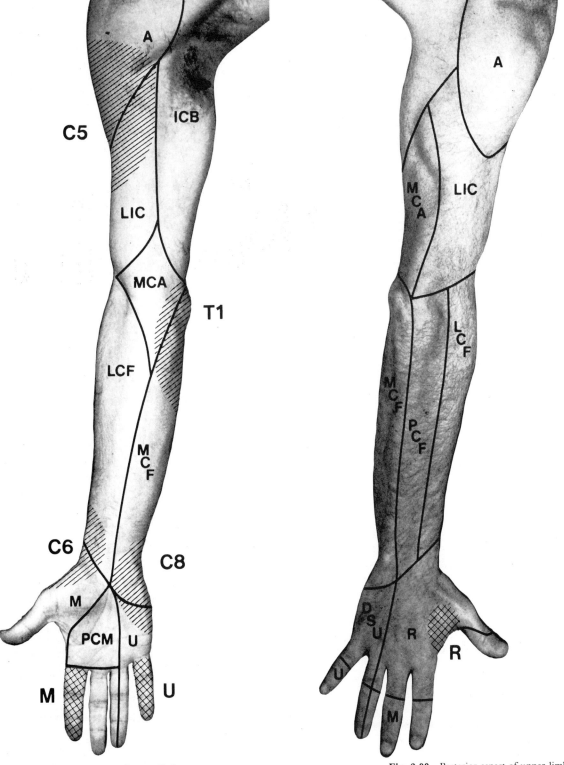

Fig. 2.89 Anterior aspect of upper limb.

Fig. 2.90 Posterior aspect of upper limb.

In these figures, the regions served by cutaneous nerves are outlined and lettered according to the abbreviations given in the table. Due to overlap these are not absolute territories of innervation, with the result that hypaesthesia, not anaesthesia, is the outcome of cutaneous nerve division. This also explains the differences to be found on comparing various anatomical texts. Areas of absolute sensory supply of the nerve roots and of the radial (R), median (M) and ulnar (U) nerves are indicated by cross-hatching.

These should be recorded for further comparison as progression of the sign indicates continued axon growth. The rate of growth varies from 1 to 4 mm per day according to the age of the patient, the size of the axons involved and the level of the injury in the limb. Henderson, in exhaustive studies on prisoners-of-war[125], found the Tinel's sign most useful for drawing conclusions as follows

Strong Tinel at injury + none distally = no chance of recovery

Reducing Tinel at injury + advancing distally = good chance of useful recovery

Strong Tinel at injury + advancing distally = poor chance of useful recovery.

SENSORY ASSESSMENT (Table 2.2, Figs. 2.89 and 2.90)

The areas of the upper limb served by its several nerves are to be found illustrated in most textbooks of anatomy and general surgery. The diagrams do not correspond exactly, which is understandable, since there is significant overlap. Clinically, this overlap results in a patient under examination reporting a large area of 'different' sensation and a small area of *absolute sensory loss*. Precise boundaries are therefore neither present nor necessary to the examiner. Rather should he be aware of areas of different sensation significant in localising the site of a nerve injury. Further confusion is sometimes caused by the failure to distinguish between diagrams of dermatomes, which strictly are areas served by one spinal nerve, and diagrams of areas of cutaneous nerve distribution, which differ because most cutaneous nerves communicate with more than one spinal nerve via the brachial plexus.

The difficulties in assessing areas of sensory loss are several:

a. *Shrinkage* of the area of reduced sensation will occur, quickly in the first few days, and slowly thereafter.

b. *Joint sense* is rarely completely lost and therefore movement of the region may be misinterpreted as cutaneous sensation.

c. Any test of sensation which requires patient responses cannot be objective and will be unreliable in the young, the mentally unfit and in patients intent upon obtaining maximum compensation for injury. (See p. 112)

d. Even in total recent nerve division, the area of *absolute sensory loss* is small compared with the total area of reduced loss. Absolute sensory loss is most commonly limited to the following areas, which have been called *autonomous zones*:

ulnar nerve	palmar aspect of small finger
median nerve	palmar aspect of index finger
radial nerve	small area on the dorsum of the MP joint of the thumb

root C5	over the belly of the deltoid
C6	the thenar eminence
C7	NIL
C8	ulnar border of the hand
T1	ulnar border of the elbow
T2	inner aspect of upper arm

Sweating

Sympathetic denervation following peripheral nerve injury results in loss of sweating. This loss is complete in the autonomous zone of the divided nerve. In the *intermediate zone* surrounding the autonomous, sweating is greatly diminished.

The presence of beads of sweat on innervated skin can be detected using the +20 dioptre lens of an ophthalmoscope. Loss of sweating is of functional importance, for the lack of the adhesion which sweat provides seriously interferes with span grasp of smooth cylindrical objects and with finger manipulations in precision or chuck grip. The latter problem can readily be appreciated by recalling the comparative difficulty of manipulating small objects with cold hands.

Smoothness is largely due to the absence of sweat, the lack of which reduces the friction between the skin and objects moved across it. While this can be detected by the examiner's finger if his hands are cold, clearly any sweat on his hands will substitute for that of the patient and the distinction may not be clear.

The tactile adhesion test[126] (p. 34). The friction on normal and denervated fingers is best tested with a smooth plastic object such as the barrel of a pen (Fig. 2.91). In the denervated areas the plastic glides smoothly and compares with the definite resistance felt on areas of normal innervation.

In the unusual situation where sweating is absent from even sensible areas, it has been stimulated for the purpose of testing by several means, including emotive conversation!

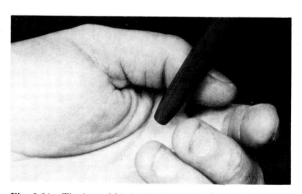

Fig. 2.91 The loss of friction in denervated fingers due to absence of sweating can be appreciated by lightly moving a plastic object over the surface. The difference in friction can best be detected by comparison with an adjacent normal finger.

a. *pneumatic tourniquet.* If applied to the upper arm at above systolic pressure for ten to fifteen minutes, the reactive hyperaemia consequent on release is accompanied by sweating in normally innervated areas.

b. *wrapping in hot blankets* is especially appropriate for children.

c. *hot room, heated bed cradle* or specially designed '*hot box*'.

d. *exercise*

One of the above methods is most often employed before conducting formal sweat pattern tests.

Sweat pattern tests have been designed, most of which depend on staining techniques and some on the fact that dry skin has a much higher resistance than moist to the passage of an electrical current[127].

Staining techniques

Iodine-starch. Iodine is painted on the area to be assessed. Starch powder is then dusted over the iodine. Sweating areas becomes dark.

Ninhydrin printing test[128-130]. The digits are pressed in turn on a strip of paper. This is then developed in acidified 1% ninhydrin in acetone, dried and heated. The sweat pattern of black dots which emerges can then be fixed in acidified copper nitrate in acetone.

Bromophenol blue. In this test the paper has been previously immersed in 5% bromophenol blue in acetone. The sweat pattern appears as blue dots on a yellow background.

Cobalt chloride. A solution of 25% cobalt chloride in 99% alcohol is painted on the injured hand; perspiration changes the solution from blue to pink.

Quinizarin. Quinizarin powder, sodium carbonate and rice starch are dusted firmly on the patient's extremity before stimulating sweating, which produces a deep violet colour.

All of these tests have the disadvantage of being time consuming, while some are messy. Seddon, who employed the quinizarin test for ten years, stated that the regular employment of one of these tests is unnecessary. They are of use where meticulous visual records are required.

Return of sweating to an area of sensory loss is one of the last cutaneous functions to return during nerve regeneration and closely parallels the return of two point discrimination. There are three exceptions to this useful rule:

1. Sweating is *not* lost in lesions of the roots of the brachial plexus proximal to the entry of the postganglionic sympathetic fibres — important in examination of patients who have suffered a brachial plexus injury (p. 168).

2. Sweating returns to distant flaps applied to the hand, even if two point discrimination does *not* return to the flap, probably due to sudomotor fibres accompanying ingrowing vessels since the sweating disappears with brachial block.

3. Patients who have undergone cervical sympathectomy.

With these rare exceptions, examination of sweating is a useful immediate guide to the patient's sensory recovery. If present, then the examiner should proceed to qualitative evaluation of the static two point discrimination. If absent, then first pin-prick and then awareness of moving and constant touch should be assessed.

Pinprick

If absence of sweating suggests dense sensory loss then the distribution of loss should be mapped out. This can be swiftly and accurately done using a pin wheel (Fig. 2.92), moving from areas of normal to abnormal sensation, marking the points of change on the skin. These should then be transferred to an outline of the hand in the patient's record. Pain perception is involved in the use of the pin wheel and the area of analgesia does not quite correspond with that of anaesthesia, being somewhat smaller. Once pinprick is present, the patient has entered the stage of 'protective sensation'.

Touch — moving and constant

If pinprick is present throughout, then moving and constant touch should be applied to the area under examination. By using his own finger the examiner can be certain that contact has been made. Some precautions should be taken to avoid misleading responses.

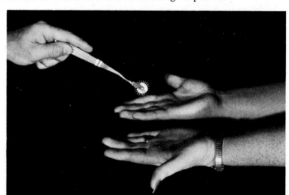

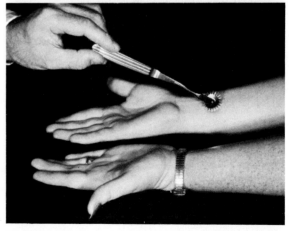

Fig. 2.92 The pinwheel provides a swift and adequate method of mapping out an area of sensory change.

1. Comparison should always be made with areas known to be normal on either the same or the other hand.
2. Occasional mock motions should be made without making contact to ensure that the patient is responding to touch and not simply to the examiner's movements.
3. Care should be taken to test known 'significant areas' such as the areas of absolute loss.

Moving touch will be appreciated before static and the presence of either is the signal to move to their qualitative equivalent, moving or static two point discrimination.

Two point discrimination (2PD) (Fig. 2.93)
This test is performed either with a calibrated caliper or, more simply, with a paper clip twisted into shape. The test should first be explained to the patient and a quick test done on the opposite hand, for rare cases of congenital absence of 2 point discrimination have been reported. The points of the caliper are set at 15 mm at first and progressively brought together as accurate responses are obtained.

As the minimum distance apart at which the patient can discriminate is approached, errors will be made. At this stage the following discipline must always be adopted.

1. An interval of 3–4 seconds should be allowed between applications of the caliper to the skin.
2. The caliper should be applied with only slight force, just less than that required to cause blanching of the skin around each point (Fig. 2.93C and 2.93D).
3. When two points are being applied they must make contact simultaneously and should be in the line of the digit.
4. The test should commence at the finger tips and should proceed across all finger tips before being carried out more proximally.
5. The same marking system should be used in all tests. Omer[131] — 2 correct out of 3 applications is a 'pass'. Moberg[132] — 10 applications of two points and 10 applications of one point are made randomly[133]. The total of *incorrect* one point applications is subtracted from the total of *correct* two point applications. An answer of five or more is considered a 'pass'.

The values for normal two point discrimination differ from one area of the hand to another[134] (Fig. 2.94). It is necessary for the surgeon to be aware of this to recognize

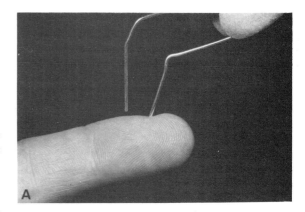

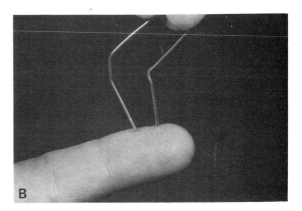

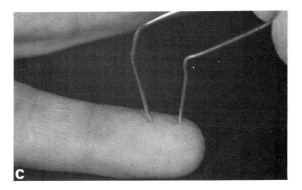

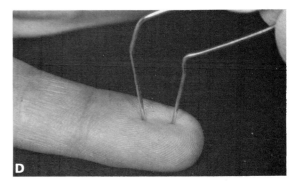

Fig. 2.93(A & B) Two point discrimination is determined by alternatively applying one or two points to the area under examination. A very satisfactory tool for this test can be produced by twisting a paper clip.

(C) Little force should be applied in testing for two points. If too much force is applied, D, the sensory receptors between the two points will be stimulated and, even in the presence of two point discrimination, the patient will feel the application of only one.

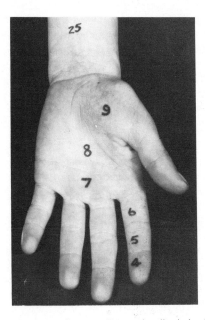

Fig. 2.94 The values for normal two point discrimination differ significantly in various areas of the hand and are shown here in millimetres.

complete recovery and to avoid wasting time using settings too close for even the normal hand.

distal phalanx	3–5 mm
middle phalanx	3–6 mm
proximal phalanx	4–7 mm
palm	
distal to distal palmar crease	5–8 mm
centre of palm	6–9 mm
thenar and hypothenar	7–10 mm
dorsum	7–10 mm
forearm	20–50 mm
arm	65–70 mm

The results of two point discrimination are seriously compromised if the hand is oedematous or callused.

This is a meticulous and time-consuming test. If the results on separate occasions, often by different observers, are to accurately assess regeneration, this care and time is necessary.

Moving[135] *and static (constant).* Moving two-point discrimination depends for its presence on the quickly adapting nerve fibres which return more quickly and in greater density than the slowly adapting fibres on which constant touch depends. Thus moving 2PD returns earlier, by some 6 months, and has a value generally 8–10 mm smaller, or better, than constant 2PD. It is a measure of the capability of the hand to feel objects provided hand motion is possible, which is the normal circumstance. Constant 2PD indicates the capacity of the hand to be aware of objects held quite still which usually returns when constant

2PD is less than 15 mm. From the above it will be realised that a hand with 10 mm of moving 2PD will be able to detect and identify objects unseen, but that once that object is lifted and held immobile, the patient will not know whether or not he still has it in his grasp.

Programme of sensory evaluation and care after nerve repair

To perform the complete battery of tests outlined above is both unnecessary and illogical. Rather should the patient progress through a series of stages. During the time normally expected for axon growth, the presence of an advancing Tinel is sufficient confirmation of progress and skin and joint care fulfill the patient's needs. Once advance and time has proceeded, pinprick and touch perception should be assessed. When moving touch returns, moving 2PD can serve as the sole criterion for recovery and the patient commences an intensive course of daily 'sensory re-education'[136,137]. Once moving 2PD falls below 10 mm the surgeon should seek the constant 2PD which once found can then serve as the monitor of the final stages.

Grading sensory recovery

Based upon the tests of light touch, pain and two point discrimination, sensory recovery can be graded according to the scale adopted by the (British) Medical Research Council:

S0	No sensation
S1	Pain sensation
S2	Pain and some touch sensation
S3	Pain and touch with no over-reaction
S3+	Some two point discrimination
S4	Complete recovery

All assessments are based on recovery of sensory faculties in the autonomous areas of the injured nerve.

This system will still be encountered in some reports and is included for that reason, but should now be superceded by a system based on a statement of the stage that a patient has reached hence,

anaesthetic
  → pin-prick (protective)
    → moving touch
      → moving 2PD of X mm
        → static 2PD of Y mm

Other clinical sensory tests

The important aspects of clinical testing are that it should advise of progress or arrest of reinnervation and that it should be as objective as possible. Quite apart from the methods of assessment detailed above many other clinical tests have been used and still are used by different clinicians. These will not all be described here because space does not allow it, because it would possibly cause confusion, because some have been found to be of questionable accuracy[138] and because the author does not use them. With one exception.

In infants

Wrinkling (Fig. 2.95)[139]. In very young children it may be difficult to perform even simple sweat tests although textile adhesion is usually detectable. If the normal hand is immersed in warm water for five minutes the digital pulps become wrinkled. It has been noted that this wrinkling occurs only in skin with some sensory innervation, remaining smooth in denervated areas. The exact stage of sensory return after injury at which this phenomenon disappears has not been established.

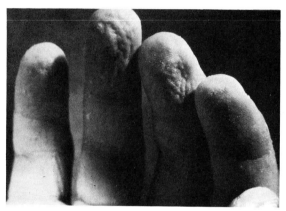

Fig. 2.95   This patient who is recovering from division and primary repair of her radial digital nerve to the index finger, shown on the right of the picture, has had the hand immersed in warm water for a period of five minutes. The very characteristic wrinkling which is produced in normal skin is seen on the small, ring, and middle fingers and is starting to reappear on the index finger.

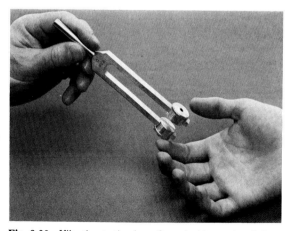

Fig. 2.96   Vibration testing is performed with a tuning fork. One of the tines should be applied to the tip of finger. Vibration sense returns at 256 cycles per second after the return of constant touch.

Vibration[140,141] (Fig. 2.96). Once wrinkling returns, the child's progress can be followed by the use of tuning forks. Most infants are entertained rather than frightened by this tool and respond perceptibly to vibration. Application of vibration at 30 cycles per second returns between pinprick and moving touch and at 256 cycles per second after the return of constant touch. Results, however, may be equivocal.

PAIN

Pain may also be elicited in the course of examination. It falls under four broad headings.

Neuroma — painful paraesthesia as described below are caused by palpating a neuroma.

Burning pain — this is sometimes present over the nerve distal to Tinel's sign.

Over-reaction (hyperpathia) — return of sensation to an area is often accompanied by hypersensitivity, which causes the patient to back away from the examining hand. Protection and disuse may result. This must be recognized and firmly discouraged for the patient has reached an important juncture. If allowed to continue protection, an established pattern of hypersensitivity and disuse will be created. If, on the other hand, the patient is exhorted to engage in 'sensory rehabilitation', recovery and full function can be anticipated. Rehabilitation requires the patient to make more contact with the previously denervated digit than others, and with as wide a variety of surfaces as possible.

Reflex sympathetic dystrophy (p. 108), of which *causalgia*[142] is a particularly intractable form resulting from nerve injury.

Neuroma

If, on palpating the scar, the patient withdraws or complains of pain of a tingling nature, this is strong evidence of a neuroma adjacent to the scar. A large neuroma may be visible or its margins palpable. The exact location of a smaller neuroma can be defined by repeating the palpation with a bluntly pointed instrument. More than one neuroma may be present when a cutaneous nerve has been divided. Probing should therefore be performed around all margins of the scar marking each neuroma with a skin pencil (Fig. 2.97). A persistently tender neuroma may respond to transcutaneous nerve stimulation but if not is an indication for nerve exploration, as the patient will be understandably reluctant to use the hand normally (Fig. 2.98). The choice of surgical procedure for relief of neuroma problems attests to the lack of universal success with any[143-145]. Certainly whichever is chosen, immediate postoperative sensory re-education contributes greatly to success.

Bowler's thumb[146,147]

In ten-pin bowling, the edge of the thumb-hold presses

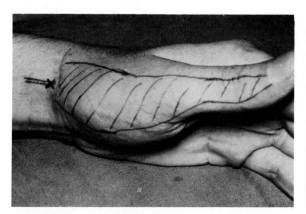

Fig. 2.97 This patient had sustained a division of the superficial branch of the radial nerve during release of de Quervain's stenosing tenovaginitis. The resultant sensory loss has been mapped out using a pinwheel and the neuroma located with a probe marked with a cross.

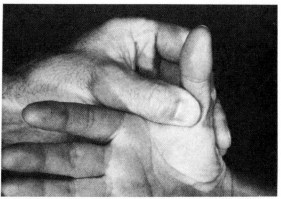

Fig. 2.99 Palpation of a firm nodule which produces paraesthesiae in the thumb. The nodule being mobile transversely but not longitudinally is diagnostic of a 'bowler's thumb'.

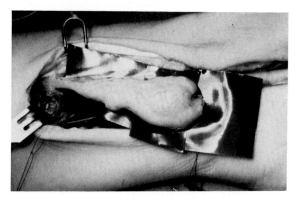

Fig. 2.98 Quite apart from loss of sensation this patient understandably had an extremely sensitive neuroma which prevented all use of the hand.

firmly against the palmar aspect of the proximal phalanx of the thumb. At the point of pressure, both digital nerves to the thumb lie close together over the sheath of flexor pollicis longus and are therefore compressed against an unyielding structure. Minor injury to the nerve or nerves results but is rarely sufficient to cause the player to give up the game. The trauma is therefore repeated and a neuroma in continuity forms.

Symptoms. The patient complains of pain on the palmar aspect of the thumb which may be associated with numbness on one or other or both aspects of the thumb pulp.

Examination. Palpation reveals a nodule, which, if the examiner is not familiar with the diagnosis, may be mistaken for a ganglion. It is more mobile than a flexor sheath ganglion in a transverse plane but not along the axis of the thumb. Firm pressure on the swelling may produce paraesthesiae in the digital nerve distribution (Fig. 2.99).

Indications. There *was* only one cure for this condition — to quit bowling. However, transfer of the ulnar digital nerve to the dorsal aspect of the adductor pollicis has been described[148].

MOTOR ASSESSMENT (see Appendix, p. 351)

All major muscles in the injured limb are tested. This is commonly not done because specific injuries produce specific muscle paralysis. However, such selectivity is not acceptable for a number of reasons:

1. Nerve injury may be partial only.
2. Recovery after repair may be only partial.
3. In multiple penetrative lacerations, such as are inflicted by shattered glass, branches of main nerves may have been divided, either alone or in combination with division of the main trunk.
4. In traction or compression injuries, the muscle loss may be of an unpredictable distribution.
5. Loss of function in isolated muscles may not be appreciated by the patient nor recognized by the surgeon unless a full systematic examination is performed and yet it may seriously reduce the patient's power or manipulative ability.
6. Innervation may be anomalous. In a small minority of patients cross-links exist between the three main nerves of the upper limb. The *Martin-Gruber anastomosis*[149,150], is an anomaly in which motor fibres, normally carried in the ulnar nerve throughout its course, join it from the median only in the forearm. The anastomosis may be from the median nerve proper or from the anterior interosseous nerve. The clinical significance is in high injuries above the link. In a complete anastomosis, the consequence will be

high ulnar nerve   no motor loss
high median nerve   total motor loss in the hand

In the first instance, low followed by high median nerve block will distinguish the anomaly from a partial ulnar nerve lesion. In the latter, exploration will reveal an intact ulnar nerve and, if done in the 48 hours after injury, stimulation of the cut median nerve distally will demonstrate its innervation of all of the small muscles of the hand.

In the course of examination, it is essential that the patient fully understands what is required of him. Several approaches may be employed.

'Bend it like this.' The patient is invited to copy with his injured limb a movement demonstrated by the examiner. While satisfactory with coarse movement such as bending the elbow, the examiner cannot always be certain whether or not the patient has fully understood.

'Do this with your good hand and then with the bad' (Fig. 2.100). A better approach, this clearly shows that the patient understands and also demonstrates his normal range in the uninjured hand as the criterion against which his injured hand is to be judged. However, it presupposes the presence of a 'good' hand and bilateral injuries are not uncommon. Further, it is often the case that patients 'forget' how to perform some movement with the injured hand and the wrong conclusion may be drawn.

'Hold your hand like that, keep it there, don't let me move it' (Fig. 2.101). The examiner places the hand or digit in the position which the muscle under test would normally produce and assesses the power it can generate. This method is the best, for the patient is not required to interpret a movement made by the examiner, it can be used in bilateral injuries and it places the limb in the required posture, reinforcing the patient's memory of how to achieve it. It also speeds the process of examination, because the examiner can record the passive range of joints while achieving each posture.

The examiner should palpate the relevant muscle belly and tendon while the patient is performing this manoeuvre (Fig. 2.102). In this way muscular activity can be detected which is not strong enough to maintain the joint position and when the joint on which the muscle acts has little or no range of motion due to injury or disease.

In conducting the muscle test it is important to determine the power which the muscle is capable of generating. This is significant not only in charting the patient's improvement but is necessary in planning a beneficial programme of tendon transfers where appropriate. The scale of power employed is

0 total paralysis — no contraction detectable on palpation
1 flicker — no movement, but contraction palpable
2 movement with gravity eliminated — this is achieved by placing the line of action of the muscle in a horizontal plane; this is not possible with all ʳuscles
3 movement against gravity

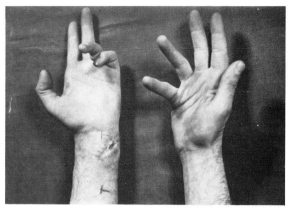

Fig. 2.100 This patient, previously seen in Figure 1.39, is demonstrating with the uninjured right hand that he is able to flex the metacarpophalangeal joint of his small finger with flexor digiti minimi but is unable to do so with the injured hand.

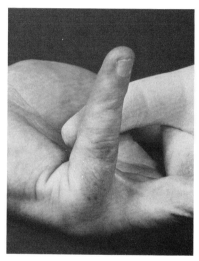

Fig. 2.101 In this instance, the patient's small finger has been placed in the position which flexor digiti minimi produces and has then been instructed to keep it in that position and resist the attempts of the examiner to move it. This demonstrates the presence of an active flexor digiti minimi.

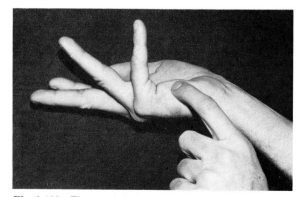

Fig. 2.102 The muscle belly under examination should be palpated as this test is performed.

4 movement against gravity and resistance

5 full power

While universally in use, this scale has serious limitations, for all weakly active muscles are graded power 4. Wherever possible a quantitative assessment should be employed. Those most used are:

Jamar grip dynamometer — this records grip power in pounds per square inch. It is important that the slot in which the adjustable bar is placed is noted (Fig. 2.103);

Pinch dynamometer (Fig. 2.104).

Clearly a large number of quantitative recording devices could be designed but it would be impractical to employ them all. In the case of certain muscles, the examiner may pit his own against that of the patient's, both normal and injured, thereby gauging the difference between them.

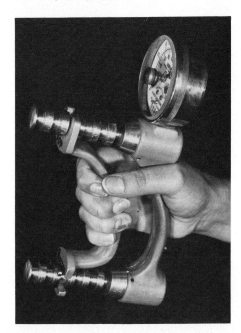

Fig. 2.103 The Jamar grip dynamometer is used to record the strength of power grasp.

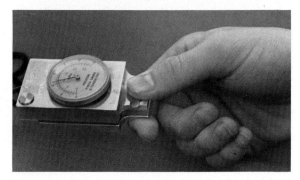

Fig. 2.104 The pinch dynamometer is employed to record pinch strength.

This can be done, for example, with abductor digit minimi, the first dorsal interosseous, the superficialis tendons and pronator teres. The reader can undoubtedly make the list more comprehensive, and the examiner's day more exhausting! This is not quantitative, however useful, and it remains that no widely applicable technique of categorizing grade 4 has been devised.

Although using similar digits the scale above has certain differences from that of the (British) Medical Research Council, and the examiner should be aware of it also to avoid confusion:

M0	No contraction
M1	Perceptible contraction in proximal muscles
M2	Perceptible contraction in both proximal and distal muscles
M3	All important muscles able to work against resistance
M4	All synergic and independent movements possible
M5	Complete recovery

This classification is more applicable in proximal nerve lesions and like the MRC sensory grading has probably outlived its usefulness.

The muscles tested, their action, and the nerve or root injury in which they are paralyzed are detailed in the Appendix (p. 351).

Reflexes (see Table 2.3)

Using a tendon hammer, reflexes should be tested with the relevant muscle contracted against moderate resistance.

Reflexes will be *absent* if the arc is interrupted, that is in lower motor neuron disorders such as division of a peripheral nerve. They will be *exaggerated* if higher control has been eliminated as in upper motor neuron injury and at certain levels in some cases of cord transection.

Having now accumulated all the necessary evidence, the precise level of a nerve lesion can be deduced in the majority of cases (see Table 2.4).

ELECTROMYOGRAPHY[151]

There are two basic groups of investigation in common use for study of muscle function following denervation and during regeneration and recovery. In the first the stimulus is applied directly to the muscle or to its nerve at the end plate and the differing response to different strengths of stimulus applied for different durations is an indication of the condition of the muscle. This group includes studies of the rheobase and chronaxie response to galvanic and faradic stimulation, strength duration curves and galvanic-tetanus ratios. The second group of tests are all based on electromyographic observation with and without stimulation of the relevant motor nerve. While both groups can provide useful information, the latter has certain advantages over the first.

Table 2.3 Reflexes

Muscle	Action	Percussion point	Level of reflex arc
Biceps (Fig. 2.105)	Elbow flexion	Biceps tendon	C5 (6)
Brachioradialis (Fig. 2.106)	Elbow flexion in neutral pronation-supination	Radial styloid	C(5) 6
Triceps (Fig. 2.107)	Elbow extension	Triceps tendon	C7
Extensor carpi ulnaris (Fig. 2.108)	Wrist extension and ulnar deviation	Base of 5th metacarpal	C8

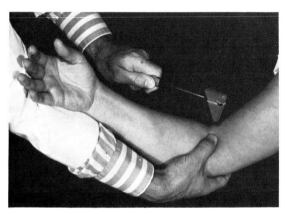

Fig. 2.105 *Biceps tendon reflex*. While palpating the tendon of biceps, the examiner's thumb nail is percussed with a tendon hammer.

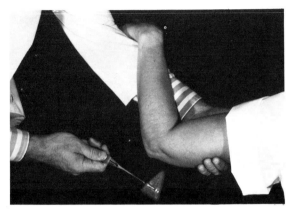

Fig. 2.107 *Triceps tendon reflex*. With the elbow flexed and relaxed over the examiner's arm, the triceps tendon is struck with the tendon hammer behind the elbow while palpating the belly of the muscWe in the upper arm.

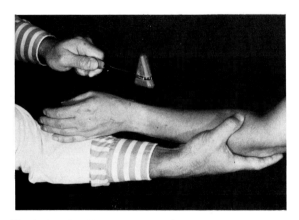

Fig. 2.106 *Brachioradialis tendon reflex*. With the arm in mid-pronation-supination and while palpating the belly of the brachioradialis the partially flexed forearm is percussed firmly with a tendon hammer proximal to the radial styloid.

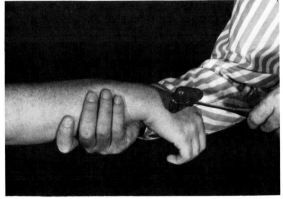

Fig. 2.108 *Extensor carpi ulnaris tendon reflex*. With the arm in pronation and the tendon of the extensor carpi ulnaris being palpated, the base of the fifth metacarpal is struck with a tendon hammer.

Table 2.4 Sensory, motor and reflex loss in differing levels or nerve injury

Abbreviations employed in table:
1. T = thumb   I = index   M = middle   R = ring   S = small
2. Muscles as in full muscle test chart (p. 351).

Nerve	Level	Loss		
		Sensory	*Motor*	*Reflex*
Median	wrist	palmar aspect TIM ½R	APB OP FPB (supf. head)	—
	above wrist	*add* 'palmar triangle'		
	elbow		*add* FCR PT FDS FDP (I and M) FPL PQ	
Ant. *interosseous*	forearm	nil	FPL FDP (I and M) PQ	
Ulnar	palm (deep branch)	nil	IO AP FPB (deep head)	
	wrist	palmar ½R S	*add* ADM FDM	
	above wrist	*add* ulnar aspect of dorsum		
	elbow		*add* FCU FDP (R and S)	
Radial	wrist	dorsum 1st web	—	—
Posterior *interosseous*	forearm	nil	ECU ED EDM EPL EI APL EPB	ECU
Radial	elbow	dorsum 1st web	*add* S	
	spiral groove	*add* dorsum of forearm	*add* ECRL BR ECRB	*add* BR
	axilla	*add* distal lateral aspect of upper arm	*add* T	*add* T
Medial cord	axilla	ulnar aspect of arm of forearm and of hand	*all* finger flexors *all* small hand muscles	nil
	subclavicular		*add* sternocostal head of PM	nil
Lateral cord	axilla	radial aspect of forearm and of hand	elbow flexion forearm pronation wrist flexion (FCR)	BB
	subclavicular		*add* clavicular head of PM	BB
Posterior cord	axilla	over deltoid posterior aspect upper arm dorsum of forearm dorsum 1st web	abduction of shoulder *all* upper limb extensors + BR	T BR ECU
	subclavicular		*add* LD	T BR ECU

Table 2.4 *(contd)*

Roots			motor loss of varying degree in isolated root lesions; increased in multiple.	
C5	posterior triangle	over deltoid	ext. rotation and abduction of shoulder	
C6	posterior triangle	thenar eminence	int. rotation and adduction of shoulder elbow flexion forearm supination	BR + BB
C7	posterior triangle	nil	elbow, wrist and finger extension forearm pronation	T ECU
C8	posterior triangle	ulnar border forearm	wrist, finger and thumb flexion	
T1	posterior triangle	inner aspect elbow	intrinsic movements	—

1. By adjusting the recording needle electrode the activity in any part of the muscle under investigation can be observed whereas direct muscle stimulation studies only the most superficial fibres.
2. The technique can be used for studying other causes of muscle weakness or paralysis such as neuropathies and compression syndromes.
3. Using the same basic equipment studies of sensory nerve activity can be performed.

For these reasons and in order to present a single, comprehensive means of investigating innervation electrically, only electromyography will be considered here.

The electrical activity in a muscle is recorded by inserting a sterile needle electrode into the appropriate muscle belly. Apart from insertion this should normally not be painful. If the discomfort persists it is possible that the needle has been inserted into the motor point — the point at which the neuromuscular end plates are situated. In this circumstance, the needle should be removed and reinserted. This should be done in any case on three or four occasions to each muscle noting the electrical activity for each successive insertion.

The activity recorded by the needle electrode is fed into an oscilloscope and it can then be appreciated both visually and by ear. Analysis of the wave form on the oscilloscope can be greatly eased by use of a storage monitor which retains each wave on a calibrated screen until it is cleared by the operator. Basically, five wave forms will be encountered (Table 2.5).

Nerve conduction studies are superimposed on this study by applying stimulating electrodes over the course of the motor nerve proximally and recording the muscle activity (Fig. 2.109). The stimulating current is gradually increased until a maximum action potential is attained. Using the storage monitor this is easily recognized and is usually achieved with a voltage of 400 V. A stimulus 20 per cent supramaximal is used thereafter. The time between the stimulus and the action potential can then be read off the calibrated scale and is referred to as *distal latency*. In

Table 2.5 **Electromyographic features**

Wave	Interpretation	Audio	Voltage
Straight line	Normal muscle at rest	Nil	Isoelectric
Motor-unit action potential	Contraction of normal muscle	Thump	10 mV
Fibrillation potential	Appears 2–3 weeks after injury Denervated muscle at rest Contraction — no effect	High pitched clicks	1 mV
Recovery action potential	Contraction of reinnervated muscle during recovery	Thump	10 mV
Recovered motor unit action potential	Recovered muscle hypertrophy of motor unit	Thump	20 mV

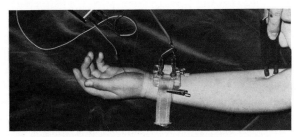

Fig. 2.109 Electromyographic nerve conduction studies in progress. A probe has been inserted in the abductor pollicis brevis and the stimulus is being applied over the median nerve at the antecubital fossa.

studying the median and ulnar nerves the electrode is inserted in abductor pollicis brevis and flexor digiti minimi respectively and the nerve stimulated at the wrist.

Normal distal motor latency
  Median 2.99 millisecs + 0.004 × age (SD ± 0.39)
  Ulnar 2.12 millisecs + 0.01 × age (SD ± 0.34)

In normal hands the distal latency of the ulnar nerve is two-thirds that of the median nerve. Latency can be affected by cold, compression and neuropathy. The test should therefore be conducted in comfortably warm surroundings and the latency should be checked in the normal limb to exclude generalized neuropathy.

If, despite adjusting the position of the stimulating electrode no action potential is recorded, then the nerve has been divided. This inability to transmit current develops distally after injury from the site of injury and therefore false positives may be obtained until 48 hours. In nerve contusion, compression and traction it is possible to differentiate between

| Axonotmesis | No distal nerve conduction after 48 hours (the lapse may be longer, see p. 72) |
| Neurapraxia | Distal nerve conduction remains normal |

This distinction cannot be made at surgical exploration except with nerve stimulation.

After nerve injury, with or without repair, distal latency will only return once the ingrowing axons have reached the neuromuscular junction but thereafter recovery action potentials will be evident some time before motor activity is evident clinically.

No estimate of the number of motor axons present can be made from the amplitude of the action potential.

Having marked the skin at the point where the nerve was stimulated at the wrist, the stimulus is reapplied at the elbow. Care should be taken that a matching wave form is obtained indicating that the same fibres have been stimulated and this is best achieved by leaving the action potential obtained at the wrist on the storage monitor. This also facilitates measurement of the difference in time taken for the potentials to appear after stimulus at the wrist and at the elbow. By also measuring the distance between the points of stimulation the conduction velocity can be calculated in metres per second (see below ★).

The minimum normal conduction velocity in nerves of the upper limb is 50–60 metres per second. Thus the above finding could indicate for example, a compression neuropathy between elbow and wrist.

After recovery of a nerve division conduction velocity across the lesion and distal to it is reduced. This improves gradually until about 18 months after repair.

Sensory studies
Sensory nerves can be stimulated *antidromically,* that is against the normal direction of current, by placing recording electrodes around each finger in turn and stimulating at the wrist as before but with a current of 50 V. This produces a large potential but considerable interference may occur due to motor activity. Therefore *orthodromic* stimulation is favoured. Two finger stimulating electrodes are placed over the digital nerve under study and the recording electrodes are strapped to the wrist (Fig. 2.110). Stimulation is applied with a current of 50 V. Unlike the motor action potential, the sensory action potential *is* quantitative, the minimum normal amplitude being 10 microvolts.

Normal distal sensory latency
  Median 3.07 millisecs + 0.01 × age (SD ± 0.94)
  Ulnar 1.78 millisecs + 0.03 × age (SD ± 0.96)

Until regrowth has occurred, of course, no sensory potentials will be detected and in one study of nerve lacerations of the wrist this was found never to occur before 10 months.[152] Thereafter the amplitude of the orthodromic action potential indicates the percentage of functioning sensory fibres and in the same study this never exceeded 40 per cent. Using similar techniques of distal stimulation and

$$\star \quad \frac{\text{distance between points (cm)}}{100} \times \frac{1000}{\text{time difference (msec)}} = \text{conduction velocity (m/sec)}$$

$$\text{e.g.} \quad \frac{13}{100} \times \frac{1000}{3.25} = 40 \text{ m/sec.}$$

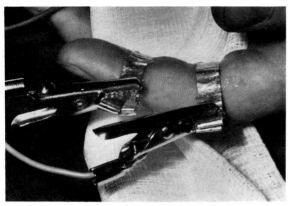

Fig. 2.110 Two stimulating electrodes have been wrapped around the left index finger of the patient in preparation for orthodromic sensory nerve studies on the median nerve.

proximal recording at the elbow, it is possible by moving the stimulus proximally along the course of the nerve to determine the site of a nerve division, no action potentials being transmitted from below the lesion to above.

In summary, what can electromyography offer to the clinician carrying out a secondary assessment of an injured limb?

1. Neurapraxia can be differentiated from axonotmesis and complete division after 48 hours by the presence or absence of action potential on stimulation of the nerve distal to the lesion.
2. After three weeks, denervation can be confirmed by the presence of fibrillation potentials.
3. A division can be localized in some cases using orthodromic sensory stimulation.
4. In brachial plexus lesions, the persistence of sensory conduction from an anaesthetic area indicates that the lesion is medial or proximal to that dorsal root ganglion and therefore not available for grafting.
5. Reinnervation can be detected prior to clinical evidence of motor return.
6. Compression neuropathies can be detected and localized.
7. In the very difficult re-exploration of the partially functioning nerve repair, evoked action potential studies during surgery may identify the transmitting, and therefore intact, fascicles.

Electromyographic interpretation clearly requires experience and clearly experienced advice is desirable. However, it is important that the hand surgeon understands the basic principles of such a useful tool and can go some way towards interpreting the results it yields.

GRADES OF NERVE DAMAGE

Especially in closed injuries or as a result of gunshot wounds, nerves may suffer less than complete transection. In 1942 Seddon[153] introduced the following classification of nerve injury.

Neurotmesis and axonotmesis

In both of these the integrity of the nerve fibres are interrupted, but in axonotmesis the *anatomical* continuity of the nerve is preserved as the Schwann cells which form the sheath are uninterrupted. The clinical and electrical findings are identical and it is therefore impossible to distinguish them clinically. Exploration is therefore required. If anatomical continuity is found, surgical repair is not necessary, as recovery, although proceeding at the same rate of 1–2 mm per day as a neurotmesis after repair, may eventually be good.

Neurapraxia

This is due to selective demyelinization of larger fibres in the nerve: no axonal degeneration occurs. The essential features which distinguish neurapraxia from the two more severe degrees of injury are:

1. sensation and sympathetic activity may be intact,
2. muscle atrophy rarely occurs although motor paralysis is complete,
3. electrically there is
   (a) no reaction of degeneration
   (b) nerve conduction distal to the lesion is preserved although voluntary action potentials disappear,
4. recovery occurs after an unpredictable interval and in no set order, that is, muscle action does not return from proximal to distal as in the other two forms.

Thus neurapraxia can often be diagnosed without surgery. If it is, conservative measures can be adopted with confident reassurance of the patient.

The delay before recovery from the different grades of nerve damage varies so greatly that only a very wide approximation can be offered to the patient. A neurapraxia should show full recovery, regardless of the level, in 1 to 4 months. Return of function from an axonotmesis depends on the level of injury and may take from 4 to 18 months. Traction injuries require significantly longer for recovery than other forms of axonotmesis.

INDICATIONS

The decision to intervene following nerve injury can be one of the more difficult which the hand surgeon has to make. Nerves which have sustained neurapraxia do not require exploration. Nerves which are known from operation reports to have been divided and not repaired should be explored.

Between these relatively clear instances lies the area of difficult decision. Problems include:

the unknown lesion

the nerve which appears to have been divided partially (anomalous innervation should be excluded by selective nerve block)

the nerve divided completely, repaired and showing only partial recovery.

The decision to explore such injuries should be made on the basis of repeated examination conducted at maximum intervals of six weeks. Indications for exploration are

1. a static Tinel's sign at the presumed site of injury (the converse is *not* true — since growth of a very small proportion of the axons can produce an advancing Tinel, such an advance is not in itself a contraindication to exploration, see p. 152),

2. absence of recovery action potentials on electromyography or, somewhat later, of clinical evidence of motor activity in the most proximal paralysed muscle by the time at which it would be expected to occur. This time can be calculated from Seddon's composite figure for rate of return in which one day is allowed for each millimeter of nerve distal to the supposed site of injury,

3. failure to recover sensation in the median nerve distribution,

4. painful neuroma formation.

The introduction of the *operating microscope* has made fascicular dissection of major nerves a practical proposition, permitting complete internal as well as external neurolysis in instances of partial nerve injury. The experimental and limited operative use of microelectrical evaluation of individual fascicular conductivity promises much for the future in these very difficult injuries[154].

Elimination of crippling neuromata and provision of sensation in median nerve distribution are the only absolute indications for exploration of partially divided or previously repaired nerves in isolated major nerve injuries. This is because good motor function can be provided by selected tendon transfers. Indeed, since full motor recovery cannot be anticipated especially in adults, appropriate transfers may be performed before motor power could be expected to return. This is the more justifiable the more proximal the lesion.

Armed with the results of the full muscle test, the examiner can select suitable motor units for transfer. While consideration of specific transfers is outwith the scope of this test, certain basic rules can be stated.

1. All joints on which the transfer is to act should have a full passive range of motion.

2. Transfer of a muscle must not cause the loss of an essential function.

3. Any transferred muscle loses at least 1 grade on the power scale — thus only grade 5 muscles are really satisfactory motors although grade 4 will suffice for certain transfers.

4. The amplitude of movement produced by the muscle for transfer should approximate to that which it is replacing. It should be remembered that the amplitude of any tendon which crosses the wrist is increased by 2–3 cm by full motion in that joint. This is invaluable in tetraplegics especially, and absolutely

contraindicates wrist fusion. The selection of a transfer has been greatly refined by the analysis of the amplitude and mass fraction of all upper extremity muscles (Brand)[155].

5. The effectiveness of certain transfers which retain their original function after transfer depends on the activity of the antagonist to that original function, which must therefore be tested. For example, brachioradialis is an effective dorsiflexor transfer to the wrist only if triceps is strong enough to resist its normal elbow flexor action.

6. Any acute angulation in the course of a transferred tendon should be avoided.

7. The correct biomechanics of insertion are usually achieved by attaching the transfer to the tendon of the paralysed muscle. Where nerve repair carries some hope of recovery in that muscle, the attachment should be done in an end-to-side manner.

While keeping a patient under review pending possible surgery, the examiner is of course responsible for keeping deterioration to a minimum by preventing deformity and joint stiffness with appropriate static and dynamic splints and by instructing the patient in basic physical therapy. Muscle bulk *may rarely* be maintained with the use of a portable galvanic muscle stimulator. Although formerly sceptical of the value of such treatment, a few obsessive patients have convinced the author of the value of regular use. However, these patients applied the stimulus hourly — such enthusiasm gives startling results after precise primary fascicular repair, but is difficult to communicate to those less devoted to their recovery.

Nerves – proximal

BRACHIAL PLEXUS INJURIES

It will be appreciated that, while C_5 and T_1 may each be injured independently by avulsion, isolated *root* lesions of C6–8 are very unlikely. The *trunks* of the brachial plexus lie in the posterior triangle where, apart from the more common traction injuries, they are also vulnerable to stab or gunshot wounds. The defects resulting from injury of the trunks are identical to the corresponding root lesions

Upper trunk	C5 and C6
Middle trunk	C7
Lower trunk	C8 and T1

It follows that it is not possible to differentiate between injuries of roots and of the trunk which they form except when the roots are damaged proximal to the posterior primary rami, the sympathetic rami communicantes or the motor nerves arising directly from the roots. This occurs most often in traction injuries of the plexus. In those instances it is important to attempt to determine at what level the root is divided, since injuries outside the spinal column can be grafted with some hope for recovery of function.

Level of root injury (considered from distal to proximal)
1. Just proximal to the trunks: rhomboids active (C5), serratus anterior active (C5,6,7) (may require EMG to detect innervation);
2. Proximal to white ramus of T1 (C8): *Horner's syndrome* — lid lag, pupillary constriction, loss of sweating in head and neck (Note: Horner's syndrome will also result from *disruption of the sympathetic chain* at any level above C8 T1); (Fig. 2.111)

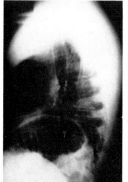
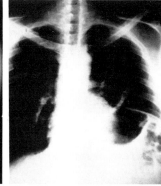

Fig. 2.112 Chest X-ray on this patient after brachial plexus injury reveals paralysis of the left diaphragm consequent upon damage to the phrenic nerve. (C3, 4 & 5).

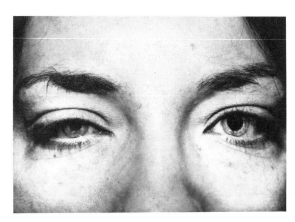

Fig. 2.111 Horner's syndrome with constriction of the pupil, conjunctival injection and ptosis of the upper lid.

3. Proximal to rami communicantes: sweating will persist in limb in areas that are anaesthetic;
4. Proximal to post primary rami: paralysis of paravertebral muscles — may be shown by posterior cervical electromyography[156];
5. Proximal to the posterior root ganglion: axon reflexes[157] will remain intact:
   a. *Histamine response.* The flare of the 'triple response' to 1% histamine is lost in peripheral lesions but preserved when the injury is proximal to the spinal ganglion.
   b. *Cold vasodilatation.* The rise in skin temperature which occurs 5–10 minutes after cold immersion in the normal digit, but is lost in peripheral nerve injury, is maintained in preganglionic lesions.

Tinel sign[158]
By percussion in the posterior triangle and distal to the clavicle, a Tinel sign should be sought. By questioning the patient, some impression of the distribution should be obtained because by identifying the dermatome(s) the surgeon will know which root neuromas are sufficiently intact to produce cortical awareness.

X-rays
Fractures of the clavicle, transverse processes of the cervical spine and neck of the first rib give some indication of the level and severity of the original injury.

Chest X-ray may reveal evidence of damage to the phrenic nerve in the form of diaphragmatic paralysis (Fig. 2.112).

Myelography may be performed in brachial plexus traction injuries. Certainly the presence of a meningocele at the level of injury strongly suggests a hopeless prognosis (Fig. 2.113). However, a number of cases have now been reported where a root suitable for grafting, showing intraoperative evoked potentials[159], has been found at the level

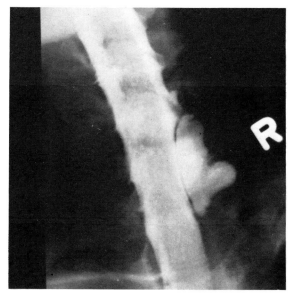

Fig. 2.113 A myelogram has been performed in a patient who had sustained a traction injury of the brachial plexus. A meningocele is demonstrated at three levels indicating avulsion of the roots from the cord.

known to have shown a pseudomyelomeningocele. For this reason, the author has abandoned routine myelography.

The majority of patients who sustain brachial plexus injuries are young and otherwise healthy. If therefore there is *any* evidence of a proximal nerve root which could be grafted, then exploration is worthwhile if only to give the patient and his family the small comfort of absolute information and of having tried all.

Partial plexus injuries

Detailed records of sensory and motor function by the techniques detailed above, must be made in such cases

1. to determine whether selected arthrodeses and transfers could restore acceptable function.
2. to locate precisely in the plexus where the lesion lies and to avoid injury to intact nerves during exploration (Fig. 2.114).
3. to monitor improvement.

Pain

Pain of a neuralgic nature may be a major complaint of the patient. This is especially true if the palsy is consequent upon irradiation for carcinoma[160], usually of the breast. If this pain is becoming more severe after a long period of quiescence, one must suspect the presence of recurrent carcinoma in the plexus. In either case, patients must be made fully aware that pain is usually a poor diagnostic sign[161]. Exploration and even grafting of the plexus carries no assurance of pain relief.

Birth palsies

An expectant course should be pursued with brachial plexus injuries resulting from delivery. An optimistic prognosis is justified, as 80%[162] make a full recovery. Muscles which will recover will all be evident by 15 months of age[163]. It is very difficult to test muscles in

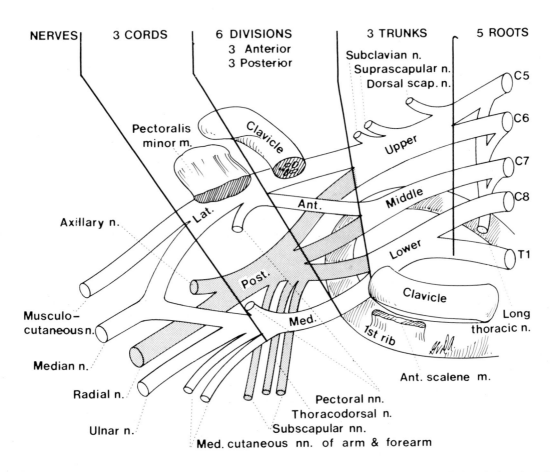

Fig. 2.114 *The brachial plexus.* It is necessary to know the ramifications of the plexus in order to deduce the location of lesions from observed peripheral loss. In addition, the relationship to the bony skeleton can provide information if fractures are evident on X-ray.

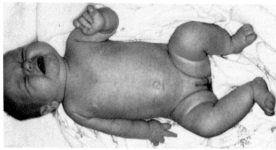

Fig. 2.115 Observation of this newborn child reveals a characteristic Erb's posture of the right upper extremity (C5, 6 (7)).

children and while the following should be tried, any or all may be fruitless on any particular visit.

1. *observation* — careful study of the child while at play, concentrating attention on one movement at a time, may reveal postural changes indicating a deficit (Fig. 2.115) or, conversely, may enable the surgeon to demonstrate convincingly to the mother motion that even she had not noticed; two-handed toys are a necessary tool.

2. *maintenance of position* — if the limb is placed in the position produced by a particular muscle, it may be held there momentarily after release.

3. *stretch-induced contraction* — conversely, if a muscle is put on full stretch and palpated, contraction may be felt or alternatively may occur on release after some thirty seconds of stretch.

CEREBRAL PALSY

Only a small percentage of children with cerebral palsy can be helped by surgery. The surgeon must spend the necessary time to evaluate those factors which serve to select those children. This may well require several visits during which the surgeon can gently but firmly make the point to the parents that even if surgery seems indicated the aim is only to provide a better 'assist hand'.

Intelligence is often severely impaired. The simple use of an arbitrary figure of Intelligence Quotient will probably result in exclusion of some who would benefit and the inclusion of some who would not. Rather should the following qualities be sought with the advice and help of parents and therapist.

interpretation	attention
collaboration	perception — both visual and auditory
motivation	emotional stability

All of these qualities are required in some measure if the child is to benefit from surgery.

Spontaneous use of the limb should be observed. If none whatsoever is seen it is unlikely that a tendon transfer will make the child aware of the hand.

Examination

If the child has not been disqualified on either of the above scores, examination should be directed at sensory and motor function.

Sensation may vary from absence to normality. In the former instance the patient is unlikely to benefit from surgery for he has no afferent input and probably displays no spontaneous use of the limb. Patients can be arbitrarily divided into 3 groups

1. No sensation, even to pinprick — no spontaneous use
   — no surgery
2. Some touch and pain;
   no proprioception; no 2PD — reluctant spontaneous use when encouraged
   — qualified prognosis
3. Proprioception, 2PD — spontaneous use
   — good prognosis for surgery

Motor function

The nature of the neurovascular disorder should be observed, for only spastic children can be helped by surgery. Significant degrees of *athetosis, tremor, ataxia* or *rigidity* therefore eliminate surgical assistance. Spasticity itself is of varying degrees which themselves change according to emotions, which may differ from day to day. The spasticity can be classified by its response to *stretch*[164]

severe — strong reflex which halts initial motion
moderate — visible response
minimum — palpable response

The more severe the stretch response, then the more that tendon requires tenotomy, and the less predictable will be its activity and antagonism if it is transferred.

The majority of patients will show the extrinsic type of spastic hand with the typical flexion-pronation deformity. The system of selection for surgery proposed by Zancolli is recommended[165]. This is based largely on the capability for finger extension relative to achievable wrist position

Group 1 finger extension *full* with wrist *neutral*
Group 2 finger extension *full* with wrist *flexed*
  (a) wrist extension with fingers flexed
  (b) *no* wrist extension even with fingers flexed
Group 3 finger extension *nil* even with wrist *flexed*

Voluntary control of possible motor for transfer should be assessed.

Indications

Group 1 patients require no surgery apart from correction of any thumb deformity which is probably mild. Group 3 shows very poor results with surgery. They may, like those disqualified on the grounds of intelligence or spontaneous use, benefit from surgery purely for cosmetic and toilet reasons. (The great majority of adult cases consequent upon cerebrovascular accidents fall into these categories.) Group 2 are good surgical candidates. Both sub-groups (a) and (b) require release of the ventral muscles at the upper part of the forearm and correction of the thumb deformities by release (Fig. 2.116) and tenodesis or transfer[166]. Group 2a requires simple tenotomy of flexor carpi ulnaris while 2b requires transfer to restore wrist extension. The best age at which to perform this evaluation and undertake the surgery is between 6 and 10.

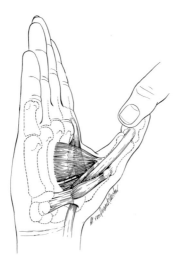

Fig. 2.116 The muscles which become contracted to form the thumb-in-palm deformity in cerebral palsy are shown in this diagram — the flexor pollicis longus, adductor pollicis, flexor pollicis brevis, and the first dorsal interosseous. All of these should be checked for spastic contracture and surgically released before undertaking transfer or tenodesis to improve thumb position.

NEURALGIC AMYOTROPHY[167,168] (= shoulder girdle syndrome = Parsonage–Turner syndrome = paralytic brachial neuritis)

This condition is of unknown aetiology, but commonly follows on an injection of some kind. It is characterised by *pain* followed by *paralysis*. The pain is sudden in onset and is usually a constant severe ache across the shoulder girdle and down into the arm. It may persist for hours to weeks but it improves markedly with the onset of paralysis. The paralysis is of a *lower motor neuron type*, with flaccidity, rapid wasting, but no fasciculations. The palsy may afflict peripheral nerves individually or in combination, nerve roots or the spinal cord itself. It may be unilateral or bilateral. The peripheral nerves most commonly involved are the long thoracic, the axillary, the radial, the anterior

interosseous, the suprascapular and the musculo-cutaneous nerves in that order. The upper roots of the plexus C5–7 are those affected in root loss. Sensation is normally not markedly reduced. The prognosis is for recovery in the majority of cases, but that may take several years.

CERVICAL CORD TRANSECTION: QUADRIPLEGIA: TETRAPLEGIA[169]

Patients who survive this injury should always be evaluated by a hand surgeon for function can be improved in the majority of patients. Formerly, these injuries were classified according either to the level of cord or of bony lesion. More recently, emphasis has been laid on residual function, both motor and sensory, which need not coincide with respect to cervical level. Freehafer[170], Lamb[171] and Zancolli[172] have introduced motor classifications which correspond except in minor detail. Zancolli has linked classification to potential surgical gain (Table 2.6) in a most practical way. Study of the Table reveals that, in his series, the majority of patients fell into the group with strong wrist extension — the so-called 'strong C6' — a group who can be helped greatly by surgery. Moberg[173] has emphasised the importance of sensibility in tetraplegia. He has classified patients as Cu = Cutaneous, being patients with useful sensory afferents from the hands and as O = Ocular, where all information available to the patient is visual. In the latter group he recommends reconstruction in only one hand since only one at a time can be controlled by visual input. Unfortunately, any attempt to rationalize the three main classifications currently in vogue (Table 2.7) reveals that there is but a poor fit. Communication therefore requires either a knowledge of all classifications, an arbitrary adoption of one or a detailed description of the individual patient.

After taking a history which determines efficiency in activities of daily living, examination is conducted as follows

1. Test sensation, using moving 2PD — in the majority, C6 will be intact and therefore sensibility will be present in thumb and index.
2. Check joint range of motion — note contractures — hyperextensibility of MP joints. The latter if present may require control by tenodesis.
3. Determine presence, spasticity and strength of muscle activity. Remember that almost all muscles are innervated from more than one root (Table 2.8) and therefore strength will increase the lower is the cervical lesion. Only power 4 and 5 muscles should be transferred.

Table 2.9 serves only as a guide to potential substitutes. For more detailed guidance and for transfers to restore intrinsic function the reader should consult Zancolli's classic text[172]. The aim of surgery should be to achieve independent transfer as from bed to chair and, in the

Table 2.6 Clinical classification of the quadriplegic upper limbs and possible function obtained by surgery

Group	Lowest functioning cord segments	Remaining motor function	Subgroups	Function regained by surgery
1 Flexor of the elbow 13%	5–6	Biceps, brachialis	A Without brachioradialis (1–A)	—
			B With bracioradialis (1–B)	Elbow extension and
2 Extensor of the wrist 74%	6–7	Extensor carpi radialis longus and brevis	A Weak and complete wrist extension (2–A)	weak lateral grip and grasping
			B Strong wrist extension (2–B), 82% — I Without pronator teres, flexor carpi radialis, and triceps (2–B: I) 76%	Elbow extension Good lateral grip and grasping
			II Without flexor carpi radials and triceps; and with pronator teres (2–B: II) 16%	
			III With pronator teres, flexor, carpi radialis, and triceps (2–B: III) 8%	Good lateral grip and better grasping than 2–B: I and 2–B: II
3 Extrinsic extensor of the finger 6.8%	7–8	Ext. digit. communis Ext. digit. quinti Ext. carpi ulnaris	A Complete extension of ulnar fingers and paralysis of radial fingers and thumb (3–A)	Good lateral and pulp grips and excellent
			B Complete extension of all fingers and weak thumb extension (3–B)	grasping (better in subgroup 3–B)
4 Extrinsic flexor of the fingers and extensor of the thumb 6.2%	8–1	Flexor digit. prof. Ext. indicis propius Ext. pollicis longus Flexor carpi ulnaris	A Complete flexion of ulnar fingers and paralysis or weakness of flexion of the radial fingers and thumb. Complete thumb extension (4–A)	Excellent lateral and pulp grips and grasping
			B Complete flexion of the fingers and thumb, with total intrinsic paralysis (4–B) I Without flexor superficialis (4–B:I) II With flexor superficialis (4–B: II)	(better in subgroup 4–B: II)

Reproduced from Zancolli, E. A. 1979 Structural and dynamic bases of hand surgery, 2nd edn. Lippincott, Philadelphia. p. 230 with kind permission of the author and publisher.

Table 2.7 Classifications of quadriplegia

	Freehafer	*Moberg*	*Zancolli*
Elbow flexion — no BR	I	O:0	1A
— + BR		O:1	1B
Weak wrist extension	II		2A
Strong BR, ECRL, and B	III	OCu:2	2B I
+ PT		OCu:3	2B II
+ triceps, FCR	IV	OCu:4	2B III
Finger extension			
— ulnar digits		OCu:5	3A
— all, including thumb		OCu:6	3B
Finger flexion			
— ulnar digits		OCu:7	4A
— all — no FDS			4B I
— + FDS	V		4B II
Intrinsics intact		OCu:8	

majority, 'strong C6' group, to restore strong grasp and lateral pinch[174,175].

The timing of reconstruction for tetraplegia should be late enough that all motors have returned to maximum strength and the patient has had time to fully understand his limitations. Conversely, it should be early enough that the patient has not completely adjusted to his life style to a degree that the time lost by surgery becomes an intrusion. In practical terms, this usually means surgery about 1 year after the cervical injury[176].

Muscles and tendons

Much of the assessment of muscle and tendon injury has been made in performing the full muscle test and examining the joints. It is necessary now to consider factors over and above the presence or absence of muscle function.

DIVISION OR PARALYSIS?

The full muscle test may have revealed total lack of function in one or more muscles. It is usually apparent

Table 2.8 The root values of muscles (after Zancolli)

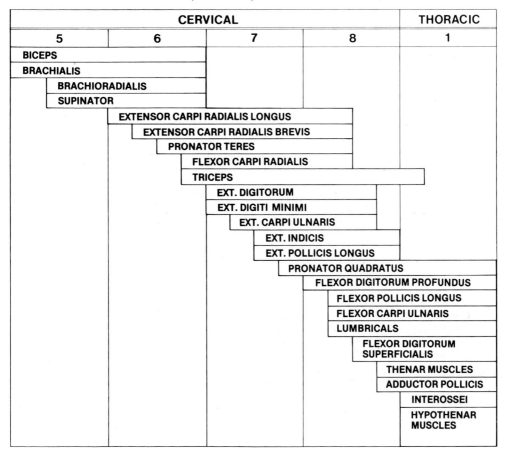

Table 2.9 Tendon transfers and tenodeses in quadriplegia

		normal motor	potential substitute
(i)	elbow flexion	biceps brachialis brachioradialis	——
(ii)	elbow extension	triceps	post. deltoid biceps
(iii)	wrist extension	ECRL ECRB	brachioradialis
(iv)	pronation	pronator teres	biceps (Zancolli 2A)
(v)	wrist flexion	FCR	——
(vi)	finger and thumb extension	ED EPL	brachioradialis or tenodesis
(vii)-	thumb flexion	FPL	brachioradialis or tenodesis
(viii)	finger flexion	FDP FDS	brachioradialis or ECRL

whether this is due to tendon division or to nerve injury by the site of the wound, the presence of muscle wasting, the pattern of motor loss and the associated sensory disturbance, but this may not be so or may require confirmation.

Posture
In the case of the long flexor tendons, for example, denervation would not produce the characteristically extended fingers of a complete tendon laceration (Fig. 2.117). By altering the position of the wrist much can be

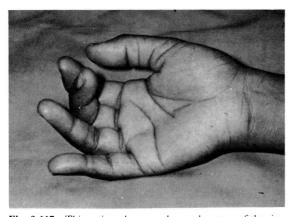

Fig. 2.117 This patient shows an abnormal posture of the ring and small fingers suggestive of adhesions or rupture of both flexor tendons to the small finger and of the entire profundus and possibly a proportion of the superficialis to the ring finger. This deduction was subsequently confirmed at surgical exploration.

learned about tendon integrity from the resulting changes in posture.

Defect
Palpation may detect the absence of a tendon from its sheath when compared with an uninjured finger or may reveal a defect in the wrist distal to the bulge of the muscle belly, which can be emphasised by attempted contraction.

Passive motion
This test is valuable in checking the integrity of long flexor tendons. Firm pressure exerted over the junction of middle and distal thirds of the forearm produces distinct flexion of the fingers in the presence of intact long flexor tendons. Similar pressure over the radius a little further distally flexes the thumb via an intact flexor pollicis longus.

CONTRACTURE
Contracture occurs most commonly in the muscle bellies of the intrinsics and of the finger flexors of the forearm.

Flexion contracture (Volkmann's)
Attempt to extend all of the fingers while also extending the forearm and hand. In the presence of a contracture the fingers will resist the attempt, remaining flexed. Flexion of the wrist will, however, allow the fingers to extend, confirming the presence of shortening, or adhesion, of the muscles above the wrist. Such flexion contracture is commonly, but not always, associated with a median nerve deficit.

Intrinsic tightness (contracture) (Fig. 2.118)
With the metacarpophalangeal joint passively hyper-extended, attempt to flex the proximal interphalangeal joint (Fig. 2.119). In the presence of intrinsic tightness, this will meet with rubbery resistance which will decrease if the metacarpophalangeal joint is now allowed to flex. If it is suspected that one or other of the radial or ulnar intrinsics is responsible for the tightness, the finger should be deviated at the metacarpophalangeal joint each way in turn. If tightness is more marked in radial deviation of the finger, the ulnar intrinsic is responsible, and vice versa.

ADHESIONS
The most common cause of inadequate range of motion in tendons, in the presence of a palpable powerful muscle belly contraction and an adequate range of passive joint motion is adhesion of the tendon, usually most firm at the site of injury.

By limiting tendon movement, adhesions produce active deficits in joint motion which exceed the passive but are also responsible for a passive deficit on the contrary movement. For example, assuming the absence of other contractures, if the flexor pollicis longus is adherent to the

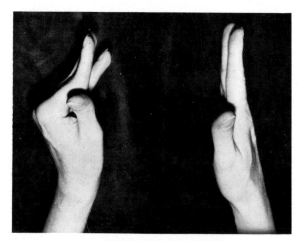

Fig. 2.118   This patient is attempting to extend both hands. In the left she shows severe advanced intrinsic contracture with metacarpophalangeal flexion contracture and hyperextension deformities of the proximal interphalangeal joints. This deformity apparently developed in the months following on a period of unexplained but severe oedema and pain in the affected hand. It can be postulated that ischaemic fibrosis of her intrinsic muscles occurred during that period of oedema.

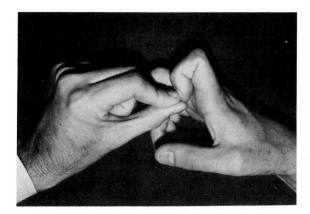

Fig. 2.119   The test for intrinsic tightness.

proximal phalanx there will be a flexion and often an extension deficit in the interphalangeal joint of the thumb. The active and the passive extension deficit will be equal because the adherent tendon acts as a check on both. However, in flexion the passive range will exceed the active since the examiner can exert more power on the joint than can the adherent tendon (Fig. 2.120).

Site of adhesion

Adhesion of muscle or tendon to the skin is easily appreciated, for each muscle contraction produces puckering of the skin. Adhesion to other tendons is indicated by mass action of normally independent tendons when the patient attempts to flex only one.

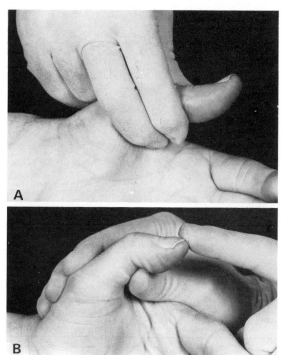

Fig. 2.120   This patient had sustained a laceration of flexor pollicis longus which at exploration subsequent to this illustration proved adherent at the site of repair.

(A) The patient is attempting active flexion but is achieving none, and, (B) the passive range of motion can be seen to considerably exceed that achieved actively.

The location of an adhesion can occasionally be accurately determined by adjusting the position of the joints. Considering the proximal interphalangeal joint with a flexion deficit, if full flexion of the metacarpophalangeal joint permits the proximal interphalangeal joint to extend, the adhesion must be proximal to the metacarpophalangeal joint. If it does not, the flexor tendon is adherent to the proximal phalanx (Fig. 2.121).

These deductions of course presuppose the absence of a contracture of the joint capsule.

BOWSTRINGING

Doyle and Blythe[177] have shown that both the A_2 and the A_4 pulleys — those at the proximal and middle phalanx respectively — are required for full flexion to be possible. If neither is divided, the flexor tendon stands out from the digital skeleton like the string on a bow. This not only markedly decreases the mechanical efficiency of the tendon but also increases the likelihood of tendon adhesion to the soft tissue. Bowstringing can be detected both on inspection and on palpating the tendon while asking the patient to flex the finger (Fig. 2.122). Such bowstringing is an indication for pulley reconstruction.

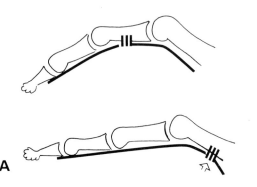

Fig. 2.121 (A) Adjustment of the joints proximal to that which appears to be the seat of contracture may reveal the primary source of that deformity. In this diagram the flexion contracture is at the proximal interphalangeal joint. Flexion of the metacarpophalangeal joint in the presence of adhesion over the proximal phalanx (upper figure) has no effect on the flexion contracture of the proximal interphalangeal joint. If, however, the adhesion of the flexor tendons lies proximal to the metacarpophalangeal joint, flexion of that will result in correction of the contracture apparently present in the proximal interphalangeal joint.

(B) This patient has a flexion contracture of the distal interphalangeal joint present when both metacarpophalangeal and proximal interphalangeal joint are extended.

(C) Flexion of the metacarpophalangeal joint has little or no effect on the flexion contracture of the distal interphalangeal joint.

(D) However, when the proximal interphalangeal is flexed, the distal interphalangeal joint can be fully extended. It can therefore be concluded that the flexion contracture is due to limitation of flexor tendon motion and further that the tendon is adherent in the region of the proximal phalanx.

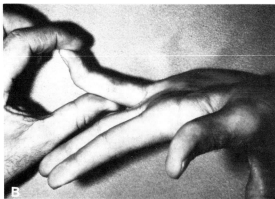

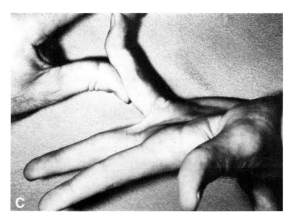

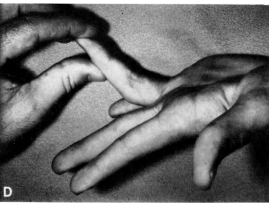

'LUMBRICAL PLUS'[178]

This disability occurs whenever the flexor digitorum profundus is released distally to a degree which causes its contraction to act through the lumbrical, causing extension of the interphalangeal joints instead of flexion. This may occur following laceration of the tendon, amputation through the finger distal to the proximal interphalangeal joint, insertion of an overlong tendon graft or the development of adhesions distal to the lumbrical. It is recognized by the occurrence of paradoxical extension on strong flexion of the fingers (Fig. 2.123). It is treated by locating and correcting the cause or, more simply, by dividing the lumbrical.

RECURVATUM (Fig. 2.124)

This hyperextension of the proximal interphalangeal joint occurs in supple patients after excision of the superficialis tendon during primary repair or tendon graft. Initially slight, it may increase to the degree where it produces a 'slow finger', flexion occuring later than in adjacent fingers. Indeed, the patient may have to help the finger around the head of the proximal phalanx before flexion can ensue. It can be avoided by not excising that portion of the superficialis distal to its chiasma. It can be cured by tenodesis or capsulodesis of the proximal interphalangeal joint.

INDICATIONS

If neither finger flexor is functioning, and no tendon repair was performed primarily, then a tendon graft should be planned and the sources of the graft checked during examination. In order of preference these are palmaris longus from either arm, one of the two tendons of extensor

Fig. 2.122 (A) This patient can clearly be seen to have no pulleys over the flexor tendon to the ring finger, the tendon standing out through the skin.

(B) The flexor tendon, although pulling through, is mechanically inefficient on account of the lack of pulleys.

(C) This patient had previously undergone a flexor tendon graft to the small finger and complained of poor range of flexion. Palpation of the palmar aspect of the small finger during flexion revealed bowstringing of the flexor tendon due to destruction or bypassing of the pulley mechanism at the time of the tendon graft.

(D) This diagram shows the placement and nomenclature of the normal pulley mechanism.

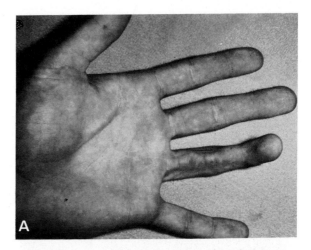

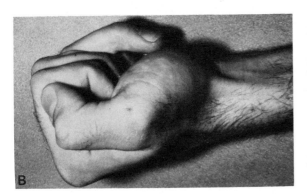

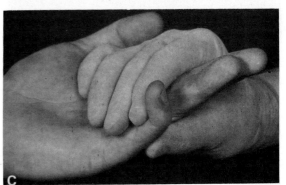

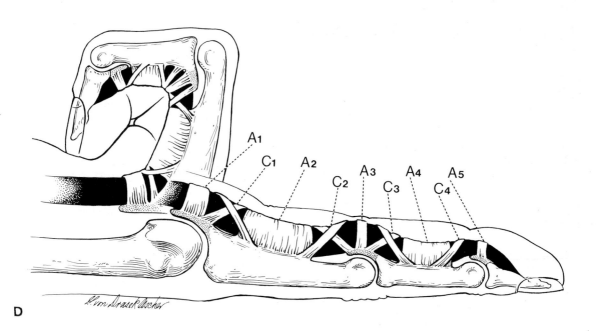

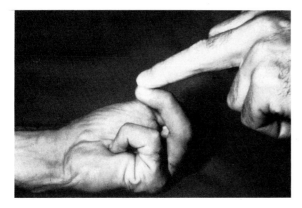

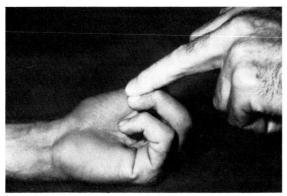

Fig. 2.123 *Lumbrical plus.* In (A) the patient is lightly flexing the hand without power. The examiner's finger is resting lightly on the distal phalanx of the ring finger. (B) With powerful grasp the small finger comes down into full flexion, but the ring finger paradoxically *extends* against the resisting finger.

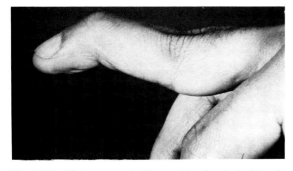

Fig. 2.124 This very supple 18-year-old patient had achieved an excellent result following flexor tendon graft to his middle finger but subsequently developed a progressive recurvatum deformity of the proximal interphalangeal joint which eventually nullified much of the value of the tendon graft, as it resulted in a 'slow finger'.

digiti minimi or one of the tendons of extensor digitorum longus from either the second, third or fourth toes. Many surgeons use the divided flexor digitorum superficialis or the plantaris. The author finds the first too thick and worries about its nutrition; the second he finds too thin and is concerned about its strength.

If flexor digitorum superficialis is intact and functioning, the choice lies between tendon graft and fixing the distal interphalangeal joint, preferably by tenodesis or capsulodesis. Littler has shown what a small proportion of the sweep of finger flexion is represented by motion of the distal interphalangeal joint and to hazard all for this small gain is indicated in only a small proportion of well-motivated patients with specialized occupations. For the great majority who have not had the benefit of a primary repair of profundus, tenodesis of the distal interphalangeal joint is the procedure of choice. If tendon graft is selected the choice must be made between sacrificing the superficialis and grafting past it. The former has been done successfully but no report exists of its consistent reliability and the latter technique certainly has a higher chance of maintaining proximal interphalangeal joint function.

The choice of motor for a tendon graft is made finally during surgery, but a preliminary selection can be undertaken at the time of examination. The surgeon should determine that the muscle can be felt contracting in the forearm and that there is prima facie evidence that the tendon crosses at least one joint. Experience has shown that this assures that the motor has adequate power and amplitude.

If primary repair or tendon graft has been performed and has resulted in adhesions, then tenolysis should be proposed preferably commencing under wrist block (Fig 2.125). In doing so, the surgeon must always warn the patient of the possibility that exploration may reveal a totally unsatisfactory tendon and graft or silastic rod insertion may be necessary.

A silastic rod is indicated in the following circumstances:
unsatisfactory skin coverage, where, for example, a cross finger flap must be done at the same procedure,
absence of pulleys, in which situation pulley reconstruction must always be performed,
limitation of passive joint motion, where capsulectomy and early motion with or without dynamic splintage is required,
a generally unsatisfactory bed, with extensive scarring and exposure of bare bone.

As previously emphasized, no tendon graft can possibly increase the range of motion in a contracted joint and this must be corrected by splintage or surgery before grafting is considered. Where secondary tendon surgery is being considered and in particular where there is a significant flexion contracture, care must be taken to evaluate the blood supply to the involved digit (Fig. 2.126). This can be

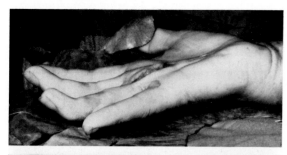

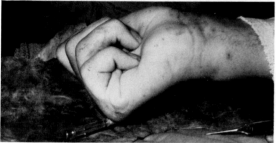

Fig. 2.125 Tendolysis under wrist block permits the patient to participate in the procedure. The intravenous cannula seen in (B) is to permit the administration of intravenous anaesthesia should forearm exploration prove necessary.

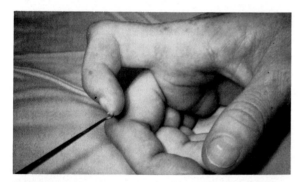

Fig. 2.126 This patient undergoing flexor tendolysis some 18 months after injury has severe scarring in a flexed position. Release was satisfactorily achieved, but when the finger was straight and the tourniquet was released, no flow was evident to the pulp. Due to inadequacy of the distal vessels, vessel reconstruction was not possible, and it was necessary to allow the finger to revert to its original position.

done by use of the *digital Allen test* or more precisely by employing a Doppler flow meter (p. 181). If flow is absent in both vessels, surgery should probably be reconsidered. If flow is present in one or even both, the patient should still be warned that release of the contracture, however meticulous, may result in no flow to the pulp necessitating return of the finger to the flexed position. As opposed to immediate replacement, late reconstruction of digital arteries is less successful largely due to poor run-off, although lengthening of shortened arteries which are carrying flow has been performed using reversed vein grafts.

Vessels

Inadequate circulation to a limb or digit, according to its degree, will declare itself by one or more of the following symptoms.

Frank necrosis. The dead part will be black or mottled brown, hard and cold (Fig. 2.127). It may be firmly adherent and the surgeon should not dislodge it until he has planned the closure of the wound and indeed prepared the patient for admission. In rare cases, mostly in young children, it may be best to leave the part to separate spontaneously, which will take several months but may leave a well-healed non-tender amputation stump.

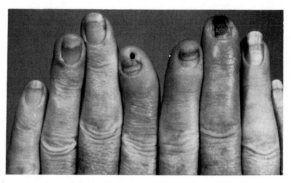

Fig. 2.127 This patient with thromboangitis obliterans demonstrates frank and incipient necrosis in several digits.

Persistent ulceration. When a wound on a digit fails to heal or minor trauma results in skin breakdown which fails to heal, the surgeon should suspect an inadequate blood supply, provided the other causes of ulceration (p. 116) have been eliminated (Fig. 2.128).

Cold intolerance. The patient who complains that any fall in ambient temperature results in pain and pallor in one or more digits has some obstruction of his vascular tree, temporary or permanent.

Colour change. The finger appears deep red with a bluish tinge. The patient may report that the finger becomes absolutely white in cold weather, and this can often be demonstrated by immersion in ice water.

Stiffness of the joints. The finger or part will be less used by the patient resulting in both oedema and stiffness, both active and passive.

Intermittent claudication. Much less common in the upper than in the lower limb, this is characterised by increasing pain with continued exercise which forces rest (not strictly 'claudication'; L. *claudicare* = to limp). Most often encountered in the forearm muscles, this is due to an obstruction of the brachial artery.

Subclavian steal syndrome[179] may present with upper extremity symptoms alone, of pain, weakness, easy fatigue and numbness. The pulse is diminished, the blood pressure is lower than in the other arm and the diagnosis is

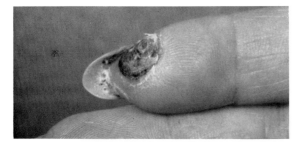

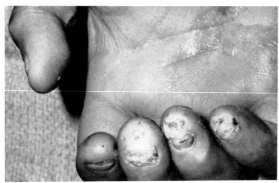

Fig. 2.128 (A) This patient had ulnar artery thrombosis resulting in poor flow to the index finger. (B) Persistent ulceration in this patient's fingertips was thought to be due to nerve injuries in the forearm.

However investigation of the vascular tree and reconstruction with reversed vein grafts resulted in satisfactory healing of the fingertips before sensation improved.

confirmed by arch angiography. 'Shunt steal' which arises in dialysis patients is considered on page 301.

The symptoms of obliterative arterial disease tend to indicate the level of obstruction[180].

Group I   proximal subclavian — steal syndrome
Group II   distal subclavian, axillary or brachial — intermittent claudication
Group III   distal disease and distal symptoms

Examination may reveal any of the following signs of vascular impairment.

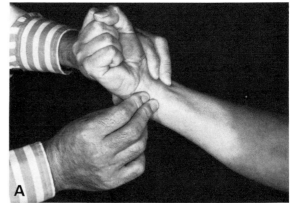

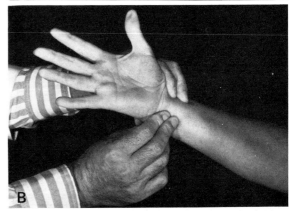

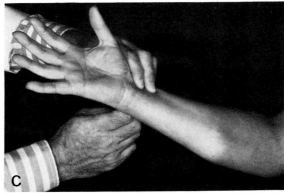

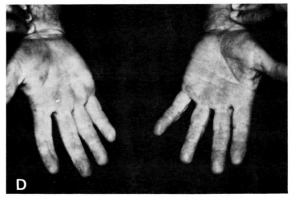

Fig. 2.129 *The Allen test.* Both radial and ulnar arteries are occluded at the wrist by the examiner. The patient is asked to firmly flex all fingers and the thumb thereby expelling blood from the hand (A).

(B) The patient is then asked to open the hand in a relatively relaxed posture and the pallor of the palm can be appreciated.

(C) Release of the compression on one or other of the arteries under test will, if that vessel is patent, result in rapid return of normal colour to the palm of the hand.

(D) If, as in this patient, one ulnar artery is thrombosed then the pallor persists when compared with the normal hand.

Slow refilling after expression. This can be detected by comparing the nail bed with that of a normal finger or by applying a digital Allen test.

Absent pulses. Only the radial pulse can be palpated with sufficient confidence to declare it absent. The ulnar artery and digital arteries can frequently be felt pulsating if the hand is warm but failure to do so is not evidence of absent flow.

Blood pressure. Recordings taken in *both arms* may reveal a significant difference due to a proximal block.

Allen test[181]. The patency of the ulnar and radial arteries at the wrist and of the two digital arteries at the base of a finger can be determined clinically by this technique. Both arteries at the wrist are occluded by the examiner's middle and index fingers of both hands (Fig. 2.129). The patient is then asked to close the hand firmly while the occlusion is maintained, thereby expelling much of the blood. With the hand then relaxed and occlusion continued, the palm appears pale. Occasionally, despite continued occlusion of both arteries, the palm will refill. This is due to a *persistent median* or other anomalous artery. Failure to observe this may lead the examiner to draw false reassurance regarding radial or ulnar artery patency, or both. It is therefore important to confirm the *persistence* of palmar pallor before

proceeding with the test. Removal of the occlusion from *one* of the vessels in the presence of a block in that vessel will result in no immediate change. By contrast, if the vessel is patent a pink blush spreads rapidly across the palm. In the event of obstruction being present the occlusion on the other vessel should be released and the response again noted. When the first vessel tested was patent the examination should be repeated for the other vessel. The Allen test has been quantified both by timing refill[182] and measuring digital systolic pressure[183].

The *digital Allen test* is performed in similar manner except that the examiner should first exsanguinate the digit by brisk proximal massage before occluding the digital arteries against the proximal phalanx (Fig. 2.130).

If either test is equivocal, warming the hand in hot water before repeating the test will eliminate doubt.

Doppler flowmeter. Flow can be detected with ease in all significant arteries in the upper extremity using ultrasound. Because of the presence of significant arches in the hand and the fingers it is important to determine the direction of flow, either by using a meter which indicates this or, more simply, by occluding any potential source of backflow while listening. Thus, while checking flow in the ulnar artery, proper or digital, the radial equivalent should be occluded, and vice versa (Fig. 2.131).

Skin temperature. While the difference in temperature between the affected hand or digit and its normal

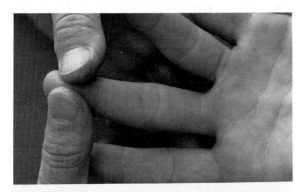

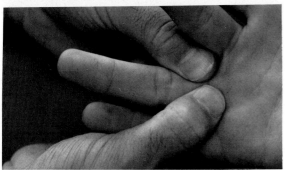

Fig. 2.130 *The digital Allen test.* (A) The thumbs of the examiner are placed on either side of the anterior surface of the digit, and (B) are swept firmly, proximally to exsanguinate the digit, coming to rest over the digital arteries on the proximal phalanx, thereby occluding inflow. As with the Allen test, release of one or other thumb will reveal the presence or absence of flow through that vessel.

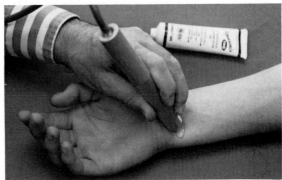

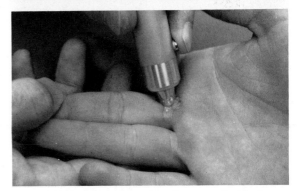

Fig. 2.131 The use of the Doppler flow meter for (A) ulnar and (B) digital arteries.

counterpart can often be detected simply by touch, a more exact record can be made by use of a portable thermocouple with digital read-out. This allows improvement to be charted and demonstrated to the patient — the basis of biofeedback techniques.

A diagnosis can be arrived at in most patients with the relatively simple office techniques which are detailed. To confirm or quantify this diagnosis or to investigate the more obscure cases, the more sophisticated techniques available in a *vascular laboratory*[184,15] may be employed —

temperature	— thermography, infra-red radiometry
perfusion	— plethysmography[186] or pulse volume record (PVR)
proximal	— Doppler wave form analysis[187] —
stenosis	velocity/time, pulsatility index

Arteriography is required to confirm, or sometimes make, a diagnosis; to determine its location and distribution; to ensure the presence of other, apparently unaffected, vessels; to gain an impression of the state of health of the vascular tree; to assist in the planning of surgical procedures.

Maximum vasodilatation is clearly desirable in these studies. By comparisons performed in the course of studying patients with bilateral disease, we have determined that this is achieved to a greater and more reliable degree after *regional nerve block* than with general anaesthesia, intra-arterial vasodilators, stellate ganglion block, sedation or with no preparation whatsoever (Fig. 2.132). Introduction of the dye is preferably made by the Seldinger technique, that is by the introduction of a catheter into the femoral artery at the groin, passing thence to the subclavian and axillary arteries. This not only permits study of the proximal portions of the vascular tree to the upper extremity where unsuspected anomalies or pathology may lie but also avoids inflicting iatrogenic insult to an arterial system already in trouble (Fig. 2.133).

Subtraction films made from the angiograms highlight the vessels very helpfully — this will become even more effective and hopefully less expensive with increasing use of *digital-enhanced,* that is, *computerised angiography.* *Magnification angiography* permits easier study of detail in the vessels but its greater cost probably outweighs any diagnostic benefit.

These various studies may reveal one of the following vascular disorders —

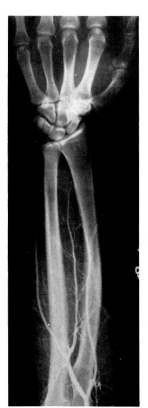
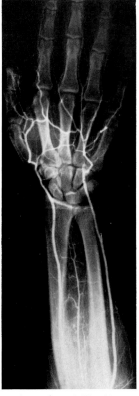

Fig. 2.132 Simultaneous arteriography performed (A) without regional block and (B) with regional block. The patient had bilateral symptoms which were more severe in (B) than in (A). As can be seen, he had an ulnar artery thrombosis, but no diagnosis could be arrived at in the arteriogram which was performed without anaesthesia.

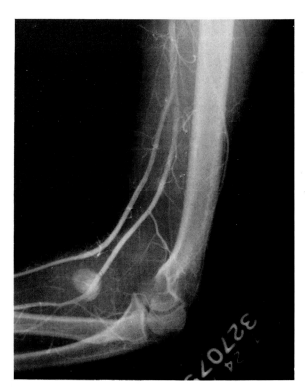

Fig. 2.133 Arteriography shows a traumatic aneurysm in the antecubital fossa. There is also a high bifurcation of the brachial artery. If the dye had been introduced below the level of the bifurcation, a faulty conclusion may have been reached regarding the circulation to this extremity.

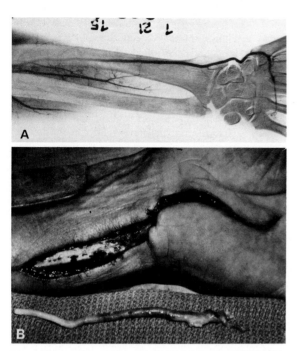

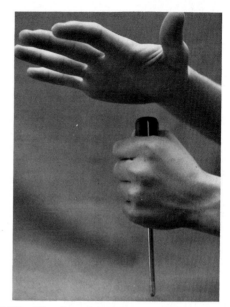

Fig. 2.135 *'Hypothenar hammer'*.

Fig. 2.134 (A) A thrombosed ulnar artery is demonstrated on arteiogram in which the radial artery is seen to provide the only blood supply to the hand. The thrombosed segment of the ulnar artery is displayed after resection (B).

Localised arterial occlusion

This is most common in the ulnar artery at the region of the canal of Guyon[188-191] (Fig. 2.134). Because thrombosis at this point probably results from the use of the butt of the hand as a blunt instrument, the condition is referred to as the *'hypothenar hammer syndrome'*[192] (Fig. 2.135). A few cases of non-thrombotic occlusion have been reported[193,194]. Usually associated with cold intolerance, pain and sometimes ulceration, most often of the ring finger, it is cured in most patients by resection of the thrombosed segment. In itself, resection is surprisingly effective probably by removing any vasospastic effects of the thrombus and also by effecting a local sympathectomy[195]. In this, as in other major vessel resections, replacement with a reversed vein graft increases the chances of a successful outcome. The difficulty in performing such a graft lies in finding a point in the vascular tree for the distal anastomosis with sufficient run-off to prevent graft failure, while not interfering appreciably with existing circulation. Such a vein graft is not itself without potential complications (Fig. 2.136).

Aneurysm (p. 303)

Generalised arterial disorders

These conditions effect many or all of the vessels in the limb and are therefore much less amenable to surgical

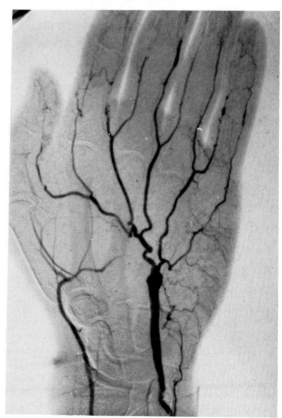

Fig. 2.136 This patient had undergone vein graft for ulnar artery thrombosis. It can be seen that multiple emboli are present throughout the digital arterial tree, probably arising from mural thrombi in the vein graft.

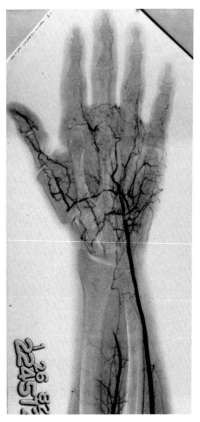

Fig. 2.137   This patient shows extensive vasospastic disease in the digital arteries with absent flow in the radial artery. (Arteriograms by courtesy of C. S. Wheeler).

correction than the localised lesions. They can be classified as

organic degenerative disease — atherosclerosis
vasospastic organic disease — e.g. thromboangiitis obliterans[196], (Fig. 2.137)
vasospastic functional disease — Raynaud's — erythromelalgia

Raynaud's disease[197] Due to small vessel spasm of unknown cause, this disorder is characterized by cyclical colour and temperature changes in the digits. The sudden onset of extreme pallor progressing to a cold, pale cyanosis, which is followed after a varying period by painful reactive hyperaemia, is diagnostic of the condition. The idiopathic disease is invariably symmetrical and bilateral and usually found in females between fifteen and forty-five. *Raynaud's phenomenon* presents in the same manner but has some underlying associated disorder[198]. Thus, the phenomenon is encountered in the following conditions: scleroderma[199], rheumatoid arthritis, cervical rib, thromboangiitis obliterans, cryoglobulinaemia, the use of vibratory

tools[200,201] and others. In both the phenomenon and the disease, a minority of cases become progressively worse, with later development of trophic changes in the affected digits, recurrent infection and even focal gangrene.

The first service that the physician can perform for any patient with vessel disease is to persuade him to *stop smoking*[202]. Indeed, the deleterious effects on flow of smoking are such as to compromise any proposed surgical procedure and the surgeon is justified in refusing to perform that surgery until the patient has abstained for six weeks. Sometimes drawing a parallel between what is happening in the digital vessels with what may be going on in the coronary and cerebral circulation serves to drive home the point.

Meanwhile, the surgeon confronted with generalised arterial disorders should institute investigations to exclude underlying systemic pathology. In those cases where none is found or where its management does not alleviate the Raynaud's phenomenon, blockade of the stellate ganglion may give temporary relief. The possible value of subsequent surgical sympathectomy can be illustrated by applying the *cold immersion test* before and after stellate block which is shown to be effective by the development of a Horner's syndrome. The hand is immersed in ice water and the time of pain onset and of removal are both noted. A significant increase in both elapsed times after stellate block indicates that a cervical sympathectomy[203,204] would provide some relief of symptoms. Recently, the merits of *local digital arterial sympathectomy*[205] have been shown, while the value of prostaglandin therapy for vasospastic disorders is under judgement.

Surgical planning

On completion of examination, the surgeon knows which of the eight basic hand functions are impaired and, of those, which are most required by the patient in pursuit of his occupation and recreation. He has also determined as fully as possible what contributions each anatomical structure makes to the impairment of hand function. Assuming that the patient is at a 'plateau' in his recovery and that all conservative aids offered by physical therapy and splintage have been exhausted, it remains for him to plan a surgical programme designed to restore the maximum hand function attainable. In doing so, efforts should be directed primarily at the functions which by their impairment prevent the patient from doing his regular job. For example, after severe injury, a hand may show loss of five of the eight basic functions (p. 108). However, of those only one, let us say power grasp in the non-dominant hand, may be essential. Having analysed the anatomical deficits, the surgeon may realize that while they are multiple only absence of flexion in the proximal interphalangeal joints of the badly injured ring and small fingers is preventing power grasp. Damage to both extensors and flexors may make the achievement of active motion unlikely but arthrodesis in a carefully selected position would result in a functional hand despite the other disabilities. In short, the reconstruction should be tailored to the individual needs of the patient. This approach is not only the most pragmatic but also serves to simplify for the surgeon what may be a bewildering complexity of structural and dynamic disturbance.

Certain general rules should assist the surgeon in reconstruction. Adequate *blood supply* must be present to ensure healing of wounds by primary intention. The *skeleton* is the structure on which all reconstruction is built. Non-union and mal-union of fractures should therefore be corrected by bone graft and osteotomy allied with internal or external fixation. *Skin cover* must be stable and sufficiently robust as to permit whatever procedure on deep structures may be necessary. These are the three basic prerequisities. If they are unsound steps should be taken to restore them. Sensation must be restored to a degree which is at the least protective. Joint motion must be secured before tendons can be expected to function. This may require not only capsulectomy in its various forms but also tendolysis and release of contractures in muscle and skin, as in adduction deformities of the thumb. Only after all these preliminaries are completed successfully, can the ultimate goal of restoration of motion be approached by appropriate tendon grafts or transfers.

Every attempt should be made to reduce the number of surgical procedures for each is an assault, however elegant technically, from which the hand must recover. Grouping of procedures is one of the intellectual pleasures of reconstructive surgery of the hand. Release of an adduction contracture of the thumb can well be combined with an opponensplasty for nought will be lost to the former by the immobilization required for the success of the transfer. If, however, the release reveals a lack of skin cover sufficient to require a distant flap, then the transfer must be postponed and the release maintained by static means. The passive motion necessary in the proximal interphalangeal joint for a tendon graft to function may require extensive work on the capsular structures, the benefit of which may only be maintained by early motion with appropriate dynamic splintage. The tendon graft must clearly wait. Many more hypothetical situations could be put forward to illustrate the point, some simple, some sufficiently problematical as to have several correct solutions — or none at all. The essence of the matter is that as many steps should be taken as possible in one procedure while being confident that the benefits of none are lost in the process.

REFERENCES

1. Kleinert H E, Cole N M, Wayne L, Harvey R, Kutz J E, Atasoy E 1973 Post-traumatic sympathetic dystrophy. Orthopaedic Clinics of North America 4: 917–927
2. Kozin F, McCarty D J, Genant H 1976 The reflex sympathetic dystrophy syndrome I. Clinical and histologic studies: Evidence for bilaterality, response to corticosteroids and articular involvement. American Journal of Medicine 60: 321–331
3. Kozin F, Genant C, Bekerman C, McCarty D J 1976 The reflex sympathetic dystrophy syndrome II. Roentgenographic and scintigraphic evidence of bilaterality and of periarticular accentuation. American Journal of Medicine 60: 332–338
4. Sudeck P 1900 Uber die akute entzundliche Knochenatropie. Arch. Klin. Chir. 11: 147
5. Colles A 1814 On fracture of the carpal extremity of the radius. Edinb. Medical Surgical Journal 10: 181. Reprinted Clinical Orthopaedics and Related Research 83: 3–5 (1972)
6. Bechtol C O 1954 Grip test: use of dynamometer with adjustable handle spacings. The Journal of Bone and Joint Surgery 36A: 820–824
7. Smith R J 1975 Factitious lymphedema of the hand. The Journal of Bone and Joint Surgery 57A: 89–94
8. Kusumi R K, Plouffe J F 1981 Gas in soft tissues of forearm in an 18-year-old emotionally disturbed diabetic. Journal of American Medical Association 246: 679–680
9. Secretan H 1901 Hard edema and traumatic hyperplasia of the dorsum of the metacarpus. Rev Med Suisse Rom 21: 409
10. Reading G 1980 Secretan's syndrome: Hard edema of the dorsum of the hand. Plastic and Reconstructive Surgery 65: 182–187
11. Saferin E H, Posch J L 1976 Secretan's disease. Post-traumatic hard edema of the dorsum of the hand. Plastic and Reconstructive Surgery 58: 703–707
12. Agris J, Simmons C 1978 Factitious (self-inflicted) skin wounds. Plastic and Reconstructive Surgery 62: 686–692
13. Phelps D B, Buchler U, Boswick J A 1977 The diagnosis of factitious ulcer of the hand: A case report. Journal of Hand Surgery 2: 105–108
14. Simmons B P, Vasile R 1980 The clenched fist syndrome. Journal of Hand Surgery 5: 420–427
15. Wallace P, Fitzmorris C 1978 The S-H-A-F-T syndrome in the upper extremity. Journal of Hand Surgery 3: 492–494
16. Spinner M 1969 Fashioned transpositional flap for soft tissue adduction contracture of the thumb. Plastic and Reconstructive Surgery 44: 345–348
17. Green D P, Dominguez O J 1979 A transpositional skin flap for release of volar contractures of a finger at the MP joint. Plastic and Reconstructive Surgery 64: 516–520
18. Joshi B.B 1972 Dorsolateral flap from same finger to relieve flexion contracture. Plastic and Reconstructive Surgery 49: 186–189
19. Lister G D 1981 The theory of the transposition flap and its practical application in the hand. Clinics in Plastic Surgery 8: 115–128
20. McCash C R 1956 Cross-arm bridge flaps in the repair of flexion contractures of the finger. British Journal of Plastic Surgery 9: 25–33
21. Matev I B 1980 Tactile gnosis in free skin grafts in the hand. British Journal of Plastic Surgery 33: 434–439

22. Porter R W 1968 Functional assessment of transplanted skin in volar defects of the digits. Journal of Bone and Joint Surgery 50A: 955–963
23. Freiburg A, Manktelow R 1972 The Kutler repair for fingertip amputations. Plastic and Reconstructive Surgery 50: 371–375
24. Joshi B B 1974 A local dorsolateral island flap for restoration of sensation after avulsion injury of fingertip pulp. Plastic and Reconstructive Surgery 54: 175–182
25. Nicolai J P A, Hentenaar G 1981 Sensation in cross-finger flaps. The Hand 13: 12–16
26. Kleinert H E, McAlister C G, MacDonald C J, Kutz J E 1974 A critical evaluation of cross-finger flaps. Journal of Trauma 14: 756–763
27. Flatt A E 1957 The thenar flap. Journal of Bone and Joint Surgery 39B: 80–85
28. Verdan C 1960 Syndrome of the quadriga. Surgical Clinics of North America 40: 425–426
29. Posner M 1979 Ray transposition for central digital loss. Journal of Hand Surgery 4: 242–257
30. Littler J W 1976 On making a thumb: One hundred years of surgical effort. The Journal of Hand Surgery 35–51
31. Verdan C 1968 The reconstruction of the thumb. Surgical Clinics of North America 48: 1033–1061
32. Miura T 1973 Thumb reconstruction using radial innervated cross-finger pedicle graft. Journal of Bone and Joint Surgery 55A: 563–569
33. Rybka F J, Pratt F E 1979 Thumb reconstruction with a sensory flap from the dorsum of the index finger. Plastic and Reconstructive Surgery 64: 141–144
34. Bunnell S 1931 Physiologic reconstruction of the thumb after total loss. Surgery, Obstetrics and Gynecology 52: 245–248
35. Matev I B 1980 Thumb reconstruction through metacarpal bone lengthening. Journal of Hand Surgery 5: 482–487
36. Reid D A C 1980 The Gillies thumb lengthening operation. The Hand 12: 123–129
37. Chase R A 1973 Atlas of hand surgery. W B Sanders Co, Philadelphia
38. Morgan L R, Stein F 1972 Method for a rapid and good thumb reconstruction. Plastic and Reconstructive Surgery 50: 131–133
39. Buck-Gramcko D 1971 Pollicisation of the index finger. Journal of Bone and Joint Surgery 53A: 1605–1617
40. Buck-Gramcko D 1977 Thumb reconstruction by digital transposition. Orthopedic Clinics of North America 8: 329–342
41. Lister, Tsai, Kalisman (in press)
42. Yoshimura M 1980 Toe-to-hand transfer. Plastic and Reconstructive Surgery 66: 74–83
43. Murray J F, Carman W, MacKenzie J K 1977 Transmetacarpal amputation of the index finger: A clinical assessment of hand strength and complications. Journal of Hand Surgery 2: 471–481
44. Kleinert H E, Putcha S M, Ashbell T S, Kutz J E 1967 The deformed fingernail, a frequent result of failure to repair nailbed injuries. The Journal of Trauma 7: 176–190
45. Watson H K, Hempton R F 1980 Limited wrist arthrodeses. I. The triscaphoid joint. Journal of Hand Surgery 5: 320–327
46. Watson H K, Goodman M L, Johnson T R 1981 Limited wrist arthrodesis. Part II: Intercarpal and radiocarpal combinations. Journal of Hand Surgery 6: 223–233
47. Inglis A E, Jones E C 1977 Proximal row carpectomy for diseases of the proximal row. Journal of Bone and Joint Surgery 59A: 460–463
48. Clendenin M B, Green D P 1981 Arthrodedis of the wrist — complications and their management. Journal of Bone and Joint Surgery 6: 253–257
49. Buck-Gramcko D 1977 Denervation of the wrist joint. The Journal of Bone and Joint Surgery 2: 54–61
50. Froimson A I 1981 Osteotomy for digital deformity. Journal of Hand Surgery 6: 585–589
51. Srinivasan H 1981 A simple method for assessing abduction of the thumb. Journal of Hand Surgery 6: 583–584
52. Kuczynski K 1974 Carpometacarpal joint of the human thumb. Journal of Anatomy 118: 119–126
53. Cooney W P, III Lucca M J, Chao E Y S, Linscheid R L 1981 The kinesiology of the thumb trapeziometacarpal joint. The Journal of Bone and Joint Surgery 63A(9): 1371–3181
54. Harris H, Joseph J 1949 Variation in the extension of the metacarpophalangeal and interphalangeal joints of the thumb. Journal of Bone and Joint Surgery 31B: 547–559
55. Smith R J, Kaplan E B 1968 Camptodactyly and similar atraumatic flexion deformities of the proximal interphalangeal joints of the fingers. Journal of Bone and Joint Surgery 50A: 1187–1203
56. Alldred A 1954 A locked index finger. Journal of Bone and Joint Surgery 36B: 102–103
57. Aston J N 1960 Locked middle finger. Journal of Bone and Joint Surgery 42B: 75–79
58. Bloom M N, Bryan R S 1965 Locked index finger caused by hyperflexion and entrapment of sesamoid bone. Journal of Bone and Joint Surgery 47A: 1383–1385
59. Charendoff M D 1979 Locking of the metacarpophalangeal joint: A case report. Journal of Hand Surgery 4: 173–176
60. Dibbell D G, Field J H 1967 Locking metacarpophalangeal joint. Plastic and Reconstructive Surgery 40: 562–564
61. Flatt A E 1958 Recurrent locking of an index finger. Journal of Bone and Joint Surgery 40A: 1128–1130
62. Flatt E A 1961 A locking little finger. Journal of Bone and Joint Surgery 43A: 240–242
63. Goodfellow J W, Weaver J P A 1961 Locking of the metacarpophalangeal joints. Journal of Bone and Joint Surgery 43B: 772–777
64. Harvey F J 1974 Locking of the metacarpophalangeal joints. Journal of Bone and Joint Surgery 56B: 156–159
65. Janecki C J, Routson G, DePapp E W 1980 Extra-articular synovial chondrometaplasia: Locking of the proximal interphalangeal joint of the finger. The Journal of Hand Surgery 5: 473–476
66. Stewart G J, Williams E A 1981 Locking of the metacarpophalangeal joints in degenerative disease. The Hand 13: 147–151
67. Yancey H A, Howard L D 1962 Locking of the metacarpophalangeal joint. Journal of Bone and Joint Surgery 44A: 380–382
68. Dupuytren G 1834 Permanent retraction of the fingers produced by an affliction of the palmar fascia. Lancet 2:222
69. Larsen R D, Takagishi N, Posch J L 1960 The pathogenesis of Dupuytren's contracture. Journal of Bone and Joint Surgery 42A: 993–1007
70. Skoog T 1963 The pathogenesis and etiology of Dupuytren's contracture. Plastic and Reconstructive Surgery 31: 258–267
71. Gabbiami G, Majho G 1972 Dupuytren's contracture: Fibroblast contraction? American Journal of Pathology 66: 131–138
72. Guber S, Rudolph R 1978 The myofibroblast. Surgery, Obstetrics and Gynecology 146: 641–649
73. Luck J U 1959 Dupuytren's contracture. Journal of Bone and Joint Surgery 41A: 635–664

74. McFarlane R M 1974 Patterns of diseased fascia in the fingers in Dupuytren's contracture. Plastic and Reconstructive Surgery 54: 31–44

75. Mikkelsen O A 1976 Dupuytren's disease — A study of the pattern of distribution and stage of contracture in the hand. The Hand 8: 265–271

76. Garrod A E 1875 Concerning pads upon the finger joints and their clinical relationships. British Medical Journal 1: 665

77. Mikkelsen O A 1977 Knuckle pads in Dupuytren's disease. The Hand 9: 301–305

78. Legge J H, McFarlane R M 1980 Prediction of results of treatment of Dupuytren's disease Journal of Hand Surgery 5: 608–616

79. Wolfe S J, Summerskill W H J, Davidson C S 1956 Thickening and contraction of the palmar fascia (Dupuytren's contracture) associated with alcoholism and hepatic cirrhosis. New England Journal of Medicine 255: 559–563

80. Short W H, Watson H K 1982 Prediction of the spiral nerve in Dupuytren's contracture. Journal of Hand Surgery 7:1 84–86

81. Elsahy N I 1976 Doppler ultrasound detection of displaced neurovascular bundles in Dupuytren's contracture. Plastic and Reconstructive Surgery 57: 104–105

82. Gordon S 1964 Dupuytren's contracture, plantar involvement. British Journal of Plastic Surgery 17: 421–423

83. Williams J L, Thomas C G 1968 Natural history of Peyronie's disease. Proceedings of the Royal Society of Medicine 61: 876–877

84. Smith R J 1971 Non-ischemic contractures of the intrinsic muscles of the hand. The Journal of Bone and Joint Surgery 53A: 1313–1331

85. Donaldson W R, Millender L W 1978 Chronic fracture-subluxation of the proximal interphalangeal joint. Journal of Hand Surgery 3: 149–153

86. Kleinert H E, Kasdan M L 1965 Reconstruction of chronically subluxated proximal interphalangeal finger joint. Journal of Bone and Joint Surgery 47A: 958–964

87. Palmer A K, Linscheid R L 1978 Chronic recurrent dislocation of the proximal interphalangeal joint of the finger. The Journal of Hand Surgery 3: 95–97

88. Mogensen B A, Mattsson H S 1980 Post-traumatic instability of the metacarpophalangeal joint of the thumb. The Hand 12: 85–90

89. Browne E Z Jr, Dunn H K, Snyder C C 1976 Ski pole thumb injury. Plastic and Reconstructive Surgery 58: 19–23

90. Smith M A 1980 The mechanism of acute ulnar instability of the metacarpophalangeal joint of the thumb. The Hand 12: 225–230

91. Redler I, Williams J T 1967 Rupture of a collateral ligament of the proximal interphalangeal joint of the finger. Journal of Bone and Joint Surgery 49A: 322–326

92. Stener B 1962 Displacement of the ruptured ulnar collateral ligament of the MCP joint of the thumb. Journal of Bone and Joint Surgery 44B: 869–879

93. Stern P J 1981 Stener lesion after lateral dislocation of the proximal interphalangeal joint — Indication for open reduction. Journal of Hand Surgery 6: 602–604

94. Osterman A L, Hauken G D, Bora F W Jr 1981 A quantitative evaluation of thumb function after ulnar collateral repair and reconstruction. Journal of Trauma 21: 854–861

95. Palmer A, Louis D 1978 Assessing ulnar instability of the metacarpophalangeal joint of the thumb. Journal of Hand Surgery 3: 542–546

96. Stothard J, Caird D M 1981 Experience with arthrography of the first metacarpophalangeal joint. The Hand 13: 257–266

97. Harrison D H 1977 The stiff proximal interphalangeal joint. The Hand 9: 102–108

98. McCue F C, Honner R, Johnson M C, Gieck J H 1970 Athletic injuries of the proximal interphalangeal joint requiring surgical treatment. Journal of Bone and Joint Surgery 52A: 937–956

99. Watson H K, Light T R, Johnson T R 1979 Checkrein resection for flexion contracture of the middle joint. The Journal of Hand Surgery 4: 67–72

100. Eaton R G, Malerich M M 1980 Volar plate arthroplasty of the proximal interphalangeal joint: A review of ten years' experience. Journal of Hand Surgery 5: 260–268

101. Engkvist O, Johansson S H 1980 Perichondrial arthroplasty. Scand. Journal of Plastic Reconstructive Surgery 14: 71–87

102. Engkvist O, Ohlsen L N 1979 Reconstruction of articular cartilage with free autologous perichondral grafts: An experimental study in rabbits. Scandinavian Journal of Plastic and Reconstructive Surgery 13: 269–274

103. Engkvist O, Skoog V, Pastacaldi P, Yormuk E, Juhlin R 1979 The cartilaginous potential of the perichondrium in rabbit ear and rib: A comparative study in vivo and vitro. Scand. Journal of Plastic Reconstructive Surgery 13: 275–280

104. Ohlsen L 1978 Cartilage regeneration from perichondrium. Experimental studies and clinical applications. Plastic and Reconstructive Surgery 62: 507–513

105. Skoog T, Johansson S H 1976 The formation of articular cartilage from free perichondral grafts. Plastic and Reconstructive Surgery 57: 1–6

106. Upton J, Sohn S A, Glowacki J 1981 Neocartilage derived from transplanted perichondrium: What is it? Plastic and Reconstructive Surgery 68: 166–172

107. Carroll R E, Hill N A 1969 Small joint arthrodesis in hand reconstruction. Journal of Bone and Joint Surgery 51A: 1219–1221

108. Moberg E 1960 Arthrodessis of finger joints. Surgical Clinics of North America 40:2 465–470

109. Robertson D C 1964 The fusion of interphalangeal joints. Canadian Journal of Surgery 7: 433–437

110. Jackson W T, Protas J M 1981 Snapping scapholunate subluxation. Journal of Hand Surgery 6: 590–594

111. Eckhardt W A, Palmer A K 1981 Recurrent dislocation of extensor carpi ulnaris tendon. Journal of Hand Surgery 6: 629–631

112. Burkhart S S, Wood M B, Linscheid R L 1982 Posttraumatic recurrent subluxation of the carpi ulnaris tendon. Journal of Hand Surgery 7: 1–3

113. Pezeshki C, Weiland A 1978 Bilateral dorsal dislocation of the distal radio-ulnar joint. Journal of Trauma 18: 673–676

114. Palmer A K, Werner F W 1981 The triangular fibrocartilage complex of the wrist — Anatomy and function. Journal of Hand Surgery 6:2 153–162

115. Joseph R B, Linscheid R L, Dobyns J H, Bryan R S 1981 Chronic sprains of the carpometacarpal joints. Journal of Hand Surgery 6: 172–180

116. Erb W H 1874 Uber eine eigenthumliche Localisation bon Lahmungen In: Plexus brachialis. Verhandl. d. Naturhist. Medical Ver. Heidelberg N.F. 2: 130

117. Brand P W 1958 Paralytic claw hand. Journal of Bone and Joint Surgery 40B: 618–632

118. Blacker G J, Lister G D, Kleinert H E 1976 The abducted little finger in low ulnar nerve palsy. The Journal of Hand Surgery 1: 190–196

119. Froment M J 1915 La Paralysie de l'adducteur du pouce et le signe de la prehension. Rev Neurol 28: 1236–1240

120. Mannerfelt L 1966 Studies on the hand in ulnar nerve paralysis. A clinical and experimental investigation in normal and anomalous innervation. Acta Orthopaedica Scandinavica Supp 87

121. Zancolli E A 1957 Clawhand caused by paralysis of the intrinsic muscles. Journal of Bone and Joint Surgery 39A: 1076–1081

122. Klumpke A 1885 Contribution a' l'etude des paralysies radiculaires du plexus brachial. Rev Med 5: 591–596

123. Tinel J 1915 Le signe du 'Fourmillement' dans les lesion des Neufs Peripheriques. Press Med 47: 388–389

124. Tinel J 1917 Nerve Wounds. Bailliere Tindal and Cox, London

125. Henderson W R 1948 Clinical assessment of peripheral nerve injuries The Lancet 801–805

126. Harrison S H 1974 The tactile adherence test estimating loss of sensation after nerve injury. Hand 6: 148–149

127. Egyed B, Eory A, Veres T, Manninger J 1980 Measurement of electrical resistance after nerve injuries of the hand The Hand 12: 275–281

128. Aschan W, Moberg E 1962 The Ninhydrin finger printing test used to map out partial lesions to hand nerves. Acta Chir Scand 123: 365–370

129. Moberg W 1958 Objective methods for determining the functional value of sensibility in the hand. Journal of Bone and Joint Surgery 40B: 454–476

130. Moberg E 1960 Examination of sensory loss by the ninhydrin printing test in Volkman's contracture. Bulletin of Hospital Joint Diseases 21: 296–303

131. Omer G E Jr 1968 Evaluation and reconstruction of the forearm and hand after acute traumatic peripheral nerve injuries. The Journal of Bone and Joint Surgery 50A: 1454–1478

132. Moberg E 1964 Evaluation and management of nerve injuries in the hand. Surgical Clinics of North America 44: 1019

133. Onne L 1962 Recovery of sensibility and sudo-motor activity in the hand after nerve suture. Acta Chir Scand Supp 300: 1–69

134. Gellis M, Pool R 1977 Two-point discrimination distances in the normal hand and forearm. Plastic and Reconstructive Surgery 59: 57–63

135. Dellon A L 1981 Evaluation of sensibility and re-education of sensation in the hand. Williams and Wilkins, Baltimore

136. Dellon A L, Curtis R M, Edgerton M T 1974 Re-education of sensation in the hand after nerve injury and repair. Plastic and Reconstructive Surgery 53: 297–305

137. Parry C B, Salter M 1976 Sensory re-education after median nerve lesions. The Hand 8: 250–257

138. Levin S, Pearsall G, Ruderman R J 1978 Von Frey's method of measuring pressure sensibility in the hand: An engineering analysis of Weinstein-Semmes pressure aesthesiometer. Journal of Hand Surgery 3: 211–216

139. O'Riain S 1973 New and simple test of nerve function in hand. British Medical Journal 3: 615–616

140. Dellon A L 1980 Clinical use of vibratory stimuli to evaluate peripheral nerve injury and compression neuropathy. Plastic and Reconstructive Surgery 65: 466–476

141. Mansat M, Delprat J, Delprat J M 1981 'The vibrometer' An electro magnetic transducer as an attempt to examine sensibility of the hand in quantitative terms. The Hand 13: 202–210

142. Mitchell S W 1872 Injuries of nerves and their consequences. Lippincott, Philadelphia

143. Herndon J, Eaton R, Littler J W 1976 Management of painful neuromas in the hand. Journal of Bone and Joint Surgery 58A: 369–373

144. Tupper J W, Booth D M 1976 Treatment of painful neuromas of nerves in the hand: A comparison of traditional and newer methods. The Journal of Hand Surgery 1: 144–151

145. Swanson A B, Boeve N R, Lumsden R M 1977 The prevention and treatment of amputation neuromata by silicone capping. The Journal of Hand Surgery 2: 70–78

146. Bodyns J H, O'Brien E T, Linscheid R L, Farrow G M 1972 Bowler's thumb: Diagnosis and treatment. Journal of Bone and Joint Surgery 54A: 751–755

147. Kisner W H 1976 Thumb neuroma: A hazard of ten pin bowling. British Journal of Plastic Surgery 29: 225–226

148. Belsky M R, Millender L H 1980 Bowler's thumb in a baseball player: A case report. Orthopedics 3: 122–123

149. Martin R 1763 Tal om Nervers allmanna Egenskaper i Manniskans kroop. L Salvius, Stockholm

150. Gruber W 1870 Uber die Verbundung des Nervus medianus mit dem Nervus ulnaris am unterarme des Meuchen und der Saugethiere. Arch Anat Physiol Med Leipzig 37: 501–522

151. Clippinger F W, Goldner J L, Roberts J M 1962 Use of the electromyogram in evaluating upper-extremity peripheral nerve lesions. The Journal of Bone and Joint Surgery 44A: 1047–1060

152. Ballantyne J P, Campbell M J 1973 Electrophysiological study after surgical repair of sectioned human peripheral nerves. Journal of Neurology, Neurosurgery and Psychiatry 36:5 797–805

153. Seddon Sir H J 1972 Surgical disorders of peripheral nerves. Williams and Wilkins, Baltimore

154. Terzis J K, Dykes R E, Hakstian R W 1976 Electrophysiological recordings in peripheral nerve surgery: A review. The Journal of Hand Surgery 1: 52–66

155. Brand P W, Thompson D E 1982 Relative tension and potential excursion of muscles in the forearm and hand. The Journal of Hand Surgery 6: 209–219

156. Bufalini C, Pescatori G 1969 Posterior cervical electromyography in the diagnosis and prognosis of brachial plexus injuries. Journal of Bone and Joint Surgery 51B: 627–631

157. Bonney G 1954 The value of axon responses in determining the site of lesion in traction injuries of the brachial plexus. Brain 77: 588–609

158. Landi A, Copeland S 1979 Value of the Tinel sign in brachial plexus lesions. Annals of the Royal College of Surgeons of England 61: 470–471

159. Landi A, Copeland S A, Parry C B, Wynn, Jones S J 1980 The role of somatosensory evoked potentials and nerve conduction studies on the surgical management of brachial plexus injuries. The Journal of Bone and Joint Surgery 62B: 492–496

160. Match R M 1975 Radiation-induced brachial plexus paralysis. Archives of Surgery 110: 384–386

161. Rorabeck C H, Harris W R 1981 Factors affecting the prognosis of brachial plexus injuries. Journal of Bone and Joint Surgery 63B: 404–407

162. Hardy A E 1981 Birth injuries of the brachial plexus. Journal of Bone and Joint Surgery 63B: 98–101

163. Hoffer M M, Braun R, Hsu J, Mitani M, Temes K 1981 Functional recovery and orthopaedic management of brachial plexus palsies. Journal of American Medical Association. 246: 2467–2470

164. Braun R M, Hoffer M M, Mooney V, McKeever J, Roper B 1973 Phenol nerve block in the treatment of acquired spastic hemiplegia in the upper limb. Journal of Bone and Joint Surgery 55A: 580–585

165. Zancolli E A 1979 Structural and dynamic bases of hand surgery 2nd edn. Lippincott, Philadelphia

166. House J H, Gwathmey F W, Fidler M O 1981 A dynamic approach to the thumb-in-palm deformity in cerebral palsy. Evaluation and results in fifty-six patients. Journal of Bone and Joint Surgery 63A: 216–225

167. Turner J W A, Parsonage M J 1957 Neuralgic amyotrophy (paralytic brachial neuritis) with special reference to prognosis. Lancet 273: 209–212

168. Parsonage M J, Turner J W A 1948 Neuralgic amyotrophy The shoulder-girdle syndrome. Lancet 973–978

169. Bedbrook G M 1979 Spinal injuries with tetraplegia and paraplegia. Journal of Bone and Joint Surgery 61B: 267–284

170. Freehafer A A, Vonhaam E, Allen V 1974 Tendon transfers to improve grasp after injuries of the cervical spinal cord. The Journal of Bone and Joint Surgery 56A: 951–959

171. Lamb D W, Lamdry R M 1972 The hand in quadriplegia. Paraplegia 9: 204–212

172. Zancolli E A 1979 Structural and dynamic bases of hand surgery 2nd edn. J B Lippincott Co, Philadelphia

173. Moberg E 1978 The upper limb in tetraplegia. Georg Thieme, Stuttgart

174. House J H, Gwathmey F W, Lundsgaard D K 1976 Restoration of strong grasp and lateral pinch in tetraplegia due to cervical spinal cord injury. The Journal of Hand Surger 1: 152–159

175. Colyer R A, Kappelman B 1981 Flexor pollicis longus tenodesis in tetraplagia at the sixth cervical level — A prospective evaluation of functional gain. Journal of Bone and Joint Surgery 63A: 376–379

176. McDowell C, Moberg E A, Smith A G 1979 International conference on surgical rehabilitation of the upper limb in tetraplagia. Journal of Hand Surgery 4: 387–390

177. Doyle J R, Blythe W 1975 The finger flexor tendon sheath and pulleys: anatomy and reconstruction. Symposium on Tendon Surgery in the Hand. AAOS. Mosby, St Louis

178. Parkes A 1971 The 'lumbrical plus' finger. Journal of Bone and Joint Surgery 53B: 236–239

179. Heath R D 1972 The subclavian steal syndrome. Cause of symptoms in the arm. Journal of Bone and Joint Surgery 54A: 1033–1039

180. Welling R E, Cranley J J, Krause R J, Hafner C D 1981 Obliterative arterial disease of the upper extremity. Archives of Surgery 116: 1593–1596

181. Allen E V 1929 Thromboangitis obliterans: methods of diagnosis of chronic occlusive arterial lesions distal to the wrist with illustrative cases. American Journal of Medical Science 178: 237–244

182. Gelberman R H, Blasingame J P 1981 The timed Allen test. Journal of Trauma 21: 477–479

183. Scavenius M, Fauner M, Walther-Larsen S, Buchwald C, Nielsen S L 1981 A quantitative Allen's test. The Hand 13: 318–320

184. Ernst D, Hurlow R, Strachan C, Chandler S 1978 The assessment of digital vessel disease by dynamic hand scanning. The Hand 10: 217–225

185. Wilgis E, Jezic D, Stonesifer G, Classen J, Sekercan K 1974 The evaluation of small-vessel flow. The Journal of Bone and Joint Surgery 56A: 1199–1206

186. Bendick P J, Mayer J R, Glover J L, Park H M 1979 A photoplethysmographic technique for detecting vascular compromise. The Journal of Trauma 19: 398–402

187. Gross W, Louis D 1978 Doppler hemodynamic assessment of obscure symptomatology in the upper extremity. Journal of Hand Surgery 3: 467–473

188. Kleinert H E, Volanitis G J 1965 Thrombosis of the palmar arterial arch and its tributaries: etiology and newer concepts in treatment. Journal of Trauma 5: 446–457

189. Koman L A, Urbaniak J R 1981 Ulnar artery insufficiency: A guide to treatment. Journal of Hand Surgery 6: 1 16–24

190. Millender L, Nalebuff E, Dasdan E 1972 Aneurysms and thromboses of the ulnar artery in the hand. Archives of Surgery 105: 686–690

191. Eguro H, Goldner J L 1973 Bilateral thrombosis of the ulnar arteries in the hands. Plastic and Reconstructive Surgery 52: 573–578

192. Conn J, Bergan J, Bell J 1970 Hypothenar hammer syndrome: Post-traumatic digital ischemia. Surgery 68: 1122–1128

193. Carneirio R S, Mann R J 1979 Occlusion of the ulnar artery associated with an anomalous muscle: A case report. The Journal of Hand Surgery 4: 412–414

194. Cho K 1978 Entrapment occlusion of the ulnar artery in the hand. Journal of Bone and Joint Surgery 60A: 841–843

195. Given K S, Puckett C L, Kleinert H E 1978 Ulnar artery thrombosis. Plastic and Reconstructive Surgery 61: 405–411

196. Hirai M, Shinoya S 1979 Arterial obstruction of the upper limb in Buerger's disease: its incidence and primary lesion. British Journal of Surgery 66: 124–129

197. Raynaud A G M 1862 De l'asphyxie locale et de la gangrene symetrique des extremites. Rignoux, Paris

198. Balas P, Tripolitis A J, Kaklamanis P, Mandalaki T, Paracharalampous N 1979 Raynaud's Phenomenon. Primary and secondary causes. Archives of Surgery 114: 1174–1177

199. Farmer R, Gifford R, Hines E 1961 Raynaud's disease with sclerodactylia. A follow-up study of seventy-one patients. Circulation 23: 13–15

200. Welsh C L 1980 The effect of vibration on digital blood flow. The British Journal of Surgery 67: 708–710

201. Teisinger J 1972 Vascular disease disorders resulting from vibrating tools. Journal of Medicine 14: 129–133

202. Mosely L H, Finseth F 1977 Cigarette smoking: Impairment of digital blood flow and wound healing in the hand. The Hand 9: 97–100

203. Arnulf G 1976 Physiological basis of sympathetic surgery for the upper limb in Raynaud's diseases. Journal of Cardiovascular Surgery 17: 354–357

204. Kirtley J A, Riddell D H, Stoney W S, Wright J K 1967 Cervicothoracic sympathectomy in neurovascular abnormalities of the upper extremity. Annals of Surgery 165: 869–879

205. Flatt A E 1980 Digital artery sympathectomy. Journal of Hand Surgery 5: 550–556

FURTHER READING

Books

Dellon A L 1981 Evaluation of sensibility and re-education of sensation in the hand. Williams and Wilkins, Baltimore

Flatt A E The care of the rheumatoid hand. Moseby In press St. Louis

Spinner M 1978 Injuries to the major branches of peripheral nerves of the forearm. Saunders, Philadelphia

Zancolli E A 1979 Structural and dynamic bases of hand surgery, 2nd edn. Lippincott, Philadelphia

Journals

Atasoy E, Ioakimidis E, Kasdan M, Kutz J E, Kleinert H E 1970 Reconstruction of the amputated fingertip with a triangular volar flap. Journal of Bone and Joint Surgery 52A: 921–926

Bowers W H, Wolf J W, Nehil J L, Bittinger S 1980 The proximal interphalangeal joint volar plate. I. An anatomical and biomechanical study. Journal of Hand Surgery 5: 79–88

Boyes J H 1980 The measuring of motions. Journal of Hand Surgery 5: 89–90

Brough M D 1977 Dermatitis artefacta. The Hand 9: 283–286

Brown P W 1979 Sacrifice of the unsatisfactory hand. The Journal of Hand Surgery 4: 417–423

Bryan R S 1977 The Moberg deltoid-triceps replacement and key-pinch operations in quadriplegia: Preliminary experiences. The Hand 9: 207–214

Camp R A, Weatherwax R J, Miller E B 1980 Chronic post-traumatic instability of the thumb metacarpophalangeal joint. Journal of Hand Surgery 5: 221–225

Carroll R E, Craig F S 1951 The surgical treatment of cerebral palsy. Surgical Clinics of North America 30: 385–396

Chait L A, Kaplan I, Stewart-Lord B, Goodman M 1980 Early surgical correction in the cerebral palsied hand. Journal of Hand Surgery 5: 122–126

Colton C L, Ransford A O, Lloyd-Roberts G C 1976 Transposition of the tendon of pronator teres in cerebral palsy. The Journal of Bone and Joint Surgery 58B: 220–223

Cooney W P, Chao E Y S 1977 Biomechanical analysis of static forces in the thumb during hand function. Journal of Bone and Joint Surgery 59A: 27–36

Cooney W P, Dobyns J H, Linscheid R L 1980 Nonunion of the scaphoid: Analysis of the results from bone grafting. Journal of Hand Surgery 5: 343–354

DeBenedetti M 1979 Restoration of elbow extension power in the tetraplegic patient using the Moberg technique. The Journal of Bone and Joint Surgery 4: 86–90

Dellon A L 1978 The moving two-point discrimination test: Clinical evaluation of the quickly adapting fiber/receptor system. Journal of Hand Surgery 3: 474–481

Earle A S, Vlastou C 1980 Crossed fingers and other tests of ulnar nerve motor function. Journal of Hand Surgery 5: 560–565

Eaton R G, Littler J W 1976 Joint injuries and their sequelae. Clinics in Plastic Surgery 3: 85–98

Eiken O, Hagberg L, Lundborg G 1981 Evolving biologic concepts as applied to tendon surgery. Clinics in Plastic Surgery 8: 1–12

Filler B C, Stark H H, Boyes J H 1976 Capsulodesis of the metacarpophalangeal joint of the thumb in children with cerebral palsy. Journal of Bone and Joint Surgery 58A: 667–670

Freehafer A A, Mast W A 1967 Transfer of the brachioradialis to improve wrist extension in high spinal-cord injury. The Journal of Bone and Joint Surgery 49A: 648–652

Gelberman R H, Menon J 1980 The vascularity of the scaphoid bone. The Journal of Hand Surgery 5: 508–513

Goldner J L, Irwin C F 1950 An analysis of paralytic thumb deformities. Journal of Bone and Joint Surgery 32A: 627–639

Grant G H 1980 The hand and the psyche. Journal of Hand Surgery 5: 417–419

Hoffer M M, Perry J, Melkonian G J 1979 Dynamic electromyography and decision-making for surgery in the upper extremity of patients with cerebral palsy. Journal of Hand Surgery 4: 424–431

Kuczynski K 1968 The proximal interphalangeal joint. Journal of Bone and Joint Surgery 50B: 656–663

Landsmeer J M F 1975 The proximal interphalangeal joint. The Hand 7: 30–45

Linscheid R L, Dobyns J H, Beabout J W, Bryan R S 1972 Traumatic instability of the wrist. The Journal of Bone and Joint Surgery 54A: 1612–1632

Lipscomb P R, Elkins E C, Henderson E D 1958 Tendon transfers to restore function of hands in tetraplegia, especially after fracture dislocations of the sixth cervical vertebra on the seventh. Journal of Bone and Joint Surgery 40A: 1071–1080

Lowry W E, Cord S A 1981 Traumatic avascular necrosis of the capitate bone — Case report. Journal of Hand Surgery 6: 245–248

Lusskin R, Campbell J B, Thompson W A L 1973 Posttraumatic lesions of the brachial plexus. Journal of Bone and Joint Surgery 55A: 1159–1176

McCue F C, Honner R, Chapman W C 1970 Transfer of the brachioradialis for hands deformed by cerebral palsy. The Journal of Bone and Joint Surgery 52A: 1171–1180

McGrath M H, Watson H K 1981 Late results with local bone graft donor sites in hand surgery. Journal of Hand Surgery 6: 234–237

McGregor I A, Morgan G 1973 Axial and random pattern flaps. British Journal of Plastic Surgery 26: 202–213

Macht S D, Watson H K 1980 The Moberg volar advancement flap for digital reconstruction. Journal of Hand Surgery 5: 372–376

May J W, Bartlett S P 1981 Staged groin flap in reconstruction of the pediatric hand. Journal of Hand Surgery 6: 163–171

Mayfield J K, Johnson R P, Kilcoyne R K 1980 Carpal dislocations: Pathomechanics and progressive perilunar instability. Journal of Hand Surgery 5: 226–241

Mital M 1979 Lengthening of the elbow flexors in cerebral palsy. Journal of Bone and Joint Surgery 61A: 515–522

Miura T, Kino Y, Nakamura R 1976 Reconstruction of the mutilated hand. The Hand 8: 78–85

Moberg E 1975 Surgical treatment for absent single hand grip and elbow extension in quadriplegia. Journal of Bone and Joint Surgery 57A: 196–206

Moberg E 1977 Reconstruction of the mutilated hand. Scand. Journal of Plastic and Reconstructive Surgery 11: 219–224

Moberg E A, Lamb D W 1980 Surgical rehabilitation of the upper limb in tetraplegia. The Hand 12: 209–213

Newman J H, Watt I 1980 Avascular necrosis of the capitate and dorsal dorsi-flexion instability. The Hand 12: 176–178

Pallin I M, Deutsch E V 1951 Death following stellate ganglion block. Annals of Surgery 133: 226–233

Palmer A, Dobyns J, Linscheid R 1978 Management of posttraumatic instability of the wrist secondary to ligament rupture. Journal of Hand Surgery 3: 507–532

Pieron A P 1972 Connection of rotational malunion of a phalanx by metacarpal osteotomy. Journal of Bone and Joint Surgery 54B: 516–519

Pulvertaft R G 1975 Psychological aspects of hand injuries. The Hand 7: 93–103

Rainsford A O, Hughes S P F 1977 Complete brachial plexus lesions. Journal of Bone and Joint Surgery 59B: 417–420

Resnick D 1974 Arthrography in the evaluation of arthritic disorders of the wrist. Radiology 113: 331–340

Richards R 1967 Causalgia. Archives of Neurology 16: 339–350

Robert P 1936 La radiographie de l'articulation trapezo metacarpienne. Les arthroses de cette jointure. Bulletins et memoires de la Societe de Radiologie medicale de France 24: 687–690

Robertson W C Jr, Eichman P L, Clancy W G 1979 Upper trunk brachial plexopathy in football players. Journal of the American Medical Association 241: 1480–1482

Rorabeck C H 1980 The management of the flail upper extremity in brachial plexus injuries. Journal of Trauma 20: 491–493

Sakellarides H T, Mital M A, Lenzi W D 1981 Treatment of pronation contractures of the forearm in cerebral palsy by changing the insertion of the pronator radii teres. Journal of Bone and Joint Surgery 63A: 645–652

Samilson R L, Morris J M 1964 Surgical improvement of the cerebral palsied upper limb. Journal of Bone and Joint Surgery 46A: 1203–1216

Samilson R L 1976 Tendon transfers in cerebral palsy. The Journal of Bone and Joint Surgery 58B: 153–154

Saveyev V, Zatevakhin I, Stepanov N 1977 Artery embolism of the upper limbs. Surgery 81: 367–375

Schmidt P E, Hewitt R L 1980 Severe upper limb ischemia. Archives of Surgery 115: 1188–1191

Sebald J R, Dobyns J H, Linscheid R L 1974 Natural history of collapse deformities of the wrist. Clinical Orthopaedics and Related Research 104: 140–148

Shelton W R, Sage F P 1981 Modified Nicoll-graft treatment of gap non-unions in the upper extremity. Journal of Bone and Joint Surgery 63A: 226–231

Smith R J 1977 Post-traumatic instability of the metacarpophalangeal joint of the thumb. Journal of Bone and Joint Surgery 59A: 14–21

Snow J W 1968 Ulnar half of extensor digiti quinti proprius tendon for flexor grafts. Plastic and Reconstructive Surgery 42: 603–604

Southcott R, Rosman M A 1977 Non-union of carpal scaphoid fractures in children. Journal of Bone and Joint Surgery 59B: 20–23

Spiegel D, Chase R A 1980 The treatment of contractures of the hand using self-hypnosis. The Journal of Hand Surgery 5: 428–432

Stark H, Zelme N, Boyes J, Ashworth C 1977 Flexor tendon graft through superficialis tendon. Journal of Hand Surgery 2: 456–461

Tranquilli-Leali E 1935 Ricostruzione dell 'apice delle falangi ungueali mediante autoplastica volare peduncolata per scorrimento. Infort traum Lavoro 1: 186–193

Weber E H 1835 Ueber den Tastsinn. Archives of Anatomy and Physiology Wissensch Med 152–160

Whitehurst L, Harrelson J M 1977 Brain-stem anesthesia. An unusual complication of stellate ganglion block. Journal of Bone and Joint Surgery 59A: 541–542

3

Compression

The pathogenesis of peripheral nerve compression is varied:

Anatomical. In certain areas, nerves pass through unyielding surroundings, as in the carpal tunnel and beneath the arcade of Frohse.

Postural. Many occupations or recreations require repetitive motions. If these are made in a posture which increases peripheral nerve compression, symptoms may develop. Examples of such positions are

(a) the flexed wrist which increases carpal tunnel compression expecially if weight is lifted in this posture,

(b) pronation of the forearm with an extended elbow and flexed wrist motion which compresses the radial nerve in its 'tunnel' at the elbow.

Developmental. Anomalous structures may overfill a tight compartment or may place a nerve on stretch, as occurs in the presence of a cervical rib or its fibrous anlage.

Inflammatory. Synovitis is the most common cause of nerve compression in the carpal tunnel. Usually non-specific, the increased bulk of inflamed synovium cannot be accommodated by the inexpansible tunnel and compression of the median nerve results. The specific synovitis of rheumatoid disease causes a much higher incidence of nerve compression amongst those so afflicted than occurs in the general population.

Traumatic. Acute carpal tunnel syndrome, requiring urgent release, may complicate any hand injury in which significant oedema occurs. Delayed nerve compression may result from trauma as in the tardy ulnar palsy following on supracondylar fractures of the humerus.

Metabolic. Alterations in fluid distribution may well precipitate or exacerbate nerve compression. This is especially common in carpal tunnel syndrome, in which the characteristic night numbness is due in part to the increased peripheral circulation which occurs during sleep, largely as a means of temperature regulation. The syndrome is more prevalent in women and is often more troublesome in the premenstrual phase and during pregnancy when water retention occurs. Certain endocrine disorders, by disturbing fluid balance, show an increased incidence of nerve compression syndromes. Thus carpal tunnel syndrome in particular is more common in myxoedema[1] and diabetes.

Swellings, by taking up already overcrowded space, may produce compression syndromes.

Iatrogenic. Acute compression may be inflicted on nerves during surgical procedures. Such injury occurs most commonly to the radial nerve travelling as it does for most of its course close to bone. It is therefore very vulnerable during internal fixation of fractures of the humerus and radius. The surgeon must identify and preserve it zealously when applying bone plates. Compression of peripheral nerves may also occur through poor positioning of the anaesthetized patient. Once again the radial nerve in the spiral groove is most at risk although the axillary nerve and ulnar nerve above the elbow[2] have been injured by this means.

When subjected to constant compression a nerve becomes narrowed. This is commonly observed in the course of relieving a carpal tunnel syndrome (Fig. 3.1). If narrowing has been present for some time, fibrosis occurs in the epineurium and between the fascicles themselves. In such circumstances, compression by fibrosis may persist even after release of the original compressing force. Curtis has demonstrated the value of splitting the epineurium and performing internal neurolysis in improving the results of carpal tunnel release.[3]

If the compressive force is applied intermittently, as in the radial tunnel syndrome, a constriction in the nerve itself is much less likely. Thus confirmation of the diagnosis at the time of surgery is less convincing and there is rarely any need to perform an internal neurolysis.

HISTORY

When a patient presents with pain or dysaesthesia he should be questioned in respect to each regarding location, radiation, duration, fluctuation and periodicity, nature and time of onset and factors which provoke or relieve the symptoms. He may be unable to give precise replies. It is then useful to ask him to record the details during an attack and report them at his next visit. For example, patients may state that numbness involves all of their digits but advised

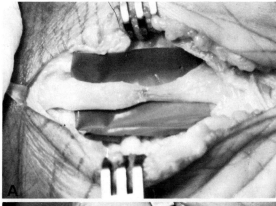

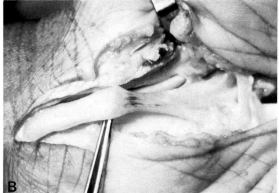

Figs. 3.1A & B This median nerve has been subjected to compression in the carpal tunnel and shows both narrowing of the nerve and hyperaemia of the narrow section.

observation reveals that only those supplied by the median nerve are affected.

Other symptoms should be recorded and a general medical history and description of occupation obtained. Particular attention should be paid to any family history of diabetes, to symptoms suggestive of other endocrine disorders, and to repetitive occupational postures which are common in production line industry. If a full physical examination has been performed in the recent past, a report should be obtained.

Symptoms and signs

Compression of peripheral nerves produces predictably one or more of four effects: pain, sensory disturbance, motor loss, electrophysiological change.

The *pain* of nerve compression may be located at the site of compression, but commonly radiates distally and proximally. Distal radiation is easily understood and knowledge of the distribution of, for example, a cervical root is necessary to localize the site of compression. Proximal radiation is more difficult to understand and may represent a generalized neuritis resulting from distal compression or referred pain to an area having a common cervical root origin with the compressed nerve. Pain occurs in compression of purely motor nerves, as in the *radial tunnel syndrome.* This is probably due to the fact that the nerve is not entirely efferent in flow, having afferent fibres from both muscles and joints.

Sensory disturbance in compression syndromes initially takes the form of intermittent numbness and tingling or paraesthesia. These are invariably within the exact sensory distribution of the compressed nerve although not necessarily throughout it. Any indisputable extension beyond the boundaries of that distribution should make the examiner beware. He may be dealing with anomalous distribution, compression of more than one nerve, or, most probably, compression located more proximally than initially suspected.

While at first present only periodically, numbness soon becomes constant. Depending upon the nerve involved, this may be a nuisance or a distinct disability. Loss of sensation in median nerve distribution causes clumsiness in fine manipulation and this may be the patient's sole or major complaint.

Examination at all stages reveals some change in sensation. This is by no means total anaesthesia or analgesia. Two point discrimination, sweating and even tactile gnosis are commonly all intact. The patient simply declares that on light touch or pinwheel testing 'it feels different' from other normal areas — this has been termed *dysaesthesia.* It follows that the area under examination must be repeatedly compared with other areas of normally similar sensibility in the same and the other hand. The boundaries of dysaesthesia should be marked out. Special attention should be paid to key areas, such as the 'palmar triangle' in median and the dorsum of the hand in ulnar nerve compression.

A Tinel's sign is often elicited at the site of compression or a little proximal to it, producing paraesthesia radiating into the sensory distribution of the nerve.

Tenderness may be present over the course of the nerve expecially when pain is the major symptom. This may be revealed by direct palpation or by the indirect compression produced by putting muscles on tension or by so positioning joints as to increase the pressure on the nerve.

Motor loss in nerve compression, unlike that following nerve section, is an insidiously progressive disability, of which the patient may be unaware. *Muscle wasting* may be far advanced but unnoticed by the patient's untrained eye. *Postural changes,* such as the development of a claw hand or abducted small finger in ulnar nerve compression may be the first feature which commands his attention or it may be *weakness and clumsiness* in certain acts. The weakness is often slight and only detectable by careful comparison with the other, supposedly normal, hand. In certain instances it is possible to pit one muscle directly against its counterpart, as with the abductor pollicis brevis of each hand (Fig. 3.2.).

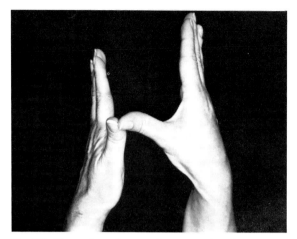

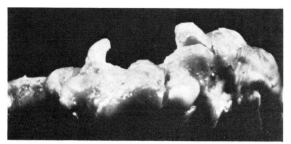

Fig. **3.3** The carpal tunnel view in relief in a dissection of the skeleton. The pisiform has been removed on the left of the photograph revealing the hook of the hamate which forms the ulnar border while on the right of the photograph the tubercle of the scaphoid and the ridge of the trapezium are seen clearly formig the radial border. Reproduced from JOHNSON, M K and COHEN M J 1975, The Hand Atlas. Thomas, Springfield with kind permission of the authors and publisher.

Fig. **3.2** The weakness in a muscle can sometimes be demonstrated by pitting it against its normal counterpart in the other hand. Here weakness of the abductor pollicis brevis in carpal tunnel syndrome is clearly demonstrated when the patient attempts to maintain both thumbs in palmar abduction while pushing out against the other.

Electrical activity may be altered in nerve compression syndromes, with a reduction in nerve conduction velocity across the area of compression. This is exemplified by the increase in distal motor or sensory latency often found in carpal tunnel syndrome. However, only a positive finding of slowing of nerve conduction is of value. Uninterrupted conduction in but a small percentage of fibres will give normal speeds of conduction for the whole nerve. Also, in those syndromes in which compression is intermittent, as in the radial tunnel, nerve conduction times are often normal. Thus a normal electrical study does not rule out a compression syndrome, while an abnormal study confirms the clinical findings. Such studies are often of greatest value in localizing the site of compression.

MEDIAN NERVE

Carpal tunnel syndrome

The carpal tunnel is a bony canal of which the margins can be palpated (Fig. 3.3).

The *scaphoid tubercle* is the bony prominence at the base of the thenar eminence just distal to the distal wrist crease. The tendon of flexor carpi radialis appears to attach to that prominence when rendered palpable by flexing the wrist against resistance — it in fact passes over the tubercle and into a groove beneath the *ridge of the trapezium,* which lies immediately adjacent distally. These two bones form the radial boundary of the carpal tunnel.

The *pisiform* is easily palpable at the ulnar end of the narrow area between the two wrist creases. Flexor carpi

ulnaris attaches to the pisiform, gaining additional purchase through the piso-hamate and piso-metacarpal ligaments which insert into the hook of the hamate and the base of the fifth metacarpal respectively.

The *hook of the hamate,* with the pisiform, forms the ulnar margin of the tunnel. More difficult to palpate, the hook of the hamate lies two centimetres distal and slightly radial to the pisiform beneath the broken skin crease which demarcates the hypothenar eminence. Over the hook the motor branch of the ulnar nerve can be rolled by the examining finger.

The *flexor retinaculum* which roofs over the tunnel is a thick, rigid, fibrous sheet which attaches to its bony boundaries. A less substantial part of the retinaculum passes superficially to blend with the hypothenar fascia. Sometimes referred to as the *volar carpal ligament,* this is the roof of *Guyon's canal* through which the ulnar nerve and artery pass, radial to the pisiform but ulnar to the hook of the hamate.

Ten structures pass through the carpal tunnel — the median nerve, flexor pollicis longus and the eight tendons to the four fingers. The tendons are enveloped by the synovium of the radial and ulnar bursae. Any volumetric increase of this synovium will compress the median nerve.

Other less common causes of median nerve compression in the carpal tunnel include

developmental — persistent median artery[4] (Fig. 3.4)

— unusually extensive lumbrical[5-7] or superficialis[8] muscle bellies (Fig. 3.5)

— anomalous muscles, of which *palmaris profundus* is the most common[9-12]

trauma[13] — the effects of trauma may be direct, as in carpal bone fractures or carpo-metacarpal dislocation (Fig. 3.6), or

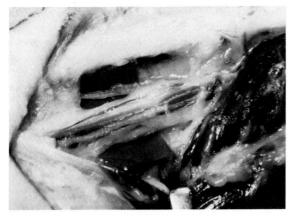

Fig. 3.4 Here a persistent median artery is seen on the surface of the median nerve. Flow has been diminished by the compression against the retinaculum.

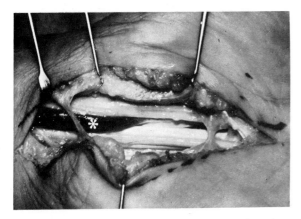

Fig. 3.5 The belly of the superficialis to the middle finger is unduly long and has produced compression in the carpal tunnel.

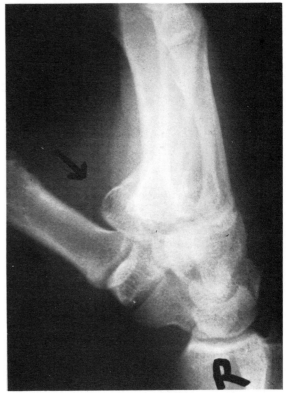

Fig. 3.6 An anterior carpometacarpal dislocation may produce pressure in the carpal tunnel resulting in acute median nerve compression. (This is the patient illustrated in Fig. 1.68.)

	indirect due to the swelling resulting from an extensive hand injury or burns[14]
swellings	— ganglion[15] or lipoma
inflammatory	— rheumatoid disease, gout and amyloidosis
metabolic	— endocrine imbalance, most common of which is pregnancy.

SYMPTOMS

Numbness is the most frequent complaint. Located in the median nerve distribution, the digits most often involved are the middle and index. Initially, the numbness is intermittent. The time of onset is characteristic in the early hours of the morning, induced by the acute wrist flexion of the 'foetal' sleeping position, by altered fluid distribution in the lying position and by increased blood flow to the limb for thermoregulation. For reasons which are obscure, symptoms are often relieved by hanging the limb dependent. Carpal tunnel syndrome may be provoked by working with the wrist flexed, while driving or reading a newspaper.

Pain in the upper limb may be due to median nerve compression in the carpal tunnel. This cause may be overlooked particularly if the pain is in the arm above the tunnel. Discomfort due to carpal tunnel syndrome may be present *as far proximal as the shoulder*[16].

Clumsiness may be due to sensory loss or to weakness in the thenar musculature.

EXAMINATION

Muscle wasting is best detected by comparison with the other hand, while viewing the thenar eminence in profile (Fig. 3.7). It may rarely affect only part of the abductor pollicis brevis, in which case it may be less pronounced.

Sensory disturbance is mapped out using light touch or, more expeditiously, by using a pin-wheel (Fig. 3.8). Loss of sensation is not commonly so advanced as to cause a detectable difference in two point discrimination. It follows that sweating is often present in which event those sensory tests based on its absence are not applicable. In performing

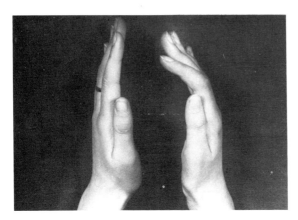

Fig. 3.7 Thenar wasting may be demonstrated best by comparing it with the opposite normal hand.

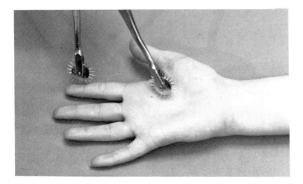

Fig. 3.8 As the pinwheel is passed from the index finger into the palm, it moves from the area of absolute innervation by the median nerve into that supplied by the palmar cutaneous. In carpal tunnel syndrome, therefore, a change will occur at some point between these two areas.

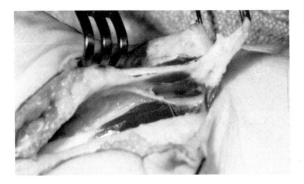

Fig. 3.9 The palmar cutaneous branch of the median nerve can be seen in this case arising just proximal to the carpal tunnel and passing through the retinaculum. This particular patient showed evidence of sensory loss in the distribution of the palmar cutaneous nerve.

the examination, repeated comparison should be made with ulnar innervated digits and with those on the other hand. The dysaesthesia does not often involve the entire median nerve distribution and this does not cast doubt on the diagnosis. However, particular attention should be paid to the 'palmar triangle' (p. 11). If sensation is lost in that area innervated by the palmar cutaneous nerve, a diagnosis of carpal tunnel compression should be made with reservations and with the knowledge that it is only tenable if

1. the 'palmar triangle' is not served by the palmar cutaneous nerve, or
2. the palmar cutaneous nerve does not arise some six centimetres proximal to the retinaculum and pass superficial to it as is normally the case, but originates, as has been described, deep to it, piercing the retinaculum to serve the palmar triangle (Fig. 3.9).

The distribution of the palmar cutaneous nerve is not limited strictly to the palmar triangle, as Erik Moberg was quick to point out to the author after the first edition of this

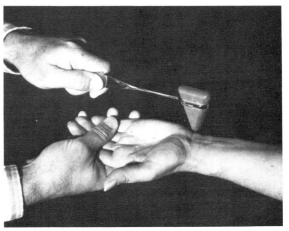

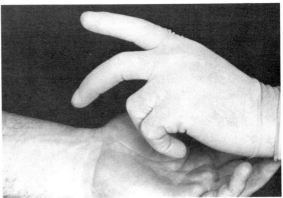

Fig. 3.10 A Tinel's sign is very frequently elicited in carpal tunnel syndrome just proximal to the tunnel. The percussion may be performed either with a tendon hammer or with the flexed middle finger as in percussing the chest.

book. Using the pinwheel from the median autonomous zone on the index finger and running towards the palm, change may occur as far distal as the middle digital crease. This *may* be due to thicker skin on the digit and the change should be compared with that on the opposite hand.

A *Tinel's sign* is detected in the majority of patients with carpal tunnel syndrome. Tapping with the flexed finger or with a tendon hammer over the course of the nerve at the retinaculum or more commonly just proximal to it produces paraesthesiae radiating into the median nerve distribution (Fig. 3.10).

The *Phalen test*[17-19] increases the compression on the median nerve by placing the wrist in acute flexion, especially in patients with carpal tunnel syndrome[20]. This is achieved by putting the dorsum of one hand against that of the other with the fingers dependent and lowering the elbows as far as possible while maintaining that contact. By doing both hands at one time the normal acts as a control

for the affected hand. However, both hands may be involved either with the patient's knowledge or subclinically. Therefore a timed Phalen test is of more value, any onset of numbness in less than one minute being considered diagnostic of carpal tunnel compression (Fig. 3.11). The patient may avoid flexing the wrist fully, knowing from experience that it is uncomfortable. For this reason, the Phalen test can probably be performed more efficiently by the examiner. The wrist is fully flexed with the forearm supinated and then maintained in that position by holding the palmar abducted thumb towards the wrist.

The *reversed Phalen test* is performed by placing the palms of the hands together and raising the elbows as high as possible. Occasionally, when the Phalen test is negative, the reverse test is positive, producing numbness and tingling in the median nerve distribution by placing the nerve on stretch (Fig. 3.12).

Abductor pollicis brevis should be tested. With the hand flat on the table, palm upwards, the patient should be asked to touch with his thumb the examiner's finger held above the hand. Strength is tested by having the patient resist downward pressure.

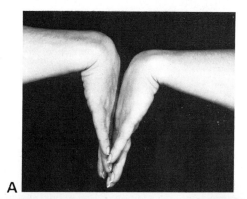
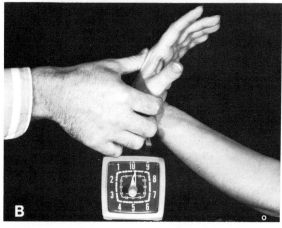

Fig. 3.11 (A) The *Phalen test* is performed by having the patient place the backs of the hands against one another and flex the wrists fully. The development of paraesthesiae in the median nerve distribution is evidence of compression of the median nerve in the carpal tunnel. (B) The test can also be performed by the examiner flexing the patient's wrist into the position as shown in (A). The test should be timed since the more rapid the onset of paraesthesiae the more definite the diagnosis.

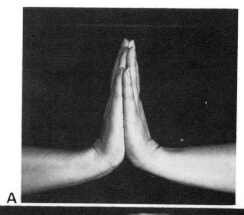
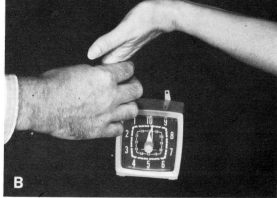

Fig. 3.12 Occasionally the reversed position with the palms together and the wrist dorsally flexed may produce paraesthesiae when the orthodox Phalen test has failed to do so.

The diagnosis of carpal syndrome in the majority of cases will be made with confidence on the basis of the above examination. In those where doubt remains *electromyography* should be undertaken. Prolongation of the distal motor latency beyond 4 ms will confirm the presence of median nerve compression. Such an increase in distal motor latency is found in approximately two thirds of patients with subsequently confirmed median nerve entrapment[21]. A normal result does not therefore rule out the diagnosis. It has been reported that orthodromic sensory nerve conduction studies are a more sensitive index of compression, 85 to 95% of surgically confirmed cases showing prolongation of the distal sensory latency beyond 3.5 ms, which is the upper limit of normal (p. 165).

All patients with carpal tunnel syndrome should have the most likely systemic causes eliminated by basic laboratory work

> sedimentation rate — if elevated this should be followed with more sophisticated tests for rheumatoid disease and collagen disorders.
> two-hour postprandial blood sugar, serum uric acid, T3 and T4 estimations.

X-rays

Standard and special views of the hand should be taken for they may reveal an unsuspected lesion producing the

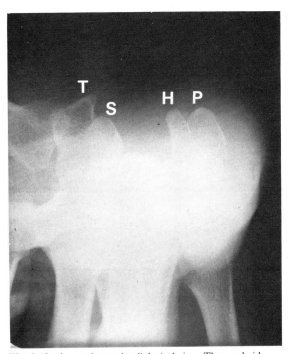

Fig. 3.13 A carpal tunnel radiological view. The scaphoid, pisiform, trapezium, and hamate are marked with initial letters. This view is of value in demonstrating the presence of abnormal radio opaque structures within the carpal tunnel.

pressure in the carpal tunnel. The specialized carpal tunnel view is most useful in this respect (Fig. 3.13)[22].

INDICATIONS

Conservative management is indicated in all patients who have only intermittent problems. While diuretics or anti-inflammatory agents may be of help, this usually consists of *injection and splintage*. The tunnel is injected with 0.5 ml of local anaesthetic and 0.5 ml of soluble steroid at a point midway between the pisiform and the scaphoid tubercle and 1 cm distal, using a short 27 gauge needle with the bevel parallel to the nerve (Fig. 3.14). Care should be taken

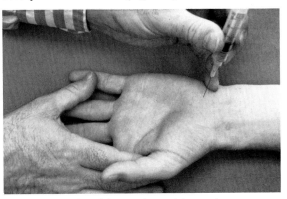

Fig. 3.14 Injection of the carpal tunnel (see text).

to ensure that the median nerve has not been impaled by asking the patient if paraesthesiae result from introduction of the needle. If they do, it should be re-inserted. The occurrence of *paraesthesiae during injection* tend to confirm the diagnosis since the addition of 1 ml of fluid should not cause significant compression of a normal nerve. The splint is worn to hold the wrist in slight dorsiflexion. Injection has been shown to cure 22-33%[23, 24] of patients with appropriate symptoms. It is especially indicated in pregnant patients in whom the compression can be expected to abate with delivery.

Surgical release of the flexor retinaculum is indicated after failed conservative management or as the first line of treatment in those patients showing *constant numbness, evident motor weakness or increased distal latency*. These are also the cases in whom internal neurolysis is required since Curtis has shown that scarring of the epineurium and around the fascicles can entirely negate the value of simple decompression. If the synovium around the flexor tendons is thickened and hypertrophied, some surgeons undertake synovectomy. Great care must be taken to protect the palmar cutaneous branch in making the incision. (Fig. 3.15[25]. The superficial palmar arch is also at risk during release of the carpal tunnel as is the motor branch of the median nerve (Fig. 3.16). The nerve may be clearly constricted as in Figure 3.1, the site of the local blood flow reduction (Fig. 3.4) or markedly hyperaemic (Fig. 3.17).

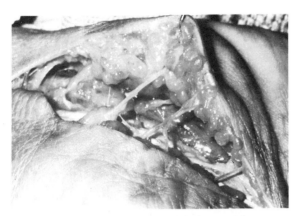

Fig. 3.15 The terminal branches of the palmar cutaneous nerve may be encountered in the process of making the incision for release of the carpal tunnel.

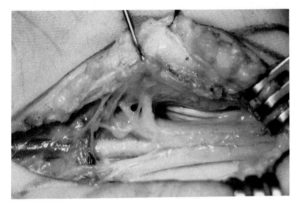

Fig. 3.16 The median nerve is seen passing beneath the superficial palmar arch which lies with one of its branches to the left end of the incision. Just proximal to the point at which it passes beneath the arch, the median nerve gives off its motor branch. Here there are two.

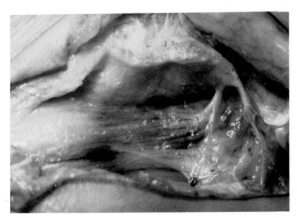

Fig. 3.17 Hyperaemia of the median nerve consequent upon compression.

Pronator syndrome[26]

On entering the forearm, the median nerve passes beneath the edge of the lacertus fibrosus of the biceps, between the two heads of pronator teres and then beneath the bridge or arch formed by the proximal edge of the flexor digitorum superficialis. The median nerve may be subjected to compression by any of these structures[27,28] or by anterior displacement of the radial head at this level. In less than one tenth of patients, the nerve may pass through the humeral head or beneath both heads of pronator teres which increases the probability of compression. The significance of the pronator syndrome is that it may easily be mistaken for carpal tunnel compression and the wrong treatment undertaken.

Points of similarity to carpal tunnel syndrome
  Numbness and paraesthesia in median innervated
  digits,
  weakness of the thenar muscles,
  pain in the wrist and forearm.
Points of contrast with carpal tunnel syndrome
  No nocturnal complaints,
  no Tinel sign at the wrist,
  nerve conduction may be delayed, but not at the wrist,
  dysaesthesia in the 'palmar triangle'.

It might be expected that the Phalen test would be negative and indeed that has been the author's limited experience. However, it was positive in 50% of patients diagnosed as having pronator syndrome at the Mayo Clinic[29].

The patient with pronator syndrome complains primarily of pain[30] in the forearm with associated dysaesthesia in the median nerve distribution and possible thenar weakness.

The *Tinel sign* is found over the median nerve either where it passes beneath the pronator teres at the junction of upper or middle thirds of the forearm or proximal to that in the antecubital fossa (Fig. 3.18).

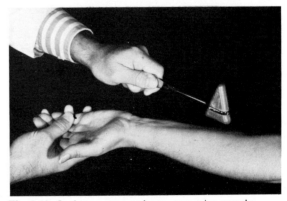

Fig. 3.18 In the pronator syndrome, percussion over the median nerve where it passes between the heads of pronator teres produces pain and paraesthesiae passing down into the median nerve distribution.

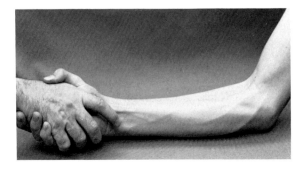

Pain and paraesthesiae into the median nerve distribution are evoked by placing stress on the three likely compressing structures.

pronator teres	— resisted pronation of the *extended* forearm (Fig. 3.19)
lacertus fibrosus	— resisted flexion of the elbow and supination of the forearm (Fig. 3.21)
arch of flexor digitorum superficialis	— resisted flexion of the proximal interphalangeal joint of the middle finger (Fig. 3.22)

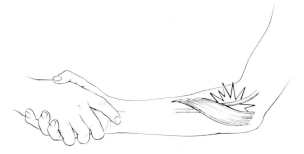

Fig. 3.19 *Pronator syndrome.* Testing pronator teres compression.

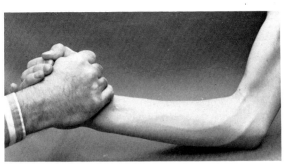

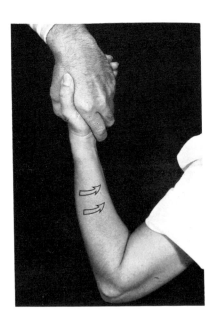

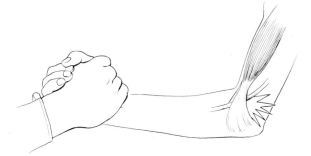

Fig. 3.21 *Pronator syndrome.* Testing for lacertus fibrosus compression.

Resisted pronation with the elbow flexed does not produce pain (Fig. 3.20), for only the ulnar head of pronator teres is rendered tense in this position, and the nerve is therefore not compressed.

Nerve conduction studies[29,31] both motor and sensory may show no change in conduction as the compression exerted by the pronator teres or superficialis is intermittent, depending upon position and muscle contraction. If, however, there is slowing it will be located in the forearm. Electromyographic studies of the muscles served by the median nerve should also be performed.

Splintage in pronation and slight wrist flexion, with or without elbow flexion, allied with a change in occupational use of the arm if possible, may relieve the symptoms. If not,

Fig. 3.20 When the resisted pronation is attempted with the elbow flexed, the patient has significantly less discomfort. In this position the humeral head of pronator teres plays little part in pronation of the forearm and therefore compression of the median nerve is not so marked.

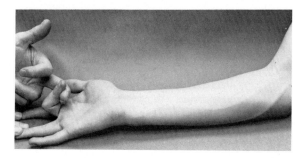

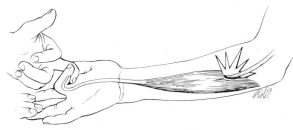

Fig. 3.22 *Pronator syndrome.* Testing for flexor digitorum superficialis compression.

exploration is indicated with decompression of the median nerve by release of the humeral head of pronator teres, the superficialis bridge and any associated compressing structures.

Anterior interosseous syndrome

The anterior interosseous nerve arises from the median nerve some 4-6 cm below the elbow. It is an entirely motor nerve, serving flexor pollicis longus, flexor digitorum profundus to the index and middle fingers and pronator quadratus.

Compression of the anterior interosseous nerve was first described by Tinel in 1918. Spinner[32], in his monograph on nerve disorders in the forearm, lists the structures which may compress the nerve:

tendinous bands — in the deep head of pronator teres
— in the origin of flexor digitorum superficialis of the middle finger
— in the origin of a palmaris profundus
accessory muscles
— from superficialis to profundus muscles
— Gantzer's muscle (an accessory head to flexor pollicis longus)
vascular — thrombosis of ulnar collateral vessels
— aberrant radial artery
other — an enlarged bicipital bursa

SYMPTOMS
Pain in the forearm is very commonly the presenting symptom. Pain is thus common to the three compression

neuropathies of the median nerve. It occurs in this purely motor nerve for reasons discussed previously (p. 193).

Weakness of pinch occurs primarily through the loss of flexor pollicis longus. The fine pinch manoeuver which requires nail to nail contact as in lifting a pin from a flat surface, is lost due to paralysis of both flexor pollicis longus and flexor digitorum profundus to the index finger.

EXAMINATION
The fine pinch posture is abnormal. The pulp of the index finger, which is extended at the distal interphalangeal joint makes contact with the pulp of the thumb just distal to its hyperextended interphalangeal joint (Fig. 3.23).

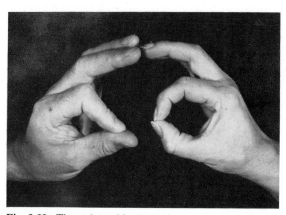

Fig. 3.23 The patient with *anterior interosseous syndrome* can flex neither the interphalangeal joint of the thumb nor the distal interphalangeal joint of the index finger. Attempted fine pinch as posed in the right hand in this photograph results in the abnormal posture seen on the left.

Muscle testing reveals

Flexor pollicis longus — absent or weak interphalangeal flexion of the thumb;
Flexor digitorum profundus — absent or weak distal interphalangeal flexion of the index and, less commonly, the middle finger;
Pronator quadratus — when compared with the normal limb pronation of the arm with the elbow flexed to reduce the power of pronator teres is weaker.

Variations — differing distribution of the anterior interosseous nerve may result in variations of this clinical picture:

Only flexor pollicis longus may be affected[33], or
In addition to flexor pollicis longus, pronator quadratus and profundus to the index and middle fingers:
1. parts of superficialis may be affected,
2. in certain instances of the Martin-Gruber anastomosis, a varying number of intrinsics normally innervated by the ulnar nerve may be affected.

INDICATIONS

Observation should be pursued for 6-12 weeks for spontaneous recovery may occur. Decompression should then be performed which, if unsuccessful, can be followed by appropriate tendon transfers some six months later.

The reported causes of median nerve compression form an impressive list. The following is an incomplete guide to the literature.

Developmental
Aberrant and anomalous lumbricals[34-36]
Anomalous superficialis[37]
Persistent median artery[38-39]
Vessel perforating nerve[40]
Supracondylar process[41]

Traumatic
'Greenstick' fracture[42-44]
Colles[46]
Hook of hamate[46]
Cut superficialis[47]
Fracture-dislocation carpo-metacarpal[48]
Elbow dislocation[49-50]
Insect sting[51]

Metabolic
Amyloid[52]
Mucopolysaccharidoses[53]

Tumours — intraneural
Lipofibroma[54-55]
Haemangioma[56]

Degenerative
Osteophyte[57]
Cyst[58]
Bursa[59]
Ganglion[60]

Iatrogenic
Opponensplasty[61]
Dialysis[62-64]
Silastic rod[65]

ULNAR NERVE

Symptoms due to compression of the median nerve are most probably due to entrapment at the wrist or in the forearm. By contrast, similar problems in ulnar nerve distribution are most often due to involvement of the nerve at the elbow or of its roots in the neck.

Guyon's canal — Ulnar tunnel syndrome[66,67]

The volar carpal ligament which roofs over the canal of Guyon is a less substantial structure than the flexor retinaculum which encloses the carpal tunnel (p. 10). Fewer structures pass through the canal, only the ulnar nerve and artery, and it contains no synovium. For these reasons, compression of the ulnar nerve is much less common than median nerve entrapment at the wrist; when it does occur, it is more frequently associated with trauma or with the presence in the canal of an abnormal structure. The configuration of the hypothenar muscle origin is probably significant.[68]

Trauma
Ulnar nerve involvement may follow on one heavy blow to the base of the hypothenar eminence but is more frequently due to repetitive occupational trauma of the type which is also responsible for thrombosis of the ulnar artery in this situation — 'hypothenar hammer syndrome' (p. 183). It may also result from the oedema following injury[69].

Abnormal structures
Swellings — a ganglion is by far the most common cause of ulnar nerve palsy in Guyon's canal, indeed four out of the first five explored by Seddon proved to be due to a ganglion (Fig. 3.24)[70].
Anomalous muscles[71-74] — reversed or accessory palmaris longus passing through the tunnel; (Fig. 3.25)
— duplication of hypothenar muscles;
— abnormal origin for the hypothenar muscles in the forearm.

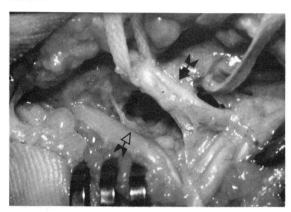

Fig. 3.24 This patient presented with loss of ulnar nerve function distal to Guyon's canal. Exploration revealed a ganglion compressing the deep branch (seen here immediately after the ganglion was opened).

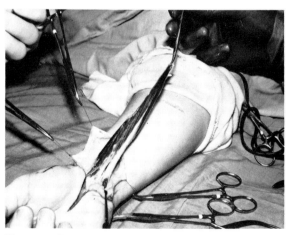

Fig. 3.25 *Guyon's canal* compression. An anomalous muscle arose from a reversed palmaris longus to pass into the canal, causing compression.

Patients will present with *pain* which may be in the hand or forearm[75], and with varying combinations of *weakness, paraesthesia* and *hypaesthesia,* for six separate patterns of involvement have been described[76].

1. Pure sensory deficit
2. Pure motor deficit involving —
   (a) all ulnar-innervated intrinsic muscles
   (b) all the above, except the hypothenar muscles
   (c) as in (a) except the abductor digiti minimi
3. Mixed motor and sensory deficit, involving
   (a) all ulnar-innervated intrinsic muscles
   (b) all the above, except the hypothenar muscles

EXAMINATION

Posture may be altered as for an ulnar nerve lesion (p.35) (Fig. 3.26).

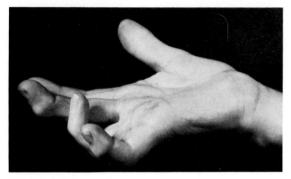

Fig. 3.26 The ulnar claw hand.

Sensory disturbance

This is the most significant part of the clinical examination and is directed at the distribution of the *dorsal sensory branch.* If this shows hypaesthesia on pinwheel testing, the compression *cannot* be in Guyon's canal. If the test is normal, it *may* be or may not. The expected sensory loss will be, as in compression of the ulnar nerve at any level, of the palmar surface of the small finger and the ulnar half of the ring.

Motor loss

Deep motor: All the interossei and adductor pollicis are weak or paralysed and this is evidenced by muscle wasting particularly noticeable in the 1st dorsal interosseous.

Complete ulnar: In addition to the above, the hypothenar muscles are weak or paralysed. Again this is demonstrated by wasting and on active testing.

Electromyography

Nerve conduction velocities will often be slowed from the wrist to the first dorsal interosseous.

INDICATIONS

Ulnar nerve entrapment at Guyon's canal more frequently results in motor loss than median nerve compression in the carpal tunnel. In all cases with such loss, exploration should be performed.

At the elbow — Cubital tunnel syndrome[77]

Traumatic ulnar neuritis, tardy ulnar palsy or cubital tunnel syndrome at the elbow was the first chronic disorder of a peripheral nerve to be described. While there is an element of compression, friction plays a greater role here than in any other of the 'compression neuropathies'. It may be due to one of several causes.

Anatomical. The aponeurosis between the two heads of flexor carpi ulnaris may be unusually tight.

Trauma - direct: any blow to the flexed elbow may injure the nerve. The exposed situation of the nerve is shown by the frequency with which the 'funny bone' is struck. If severe, such a blow may lead to a chronic neuritis.

Trauma — indirect: injuries to the bones of the elbow joint, especially in childhood, may result in 'tardy ulnar palsy' at a much later date.

$$\left. \begin{array}{l} \text{fractures of lateral condyle} \\ \text{dislocation of radial head} \end{array} \right\} \rightarrow \text{cubitus valgus}$$

fractures of medial condyle → irregular ulnar groove

The latter has its effect by direct impingement on the nerve, the former by placing the nerve on undue stretch.

Recurrent dislocation of the nerve. Normally firmly seated in the ulnar groove, or cubital tunnel as it is also named, the ulnar nerve in some instances dislocates over the medial epicondyle on flexion. This movement in itself is sufficient to produce neuritis and also further exposes the nerve to trauma. It is important to remember nonetheless that recurrent dislocation of the nerve was found in 16.2% of one series of entirely asymptomatic volunteers[78].

Arthritis. Osteoarthritis or rheumatoid disease of the humero-ulnar joint may result in cysts[79] or bone spurs (Fig. 3.27). These bone spurs may impinge upon the ulnar nerve.

Swellings. The ubiquitous ganglion is again the swelling most likely to embarrass the nerve.

Abnormal muscle. Anconeus epitrochlearis passes from the medial border of the olecranon to the medial epicondyle and may compress the ulnar nerve.

SYMPTOMS

Pain in the upper extremity, often of an ill-defined nature, may be the major complaint.

Paraesthesiae and numbness involving the ulnar innervated digits are usually present. The numbness and tingling may be similar to that of carpal tunnel compression, initially nocturnal and infrequent, but that of cubital tunnel neuropathy from the onset tends to be more progressive in nature. Vigorous use is likely to make both

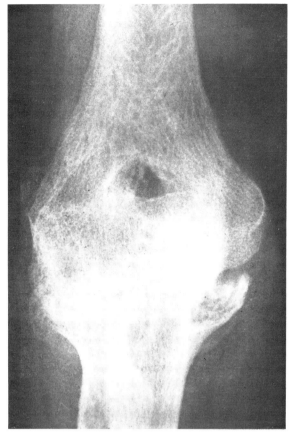

Fig. 3.27 Spurs around the elbow joint in association with rheumatoid arthritis may produce compression of the ulnar nerve in the cubital tunnel.

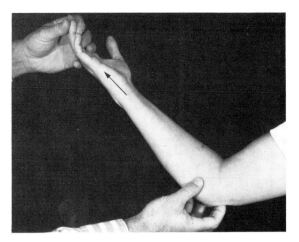

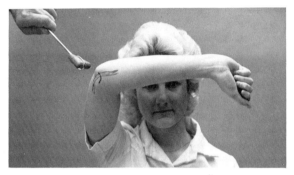

Fig. 3.28A Palpation of the ulnar nerve in the cubital tunnel will produce paraesthesiae radiating down to the small finger in the presence of ulnar neuropathy at the elbow. It is important to compare this with the unaffected limb as the ulnar nerve frequently shows a positive Tinel's sign in this position. (B) Percussion of the ulnar nerve at the cubital tunnel can be more easily undertaken with the shoulder flexed and internally rotated, bringing the arm in front of the head.

pain and paraesthesiae more troublesome, but there is otherwise no cyclical pattern.

Weakness in the ulnar innervated musculature in the hand is common. The muscles in which weakness is most noticed by the patient are the adductor pollicis and the first dorsal interosseous, due to reduction in pinch strength.

EXAMINATION

Distinction between cubital tunnel neuritis and involvement of the ulnar nerve in Guyon's canal or more proximal compression of cervical roots C8 and T1 at the neck is of course mandatory if surgical relief is to be obtained. This distinction is not easily made.

Sensory disturbance

As in carpal tunnel syndrome, this is not always sufficiently severe to reduce two point discrimination or sweating.

Dysaesthesia is more likely, involving the small and ring fingers, hypothenar eminence and the ulnar half of the dorsum of the hand. The last is of great diagnostic

significance in eliminating Guyon canal compression as the cause of the patient's complaints.

Tinel's sign is invariably positive over the ulnar nerve in the cubital tunnel, producing tingling radiating into the ulnar two fingers (Fig. 3.28). However, the normal ulnar nerve often 'Tinel's' in this situation and therefore only a difference from the unaffected side is significant.

Flexion of the elbow produces pain and paraesthesiae in the ulnar nerve distribution in some patients. When this occurs it is virtually diagnostic of cubital tunnel syndrome (Fig. 3.29). It is something akin to the Phalen test in carpal tunnel syndrome, and, like that, can be timed to give some measure of severity.

Motor loss

Weakness or paralysis and *wasting* of the ulnar innervated muscles in the hand occurs in established ulnar neuropathy

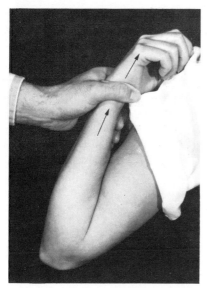

Fig. 3.29 If the paraesthesiae and pain are produced by forceful flexion of the elbow, this is virtually diagnostic of an ulnar neuropathy in the cubital tunnel.

at the elbow. Active testing should be performed on all the intrinsic muscles. Froment's sign may be present (p. 150) and also clawing may result, affecting only the ring and small fingers.

The nerve supply to flexor digitorum profundus of the ring and small fingers comes from the ulnar nerve five or six centimeters distal to the cubital tunnel. Paralysis of these muscles may therefore be encountered in ulnar nerve compression at the elbow but is surprisingly rare. So also is palsy of flexor carpi ulnaris and this may be for the same reason, namely that the fascicles to these muscles are located on the deep surface of the nerve in the cubital tunnel. Active testing will reveal this loss. If flexor digitorum profundus is affected it will have two consequences

1. clawing will not occur, as the imbalanced pull of the flexor on the interphalangeal joint will have been eliminated;
2. the examiner will have further confirmation that the lesion lies proximal to the canal of Guyon, indeed certainly lies at or above the elbow.

However, as emphasized above, flexor digitorum profundus is often unaffected even in the presence of complete paralysis of ulnar innervated intrinsics.

Electrophysiological changes
These are often present, indeed they help to determine the need for surgery and the level at which the exploration is indicated much more in ulnar neuropathy than in affections of the median nerve. Slowing of the nerve conduction velocity across the elbow suggests the need for exploration of the cubital tunnel.

X-ray
The elbow should be X-rayed, both standard anteroposterior and lateral and also a cubital tunnel view, taken with the elbow flexed (Fig. 3.30).

The features of ulnar neuropathy at the elbow by which it is distinguished from compression at Guyon's canal and at the thoracic outlet are summarized below.

1. Dysaesthesia in the distribution of the dorsal sensory branch of the ulnar nerve.
2. A strongly positive Tinel at the cubital tunnel especially if it is elicited by elbow flexion.
3. Slowing of nerve conduction across the elbow.
4. Absence of wasting or weakness in the thenar muscles.
5. Lack of dysaesthesia in the T1 dermatome, that is, the inner aspect of the elbow region.

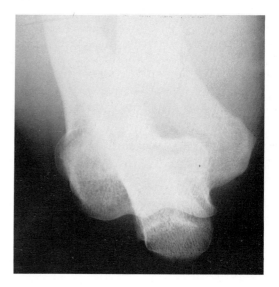

Fig. 3.30 Cubital tunnel view.

INDICATIONS
The results of surgical release are less predictable than one would wish. For this reason, provided no impinging pathology is suspected in the tunnel, a trial of splintage should be discussed with the patient. The splint should be long arm with the elbow set at whatever angle less than 90° suits the patient. The wrist should be supported. The splint serves to protect the nerve from direct contact and from the friction of flexion. It should be worn at all times apart from bathing until one week after all symptoms have resolved.

Where this fails, then the surgeon has the problem of selecting the appropriate surgical procedure. Transposition of the nerve with or without medial epicondylectomy has been widely practised but is not without morbidity, expecially in heavy manual workers. Osborne[80,81] has shown that simple neurolysis with division of the aponeurosis which joins the humeral and ulnar origins of the flexor carpi ulnaris is effective treatment in many cases (Fig. 3.31). If the nerve appears to be subject to fibrosis, internal neurolysis should also be performed, but great care must be exercised in doing interfascicular dissection for there are many more cross connections here than in the median nerve at the carpal tunnel.

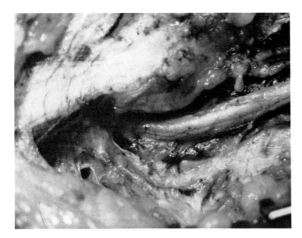

Fig. 3.31 The ulnar nerve is seen here in the cubital tunnel passing beneath the aponeurosis of the flexor carpi ulnaris to enter the forearm.

Anterior transposition is indicated in the following instances: cubitus valgus, arthritis, recurrent dislocation of the nerve, pain and recurrent symptoms after simple neurolysis, provided other causes have been eliminated.

When performed, transposition beneath the entire flexor mass as described by Learmonth[82], subcutaneous and intramuscular translocation and medial epicondylectomy[83-85] all have their advocates and their critics. Whatever procedure is selected, the medial intermuscular septum must be split above the elbow at the point where the ulnar nerve passes posteriorly through the septum or the angulation compression may simply be moved a little proximally[86].

Other reported causes of ulnar nerve compression

Developmental and anatomical
Triceps[87, 89]
Flexor carpi ulnaris — mid-forearm[89]
Adductor pollicis[90]
Epitrochleo-anconeus[91]
Supracondylar process[92]
Trochlear hypoplasia[93, 94]

Traumatic
Wrist fractures[95-97]
Carpometacarpal dislocation[98]

Tumours
Giant cell[99-100]
Lipoma[101]
Intraneural cyst[102]
Synovial osteochondromatosis[103]

Rheumatoid
At the wrist[104,105]

Thoracic outlet syndrome

The brachial plexus and the subclavian artery emerge from the neck and the thorax into the supraclavicular region through a narrow, triangular space bounded

below by the first rib,
anteriorly by scalenus anterior,
behind by scalenus medius.

They then pass beneath the clavicle and coracoid process[106] in turn, with the rib cage, in the form of the first and second ribs, lying immediately below the neurovascular structures. To join the plexus and proceed through this course the cervical root T1 passes upwards through the thoracic outlet, across the first rib to turn down again towards the arm. Just medial to the rib it is joined by the C8 root to form the lower trunk.

Any structure which encroaches on this narrow space or any process which in some other way reduces its dimension will be likely to compress the roots or the trunks of the brachial plexus and may also narrow the subclavian artery. From whatever sources comes the compression, T1 and the lower trunk bear the brunt of problems. Such compression has been described in association with

Cervical rib[107] — while this may indeed produce compression it is often innocent, but may delude the surgeon into undertaking its removal to no avail (Fig. 3.32).

Fibromuscular, tendinous or ligamentous bands — Roos[108], in the course of over 1000 operations, has identified 9 types of band associated with the first rib, scalenus anterior and scalenus medius. He believes them to be the major cause of the syndrome. No direct evidence of their presence is available preoperatively other than a C7 transverse process extending beyond that of T1 in AP or oblique cervical spine views.

Swellings — Seddon described a chondroma causing a thoracic outlet syndrome.

Trauma — severe fractures of the clavicle may cause costo-clavicular compression of the plexus and artery (Fig. 3.33). In addition, relatively minor trauma to the neck or shoulder may induce the syndrome through muscle spasm which causes the outlet to narrow and bands to impinge on the plexus.

Postural changes — the 'military brace' position, in which the shoulders are held back in an exaggerated posture, has been shown to produce thoracic outlet

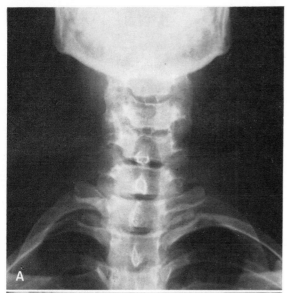

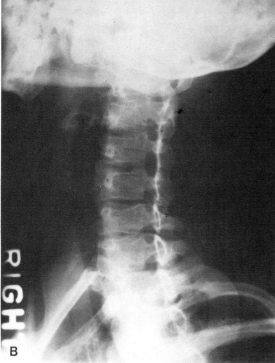

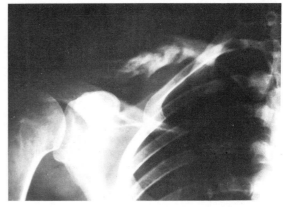

Fig. 3.33 This patient had sustained a severe fracture of the clavicle in falling from a horse and this came to non-union. Severe compression of the lower cords of the brachial plexus resulted and were relieved by removal of the excess callus from the clavicle.

Figs. 3.32A & B This patient shows a cervical rib, more evident in the oblique view. In this instance, the rib was responsible for thoracic outlet syndrome which resolved after its removal.

syndrome. The opposite extreme of posture, namely slumping of the shoulders, is believed to contribute to the increased incidence of thoracic outlet syndrome in patients in their fourth decade, with or without the presence of a cervical rib. Any sustained activity of the arm may aggravate the patient's symptoms. Examples of such troublesome actions include holding a steering wheel and combing and setting the hair.

SYMPTOMS

Pain is usually present and is described as being of a persistent, 'gnawing' or 'burning' nature. More aching than sharp in quality, it is usually located in the shoulder and inner aspect of the upper arm, radiating down into the hand. Unlike root compression at the intervertebral foramen, the pain rarely radiates upwards into the head. It becomes worse in the course of a day's work, especially if the patient's occupation demands repetitive movements of the hands with the shoulders in an exaggerated position, either reaching forward or upwards. The pain may then be relieved briefly by shrugging the shoulders and exercising the hands, but return to the prevailing posture produces renewed discomfort.

The pain may be worse at night, expecially if the patient is accustomed to sleeping on the affected side, and may be relieved by swinging the arm around.

Sensory disturbance

Tingling and numbness are common, usually in the C8 and T1 distribution, although they may involve the entire hand. The symptoms in the ulnar two fingers and on the ulnar dorsum of the hand may be confused with ulnar nerve compression. If the numbness can clearly be shown to extend on to the ulnar border of the forearm or upper arm then the likelihood of a thoracic outlet or root aetiology is increased, since these are the territories of the medial cutaneous nerves of forearm and arm respectively, not of the ulnar nerve.

Motor loss

Heralded by a complaint of *swift fatigue* in the arm, wasting and weakness affects mainly those muscles innervated by the first thoracic root, namely the intrinsic muscles of the hand and the patient will complain of incoordination in all fine movements, especially pinch manoeuvres.

Vascular changes

A minority of patients may present because of the vascular effects of the thoracic outlet syndrome. These may be due to direct compression of the vessel or due to thrombosis in or embolization from a poststenotic aneurysm just distal to the point of compression. In vascular compression patients may complain of:

venous congestion[109] in the form of swelling, heaviness and cyanosis

cold intolerance

colour changes in the digits occurring most commonly in the index finger but often involving all. These may take the form of attacks of complete pallor, followed by painful hyperaemia or cyanosis, characteristic of *Raynaud's phenomenon* (p. 184).

If significant thrombosis or embolization ensues *necrosis* of the tips of the digits will result.

EXAMINATION

Sensory disturbance

Localization of areas of dysaesthesia, that is where sensation 'feels different' from adjacent regions, should be made using light touch or a pinwheel. Commonly the usual distribution of the ulnar nerve will be involved. To differentiate thoracic outlet syndrome from ulnar neuropathy, particular attention should be paid to the forearm and upper arm (Fig. 3.34). Sensitivity here is much less acute than in the hand and time should be allowed for the patient to be clear which areas are involved. This may require repeated tests and comparison should be made with the other upper limb, while remembering that thoracic outlet syndrome may well be bilateral.

   Dysesthesia of the ulnar nerve
   　+medial cutaneous of arm
   　　+medial cutaneous of forearm

   suggests thoracic outlet syndrome.

Tingling and pain may be elicited by direct palpation or *percussion over the brachial plexus* which can be felt in the posterior triangle as it emerges from behind scalenus

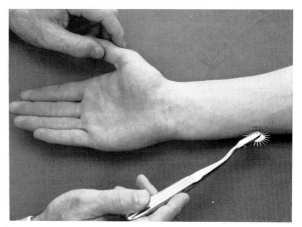

Fig. 3.34 In testing for sensory disturbance in possible thoracic outlet syndrome, particular attention should be paid to the ulnar aspect of the upper arm and forearm since the cutaneous supply while deriving from a lower cervical root does not pass distally in the ulnar nerve but rather as the medial cutaneous nerves of arm and forearm. Dysaesthesia in this situation, therefore, serves to eliminate the possibility of ulnar neuropathy.

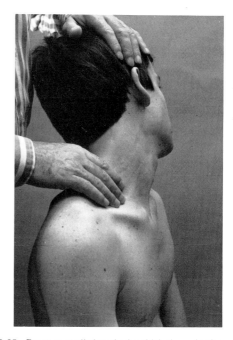

Fig. 3.35 Pressure applied to the brachial plexus in the posterior triangle will produce symptoms in the form of paraesthesia and discomfort in the appropriate dermatome in thoracic outlet syndrome.

anterior (Fig. 3.35). These paraesthesiae radiate into the distribution of which the patient complains and should be compared with the contralateral side. They may also be produced by movements of the neck, in which event distinction must be made from cervical root, as opposed to trunk, compression. As classically described lateral flexion can distinguish between thoracic outlet and root compression syndromes —

Symptoms on lateral flexion towards the affected side are due to root compression.

Symptoms on lateral flexion away from the affected side are due to thoracic outlet syndrome (Fig. 3.36).

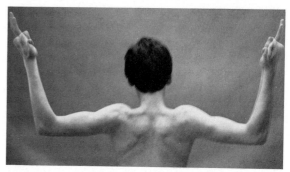

Fig. 3.37 *Roos test.* The shoulders are braced, the arms elevated, and the hands exercised. In thoracic outlet syndrome, the patient is unable to continue this for three minutes.

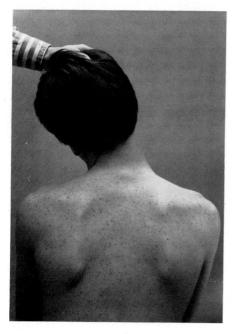

Fig. 3.36 *Thoracic outlet syndrome.* Flexion of the neck away from the affected side produces discomfort by stretching the compressed nerves.

Motor loss

Wasting is detected by inspection.

Weakness is detected by active muscle testing.

In both instances particular attention should be paid to the thenar muscles for therein lies an important distinguishing feature from ulnar neuropathy: palsy of the intrinsic muscles of the hand *including* the median-innervated thenar muscles suggests thoracic outlet syndrome.

Commonly the triceps (C7) is weak but the reflexes are normal. This may be a point of distinction from the patient with cervical disc disease in whom strength may be normal but reflexes not.

3-minute elevated arm exercise test[108] (Fig. 3.37). This simple test has proved the most reliable in diagnosing thoracic outlet syndrome. With the patient sitting with the arms abducted to 90° and the elbow flexed to 90°, he is asked to open and close his hands repeatedly while keeping

the shoulders gently braced backwards. The patient with thoracic outlet syndrome will be quite unable to complete this test due to recurrence of all the symptoms of which he complains. If he is able to complete 3 minutes, he does not have outlet compression.

Vascular compromise

In those few cases with peripheral evidence of circulatory disturbance of some magnitude, vascular signs will be detected

colour and temperature difference — when compared with the opposite limb, the affected hand may clearly be pale, blue or cold;

diminished pulses — the radial pulse may be more difficult to palpate and an *Allen test* (p. 181) may show significantly slower filling than in the opposite limb;

lower blood pressure — the blood pressure should be recorded in both limbs for comparison. When the possibility of bilateral involvement exists, the pressure should be taken in the lower limbs also, using an oscillometer;

thrill and bruit — gentle palpation over the subclavian artery in the posterior triangle may reveal a palpable thrill. More often a bruit may be heard in the same site though the stethoscope.

Vascular compromise through change of position

Several other tests have been described to demonstrate neurological and vascular compromise due to thoracic outlet syndrome. *These have proved unreliable and misleading and the author never uses them.* They are included here because they are still widely practised. It should be emphasized that if performed, the most significant finding in any of these tests is reproduction of the symptoms of which the patient complains.

Adson's sign[110, 111]. The patient is asked to brace the shoulders backwards, rotate his head to the affected side, elevate the chin and hold his breath in full inspiration. The radial pulse may disappear in this position or be palpably reduced in volume. This may be evidence of thoracic outlet syndrome but the examiner must be aware that this test is positive in one out of every four or five normal subjects.

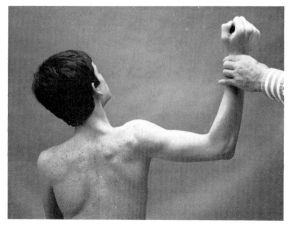

Fig. 3.38 *Hyperabduction test.* The arm is hyperabducted, the patient's head is turned towards the side of the lesion and the chin tilted upwards. Disappearance of the pulse represents a positive hyperabduction test but may be present in as many as 25 per cent of the normal population.

Hyperabduction (Wright) test[112] (Fig. 3.38). With the patient in the same posture as for the Adson test, the arm is abducted to 90° in full external rotation of the shoulder. Diminution or disappearance of the radial pulse should again be sought. In this position auscultation over the subclavian artery may reveal a bruit due to partial occlusion (Fig. 3.39).

Claudication. Keeping the patient in the same position, but allowing him to breathe normally, he is asked to exercise the hand vigorously. Forearm pain and tingling will ensue within a few seconds in the presence of compression and the patient will soon lower the arm, complaining of considerable discomfort. An extremity without neurovascular compression, by contrast, can be exercised for over a minute with little or no distress.

Costoclavicular compression (Fig. 3.40). The patient is asked to stand, allow his shoulders to slump and put his extended, supinated arms down alongside and a little behind his thighs. While palpating both radial arteries, the surgeon applies gentle downward traction to the arms. The pulse may be diminished or occluded and the patient may complain of pain and tingling in the affected limb.

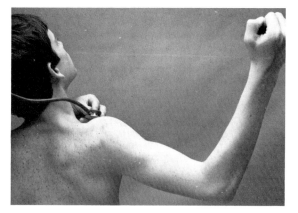

Fig. 3.39 While maintaining the arm in the hyperabducted position auscultation over the subclavian artery may reveal a distinct bruit.

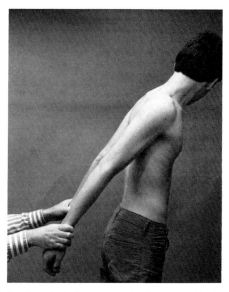

Fig. 3.40 Costoclavicular compression is produced by having the patient relax the shoulders completely while the examiner draws the arms downward and posteriorly while palpating the radial pulses. The pulse may be diminished or disappear and the patient may complain of numbness and tingling.

SPECIAL STUDIES

All patients suspected of having a thoracic outlet syndrome should have the following studies performed.

X-rays of cervical spine: AP and both obliques, lateral views in flexion and extension. The presence of a cervical rib, as emphasized above, does not necessarily mean that it is the cause of the patient's complaints. Vague symptoms and imprecise signs are most unlikely to be cured by resection of a cervical rib simply because it is there. Cervical spondylosis and osteoarthritis especially with encroachment on the inter-vertebral foramen by osteophytes may lead the surgeon to revise his diagnosis from trunk to root compression and he should review his records with this possibility in mind. Spasm of the paravertebral muscles which may result from, or predispose to, outlet compression — hence creating a vicious cycle — may be evidenced by loss of the normal lordotic curve on the otherwise normal lateral X-ray. (Fig. 3.41)

Electrophysiological studies may well reveal slowing of nerve conduction velocities across the supraclavicular fossa. Even when this is not the case, such studies are necessary to eliminate more peripheral neuropathies which may remain a possible cause of symptoms. There is some evidence that slowing may be precipitated in outlet compression by adopting the abducted position during testing[113]. This is true of other intermittent compression such as pronator syndrome and radial tunnel syndrome. In all, relaxed and provocative conduction studies should be performed.

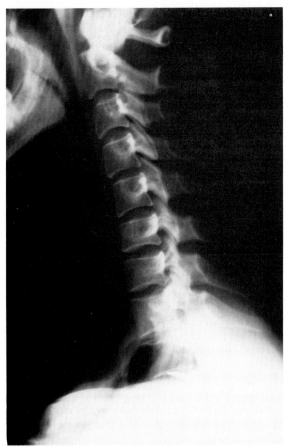

Fig. 3.41 Loss of the normal lordotic curve in an otherwise normal cervical spine is evidence of paravertebral muscle spasm which often occurs in thoracic outlet syndrome.

Transfemoral subclavian angiography is indicated only in the small minority of cases showing predominantly vascular signs. It may reveal narrowing of the subclavian artery, poststenotic dilatation, vascular anomalies (Fig. 3.42) or vascular occlusion. Narrowing may not be evident on standard studies and it is important that angiograms be obtained in the posture in which the patient normally experiences symptoms (Fig. 3.43).

[Note: emphasis has been laid in examination on distinguishing ulnar neuropathy from thoracic outlet syndrome producing compression of the lower trunk of the plexus, by far the most frequent involvement and certainly the most difficult diagnostic problem. The 'military brace syndrome'[114,115] may produce an Erb's palsy by compressing the upper trunk and also a cervical rib, scalenus medius band or swelling may compress the middle trunk.

The characteristics of such compressions have been detailed in the chapter on Reconstruction (p. 163) and do not present any diagnostic confusion with a more peripheral lesion as does the more common lower trunk compression.]

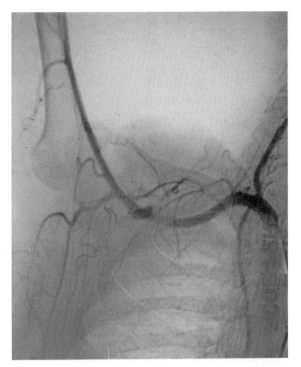

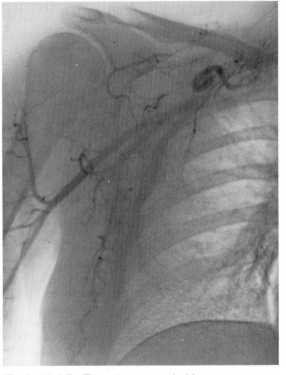

Fig. 3.42A & B The patient presented with severe symptoms and signs of thoracic outlet compression. Hyperabduction angiogram was performed which revealed normal flow but an abnormal vascular structure which filled late (B) and remained filled. Exploration revealed a hamartoma in the region of the plexus causing severe compression.

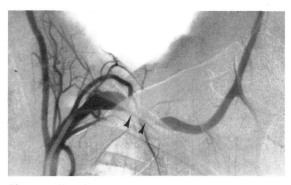

Fig. 3.43 Transfemoral subclavian angiography here reveals total occlusion of the subclavian artery in the hyperabducted position.

INDICATIONS[117]

Conservative measures include postural and stretching exercises, weight loss and a period of rest from provoking occupation[118]. Intensively followed under encouraging supervision, this regime cures more than half of the patients with outlet disease. If it fails or if vascular compromise is a major element of the disorder, surgical intervention is indicated.

Anterior scalenotomy[119], originally favoured by Adson, has not proved as successful as he first reported. However, the procedure allows visualization of the entire plexus and may reveal unexpected causes of compression including soft tissue tumors and more commonly fascial bands passing to the first rib. *Resection of a cervical rib* seen to be impinging on the plexus can be performed through the scalenotomy incision. Release of the anterior scalene is easily undertaken together with removal of all fibromuscular bands which can be found. It is important that these be sought with the arm held in a variety of positions.

All patients to whom this procedure is recommended should be warned of the possibility of failure to relieve the presenting symptoms. In the event of failure or recurrence *first rib resection*[120], best performed by the transaxillary route, may well prove effective.

Cervical root compression

We have progressed well outwith the domain of the hand surgeon in pursuit of the cause of symptoms in the ulnar nerve distribution in the upper extremity. Although we are about to abandon the chase with a few cautionary words regarding our responsibility to pass on the task to others where appropriate, complaints relative to the hand so commonly come from the neck that cervical root compression must be briefly considered.

Root compression may arise from a tumor of the cervical cord, acute herniation of a disc, chronic herniation with associated spondylosis or intervertebral foraminal osteophyte formation.

In dealing with any neurological disorder radiating from neck to forearm the possibility of a space-occupying lesion should always be remembered and investigated appropriately.

Acute herniation of a cervical disc is usually associated with a definite injury, which may be a vertebral compression or less frequently a 'whip lash' type of road traffic accident. Pain is the predominant symptom. It is very severe, producing marked limitation in neck motion and radiating into the upper limb. Usually one root alone is involved and paraesthesia, motor weakness and alteration in reflexes help to localize that one involved. This patient rarely presents to the hand surgeon.

Chronic cervical root compression by slow disc extrusion or by bony encroachment on the intervertebral foramen may produce symptoms predominantly in the forearm and hand and therefore requires more detailed consideration.

SYMPTOMS

Pain is a major complaint. This usually commences in the neck, involving in turn shoulder, forearm and hand, often becoming sufficiently severe distally as to completely mask more proximal components. The pain is aching in character, made worse by extreme neck movements, by poor sleeping posture and by maintaining one position for prolonged periods as is commonly required in industry. It is typically subject to acute exacerbations, when pain may be excruciating. Such exacerbations may be brought about by uncontrolled movements such as coughing or sneezing, which also act by raising the spinal fluid pressure.

Radiation into the occipital region is commonly present and distinguishes radicular pain from more peripheral compression.

Dysaesthesia, wasting and weakness may present and all show a specific root distribution. The points of greatest strain in the cervical spine are discs C5–6 which produces C6 root compression, and C6–7 which produces C7 root compression. Knowledge of this arrangement which differs from the thoracic and lumbar spine is necessary if X–ray changes and clinical findings are to be correlated.

EXAMINATION

Sensory disturbance

In more advanced cases typical dermatome dysaesthesia may be found. Clinical evidence of sensory loss may, however, be completely absent despite the patient's complaints of numbness. In these cases the symptoms may be reproduced by *Spurling's test*[121] in which the head is tilted toward the involved side and pressure applied to the top of the head (Fig. 3.44).

Tenderness posteriorly over the vertebra involved may be present. Percussion over the appropriate spinous process may produce radicular pain (Fig. 3.45).

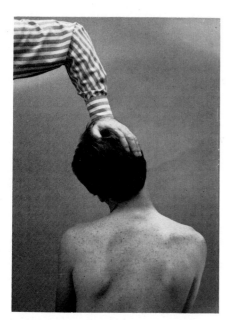

Fig. 3.44 *Spurling test.* The head is tilted towards the affected side and direct compression on the vertex is applied. If increase in symptoms results the test is positive.

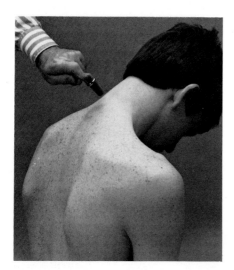

Fig. 3.45 Percussion over the spinous process of the affected vertebrae may produce root pain in cervical root compression.

Motor weakness may be present and this shows a specific root distribution as does any reduction in tendon jerks:

C5–6 disc — weakness of biceps, reduced biceps jerk;
C6–7 disc — weakness of triceps, reduced triceps jerk.

Special studies

X-ray of the cervical spine, especially the oblique views, may well show significant narrowing of the intervertebral foramina (Fig. 3.46). The lateral view may show loss of

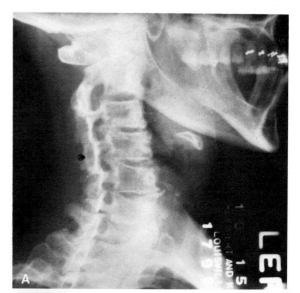

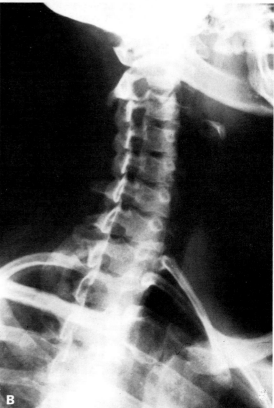

Fig. 3.46 Oblique views of the cervical spine in this patient show significant narrowing of the interverbal foramina together with narrowing of the disc spaces and beaking of the anterior aspect of the vertebral bodies. A normal oblique view is shown for comparison (B).

intervertebral disc space with loss of the normal lordotic curve even in the hyperextended position and 'beaking' of the vertebral bodies anteriorly.

Electromyography, apart from implicating the muscle of the appropriate myotome, has been reported as providing absolute evidence of root involvement as opposed to more peripheral lesions by showing denervation patterns in the paraspinal muscles for this can only occur if the neuropathy lies proximal to the posterior primary ramus. It is, however, difficult to perform and interpret on account of significant interference.

Myelography is essential in root lesions to eliminate cervical cord tumors. It also commonly confirms the presence of a herniated disc by revealing obliteration of the axillary sleeve which is normally seen passing into the intervertebral foramen.

Discography and nerve root infiltration[122] help localize cervical disc degeneration.

Computerised tomography can be of value in studying the bony elements of the cervical spine and can delineate soft tissue lesions, when used in conjunction with subarachnoid water soluble contrast medium.

RADIAL NERVE

The radial nerve arises from the posterior cord of the brachial plexus and gains the posterior aspect of the humerus by passing through the triangular space created by the teres major above the long head of triceps medially and the humerus laterally. It comes to lie in the spiral radial groove beneath the lateral head of triceps and immediately proximal to the origin of the medial head. It then gains the anterior aspect of the arm by piercing the lateral intermuscular septum 10 – 12 cm proximal to the lateral epicondyle where it can be easily rolled against the humerus by the finger in most limbs. It then lies between the brachialis and biceps tendon medially and the muscles arising from the lateral supracondylar ridge laterally, brachioradialis, extensor carpi radialis longus and brevis. The nerve passes directly over the anterior ligament of the elbow joint or, more specifically, the articulation between the capitulum of the humerus and the head of the radius. At some point between 3 cm above and below that joint the nerve divides into the sensory superficial radial nerve and the motor posterior interosseous nerve. The two diverge gradually at first but to a degree which bodes ill for the motor nerve. While the superficial radial nerve adheres securely to the deep surface of the brachioradialis, the posterior interosseous nerve passes deep and laterally to gain the extensor surface of the forearm, encountering as it does so three potentially constricting structures.

Extensor carpi radialis brevis, arising from the common extensor origin often has a sharp fibrous medial border which overlies the posterior interosseous nerve;

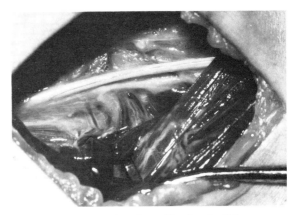

Fig. 3.47 *Radial tunnel syndrome.* The fan of radial recurrent vessels which crosses the deep posterior interosseous nerve is clearly demonstrated after splitting the brachioradialis muscle. Superficially, the sensory radial nerve is seen overlying the vessels.

A 'fan' of vessels from the radial recurrent artery crosses the nerve to supply the structures lateral to it (Fig. 3.47);

The arcade of Frohse[123] is the free, fibrous proximal margin of the superficial portion of the supinator beneath which the posterior interosseous nerve passes (Fig. 3.48). Spinner[124], whose studies of this area are definitive, states that the size of the space beneath the arcade varies greatly and that the arch is thickened and fibrous in 30% of adults examined. He also notes that it is never fibrous in infants. In the release of over fifty radial tunnels, this author has always found the arch to be largely fibrous. Whether this is a developmental feature or an occupational adaptation it is impossible to say. Certainly it would appear to be a prerequisite to the onset of nerve compression.

The radial nerve and its posterior interosseous termination run close to bone throughout much of their

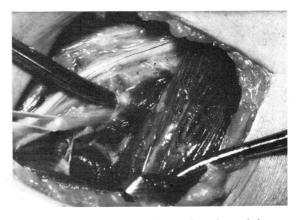

Fig. 3.48 The scissors in this photograph are inserted along the posterior interosseous nerve beneath the arcade of Frohse in the supinator.

These anatomical structures compress the nerve only when the wrist is passively flexed and pronated or conversely when the wrist is extended or supinated against resistance. Occupation therefore plays a major role, since employment requiring frequent repetitive movements of the wrist and forearm in this position may well cause compression. For example, one of the author's patients repeatedly reached over into the back of his car to lift out a heavy case of sample materials. When encouraged to keep the case on the passenger seat and lift it with a supinated arm with the wrist in neutral position, his symptoms regressed.

Men and women appear to be affected equally, mainly between the ages of 30 and 50 and in the dominant hand in the great majority of cases.

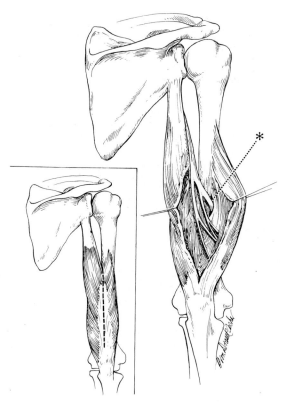

Fig. 3.49 Compression of the radial nerve beneath a fibrous arch in the lateral head of the triceps.

course, the former on the humerus[125, 126], the latter on the radius. They are thus prone to injuries of all degrees in fractures and the management[127] thereof.

While radial palsy has been ascribed to compression of the nerve by a fibrous arch in the lateral head of triceps[128, 129] — the author has operated on one in ten years (Fig. 3.49) — and by the lateral intermuscular septum[130] the major compression syndromes of the radial nerve without fracture are related to the posterior interosseous nerve in the region of the supinator.

While two distinct such syndromes have been described, as Roles and Maudsley[131] emphasized in describing the radial tunnel syndrome, they are simply two points in a spectrum extending from simple 'tennis elbow' (p. 244) to irreversible paralysis of the muscles supplied by the posterior interosseous nerve.

Radial tunnel syndrome (pain)[132]

The compressive factors in radial tunnel syndrome are all anatomical:

fibrous bands tethering the nerve to the radiohumeral joint,
extensor carpi radialis brevis,
the radial recurrent 'fan' of vessels,
the arcade of Frohse.

SYMPTOMS

Pain is usually the *only* presenting symptom. Well localized to the extensor mass just below the elbow, the pain may radiate to the wrist dorsally. Described as aching in character, it can be made more severe by certain movements. Analysis of those movements always reveals wrist flexion and forearm pronation. Typically the pain is absent on awakening but becomes progressively more severe as the arm is used leaving the patient with a persistent ache in the evening.

The patient has very frequently been diagnosed as having 'tennis elbow' and may have had several injections to or surgical procedures on the lateral epicondylar region with temporary relief. Werner in a thorough study of the relationship between lateral elbow pain and nerve entrapment, found it to be present in 5% of 'tennis elbows'[133].

Weakness may be a complaint, when it will be in extending the wrist and fingers. The wrist extension weakness may result in *reduced grip strength,* a troublesome problem especially for manual workers. This extensor weakness may be due entirely to the pain which these movements elicit or may be early evidence of a posterior interosseous nerve syndrome.

EXAMINATION

In radial tunnel syndrome,, there is *no sensory disturbance or motor loss.*

Tenderness is located along the line of the radial nerve over the radial head. The nerve winds around the neck so pressure can be applied over the head anteriorly through the muscles of the 'mobile wad' of Henry[134], or over the neck laterally behind those muscles (Fig. 3.50). This tenderness should always be compared with the opposite side since the region of the radial tunnel is sensitive to pressure even in normal limbs. Tenderness is often also located over the laterla epicondyle but, unlike tennis elbow, is less severe than over the course of the nerve.

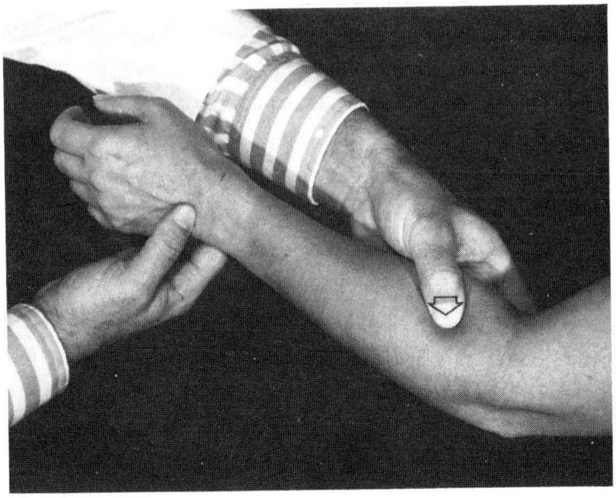

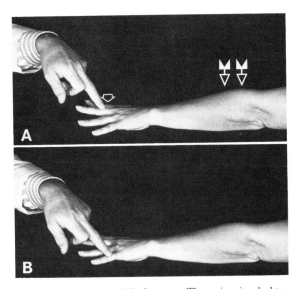

Full passive wrist and finger flexion with the elbow extended usually produces pain but, unlike lateral epicondylitis it is less severe in radial tunnel syndrome than that elicited by the 'middle finger' test (Fig. 3.52).

Resisted supination of the extended arm may also produce pain over the radial tunnel (Fig. 3.53). The arm should be extended during this test to elimate the powerful supinating effect of biceps and place all the load on the supinator proper.

Fig. 3.50 Palpation along the course of the radial nerve in the region of the anterior aspect of the radial head in the 'mobile wad' may show tenderness over the radial tunnel.

Middle finger test (Fig. 3.51). If the patient is asked to extend each finger in turn against resistance with the elbow fully extended pain is experienced over the radial tunnel, sometimes in all fingers but always and most severely on stressing the middle finger. This is accounted for by the fact that extensor carpi radialis brevis inserts into the base of the metacarpal of the middle finger, and the stress drives its fibrous medial edge down on to the posterior interosseous nerve.

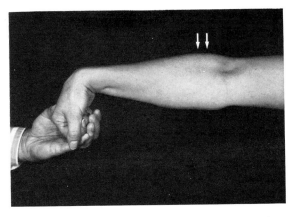

Fig. 3.52 With the elbow extended, the examiner carries the wrist and fingers into full flexion. In radial tunnel syndrome, this may well produce pain but this is less than that experienced with the middle finger test.

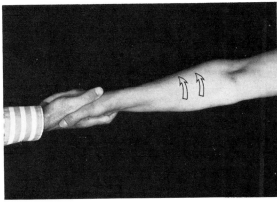

Fig. 3.53 *Radial tunnel syndrome.* Resisted supination may also produce pain in the patient with compression of the radial nerve in its tunnel.

Figs. 3.51A & B *The middle finger test.* The patient is asked to maintain the elbow, wrist, and all fingers in full extension against counter-pressure exerted by the examiner. In the radial tunnel syndrome, the pain experienced on this manoeuvre is significantly greater when pressure is exerted on the middle finger than on any other digits.

Electrophysiological changes were described in those patients in whom Roles and Maudsley performed nerve conduction studies. They took the form of a significant delay in motor latency in the radial nerve from the spiral groove to the extensor digitorum. The proportion of patients in whom such tests were performed was not stated. Changes may also be provoked by resisted supinator contraction during the study.[135] The author has found that several patients with convincing clinical signs subsequently relieved by surgery showed no electrophysioligical changes whatsoever. This would be compatible with the intermittent nature of the stress.

INDICATIONS

Surgical exploration is indicated on entirely clinical grounds and the examiner comes to depend heavily on accurate localization of the tenderness and the 'middle finger' test.

Even when these are present conservative measures should be adopted initially. These include rest from repetitive movements likely to stress the nerve, the wearing of a wristlet to prevent wrist flexion and judicious injection of limited quantities of steroid into the common tendinous origin of the extensor muscles to eliminate any element of lateral epicondylitis. If the clinician is convinced of the diagnosis and these measures fail, exploration of the radial tunnel with release of the medial border of extensor carpi radialis brevis and the arcade of Frohse together with ligation and division of the 'fan' of vessels can give dramatic relief. No macroscopic evidence of compression is found in most cases, although there are always microscopic changes.[136]

Posterior interosseous nerve syndrome (palsy)

This entity has become recognized increasingly since four papers on the topic appeared in the November 1966 issue of the Journal of Bone and Joint Surgery.[137-40]: However, the possibility of paralysis through compression of this nerve had been recorded over one hundred years previously and the various cases reported during that century are well documented in those four papers. Unlike the radial tunnel syndrome, many causes of posterior interosseous nerve syndrome other than the purely anatomical have been inculpated:

Trauma — dislocation of the elbow or, more commonly, fracture or dislocation of the radial head as in the lateral displacement encountered in the Monteggia fracture of the forearm.[141] The palsy may be immediate or delayed.[142, 143]

Inflammation — synovitis associated with rheumatoid disease commonly affects the radiohumeral joint.[144, 145] Compression of the posterior interosseous nerve and the resultant paralysis of the extensors by the synovium or by subluxation of the radial head (Fig. 3.54) may be mistaken for rupture of the tendons at the wrist (p. 264). Inflammatory swelling of the bicipital bursa which lies between the tendon and the radius was the first cause of this syndrome described, by Agnew at the Pathological Society of Philadelphia in 1863.[146]

Swelling — benign swelling of any kind may compress the nerve in the region of the radial tunnel. Those reported include ganglion,[147] lipoma[148] and fibroma.

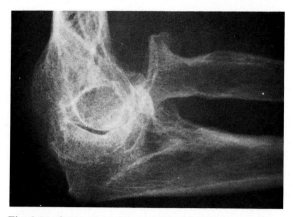

Fig. 3.54 Subluxation of the radial head in this rheumatoid patient produced compression of the posterior interosseous nerve.

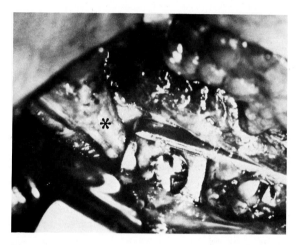

Fig. 3.55 This patient had previously sustained a fracture of the radius. Postoperative development of radial palsy following compression plating brought the patient to exploration of the radial nerve (*) which was found caught beneath the compression plate which had been used in internal fixation.

Anatomical, postural and *occupational* as described in radial tunnel syndrome.

Iatrogenic — injections in the region of the radial tunnel for tennis elbow have caused temporary, and rarely permanent, posterior interosseous nerve paralysis. Compression may also result from plating of fractures of the radius (Fig. 3.55).

SYMPTOMS

Pain is frequently the first complaint and is similar in nature to that of radial tunnel syndrome. This is later accompanied or replaced by *weakness and paralysis* which may develop slowly over a period of two to six weeks or dramatically overnight, usually after a bout of un-accustomed exercise. The sequence in which muscles are affected follows no pattern, the ulnar three fingers, the index finger and the thumb all having been reported as first affected. When fully developed the patient complains of inability to extend the fingers and weakness in extension of the wrist.

In no instance does sensory disturbance occur. This serves to distinguish this syndrome symptomatically from higher lesions of the radial nerve.

EXAMINATION
Sensory disturbance
Dysaesthesia should be carefully excluded, particular attention being paid to the area of absolute radial nerve innervation over the dorsum of the first web and the thumb. Its presence would indicate a more proximal radial nerve lesion.

Motor loss
Wasting of the extensor mass may be evident, contrasting with the normal bulk of the 'mobile wad' of Henry which consists of brachioradialis and the radial extensors of the wrist supplied by the radial nerve before its division.

The posture of the hand is affected little when compared with complete radial palsy for the wrist can be extended. However, the extension is weak and the attitude diagnostic, the wrist being radially deviated in neutral position on attempted full extension (Fig. 3.56).

Attempted extension of the fingers produces a characteristic posture in which the interphalangeal joints are fully extended but the metacarpophalangeal joints cannot be extended beyond 45° and often not that far. This posture may mimic intrinsic tightness and indeed the posture is produced by intrinsic action unaided by long extensor pull — an 'extrinsic minus' rather than an 'intrinsic plus' hand. True intrinsic tightness can be quickly excluded by testing (p. 138).

Partial paralysis of the muscles supplied by the posterior interosseous nerve may result in lack of extension of the joints of the ring and little fingers alone. This produces the appearance of a 'false ulnar claw hand'. The metacarpophalangeal joints are not hyperextended as in the true ulnar claw and the ulnar innervated intrinsics function normally.

Radial abduction of the thumb is also weakened. Some modest extension of the interphalangeal joint may be retained by virtue of the contributions made via the lateral bands by abductor pollicis brevis and adductor pollicis.

Active testing shows weakness or paralysis in some or all of the muscles innervated by the branches of the posterior interosseous nerve

short	— extensor digitorum
	extensor carpi ulnaris
	extensor digiti minimi
long—lateral	— abductor pollicis longus
	extensor pollicis brevis

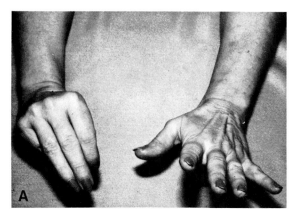
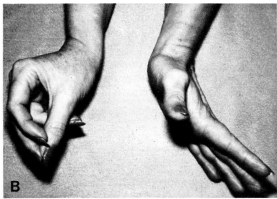

Fig. 3.56 (A, B) On the morning after moving some heavy furniture, this patient woke with pain over the extensor aspect of her forearm and associated loss of extension of her fingers and of her thumb. Wrist extension was still present but less strongly with quite evident radial deviation when compared with the normal hand. In each photograph the patient is attempting full extension of both wrist and fingers with the involved and the normal hand.

—medial	— extensor pollicis longus
	extensor indicis

Rarely the long branch passes over rather than through supinator and if the cause of compression lies therein, the relevant muscles are spared.

Electrophysiological changes will show denervation of paralysed muscles and increased distal latency in the radial nerve in patients showing weakness.

INDICATIONS
Appropriate splintage should be provided to support the paralysed muscles and permit something approaching normal function. Many will show recovery with time and repeated evaluation should be performed. It will often demonstrate progressive return of individual muscles. Surgical exploration is indicated in all persistent cases of posterior interosseous nerve syndrome.

Differential diagnosis from *high radial nerve lesions* is made by the lack of sensory disturbance and normal strength of brachioradialis, the radial wrist extensors and the supinator. *Lead poisoning* may produce radial palsy with no sensory loss but it is a high lesion, showing paralysis of brachioradialis and the radial wrist extensors. The diagnosis can be confirmed by seeking the characteristic gingival discoloration and by haematological and urinary studies. *Hysterical drop wrist* shows persistent inability to extend the interphalangeal joints of the fingers even with the metacarpophalangeal joints held in flexion.

Other reported causes of radial nerve compression

Anatomical	— distal edge of supinator[149]
Tumour	— Hamartoma[150]
	Angioleiomyoma[151]
	Synovial chondromatosis[152]

Polyarteritis[153]

Nerves, other than radial, ulnar and median, have rarely been reported as compressed — the suprascapular[154-156], the long thoracic[157] and the supraclavicular[158]. All were the cause of pain and the compression of the first two were associated with appropriate muscular weakness and paralysis.

Muscle compression syndromes

Some of the nerve compression syndromes described above may be caused by the presence of an anomalous muscle in the nerve tunnel, such as a reversed palmaris longus, palmaris profundus or an origin in the forearm of the abductor digiti minimi.

Anomalous muscles may in themselves produce discomfort, mainly with use. This difficulty usually arises in the fourth and fifth decades and much more commonly in females, which may be due to occupational stress or hormonal fluid retention.

That apart, compression syndromes have been described in which nerves are not involved, but in which a normal or anomalous muscle becomes hypertrophied or inflamed within a tight tunnel, resulting in pain and discomfort.

EXTENSOR INDICIS SYNDROME

Originally described by Ritter and Inglis in 1969[159], this syndrome is due to inflammation associated with a normal or anomalous extensor indicis at the point at which it passes through the fourth dorsal compartment beneath the extensor retinaculum.

Symptoms

Pain in the wrist, which shows a normal pain-free range of motion is characteristic of the disorder. Point tenderness over the fourth compartment at the wrist has often been localised by the patient before presentation.

Examination

Extensor indicis test (Fig. 3.57). Spinner[160] reported in 1973 that if, with the wrist fully flexed, the patient is asked to extend the proximal phalanx of the index finger against resistance, he will complain of sharp pain well localized to the fourth compartment at the wrist. If the tender area is palpated during this resisted extension, crepitation can frequently be felt.

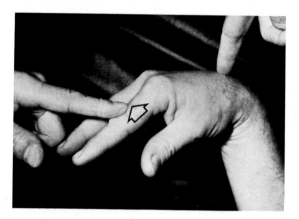

Fig. 3.57 This patient presented with a complaint of pain over the dorsal aspect of the right wrist. Examination revealed a full painfree range of motion in the wrist but when extension of the index finger was attempted against resistance, he experienced pain in the site indicated by the examiner's other finger. This discomfort was associated with crepitus in the region of the fourth dorsal compartment.

Surgical release of the tunnel is indicated only if splintage, local steroids and anti-inflammatory agents fail to produce relief.

EXTENSOR DIGITI MINIMI PROPRIUS[161]

A syndrome similar to the extensor indicis syndrome, but related to the extensor digiti minimi in the fifth compartment has recently been reported. The muscle was anomalous in that it had a musculotendinous slip to the ring finger. Pain, elicited on movement of the small finger, was the presenting symptom, and excision of the anomalous slip resulted in improvement.

EXTENSOR DIGITORUM BREVIS MANUS[162, 3]

This anomalous muscle was first named by Wood in the Proceedings of the Royal Society of London in 1864[164]. Originating on the carpus and wrist capsule a little distal to the extensor retinaculum, it may become troublesome because of pain or swelling. Often mistaken for a ganglion, it is recognized if the surgeon is aware of the entity, for it quite evidently contracts on resisted extension of the fingers. The correct treatment is surgical excision.

Non-compressive causes of neuropathy

Because their symptoms are confined to the upper limb, many patients with conditions outwith the realm of the hand surgeon will nonetheless understandably present themselves to him for help. A considerable responsibility rests on him to remain aware of the other possibilities, which are legion:

Generalised neuropathy
Spinal cord disease
Spinal tumours
Intracranial disorders
Intrathoracic pathology — 'Pancoast's syndrome'.[165]

The hand surgeon should keep a high index of suspicion in talking to and examining any patient complaining of pain, weakness or paralysis of the upper limb. The history should seek out evidence of familial disorders, of metabolic disturbance, of weakness elsewhere, of visual or cranial nerve disorder or other symptoms apparently unrelated in the patient's estimation. In examination, the signs of upper motor neurone involvement should be sought in the form of increased reflexes and spasticity, the muscles should be observed for fibrillation, the blood pressure should always be recorded and the urine subjected to analysis.

If careful examination suggests that the source lies proximal to the shoulder all patients should undergo chest X-ray, including apical lordotic views, X-rays of the cervical spine and neurological consultation, pending appropriate study by electroencephalography, brain scan or myelography. Only by remaining constantly mindful of where the nerves which are disturbed in the hand and arm come from and go to can the hand surgeon avoid the tragedy of a missed diagnosis compounded by inappropriate treatment.

REFERENCES

1. Frymoyer J W, Bland J 1973 Carpal tunnel syndrome in patients with myxedematous arthropathy. The Journal of Bone and Joint Surgery 55A: 78-82
2. Ekerot L 1977 Postanesthetic ulnar neuropathy at the elbow. Scandinavian Journal of Plastic and Reconstructive Surgery 11: 225-229
3. Curtis R M, Eversmann W W 1973 Internal neurolysis as an adjunct to the treatment of the carpal tunnel syndrome. The Journal of Bone and Joint Surgery 55A: 733-740
4. Lavey E B, Pearl R M 1981 Patent median artery as a cause of carpal tunnel syndrome. Annals of Plastic Surgery 7:3 236-238
5. Barton N J 1979 Another cause of median nerve compression by a lumbrical muscle in the carpal tunnel. Journal of Hand Surgery 4: 189-191
6. Schultz R J, Endler P M, & Huddleston H D 1973 Anomalous median nerve and an anomalous muscle belly of the first lumbrical associated with carpal tunnel syndrome. Journal of Bone and Joint Surgery 55A: 1744-1746
7. Butler B, Bigley E C 1971 Aberrant index (first) lumbrical tendinous origin associated with carpal tunnel syndrome. The Journal of Bone and Joint Surgery 53A: 160-162
8. Smith R J 1971 Anomalous muscle belly of the flexor digitorum superficialis causing carpal tunnel syndrome. Journal of Bone and Joint Surgery 53A: 1215-1216
9. Backhouse K M Churchill-Davidson D 1975 Anomalous palmaris longus muscle producing carpal tunnel-like compression. The Hand 7: 22-24
10. Brones M, Wilgis E 1978 Anatomical variations of the palmaris longus, causing carpal tunnel syndrome. Plastic and Reconstructive Surgery 62: 798-800
11. Carroll M P, Montero C 1980 Rare anomalous muscle cause of carpal tunnel syndrome. Orthopaedic Review 9: 83-85
12. Still J M, Kleinert H E 1973 Anomalous muscles and nerve entrapment in the wrist and hand. Plastic and Reconstructive Surgery 52: 394-400
13. Adamson J E, Srouji S J, Horton C E, Mladick R A 1971 The acute carpal tunnel syndrome. Plastic and Reconstructive Surgery 47: 332-336
14. Fissette J, Onkelinx A, Fandi N 1981 Carpal and Guyon tunnel syndrome in burns at the wrist. Journal of Hand Surgery 6: 13-15
15. Harvey F J, Bosanquet J S 1981 Carpal tunnel syndrome caused by simple ganglion. The Hand 13: 164-166
16. Kummel B M, Zazanis G A 1973 Shoulder pain as the presenting complaint in carpal tunnel syndrome. Clinical Orthopaedics and Related Research 92: 227-230
17. Phalen G S 1951 Spontaneous compression of the median nerve at the wrist. Journal of American Medical Association 145: 1128-1133
18. Phalen G S 1966 The carpal tunnel syndrome. Journal of Bone and Joint Surgery 48A: 211-228
19. Phalen G S 1968 The carpal tunnel syndrome: 17 years experience in diagnosis and treatment of 654 hands. Journal of Bone and Joint Surgery 48A: 211-228
20. Gelberman R H, Hergenroeder P T, Hargens A R, Lundborg G N, Akeson W H 1981 The carpal tunnel syndrome – Study of carpal canal pressures. Journal of Bone and Joint Surgery 63A: 380-383
21. Melvin J L, Schuchmann J A, Lanese R R 1973 Diagnostic specificity of motor and sensory nerve conduction variables in the carpal tunnel syndrome. Archives of Physical and Medical Rehabilitation 54: 69-74
22. Hart V L, Gaynor V 1941 Roentgenographic study of the carpal canal. Journal of Bone and Joint Surgery 23: 382-383
23. Wood M R 1980 Hydrocortisone injections for carpal tunnel syndrome. The Hand 12: 62-64
24. Gelberman R H, Aronson D, Weisman M H 1980 Carpal tunnel syndrome. Journal of Bone and Joint Surgery 62A: 1181-1184
25. Nalebuff E A, Smith J 1979 Preservation of terminal branches of the median palmar cutaneous nerve in carpal tunnel surgery. Orthopaedics 2: 369-372
26. Seyffarth H 1951 Primary myoses in the m. pronator teres as a cause of lesion of the n. medianus (the pronator syndrome). Acta Psychiatria Scandinavica Supp 74: 251
27. Vichare N A 1968 Spontaneous paralysis of the anterior interosseous nerve. The Journal of Bone and Joint Surgery 50B: 806-808
28. Johnson R K, Spinner M, Shrewsbury M M 1979 Median nerve entrapment syndrome in the proximal forearm. The Journal of Hand Surgery 4: 48-52
29. Hartz C R, Linscheid R L, Gramse R R, Daube J R 1981 The pronator teres syndrome: Compressive neuropathy of the median nerve. The Journal of Bone and Joint Surgery 63A: 885-890

30. Farrell H F 1979 Pain and the pronator teres syndrome. Bulletin of the Hospital for Joint Diseases 37: 59-62

31. Buchthal F, Rosenfalck A, Trojaborg W 1974 Electrophysiological findings in entrapment of the median nerve at wrist and elbow. Journal of Neurology, Neurosurgery and Psychiatry 37: 340-360

32. Spinner M 1978 Injuries to the major branches of peripheral nerves of the forearm 2nd edn. W B Saunders Co, Philadelphia

33. Maeda K, Miura T, Komada T, Chiba A 1977 Anterior interosseous nerve paralysis. Report of 13 cases and review of Japanese literature. The Hand 9: 165-171

34. Jabaley M E 1978 Personal observations on the role of the lumbrical muscles in carpal tunnel syndrome. The Journal of Hand Surgery 3: 82-84

35. Nather A, Pho R W H 1981 Carpal tunnel syndrome produced by an organising haematoma within the anomalous second lumbrical muscle. The Hand 13: 87-91

36. Wiss D 1979 Aberrant lumbrical muscles causing carpal tunnel syndrome. Orthopedics 2: 357-358

37. Hutton P, Kernohan J, Birch R 1981 An anomalous flexor digitorum superficialis indicis muscle presenting as carpal tunnel syndrome. The Hand 13: 85-86

38. Chalmers J 1978 Unusual causes of peripheral nerve compression. The Hand 10: 168-175

39. Levy M, Pauker M 1978 Carpal tunnel syndrome due to thrombosed persisting median artery. A case report. Hand 10: 65-68

40. Spinner M 1976 Cryptogenic infraclavicular brachial plexus neuritis. Bulletin of the Hospital for Joint Diseases 37: 98-104

41. Laha R K, Dujovny M, DeCastro S C 1977 Entrapment of median nerve by supracondylar process of the humerus. Journal of Neurosurgery 46: 252-255

42. Wolfe J S, Eyring E J 1974 Median nerve entrapment within a greenstick fracture. The Journal of Bone and Joint Surgery 56A: 1270-1272

43. Nunley J A, Ubaniak J R 1980 Partial bony entrapment of the median nerve in a greenstick fracture of the ulna. Journal of Hand Surgery 5: 557-559

44. Macnicol M 1978 Roentgenographic evidence of median nerve entrapment in a greenstick humeral fracture. Journal of Bone and Joint Surgery 60A: 998-1000

45. Lewis M H 1978 Median nerve decompression after Colles' fracture. Journal of Bone and Joint Surgery 60B: 195-196

46. Manske P 1976 Fracture of the hook of the hamate presenting as carpal tunnel syndrome. The Hand 10: 181-183

47. Sturim H S, Edmond J A 1980 Carpal tunnel compression syndrome secondary to a retracted flexor digitorum sublimis tendon. Plastic and Reconstructive Surgery 66: 846-848

48. Weiland A J, Lister G D, Villarreal-Rios A 1976 Volar fracture dislocations of the second and third carpometacarpal joints associated with acute carpal tunnel syndrome. Journal of Trauma 16: 672-675

49. Matev I 1976 A radiological sign of entrapment of the median nerve in the elbow joint after posterior dislocation. Journal of Bone and Joint Surgery 58B: 353-355

50. Hallett J 1981 Entrapment of the median nerve after dislocation of the elbow: A case report. Journal of Bone and Joint Surgery 63B: 408-412

51. Lazaro L 1972 Carpal tunnel syndrome from an insect sting. Journal of Bone and Joint Surgery 54A: 1095-1096

52. Short W H, Palmer A K 1981 Amyloidosis and the carpal tunnel syndrome. Orthopaedic Review 10: 89-94

53. MacDougal B, Weeks P M, Wray R C 1977 Median nerve compression and trigger finger in the mucopolysaccharidoses and related disease. Plastic and Reconstructive Surgery 59: 260-263

54. Johnson R J, Bonfiglio M 1969 Lipofibromatous hamartoma of the median nerve. Journal of Bone and Joint Surgery 51A: 984-990

55. Louis D S, Dick H M 1973 Ossifying lipofibroma of the median nerve. Journal of Bone and Joint Surgery 55A: 1082-1084

56. Kojima T, Ide Y, Marumo E, Ishikawa E, Yamashita H 1976 Haemangioma of median nerve causing carpal tunnel syndrome. The Hand 8: 62-65

57. Engel J, Zinneman H, Tsur H, Farin I 1978 Carpal tunnel syndrome due to carpal osteophyte. The Hand 10: 283-284

58. Pritsch M, Engel J, Horowitz A 1980 Cystic change in the wrist, causing carpal tunnel syndrome. Plastic and Reconstructive Surgery 65: 494-495

59. Linscheid R L 1979 Carpal tunnel syndrome secondary to ulnar bursa distention from the intercarpal joint: Report of a case. Journal of Hand Surgery 4: 191-193

60. Seddon H J 1952 Carpal ganglion as a cause of paralysis of the deep branch of the ulnar nerve. The Journal of Bone and Joint Surgery 34B: 386-390

61. Wood V E 1980 Nerve compression following opponensplasty as a result of wrist anomalies: Report of a case. Journal of Hand Surgery 5: 279-280

62. Mancusi-Ungaro A, Corres J J, Di Spaltro F 1976 Case reports: Median carpal tunnel syndrome following a vascular shunt procedure in the forearm. Plastic and Reconstructive Surgery 57: 96-97

63. Kenzora J E 1978 Dialysis carpal tunnel syndrome. Orthopaedics 1: 195-203

64. Jain V K, Cestero R V M, Baum J 1979 Carpal tunnel syndrome in patients undergoing maintenance hemodialysis. Journal of American Medical Association 242: 2868-2869

65. DeLuca F N, Cowen N J 1975 Median nerve compression complicating a tendon graft prosthesis. The Journal of Bone and Joint Surgery 57A: 553

66. Hunt J R 1908 Occupation neuritis of the deep palmar branch of the ulnar nerve. Journal of Neurological and Mental Diseases 35: 673-689

67. Kleinert H E, Hayes J E 1971 The ulnar tunnel syndrome. Plastic and Reconstructive Surgery 47: 21-24

68. Hayes J R, Mulholland R C, O'Connor B T 1969 Compression of the deep palmar branch of the ulnar nerve. Journal of Bone and Joint Surgery 51B: 469-472

69. Leslie I J 1980 Compression of the deep branch of the ulnar nerve due to edema of the hand. The Hand 12: 271-272

70. Seddon H J 1952 Carpal ganglion as a cause of paralysis of the deep branch of the ulnar nerve. Journal of Bone and Joint Surgery 34B 386

71. Salgeback S 1977 Ulnar tunnel syndrome caused by anomalous muscles. Scand. Journal of Plastic and Reconstructive Surgery 11: 255-258

72. Turner M S, Caird D M 1977 Anomalous muscles and ulnar nerve compression at the wrist. The Hand 9: 140-141

73. Weeks P M, Young V L 1982 Ulnar artery thrombosis and ulnar nerve compression associated with an anomalous hypothenar muscle (Case Report) 69: 130-131

74. Jeffery A K 1971 Compression of the deep palmar branch of the ulnar nerve by an anomalous muscle. Journal of Bone and Joint Surgery 53B: 718-723

75. Fahrer M, Millroy P J 1981 Ulnar compression neuropathy due to an anomalous abductor digiti minimi – Clinical and anatomic study. Journal of Hand Surgery 6: 266-268

76. Uriburu I J F, Morchio F J, Marin J C 1976 Compression syndrome of the deep motor branch of the ulnar nerve (Piso-Hamate Hiatus syndrome). Journal of Bone and Joint Surgery 58A: 145-147

77. Panas J 1878 Sur une case pas connue de paralysie du neuf cubital Archives Generales de Medicine 2: 5-22
78. Apfelberg D B, Larson SJ 1973 Dynamic anatomy of the ulnar nerve at the elbow. Plastic and Reconstructive Surgery 51: 76-81
79. Leffert R D, Dorfman H D 1972 Antecubital cyst in rheumatoid arthritis – surgical findings. Journal of Bone and Joint Surgery 54A: 1555-1557
80. Osborne G 1957 The surgical treatment of tardy ulnar neuritis. Journal of Bone and Joint Surgery 39B 782
81. Osborne G 1970 Decompression of ulnar nerve at elbow. Hand 2: 10-13
82. Learmonth J R 1942 A technique for transplanting the ulnar nerve. Surgery Gynecology and Obstetrics 75: 792-793
83. Craven P R, Green D P 1980 Cubital tunnel syndrome. Treatment by medial epicondylectomy. Journal of Bone and Joint Surgery 62A: 986-989
84. Froimson A I, Zahrawi F 1980 Treatment of compression neuropathy of the ulnar nerve at the elbow by epicondylectomy and neurolysis. Journal of Hand Surgery 5: 391-395
85. Neblett C, Ehni G 1970 Medial epicondylectomy for ulnar palsy. Journal of Neurosurgery 32: 55-62
86. Spinner M, Kaplan E B 1976 The relationship of the ulnar nerve to the medial intermuscular septum in the arm and its clinical significance. Hand 8: 239-242
87. Reis N D 1980 Anomalous triceps tendon as a cause for snapping elbow and ulnar neuritis: A case report. Journal of Hand Surgery 5: 361-362
88. Rolfsen L 1970 Snapping triceps tendon with ulnar neuritis. Acta Orthopaedic Scandinavia 41: 74-76
89. Harrelson J M, Newmann M 1975 Hypertrophy of the flexor carpi ulnaris as a cause of ulnar nerve compression in the distal part of the forearm. Journal of Bone and Joint Surgery 57A: 554-555
90. Comtet J, Quicot L, Moyen B 1978 Compression of the deep palmar branch of the ulnar nerve by the arch of the adductor pollicis. The Hand 10: 176-180
91. Hirasawa Y, Sawamura H, Sakakida K 1979 Entrapment neuropathy due to bilateral epitrochleoanconeus muscles: A case report. Journal of Hand Surgery 4: 181-185
92. Thomsen B 1977 Processus supracondyloidea humeri with concomitant compression of median nerve and ulnar nerve. Acta Orthopaedic Scandinavica 48: 391-393
93. Murakami Y, Komiyama Y 1978 Hypoplasia of the trochlea and the medial epicondyle of the humerus associated with ulnar neuropathy. Journal of Bone and Joint Surgery 60B: 225-227
94. Hirotani H 1975 An unusual cause of ulnar nerve compression. The Hand 7: 266-268
95. Vance R, Gelberman R 1978 Acute ulnar neuropathy with fractures at the wrist. Journal of Bone and Joint Surgery 60A: 962-965
96. Poppi M, Padovani R, Martinelli P, Pozzati E 1978 Fracture of the distal radius with ulnar nerve palsy. Journal of Trauma 18: 278-279
97. Howard F M 1961 Ulnar nerve palsy in wrist fractures. Journal of Bone and Joint Surgery 43A: 1197-1201
98. Gore D R 1971 Carpometacarpal dislocation producing compression of the deep branch of the ulnar nerve. Journal of Bone and Joint Surgery 1387-1390
99. Milberg P, Kleinert H E 1980 Giant cell tumor compression of the deep branch of the ulnar nerve. Annals of Plastic Surgery 4: 426-429
100. Hayes C 1978 Ulnar tunnel syndrome from giant cell tumor of tendon sheath: A case report Journal of Hand Surgery 3: 187-188

101. McFarland G B, Hoffer M M 1971 Paralysis of the intrinsic muscles of the hand secondary to lipoma in Guyon's canal. Journal of Bone and Joint Surgery 53A: 375-376
102. Bowers W, Doppelt S 1979 Compression of the deep branch of the ulnar nerve by an intraneural cyst. Case report. Journal of Bone and Joint Surgery 61A: 612-613
103. Fahmy N R M, Noble J 1981 Ulnar nerve palsy as a complication of synovial osteochondromatosis of the elbow. The Hand 13: 308-310
104. Taylor A R 1974 Ulnar nerve compression at the wrist in rheumatoid arthritis. Journal of Bone and Joint Surgery 56B 142-143
105. Dell P C 1979 Compression of the ulnar nerve at the wrist secondary to a rheumatoid synovial cyst: Case report and review of the literature. Journal of Hand Surgery 4: 468-473
106. McIntyre, D I 1975 Subcoracoid neurovascular entrapment. Clinical Orthopaedics 108: 27-30
107. Brannon E W 1963 Cervical rib syndrome. Journal of Bone and Joint Surgery 45A: 977-998
108. Roos D B 1979 New concepts of thoracic outlet syndrome that explain etiology, symptoms, diagnosis, and treatment. Vascular Surgery 13: 313-321
109. Siegel R S, Steichten F M 1967 Cervicothoracic outlet syndrome. Journal of Bone and Joint Surgery 49A: 1187-1192
110. Adson A W 1947 Surgical treatment for symptoms produces by cervical ribs and the scalenus anticus muscle. Surgery, Gynecology and Obstetrics 85: 687-700
111. Adson A W 1951 Cervical Ribs: Symptoms, differential diagnosis and indications for section of the insertion of the scalenus anticus muscle. Journal of the International College of Surgeons 16: 546-559
112. Wright I S 1945 The neurovascular syndrome produced by hyperabduction of the arms. American Heart Journal 29: 1-19
113. Rainer W G, Mayer J, Sadler T R, Dirks D 1973 Effect of graded compression on nerve conduction velocity. Archives of Surgery 107: 719-721
114. Lain T M 1969 The military brace syndrome. Journal of Bone and Joint Surgery 51A: 557-560
115. Lain T M 1969 The military brace syndrome: A report of sixteen cases of Erb's palsy occuring in military cadets. Journal of Bone and Joint Surgery 51A: 557-560
116. Bonney G 1965 Scalenus medius band. Journal of Bone and Joint Surgery 47B: 268-272
117. Urschel H C, Razzuk M A 1972 Management intelligence. Management of the thoracic outlet syndrome. The New England Journal of Medicine 286: 1140-1143
118. Smith K F 1979 The thoracic outlet syndrome: A protocol of treatment. Journal of Orthopaedic and Sports Physical Therapy 2: 89-99
119. Adson A W, Coffey J R 1927 Cervical Rib. A method of anterior approach for relief of symptoms by division of the scalenus anticus. Annals of Surgery 85: 839-857
120. Roos D B 1966 Experience with first rib resection for thoracic outlet syndrome. Annals of Surgery 163: 354-358
121. Spurling R G, Scoville W R 1944 Lateral rupture of the cervical intervertebral discs. Surgery Gynecology and Obstetrics. 78: 350-357
122. Kikuchi S, Macnab I, Moreau P 1981 Localisation of the level of symptomatic cervical disc degeneration. Journal of Bone and Joint Surgery 63B: 272-277
123. Frohse F, Frankel M 1908 Die Muskaln des Menschlichen Aunes. Bardelehen's Handbuch der Anatomie des Manschlichen. Fischer, Jena
124. Spinner M 1968 The arcade of Frohse its relationship to posterior interosseous nerve paralysis. Journal of Bone and Joint Surgery 50B: 809-812

125. Pollock F H, Drake D, Bovill E G, Day L, Trafton P G 1981 Treatment of radial neuropathy associated with fractures of the humerus. Journal of Bone and Joint Surgery 63A: 239-243

126. Kaiser T E, Sim F H, Kelly P J 1981 Radial nerve palsy associated with humeral fractures. Orthopedics 4: 1245-1251

127. Strachan J C H, Ellis B W 1971 The vulnerability of the posterior interosseous nerve during radial head resection. Journal of Bone and Joint Surgery 53B: 320-323

128. Lotem M, Fried A, Levy M, Solzi P, Najenson T, Nathan H 1971 Radial palsy following muscular effort. Journal of Bone and Joint Surgery 53B: 500-506

129. Manske P R 1977 Compression of the radial nerve by the triceps muscle. Case report. Journal of Bone and Joint Surgery 59A: 835-836

130. Wilhelm A 1976 Radialis kompressions syndrome. Handchirurgie 8: 113-116

131. Roles N C, Maudsley R 1972 Radial tunnel syndrome: Resistant tennis elbow as a nerve entrapment. Journal of Bone and Joint Surgery 54B: 499-508

132. Lister G D, Belsole R B, Kleinert H E 1979 The radial tunnel syndrome. The Journal of Hand Surgery 4: 52-60

133. Werner C 1979 Lateral elbow pain and posterior interosseous nerve entrapment. Acta Orthopaedic Scandinavica Supp 174

134. Henry A K 1973 Extensile exposure, 2nd edn. Churchill Livingstone, Edinburgh

135. Rosen, I, Werner C 1980 Neurophysiological investigation of posterior interosseous nerve entrapment causing lateral elbow pain. Electroencephalography & Clinical Neurophysiology 50: 125-133

136. Hagert C G, Lundborg G, Hansen T 1977 Entrapment of the posterior interosseous nerve. Scandinavian Journal of Plastic and Reconstructive Surgery 11: 205-212

137. Bowen T L, Stone K H 1966 Posterior interosseous nerve paralysis caused by a ganglion at the elbow. Journal of Bone and Joint Surgery 48B: 774-776

138. Mulholland R C 1966 Nontraumatic progressive paralysis of the posterior interosseous nerve. Journal of Bone and Joint Surgery 48B: 781-785

139. Capener N 1966 The vulnerability of the posterior interosseous nerve of the forearm. The Journal of Bone and Joint Surgery 48B: 770-783

140. Sharrard W J W 1966 Posterior interosseous neuritis. Journal of Bone and Joint Surgery 48B: 777-780

141. Agnew D H 1863 Bursal tumour producing loss of power of forearm. American Journal of Medical Science 46: 404-405

142. Spinner M, Freundlich B D, Teicher J 1968 Posterior interosseous nerve palsy as a complication of Monteggia fractures in children. Clinical Orthopaedics 58 141-145

143. Lichter R L, Jacobson T 1975 Tardy palsy of the posterior interosseous nerve with a Monteggia fracture. Journal of Bone and Joint Surgery 57A: 124-125

144. Austin R 1976 Tardy palsy of the radial nerve from a Monteggia fracture. Injury 7: 303-304

145. Popelka S, Vainio K 1974 Entrapment of the posterior interosseous branch of the radial nerve in rheumatoid arthritis. Acta Orthopedic Scandinavica 45: 370-372

146. Millender L H, Nalebuff M D, Edward A, Holdsworth D E 1973 Posterior interosseous nerve syndrome secondary to rheumatoid synovitis. The Journal of Bone and Joint Surgery 55A: 753-757

147. Mass D P, Tortosa R, Newmeyer W L, Kilgore Jr E S 1982 Compression of posterior interosseous nerve by a ganglion. Case report. Journal of Hand Surgery 7: 92-94

148. Blakemore M E 1979 Posterior interosseous nerve paralysis caused by a lipoma. Journal of the Royal College of Surgeons of Edinburgh 24: 113-117

149. Derkash R S, Niebauer J J 1981 Entrapment of the posterior interosseous nerve by a fibrous band in the dorsal edge of the supinator muscle and erosion of a groove in the proximal radius. Journal of Hand Surgery 6: 524-526

150. Herrick R T, Godsil R D, Widener J H 1980 Lipofibromatous hamartoma of the radial nerve. A case report. Journal of Hand Surgery 5: 211-213

151. Sunram F, Hippe P 1979 Radial nerve paralysis by congenital angioleiomyoma. Hand Chirurgia 11: 27-29

152. Field J H 1981 Posterior interosseous nerve palsy secondary to synovial chondromatosis of the elbow joint. Journal of Hand Surgery 6: 336-338

153. Belsole R, Lister G, Kleinert H 1978 Polyarteritis: A cause of nerve palsy in the extremity. Journal of Hand Surgery 3: 320–325

154. Garcia G, McQueen D 1981 Bilateral suprascapular nerve entrapment syndrome. Case report and review of the literature. Journal of Bone and Joint Surgery 63A: 491-492

155. Rask M R 1977 Suprascapular nerve entrapment: A report of two cases treated with suprascapular notch resection. Clinical Orthopaedics 123: 73-75

156. Swafford A R, Lichtman D H 1982 Suprascapular nerve entrapment. Case report. Journal of Hand Surgery 7: 57-60

157. Gozna E R, Harris W R 1979 Traumatic winging of the scapula. Journal of Bone and Joint Surgery 61A: 1230-1233

158. Gelberman R H, Verdeck W N, Brodhead W T 1975 Supraclavicular nerve-entrapment syndrome. Journal of Bone and Joint Surgery 57A: 119

159. Ritter M A, Inglis A E 1969 The extensor indicis proprius syndrome. Journal of Bone and Joint Surgery 51A: 1645-1648

160. Spinner M, Olshansky K 1973 The extensor indicis proprius syndrome. Plastic and Reconstructive Surgery 51: 134-138

161. Ambrose J, Goldstone R 1975 Anomaous extensor digiti minimi proprius causing tunnel syndrome in the dorsal compartment. The Journal of Bone and Joint Surgery 57A: 706-707

162. Hart J A L 1972 Extensor digitorum brevis manus. The Hand 4: 265-267

163. Reef T C, Brestin S G 1975 The extensor digitorum brevis manus and its clinical significance. The Journal of Bone and Joint Surgery 57A: 704-706

164. Wood J 1864 On some varieties in human myology. Proceedings of the Royal Society London 13: 299-303

165. Pancoast H K 1932 Superior pulmonary sulcus tumor. The Journal of the American Medical Association 99: 1391-1396

FURTHER READING

Aghasi M K, Rzetelny V, Axer A 1980 The flexor digitorum superficialis as a cause of bilateral carpal tunnel syndrome and trigger wrist. A case report. Journal of Bone and Joint Surgery 62A: 134–135

Bentley F H, Schlapp W 1943 The effects of pressure on conduction in peripheral nerves. Journal of Physiology 107: 72–82

Childress H M 1975 Recurrent ulnar-nerve dislocation at the elbow. Clinical Orthopaedics and Related Research 108: 168–173

Danielsson L G 1980 Iatrogenic pronator syndrome. Scand. Journal of Plastic and Reconstructive Surgery 14: 201–203

Das S K, Brown H G 1976 In search of complications in carpal tunnel decompression. The Hand 8: 243–249

Denman E E 1982 The anatomy of the incision for carpal tunnel decompression. The Hand 13: 17–28

Dupont C, Cloutier G E, Prevost Y, Dion M A 1965 Ulnar-tunnel syndrome at the wrist. A report of 4 cases of ulnar-nerve compression at the wrist. Journal of Bone and Joint Surgery 47A: 757–761

Eisen A, Schomer D, Melmed C 1977 The application of F-wave measurements in the differentiation of proximal and distal upper limb entrapments. Neurology 27: 662–668

Entin M A 1968 Carpal tunnel syndrome and its variants. Surgical Clinics of North America 48: 1097–1112

Eversmann W W Jr, Tirsick J W 1978 Intraoperative changes in motor nerve conduction latency in carpal tunnel syndrome. The Journal of Hand Surgery 3: 77–81

Fitzgerald B 1978 St. Anthony's fire or carpal tunnel syndrome. A case of iatrogenic ergotism. The Hand 10: 82–86

Freshwater M F, Arons M S 1978 The effect of various adjuncts on the surgical treatment of carpal tunnel syndrome secondary to chronic tenosynovitis. Plastic and Reconstructive Surgery 61: 93–96

Gilliatt R W, Ochoa J, Rudge P, Neary D 1974 The cause of nerve damage in acute compression. Transactions of the American Neurologic Association 99: 71–74

Greene M H, Hadied A M 1981 Bipartite hamulus with ulnar tunnel syndrome — Case report and literature review. Journal of Hand Surgery 6: 605–609

Hagstrom P 1977 Ulnar nerve compression at the elbow. Scandinavian Journal of Plastic and Reconstructive Surgery 11: 59–62

Harris C M, Tanner E, Goldstein M N, Pettee D S 1979 The surgical treatment of the carpal-tunnel syndrome correlated with preoperative nerve-conduction studies. Journal of Bone and Joint Surgery 61A: 93–98

Hecht O, Lipsker E 1980 Median and ulnar nerve entrapment caused by ectopic calcification: Report of two cases. Journal of Hand Surgery 5: 30–31

Hoehn J G 1980 Neurolysis in the treatment of carpal tunnel syndrome. Orthopaedic Review 9: 103–107

Kane E, Kaplan E B, Spinner M 1973 Observations of the course of the ulnar nerve in the arm. Annals de Chirurgie 27: 487–496

Karpati G, Carpenter S, Eisen A, Feindel W 1973 Familial multiple peripheral nerve entrapments — An unusual manifestation of a peripheral neuropathy. Transactions of the American Neurological Association 98: 267–269

Knight C R, Kozub P 1979 Anterior interosseous syndrome. Annals of Plastic Surgery 3: 72–76

McGrath M H, Polayes I M 1979 Post-traumatic median neuroma: A cause of carpal tunnel syndrome. Annals of Plastic Surgery 3: 227–230

Mills R A B, Mukheyee K, Bassett I B 1969 Anterior interosseous nerve palsy. British Medical Journal 2: 555

Mittal R, Gupta B 1978 Median and ulnar-nerve palsy: An unusual presentation of the supracondylar process. Report of a case. Journal of Bone and Joint Surgery 60A: 557–558

Moldaver J 1954 Tourniquet paralysis syndrome. Archives of Surgery 68: 136–144

Morris H H, Peters B H 1976 Pronator syndrome: clinical and electrophysiological features in seven cases. Journal of Neurology, Neurosurgery, and Psychiatry 39: 461–464

Neary D, Ochoa J, Gilliatt R W 1975 Sub-clinical entrapment neuropathy in Man. Journal of the Neurological Sciences 23: 283–298

Nelson R M 1980 Effects of elbow position on motor conduction velocity of the ulnar nerve. Phys Therapy 60: 780–783

Pechan J, Julis I 1975 The pressure measurement in the ulnar nerve. A contribution to the pathophysiology of the cubital tunnel syndrome. Journal of Biomechanics 8: 75–79

Posch J L, Marcotte D R 1976 Carpal tunnel syndrome. An analysis of 1,201 cases. Orthopaedic Review 5: 25–35

Richmond D A 1973 Uncommon causes of nerve compression with hand symptoms. The Hand 5: 209–213

Roos D R, Owens J C 1966 Thoracic outlet syndrome. Archives of Surgery 93: 163, 354

Rydevik B, Lundborg G 1977 Permeability of intraneural microvessels and perineurium following acute, graded experimental nerve compression. Scand. Journal of Plastic and Reconstructive Surgery 11: 179–187

Rydevik B, Lundborg G, Bagge U 1981 Effects of graded compression on intraneural blood flow. Journal of Hand Surgery 6: 3–12

Schorn D, Hoskinson J, Dickson R A 1978 Bone density and the carpal tunnel syndrome. The Hand 10: 184–186

Schuler F, Adamson J 1978 Pacinian neuroma, an unusual cause of finger pain. Plastic and Reconstructive Surgery 62: 576–579

Spinner M, Spencer P S 1974 Nerve compression lesions of the upper extremity. Clinical Orthopaedics 104: 46–67

Stern P J, Kutz J E 1980 An unusual variant of the anterior interosseous nerve syndrome: A case report and review of the literature. Journal of Hand Surgery 5: 32–34

Sunderland S 1976 The nerve lesion in the carpal tunnel syndrome. Journal of Neurology, Neurosurgery and Psychiatry 39: 615–626

Symeonides P P, Paschaloglou C, Pagalides T 1975 Radial nerve enclosed in the callus of a supracondylar fracture. Journal of Bone and Joint Surgery 57B: 523–524

Zweig J, Burns H 1968 Compression of digital nerves by Pacinian corpuscles. Journal of Bone and Joint Surgery 50A: 999–1001

Inflammation

4

ACUTE INFLAMMATORY CONDITIONS

Infection

With the discovery of antibiotics infections of the hand, formerly crippling and even life-endangering, have become less significant. The classic work of Kanavel[1] published in 1912 still holds good with regard to diagnosis and conservative management. His formal incisions, designed to decompress extensive areas, have however been supplanted by more simple rules of drainage.

1. Do not wait for a fluctuant swelling in hand infections.
2. Pus is present, even when it cannot be seen, if
   (a) the patient complains of throbbing pain,
   (b) he has lost a night's sleep.
3. In the presence of pus, always incise over the point of maximum tenderness. If pus cannot be seen through the skin, the point of maximum tenderness should be sought by the gentlest pressure with a blunt probe.

Abscesses may develop at differing levels in the tissue:
subcuticular — lying immediately beneath the epidermis this is easily recognized, being a thinly covered pocket of pus under very little tension
intracutaneous — most common on the dorsum of the fingers in the form of a boil
subcutaneous
subfascial — beneath the palmar aponeurosis.

The deeper abscesses may, in the necrotic process of the overlying tissue known as 'pointing', communicate with more superficial layers. *Collar-stud abscesses* are so formed. The term indicates that two loci of pus communicate with one another through a narrow channel. In the case of subfascial abscesses, there may develop an abscess with three pockets, one beneath the fascia, one subcutaneous and one subcuticular. The implications surgically are quite clear — the more superficial abscess may be drained and the deeper not recognized, resulting in continued infection (Fig. 4.1).

Anatomical compartments
The palmar surface of the hand and the tissues around the

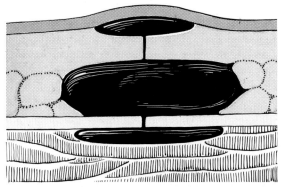

Fig. 4.1 *Collar-stud abscess.* In this, the accumulation of pus is at two or more sites between natural tissue layers (see text).

distal phalanx, are divided into compartments which serve to limit the spread of infection.

Nail fold. The eponychium, which is the fold of skin overlying the root of the nail, is defined distally by its free margin and proximally by the fascial attachment of the skin to the base of the distal phalanx just distal to the insertion of the extensor tendon. Laterally, the area is defined by the firm attachment of the margin of the nail to the lateral interosseous ligament of the distal phalanx[2].

The nail-fold is especially susceptible to injury, often in the course of manicuring or in the form of a 'hangnail'. Infection of such minor wounds is very common, probably because they are initially neglected and the area is subjected to repeated trauma. Infections of the nail-fold are called paronychia.

Apical spaces. The skin of the very tip of the finger is very firmly attached to the distal phalanx by numerous fibrous septa which divide the soft tissue immediately beneath the nail into a large number of virtually closed compartments.

Digital pulps. The middle and distal digital creases which overlie the joints are attached to the cruciate portions of the tendon sheath. This can be confirmed at surgery or more simply by observing the relative immobility of the creases to tangential movement when compared with the adjacent pulps. The pulps therefore become relatively confined compartments. Infection in these pulps remains localized, rarely extending into adjacent compartments. Indeed, soft tissue necrosis and phalangeal osteitis will develop sooner.

Tendon sheaths. The cruciate portion of the sheath is much more flimsy than the annular. In addition it is attached to skin with no intervening fat to absorb puncture wounds. Injuries to the digital creases are therefore more likely to result in tendon sheath infections.

In over 80% of hands the tendon sheath of the small finger communicates with the ulnar bursa. That of the thumb almost invariably is continuous with the radial bursa. Infection involving the sheaths of these digits may easily communicate with the wrist and lower forearm. They may also connect one with the other, creating the so-called 'horseshoe' abscess which involves the tendon sheaths of both thumb and small finger. The tendon sheaths of the other fingers may communicate with the ulnar bursa — 2.7 to 3.5% in different fingers, other than the small — but more commonly end proximally at the metacarpophalangeal joint, that is, beneath the palmar creases.

Distally the tendon sheaths end at the insertion of the flexor digitorum profundus, encroaching very little on the terminal pulp.

Web space. Less well-defined anatomically than the other compartments, the web space is nonetheless clearly circumscribed when infected. It is bounded by the margin of the web containing the natatory or superficial transverse palmar ligament distally, by the deep attachments of the palmar fascia proximally and by its attachment to the tendon sheaths laterally. The deep transverse metacarpal ligament forms the floor of the space which extends dorsally between the fingers around the distal edge of that ligament.

Deep palmar space. This lies deep to the palmar fascia. The rigid nature of the fascia allied to its resistance to penetration by pus results in considerable tension, and consequent pain, in the relatively rare infection of this space. Kanavel described 'thenar' and 'mid-palmar' spaces. While these can be defined anatomically, deep infection is not always confined to one or other.

The dorsum of the hand has no anatomical compartments of significance in containing sepsis. In the matter of infection it behaves like the skin elsewhere in the body. Thus, sepsis is most common in those areas which are hairbearing, one or more follicles becoming involved, a boil or carbuncle developing accordingly. The carbuncle of the dorsum of a finger is also known as a *whitlow* (Fig. 4.2).

Dorsal infections are of significance mainly when they develop over a joint. Unlike boils and carbuncles these infections usually follow recognized injuries, often puncture wounds, often inflicted by animal or human teeth. They carry the danger of *septic arthritis*.

In summary, localized hand infections can be classified as follows

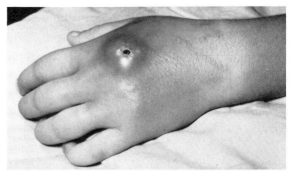

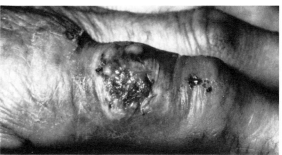

Fig. 4.2A & B Infection on the dorsum of the hand forms a *whitlow*. The pus-filled cavities are multilocular, and care must be taken to evacuate all pockets.

Palmar	Dorsal
Apical	*Paronychia*
Pulp (felon)	*Boil*
Web space	*Carbuncle (whitlow)*
Deep palmar space	
Tendon sheath	

Generalized infection occurs in the form of *cellulitis*.

History

Injury. With the notable exception of those with boils or carbuncles, the majority of patients will recall the injury which preceded the infection. In most cases it was trivial and received little or no treatment. Nonetheless, its position and type will indicate the exact diagnosis.

In certain less common infections, the surroundings and occupation in which the injury occurred are important, giving the clue to the nature of the infection, e.g.

injuries in contaminated water — *Mycobacterium marinum*

in an animal slaughterhouse — *Erysipelothrix rhusiopathiae, orf*

in dentists and nurses — *Herpes simplex*

in barbers — interdigital pilonidal sinus[3]

Time lapse since injury will often differ according to the infection

cellulitis	within 24 hours
tendon sheath	within 48 hours
web deep palmar	days
paronychia pulp	4–5 days
septic arthritis	up to 2 weeks after injury

Symptoms

Pain and loss of function are two of the five cardinal signs of inflammation and are always present in the patient with a hand infection. If pus is present within a confined compartment, the pain will be of a throbbing nature. Accurate localization of pain will already have been made by the patient. This should be determined by questioning. It will invariably correspond with the point of maximum tenderness. While function will be impaired wherever the infection is seated, the disability is greatest in tendon sheath infection, where no movements whatsoever of the involved digit can be tolerated.

Tenderness radiating up the arm even to the axilla is evidence of ascending lymphangitis. Usually associated with streptococcal infection, this is often present in cases of cellulitis and sometimes in tendon sheath infections and septic arthritis.

General malaise, often with associated *pyrexia*, as a general rule accompanies only those hand infections which show ascending lymphangitis. It is particularly marked in those with cellulitis.

Loss of sleep is an important symptom to seek, for it invariably indicates pus gathering in the tissues.

Coincident symptoms suggestive of predisposing or causative factors, should also be sought, e.g.

diabetes[4,5] — somewhat surprisingly, in Sneddon's series the incidence of hand infections in diabetics was identical with that in the population at large[6,7]

gonococcus — history of exposure, skin lesions, fever

Reiter's — urethritis, conjunctivitis.

Examination

The three other cardinal signs of inflammation are found on examination, the affected part being red, swollen and hot.

Paronychia (Fig. 4.3) presents as a typical lesion usually confined to one or other corner of the nail fold. Where it runs around to the other corner it is known as just that — a 'run-around'. Later a paronychia may pass beneath the nail around the cul-de-sac of the nail bed and pus will be evident beneath the nail.

A subungual haematoma may produce inflammation in the eponychium and therefore be mistaken for a paronychia in its early stages.

A *chronic paronychia*[8] is characterized by swollen, red, indurated eponychium with loss of the cuticle which

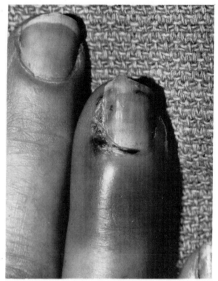

Fig. 4.3 *Paronychia,* with inflammation around the full extent of the eponychium.

normally adheres to the superficial surface of the nail. From the resultant open cul-de-sac small quantities of pus can be expressed. Such chronic paronychia are often encountered in those whose employment involves repeated and prolonged immersion in water.

Apical pulp infections show a very small area of acute tenderness immediately beneath the free margin of the nail. This may be overlooked and a mistaken diagnosis of a full blown, but as yet unlocalized, terminal pulp infection may be made and observation instituted. Later apical pulp infection tracks beneath the nail which may be completely detached by a pocket of pus (Fig. 4.4).

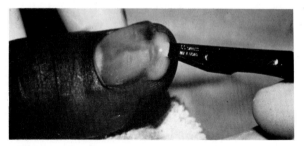

Fig. 4.4 *Apical abscess.* This is localized to the tip just beneath the nail, and, if advanced, dissects under the nail. Here the track can be seen passing all the way up to the lunula.

The *terminal pulp* of the normal digit is fluctuant. When infection develops in this closed compartment, fluctuation is lost initially and does not appear until sepsis has destroyed the fibrous septa which bind the skin to the periosteum of the terminal phalanx. If neglected until that

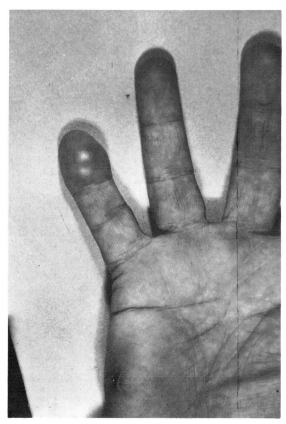

Fig. 4.5 A terminal pulp infection of the right small finger. It is important to note that while the inflammation is very marked in the terminal pulp, there is little evidence of involvement of the digit over the middle phalanx.

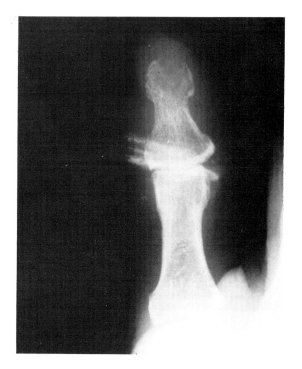

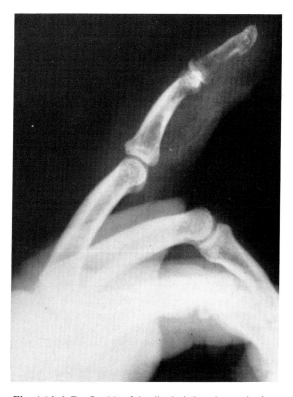

stage, terminal pulp infection (Fig. 4.5) is often associated with osteitis and destruction of the terminal phalanx (Fig. 4.6).

A crush injury of the finger tip with fracture of the distal phalanx may be mistaken for a pulp infection in its early stages.

Web space infections (Fig. 4.7), like those of the deep palm, are located primarily on the palmar surface but are most easily recognized from the dorsal aspect. Oedema is very evident on the dorsum and the infection understandably forces the adjacent fingers apart. This fixed separation is absolutely diagnostic of a web space infection.

Deep palmar space infections (Fig. 4.8) are characterized by severe pain, gross dorsal oedema, loss of normal palmar concavity, and fixed posture of the fingers. This results from oedema in the periarticular structures of the metacarpophalangeal joints and from the splinting which this partly voluntary posture provides to the extremely painful hand. Despite their fixed posture, the fingers can be moved at the interphalangeal joints without undue pain, distinguishing deep palmar from tendon sheath infections.

Fig. 4.6A & B Osteitis of the distal phalanx is seen in these two cases with destruction in (A) of the distal tuft, and in (B) of the juxta articular region. (The opacity across the interphalangeal joint in (A) is ingrained dirt in an old wound)

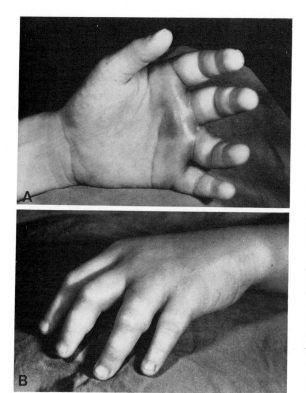

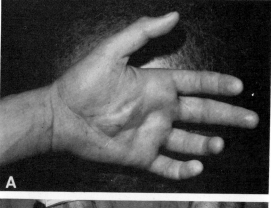

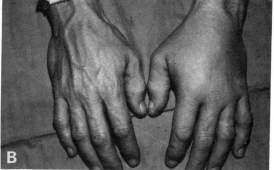

Fig. 4.7 (A) *Web space infection.*
(B) This diagnosis is emphasized by the unnatural separation of middle from ring fingers when viewed from the dorsum.

Fig. 4.8 (A) A deep palmar space infection producing fullness of the radial aspect of the palm with alteration of posture in the middle finger.
(B) The major part of the oedema in a deep palmar space infection is to be seen on the dorsum.

Tendon sheath infections (Fig. 4.9) invariably show the four classical signs as stated by Kanavel

1. the finger is held fixed in slight flexion, the hand being well guarded,
2. the finger is uniformly swollen and red,
3. there is intense pain on attempted extension,
4. tenderness is present along the line of the sheath.

The tenderness is very accurately localized, little being evident in the distal digital pulp while the metacarpophalangeal joint can be moved with little pain, albeit through a limited range.

In all of these palmar infections, the point of maximal tenderness should be carefully and gently sought with a blunt probe.

Dorsal infections are easily recognized by the presence of all the cardinal signs and by their location.

Septic arthritis should be suspected in the presence of a wound overlying the finger joints dorsally. If such a wound continues to discharge small quantities of sero-purulent fluid more than a week after the original injury then suspicion should approach certainty.

By far the most common cause of septic arthritis is a human 'bite' (p. 231). Septic arthritis can develop without such a wound or indeed any recent injury. In such a situation, the surgeon should be mindful of less common causes of septic arthritis, such as gonorrhea, and of the non-infective causes of acute arthritis, including gout and rheumatoid disease (see Chapter 5). The clinical features of septic arthritis are

swelling out of proportion to the inflammation present in the skin around the wound and, at later stages;

restricted motion in the joint; this is often surprisingly slow to develop but eventually both flexion and extension will produce pain;

instability will be evidenced latterly by increased laxity in the collateral ligaments; this motion may be accompanied by crepitus;

discharging sinuses will develop if drainage is not instituted;

radiological changes (Fig. 4.10), only the first of which is apparent in the initial two weeks, are, in sequence,
   — dorsal soft tissue swelling evident on lateral views
   — decalcification of the juxta articular bone
   —narrowing of the joint space
   — progressive fragmentation of the bone ends.

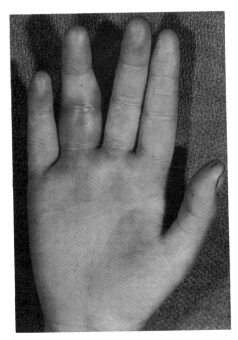

Fig. 4.9 *Tendon sheath infection.* The ring finger is uniformly swollen and red. Intense pain was present on any attempt to extend the finger.

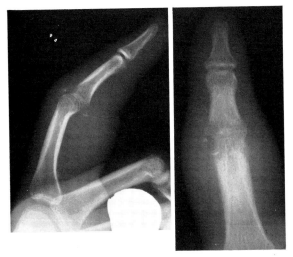

Fig. 4.10A & B The X-ray of this patient with septic arthritis of the proximal interphalangeal joint demonstrates extensive soft tissue swelling, decalcification of the bone adjacent to the joint, and narrowing of the joint space with early fragmentation of the bones.

It should be emphasized that instability, sinuses, X-ray changes and even severe pain on motion may not be present at the stage when the patient with septic arthritis can best be helped[9]. The surgeon therefore must have a high degree of awareness when disproportionate swelling accompanies a wound in the appropriate site and which continues to discharge long after injury. Culture of the effusion from the wound and also of the synovial fluid when the wound is explored is mandatory.

It is not always easy to distinguish septic arthritis from non-infective disorders, particularly if no wound is evident. The differential diagnosis includes osteoarthritis, gout and rheumatoid arthritis. These present a problem mainly when they are monoarticular since inspection of other joints in polyarthritic forms will reveal characteristic signs. X-ray, while not showing evidence of infective arthritis for more than two weeks after onset may identify any of the non-infective alternatives.

Cellulitis in the hand is dramatic in onset. The patient presents with a history of very acute onset of swelling, redness and pain following often a minor injury. He arrives within 12 to 24 hours of the start of infection.

Examination shows that the patient appears ill, pale and sweating often with a marked elevation of temperature. The most striking feature in the hand is the extensive puffy redness with streaks of lymphangitis often obvious in the forearm. The axillary nodes are enlarged on occasion, but are more often simply tender in the early stages. There may be a *haemorrhagic blister* present which can be removed without pain. If a wound is present it is usually unremarkable, exuding only a few drops of serous fluid. Culture of the serous fluid from either the blister or the wound usually yields haemolytic streptococcus.

Incision and drainage is never indicated in cellulitis and is indeed meddlesome.

Special problems

Blistering distal dactylitis, probably the forerunner of full-blown streptococcal cellulitis presents as a subcuticular blister over the terminal phalanx. Associated with very little local or generalized reaction, the blister contains whitish, watery pus which grows streptococcus on culture. Easily treated — for the blister can be trimmed away painlessly without anaesthesia (Fig. 4.11) — its significance lies in the need for a full course of penicillin therapy to ensure that no cellulitis, or worse, rheumatic fever or acute glomerulonephritis follows this otherwise minor disorder.

Herpetic whitlow[10-12] (Fig. 4.12), despite its name, occurs mainly on the digital pulp. Commencing with pain, redness and swelling, it may be mistaken for a distal pulp infection in its initial stages. After 24–36 hours, the characteristic vesicles appear, clear at first, quickly becoming opaque and apparently purulent. Culture is sterile but the causative virus can be demonstrated within six hours if there is cause for doubt. The importance is to recognise the nature of the

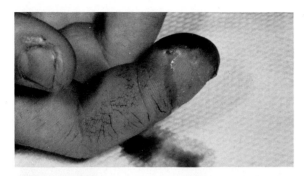

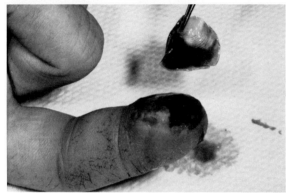

Fig. 4.11A & B *Blistering distal dactylitis.* This streptococcal infection is subcuticular and can be evacuated without anesthesia simply by trimming away the skin.

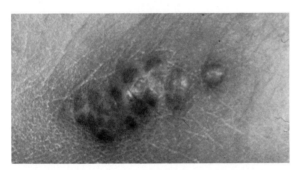

Fig. 4.12 *Herpetic whitlow.* The characteristic vesicles are pathognomonic of herpes simplex.

condition, for incision and drainage is contraindicated. With observation the lesion will regress spontaneously.

Gonorrhea[13-15] may cause a septic arthritis or acute tendon sheath infection. In a more chronic form it may involve the synovium around the extensors on the wrist, resembling rheumatoid disease. In either event, the importance to the hand surgeon is to remember the possibility and to seek evidence in the form of cultures from either the pus released by incision, which may however fail to reveal the gonococcus, or from skin lesions, prostatic smears, vaginal or rectal swabs. Gonococcal complement fixation tests should provide confirmation, although these may be weakly

positive in rheumatoid patients also and obviously care must be taken to make firm the diagnosis before discussing the matter with the patient.

Cat scratch disease[16,17] should be considered when the patient, usually a child, develops papules or vesicles at the site of a cat scratch or bite which are in themselves unimpressive but are associated with significant epitrochlear and axillary lymphadenitis and often with high fever.

Human[18-22] *and animal bites,* because of the organisms encountered in the oral cavity, are serious injuries which require vigorous treatment. The majority of human 'bites' are not in fact bites but are rather tooth wounds sustained while punching the 'biter' in the mouth! For this reason patients may be late in seeking treatment and may lie about how the injury was sustained. It should always be assumed that a wound over the knuckle communicates with the joint space and it should be explored with that in mind. The wound should be excised at each level, remembering that the posture at exploration is entirely different from that at the time of the blow. For this reason the successive wounds in skin, extensor apparatus, joint capsule and metacarpal head do not correspond, indeed are far removed one from the other (Fig. 4.13). The injury to the metacarpal head will not be seen on X-ray for it is a *chondral 'divot' fracture.* In the author's experience such a chondral injury is found in the large majority of human fist bites (Fig. 4.14). With early adequate excision and a period of wound irrigation bite injuries do not live up to their evil reputation[23].

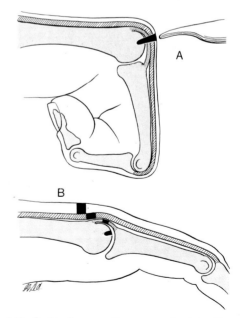

Fig. 4.13 In this diagrammatic representation it can be seen (A) that the tooth pierces the clenched fist of the attacker penetrating skin, tendon, joint capsule, and the metacarpal head. (B) When the finger is extended by swelling and at surgery, the four puncture wounds do not correspond.

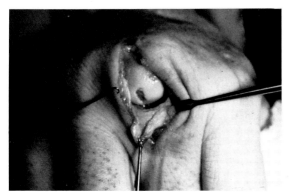

Fig. 4.14   A cartilaginous 'divot' fracture resulting from a human bite.

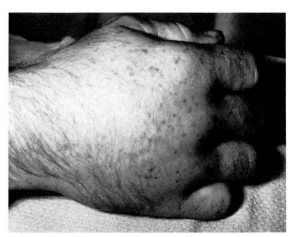

While the organisms may vary, and routine cultures should always be supplemented by anaerobic[24] and 10% carbon dioxide[25] preparations, the most likely growth in human bites is *Eikenella corrodens*[26] and in animal bites *Pasteurella multocida*[27-30]. By happy coincidence, both are sensitive to crystalline penicillin, which should therefore be given in appropriate doses[31].

Drug addiction has become an increasing source of infection and for similar reasons of guilt to those above, enhanced by the effects of drug abuse, the patient presents late and gives an inaccurate history[32]. Dorsal abscesses are most common, but septic arthritis may be the presenting disorder, cases due to *Serratia* and *Pseudomonas* having been reported[34]. It is very unlikely that the infection will follow the first use of intravenous or 'main-line' drugs by the patient and therefore extensive soft tissue changes will be present in the limb due to previous insults. The typical hand of the established addict shows extensive indurated puffy oedema, chronic tenosynovitis or inflexible ankylosis of the small joints.

Persistent infection
Apart from unusual organisms, there are several factors which cause infection to persist despite treatment.

Inadequate drainage is by far the most common and is most likely to occur

1. when incision has been performed too early, that is, before throbbing and sleep loss indicated pus accumulation,
2. when the incision has not been made over the point of maximum tenderness,
3. when all pockets have not been drained — this is especially common when a collar-stud abscess has developed,
4. where the drainage incision has been allowed to heal too soon, leaving a cavity. This is prevented by copious, repeated irrigation through an indwelling catheter introduced through adjacent healthy skin[35,36] (Fig. 4.15).

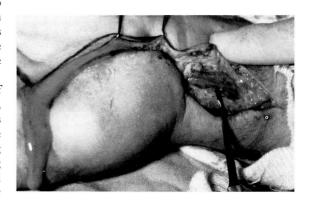

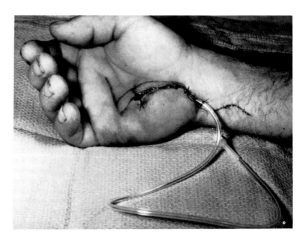

Fig. 4.15   (A) This patient presented with the characteristic features of pus in the hand, and the dorsal swelling was marked. (B) The point of maximal tenderness was over the Guyon's canal, and for this reason exploration was commenced by proximal exposure of the ulnar nerve and artery. Pus was released from the region of the canal, and (C) an irrigating catheter was inserted to wash out the cavity at regular intervals during the subsequent three days.

Presence of a foreign body, sequestrum of bone or slough
Ischaemia of the limb

Continued trauma to the part — this may be iatrogenic, unintentional or factitious

Generalized systemic disorders sufficiently severe to prevent wound healing should be immediately apparent. However, a full physical examination with special laboratory studies should be undertaken in all persistent infections where no cause is located.

Uncommon organisms[37] have been recorded as causing hand infections:

Mycobacterium[38] *(fortuitum,*[39] *kansasii,*[40-43] *marinum,*[44] and others) have been reported in recent years involving tendon sheaths, bursae, joints, fascia and bone in that order of frequency. The more chronic forms may be mistaken for gout or rheumatoid disease. Difficult to culture — *marinum* for example, grows at 30°–32°C — the diagnosis may be suspected if the tuberculin skin tests are strongly positive.

Histoplasmosis[45]
Coccidioidomycosis[46,47] both of the tendon sheath.
These are merely examples of a much wider range of uncommon flora which may complicate the management of a hand infection. In all instances of infection resistant to treatment the active guidance and participation of the bacteriologist should be sought in establishing the diagnosis.

Other uncommon 'organisms' reported in hand infections
    Bacteria
    Aeromonas hydrophila[48,49]
    Bacteroides fragilis (arthritis)[50]
    Clostridium welchii (arthritis)[51]
    — Gas gangrene[52]
    — Non-clostridial gas gangrene[53,54]
    Haemophilus influenzae (cellulitis)[55]
    Mycobacterium tuberculosis[56-59]
    Serratia perfringens (arthritis)[60]
    Fungi
    Actinomycosis[61-63]
    Aspergillosis[64]
    Chromohyphomycosis[65]
    Maduromycosis[66]
    Mucormycosis[67]
    Nocardia[68-70]
    Sporotrichosis[71]
    Alga — prototheca[72,73]
    Larva[74]
    Parasite — onchocerciasis[75]

Non-infective causes of acute inflammation

Calcific deposits[76] are well known to produce acute inflammation in regions other than the hand but that they may do so in the hand is less well recognized. The patient presents with a complaint of pain and consequently reduced function. Examination reveals a tense, red, shiny, warm area which is acutely tender. The location of the calcium deposits varies but it often presents as an acute calcific tendinitis. Unless aware of the possibility, the surgeon may resort to incision to no avail.

X-rays so taken as to throw the inflamed area into relief may show calcium deposits as flecks of radio-opaque material in the soft tissues. Rest and support are indicated.

Acute gout may show all the symptoms and signs of septic arthritis. Suspicion should be aroused by the great severity of the pain which is unrelieved by immobilization. A positive history of gout, evidence of chronic disease in other joints or an elevated serum uric acid will confirm the diagnosis in the majority of cases. In the remainder, however, diagnosis is possible only by the detection of birefringent needle-like crystals of monosodium urate monohydrate in the joint fluid or synovium, usually within polymorphonuclear leucocytes.

CHRONIC INFLAMMATORY DISORDERS

The patient with any of the chronic inflammatory disorders presents with a complaint of pain, made worse by use and always relieved by total rest of the afflicted part. The pain may not be present at all times, showing flares of activity, often initiated by unremembered minor trauma. Depending upon the patient's occupation and on the severity or frequency of the attacks of pain, the disorder may be simply a nuisance or may force the patient to forsake his employment increasingly, often resulting in his being labelled a malingerer or in the loss of his job. Chronic inflammation, therefore, constitutes a major cause of loss of work time and may result eventually in social dependency. While specific causes may be identified, such as gout, rheumatoid disease or any of the rheumatoid variants (Chapter 5) the majority of cases come about as the result of trauma. The injury may be clearly remembered and may have been adequately treated. More commonly, the afflicted part has been repeatedly subjected to forgotten minor stresses to which it has not proved equal.

The structures affected by these 'chronic inflammatory disorders' are most commonly the joints and the musculo-tendinous units.

Joints – osteoarthritis

Any joint in the hand may be affected by chronic inflammation. Some may proceed to full-blown osteoarthritis, but the majority do not. Those joints which do would appear to be subjected to unavoidable daily stress, while the others are either very well supported or it is possible for the patient to protect them during use.

Joints which are chronically inflamed cause *pain on stress*. Characteristically, the patient states that he has no problems in the morning on rising, in contrast to the rheumatoid patient, but as the day progresses his discomfort increases. In the evening the affected joint is the seat of a dull ache, which may interfere with sleep.

Examination of such patients should be directed at locating the point of maximal tenderness and detecting any laxity in supporting ligamentous structures. Pain or crepitus on grinding movements of the joint, early evidence of ensuing osteoarthritis, should also be sought.

Laboratory studies should be performed on all such patients to exclude rheumatoid disease or variants (see Chapter 5). X-rays will show any early osteoarthritic changes. Stress films should be taken to detect any ligamentous instability.

Even in patients who have no clear evidence of frank osteoarthritis, surgery is indicated where marked laxity of ligaments is present or where pain is preventing work, is clearly localized to one joint and has not responded to conservative therapy. A common example of such chronic inflammation due to instability which later progresses to established osteoarthritis is found in the basal joint of the thumb. Where the joint surface is still good but a ligament is incompetent it can frequently be replaced by tendon graft or transfer. Where the surface is irretrievably damaged, the choice lies between arthrodesis and arthroplasty.

It is estimated that 40% of the adult population are afflicted by osteoarthritis in one form or another, but that of these only 10% seek medical advice and only 1% are severely disabled.

It is probable that multiple genetic factors predispose certain patients to the development of osteoarthritis, factors which influence the structure and maintenance of articular cartilage. However, the development of osteoarthritis is mainly due to ageing, major injuries and the microtrauma of daily stress.

The primary disorder in osteoarthritis is loss of articular surface, which is seen on X-ray as narrowing of the joint space. Increasingly the bare bones denuded of cartilage make contact with one another. This causes pain, the bone becomes more dense or eburnated and this is shown by sclerosis on X-ray. Cystic erosions occur in the bone ends and bone spurs, osteophytes or exostoses build up around the bony margins of the joint. The synovium in such joints is subject to inflammatory proliferation. When fully advanced, the osteoarthritic joint is disturbed by the most minor trauma and suffers repeated bouts of acute inflammation. While osteoarthritis may develop in any of the joints in the hand, those most commonly affected and which most come to surgical treatment are certain carpal articulations and the distal interphalangeal joints.

TRAPEZIUM

Problems with the basal joints of the thumb are common to a degree not always appreciated and they commence before any of the characteristic features of osteoarthritis are present.

The key structures in the trapeziometacarpal joint are the palmar or ulnar ligament which holds the beak of the thumb metacarpal down to the ridge on the trapezium and the dorsal intermetacarpal ligament which holds the first to the second metacarpal[77]. The alternative names for the first ligament emphasize the differing relationships of the ligament to the planes of the thumb and the hand, respectively. The ligament is on the palmar aspect of the thumb, that is directly opposite the thumb nail, but because the plane of the relaxed thumb lies at right angles to that of the hand, the ligament is ulnar when the plane of the hand is taken as reference. In normal flexion and extension of the thumb, the joint and the two ligaments are little stressed. In opposition and power pinch however, the joint surfaces twist one on the other, threatening to come apart, only the ligaments preventing them[78]. In this position, stresses are unequally distributed over the joint surfaces. With time wear results. If, in addition, injury damages the joint surface making it incongruous or, worse still, disrupts the ligaments, arthrosis — as the initial stage of the disorder is called — and osteoarthritis become inevitable.

Use of the thumb is unavoidable in the human hand and therefore arthrosis and osteoarthritis of the trapezio-metacarpal joint develop relatively early in life, usually in the fifth decade. Disease in this joint is much more common in the female than in the male patient. It may follow recognized trauma, develop as a consequence of rheumatoid arthritis, or, in most instances, arise for no apparent reason. To quote Eaton and Littler, 'whatever the underlying cause, once hypermobility is present a painful synovitis is common and the possibility of accelerated articular attrition is increased'[79].

Symptoms
Pain with use is the patient's one complaint in the early stages. The pain is localized to the base of the thumb, the patient usually pointing to the radial aspect of the thenar eminence just anterior and distal to the anatomical snuff box. Later marked instability with resultant weakness of pinch grip further reduces the patient's capacity to use the affected hand.

Examination
Tenderness is well localised with thumb or fingertip pressure applied exactly over the joint on its anterior aspect. The joint is located at the proximal margin of the thenar eminence 1 to 2 cm radial and slightly distal to the scaphoid tubercle (p. 10).

The *torque test* serves further to distinguish basal joint arthrosis from other disorders. Axial rotation is applied to the thumb with the basal joint alternately distracted and compressed and the metacarpophalangeal joint gently flexed. Pain on this manoeuvre is pathognomonic. Later, instability of the joint is evidenced by the prominence of the metacarpal base when compared with a normal thumb. It can be confirmed by applying intermittent pressure to the base while asking the patient to pinch strongly. Considerable motion and often crepitus will be detected. Finally stress applied to the dorsal intermetacarpal ligament will sometimes reveal marked laxity and will always be painful. This is achieved by fixing the first metacarpal with a thumb on the radial side of its head and then applying radially directed force to the ulnar border of the shaft with the middle finger of the same hand (Fig. 4.16).

Collapse of the thumb may eventually occur with adduction of the first metacarpal and hyperextension of the metacarpophalangeal joint. This produces a 'swan-neck' deformity, similar to a rheumatoid Nalebuff Type III thumb (p. 268) (Fig. 4.17).

Pinch strength will progressively decrease and should be recorded with a dynamometer.

X-ray

While the basal joint can be seen on standard anteroposterior views, it and the other articulations of the trapezium are best studied on a Robert view (p. 48). Radiological changes have been divided into four stages:

Stage I — widening of the joint space, (evidence of effusion); less than one-third subluxation in any projection.

Stage II — more than one-third subluxation demonstrated especially on stress films; small bone or calcific deposits 2 mm in diameter are to be seen (Fig. 4.18).

Stage III — larger fragments present; joint space narrowing evident (Fig. 4.19).

Stage IV — advanced changes: major subluxation, cystic and sclerotic bone changes, lipping and osteophyte formation (Fig. 4.20).

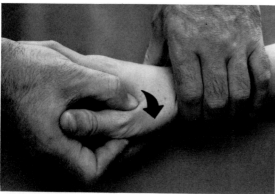

Fig. 4.16 The basal joint of the thumb is stressed by blocking the metacarpal head and applying pressure to the shaft.

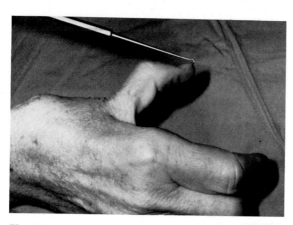

Fig. 4.17 A hyperextension deformity of the metacarpophalangeal joint is demonstrated. The subluxation of the basal joint can be seen to the left of the first metacarpal.

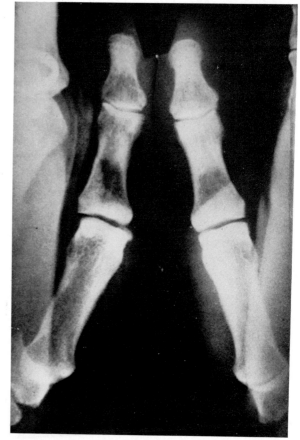

Fig. 4.18 Employing the Eaton stress view in which the two thumbs are driven firmly against one another, subluxation of the basal joint on the left can be seen (Stage II).

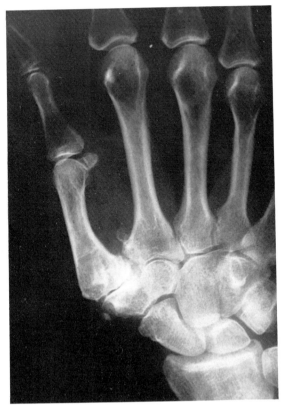

Fig. 4.19 Stage III Carpometacarpal arthritis (see text).

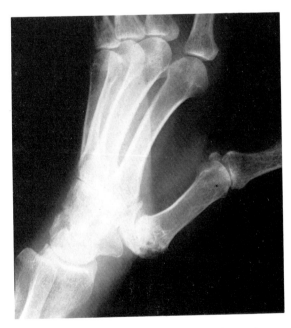

Fig. 4.20 Stage IV Carpometacarpal arthritis (see text).

Involvement of other trapezial joints
While description has thus far been confined to trapeziometacarpal joint, Swanson has pointed out that osteoarthritis is confined to that joint in only a minority of cases[80]. In his series, the other articulations of the trapezium were involved as follows

with the second metacarpal	86.2%
with the scaphoid	48.3%
with the trapezoid	34.6%

Such involvement cannot be diagnosed clinically but can be seen clearly on X-ray. Careful study is therefore necessary if the correct treatment is to be prescribed to relieve the patient's symptoms (Fig. 4.21).

Infrequently patients will be seen in whom changes are entirely limited to a trapezial articulation other than that with the first metacarpal, most commonly that with the scaphoid (Fig. 4.22).

Indications
At any point in the deterioration of the joint, relief can be provided by fitting the patient with a hand-based, or better forearm-based, thumb support splint. Most patients eventually come to surgery.

In the early stages, before any evidence of loss of articular cartilage is present, discomfort can be eliminated and further deterioration prevented or at least postponed by stabilizing the joint. The most used procedure has been that of Eaton and Littler[79] in which half of the flexor carpi radialis, left attached distally, is passed through the base of the metacarpal to replace the attenuated ulnar collateral ligament (Fig. 4.23). Recently, the author has been strengthening the attenuated dorsal intermetacarpal ligament with a strip of extensor carpi radialis longus — a simpler and so far effective procedure.

In late stages with established osteoarthritis the choice lies, as in other joints so afflicted, between arthrodesis[81,82] and arthroplasty. If arthritis clearly involves other trapezial joints, arthrodesis of the trapeziometacarpal joint will give only limited, if any, relief of symptoms, as will any interpositional arthroplasty of that joint alone[83]. Excision of the trapezium becomes necessary and good results have been reported from that alone[84,85]. However, others found that simple excision relieved pain but gave an unstable and therefore weak thumb. Replacement of the excised trapezium by rolled tendon[86] or fascia[87] or with a silastic prosthesis[88-92] is therefore increasingly practised. Whatever excisional procedure is selected, it is important to correct any Z hyperextension deformity of the metacarpophalangeal joint by simultaneous tenodesis, capsulodesis or arthrodesis. Otherwise, subluxation will occur at the basal joint with recurrence of pain and weakness (Fig. 4.24).

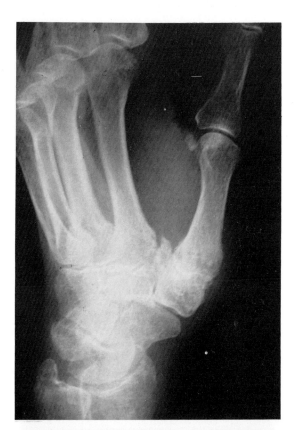

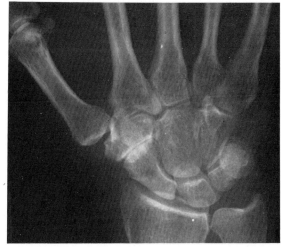

Fig. 4.21 These patients have been treated (A) by fusion and (B) interpositional arthroplasty of the basal joint. Their pain persists because of evident osteoarthritis between the trapezium and the first metacarpal, the trapezoid, and the scaphoid.

Fig. 4.22 *Scaphotrapezial arthritis.* This patient presented with symptoms similar to those of trapeziometacarpal disease. X-ray, however, revealed that the arthritis existed only between the scaphoid and trapezium. Intercarpal fusion cured her symptoms.

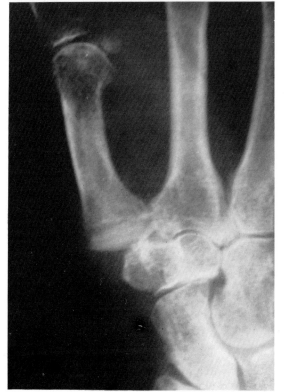

Fig. 4.23 This patient has undergone an Eaton-Littler reconstruction shown on the left for the stage two subluxation shown on the right.

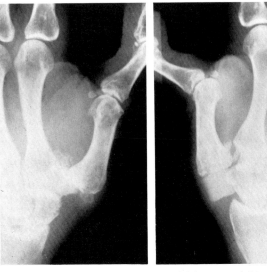

Fig. 4.24 This patient had bilateral basal joint osteoarthritis with severe hyperextension of the metacarpophalangeal joints. The significance of correcting the latter deformity was not appreciated when the trapezial implant was placed in the right. The resulting deformity was worse than the original problem, and pain and weakness persisted.

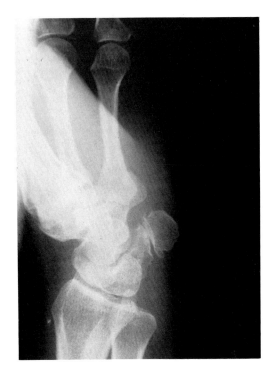

Fig. 4.25 Piso-triquetral osteoarthritis (see text).

OTHER CARPAL JOINTS

Osteoarthritis of other carpal and carpometacarpal articulations is much less frequent[93]. It is characterised by similar symptoms of pain and weakness, diagnosed by the same findings of localized tenderness and radiological findings. In most instances, such as the isolated scaphotrapezial disease mentioned above, they are treated by appropriate intercarpal fusion or interpositional arthroplasty[94,95].

Piso-triquetral arthritis[96] causes wrist pain which may be largely referred to the dorsum of the hand. The earlier stages, arthrosis and chondromalacia of the joint, may result from the use of a racquet[97] or club or, rarely, following carpal tunnel release. The diagnosis is made by *tenderness* produced by stressing the joint. This can be done in two ways

i.   direct radial pressure over the ulnar aspect of the pisiform
ii. resisted combined flexion and ulnar deviation of the wrist.

X-Ray of the joint is taken with the hand supinated 30°–40° from true lateral (Fig. 4.25). Mild problems can be alleviated by injection with local anaesthetic and soluble steroid; more severe are cured by excision of the pisiform.

ASEPTIC NECROSIS

This disorder afflicts any bone which loses its blood supply, but suffers no superadded infection, as its name implies. The bone collapses and its presence, and that of the osteoarthritis which ensues in surrounding joints, causes pain. In the carpus, it is seen in the following

Scaphoid fracture (p. 127) — invariably of the proximal pole

Kienbock's disease[98,99] (lunatomalacia) This probably results from microfractures of the lunate interfering with its blood supply[100,101] and is more common when the ulna is short relative to the radius — *ulnar minus variant*[102]. The stages have been classified as follows:

I.   acute, with no changes on X-ray apart from a possible linear or compression fracture; radionuclide scanning usually shows increased uptake,

II. definite increase in density with no change in shape apart from some loss of height on the radial side of the lunate,

III. collapse and sclerosis of the entire lunate with disruption of the carpal architecture (Fig. 4.26)

IV. generalised degenerative arthritis of carpus due to Stage III.

Early cases have been effectively treated by correcting the variant, either by lengthening the ulna or shortening the radius[103,104]. Established collapse, with or without associated arthritis confined to the lunate articulations is treated by excision and silastic replacement[105,106].

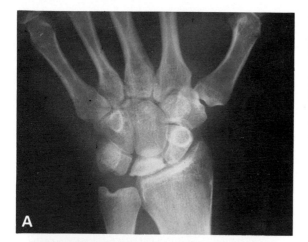

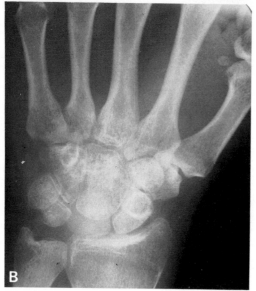

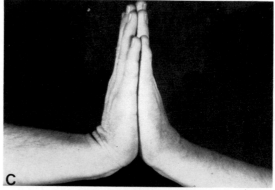

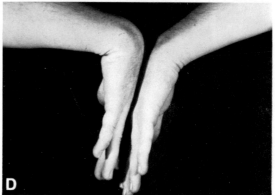

Fig. 4.26 (A) This patient presented with aseptic necrosis of the lunate (Kienbock's disease) which was producing associated osteoarthritis of the radiocarpal joint. He complained of severe pain on vigorous exercise and an aching discomfort at other times.

(B) He was treated with silastic replacement of the lunate and achieved a painfree though somewhat reduced range of motion in the wrist some three months later, C and D. He returned to heavy construction work despite some misgivings on the part of his surgeon.

Preiser's disease[107] — a much more rare but identical disorder of the scaphoid.

(Non-German scholars can remember the correct pronunciation of these eponyms by the phrase 'A keen price').

Avascular necrosis has also been reported in the pisiform[108].

ISOLATED CARPAL CYSTS

Occasionally a patient may be seen complaining of poorly localized wrist pain in whom the only positive finding is a cyst in a carpal bone (Fig. 4.27). In a characteristically thorough review[109], Eiken has determined that such bone cysts are the cause of pain only if they have *sclerotic margins* or they *communicate with the joint space*. Such cysts are most common in the scaphoid and lunate and are treated by curettage and bone grafting, providing the joint surfaces are otherwise in good condition.

THE DISTAL INTERPHALANGEAL JOINT

The patient with distal interphalangeal joint disease may present during the initial phases but more commonly has full-blown osteoarthritis when she consults the surgeon.

The symptoms are those of pain on use, worsening as the day progresses, and instability of the joint.

Examination in the fully developed case is conclusive. The development of *exostoses* is especially florid around the distal interphalangeal joint and these are immediately apparent, giving a knobbly appearance to the joint. Heberden (1710-1801)[110] first described these osteophytes 'Little hard knobs, the size of a small pea, frequently seen upon the fingers, particularly a little below the top, near the joint' and they are named for him — *Heberden's nodes* (Fig. 4.28). (In the much less frequent osteoarthritis of the proximal interphalangeal joint, the osteophytes are known as *Bouchard's nodes*)[111].

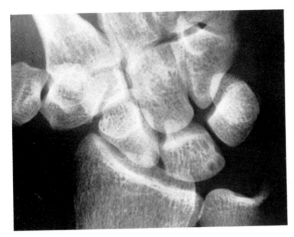

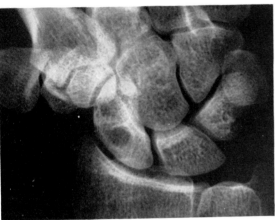

Fig. 4.27 *Isolated carpal cysts.* (A) in the lunate, and (B) in the scaphoid (see text).

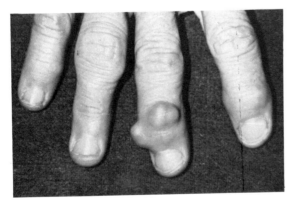

Fig. 4.28 *Heberden's nodes.* Osteoarthritis of the distal interphalangeal joint with gross osteophyte formation.

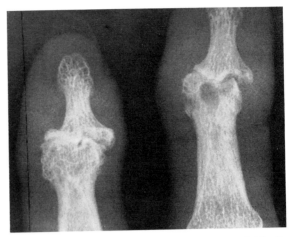

Fig. 4.29 Characteristic X-ray appearance in osteoarthritis of the distal interphalangeal joints, with loss of joint space, formation of exostoses and associated soft tissue swelling.

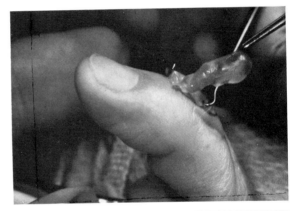

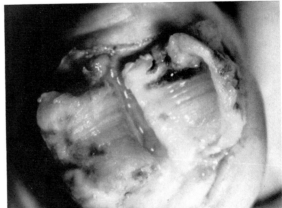

Fig. 4.30 (A) A ganglion of the distal interphalangeal joint which had developed in association with osteoarthritis, this presented as a 'mucous cyst' with grooving of the nail. Care is taken at surgery to trace the ganglion down to its origin in the joint.

(B) This joint shows marked osteoarthritic grooving in association with a ganglion cyst of the distal interphalangeal joint.

Exostoses develop at an early phase in the distal interphalangeal joints and some articular cartilage may still remain despite their presence. Its loss should be confirmed by attempting to elicit crepitus, moving the joint while applying longitudinal compression. The joint often shows additional deformity, with lateral instability or the development of a mallet finger deformity due to erosion of the extensor tendon. The stability of the joint should be checked by stressing the joint laterally using three point leverage.

X-ray examination confirms the diagnosis (Fig. 4.29).

Ganglion — the 'so-called' mucous cyst[112]. Until recently the pathogenesis of these lesions was disputed. However, it is now evident that the 'mucous cyst' is always a ganglion arising from the distal interphalangeal joint, usually in association with osteoarthritis of that joint (Fig. 4.30). Small ganglions may be mistaken for osteophytes.

Indications

By the time most patients present for help with interphalangeal osteoarthritis, surgery is necessary to give relief. Most surgeons recommend arthrodesis and this is certainly the only treatment in the presence of gross instability or significant bone destruction (Fig. 4.29). In cases where the joint is stable and the bone ends of good contour, however, some have adopted a more conservative approach, performing osteophytectomy and synovectomy, with an acceptable pain-free range of motion resulting[113]. When a ganglion cyst is the reason for surgery, great care must be taken to track the neck of the cyst back to the joint and to perform an adequate synovectomy. Only thus can recurrence be minimized.

Chronic gout

Gout is a disorder primarily of middle-aged and older men and of postmenopausal women. There is often a family history of affliction. It develops as a result of prolonged periods of hyperuricaemia. Uric acid is only sparingly soluble in tissue fluids and is therefore precipitated as monosodium urate monohydrate crystals.

Acute gouty arthritis occurs when these crystals form in the synovial fluid. As the disease progresses, gross deposits of sodium urate, known as *tophi*, appear in the joints, in the periarticular tissues, in the kidneys and in ectopic deposits beneath the skin. One classical site for such ectopic trophi is around the helical margin of the ear.

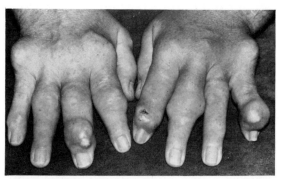

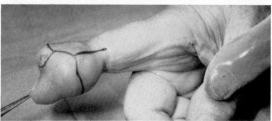

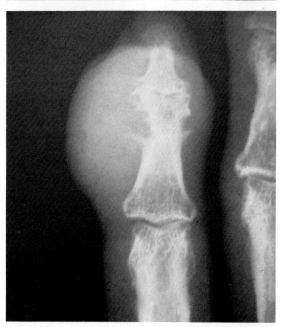

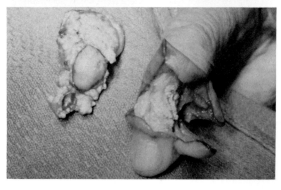

Fig. 4.31 (A) Extensive gouty deposits involving many of the joints in the hand.

(B) In another patient the circumferential nature of the gouty deposit can be seen. (C) The uric acid is entirely radiolucent. (D) Excision involved dissection around the circumference of the joint. Not all material could be removed, and arthrodesis was necessary.

While early acute monarticular gout may be difficult to distinguish from septic arthritis (p. 229), the established case has no mimics. The history is one of an onset of monoarticular arthritis usually in the lower extremity, followed by increasingly severe and frequent attacks of joint pain affecting more and more regions. In the upper limb these include the elbow, wrist and fingers. Although at first appearing to return to normal after each attack, the swelling and disability persist for longer periods, eventually becoming permanent.

Examination of the upper limbs of the patient with chronic gout reveals tophi, earliest around the olecranon and on the extensor surface of the forearms and later as tumour-like swellings around the joint (Fig. 4.31). These may cause ulceration of the skin and discharge white material with the consistency of wet cement. Tophaceous deposits may also form in the tendon sheaths.

Considerable limitation of motion results and this, or ulceration, may be an indication for surgical intervention, as much of the sodium urate being removed as possible[114]. This is a messy operation, which provokes some anxiety when performed on the interphalangeal joints, for the white material is often all around the finger encasing and camouflaging all structures, including both neurovascular bundles. Arthrodesis is often necessary to stabilize the joint.

Radiological changes are typical, the bone ends adjacent to the joints showing translucent defects which are deposits of sodium urate, with the later development of an appearance similar to osteoarthritis.

The serum uric acid is consistently elevated in most patients, but not in all.

Musculotendinous units

Considering the significant distances travelled daily around pulleys and through tunnels by the tendons of the upper limb, *chronic tendinitis* is surprisingly uncommon.

The shoulder will not be considered since it is more the province of the orthopaedic than of the hand surgeon. Musculotendinous units become painful primarily at two sites — when they pass through tight tunnels and are therefore lubricated by synovium and where they attach to bone. There are four sites which frequently give trouble: abductor pollicis longus — de Quervain's disease; flexor tenosynovitis — trigger finger; flexor carpi radialis tendinitis and tennis elbow; and three others which rarely do: the tendon sheaths of the radial wrist extensors[115,116], the extensor pollicis longus[117] and the extensor digiti minimi[118].

STENOSING TENOVAGINITIS AT THE RADIAL STYLOID — DE QUERVAIN'S DISEASE[119]

The abductor pollicis longus and extensor pollicis brevis pass through the first dorsal compartment beneath the extensor retinaculum. The first compartment is more radial than dorsal in position and can be located on the examiner's own hand by tracing the two tendons back on to the radius from their prominent position as the anterior boundary of the anatomical snuff box. Each compartment is lined by synovium and that in the first compartment is particularly prone to become inflamed.

Symptoms

Acute pain on any movement of the thumb is the primary symptom. The pain is located over the tunnel but often radiates into the forearm. Weakness of any hand function involving the wrist or thumb accompanies the pain.

Examination

Tenderness over the first dorsal compartment in the acute phase is well localized. In less severe cases it may be difficult to distinguish de Quervain's from arthrosis of the basal joint of the thumb and from flexor carpi radialis tendinitis.

The *Finkelstein test*[120] (Fig. 4.32) is performed by asking the patient to grasp the thumb firmly in the palm of his hand. The examiner then abruptly deviates the hand in an

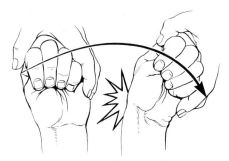

Fig. 4.32 *The Finkelstein test.* The patient's thumb is enclosed in the palm. The wrist is then abruptly deviated ulnarwards by the examiner. In a positive test pain is produced on the radial border of the wrist.

ulnar direction. This places maximum stress on the involved tendons and produces severe pain in de Quervain's disease. The test should be interpreted with some caution. The examiner can confirm on his own hand that the Finkelstein manoeuvre is not comfortable and therefore anxious patients may over-react to normal discomfort. Comparison with the opposite limb should aid in confirming a positive test. The Finkelstein test may also be positive in basal joint arthrosis. This can be differentiated from de Quervain's disease by precise localisation of tenderness and by X-ray (p. 235). Inflammation in the radial aspect of the wrist proper may also produce a falsely positive test but will produce identical pain if the test is repeated with the thumb *excluded* during ulnar deviation.

Abductor pollicis longus bursitis[121] may mimic de Quervain's disease. It presents as a tender swelling localized to the region where the abductor pollicis longus crosses the radial wrist extensors on the radiodorsal aspect of the wrist. Distinct *crepitance* can be felt in the swelling. The Finkelstein test produces pain, referred to the area of the bursitis. Injection and splintage cures most, but some require exploration.

Indications

If injection with steroids and splintage fail to give permanent relief in de Quervain's then surgical release of the first compartment should be performed. Abductor pollicis longus commonly has multiple tendons. On occasion, one or more of them or the tendon of extensor pollicis brevis may have a separate compartment. Failure to release this may result in a persistence of symptoms. While technique is outwith the scope of this text, a cautionary word on the radial nerve in de Quervain's release is always appropriate. Division of the radial nerve in the process of this procedure is probably the most common error of commission in hand surgery and is certainly the iatrogenic disorder most frequently seen by the hand surgeon. Radial nerve neuroma at the wrist can be a most crippling disorder and one very difficult to treat. The lesson, of course, is to carefully identify all branches of the nerve — and there may be several — and preserve them during this otherwise simple procedure.

FLEXOR TENOSYNOVITIS

Synovitis of the flexor tendons occurs most frequently in rheumatoid patients or those suffering from variants of that disease. It may also occur in other patients for no clear reason, although a higher incidence is recognized in the diabetic patient. The patient does not present with symptoms of chronic synovitis but rather with the consequence — *trigger finger*.

The triggering comes about by the formation of a nodule on the tendon which passes through the proximal pulley of the tendon sheath in a proximal direction with some discomfort (Fig. 4.33). When the extensors, weak relative to the finger flexors, attempt to straighten the digit the

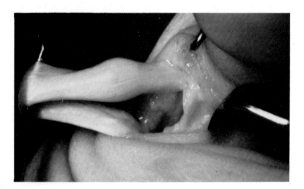

Fig. 4.33 A nodule on the flexor tendon producing trigger finger.

nodule jams in the pulley, arresting motion of that finger. It may release suddenly as further extensor force is applied — hence the name.

Trigger thumb also occurs, but a large minority are congenital in origin[122] (p. 328). When so, trigger thumb must be distinguished from congenital shortness of flexor pollicis longus.

Symptoms

Locking in flexion is the major complaint. Initially present merely as a 'slow finger', in time this comes to the stage where it is necessary to release the locked finger with an adjacent digit or even with the opposite hand. In either event release is painful and may in time prove impossible. The patient then presents with one finger acutely flexed into the palm. Alternatively, the patient becomes understandably more reluctant to bend the digit and may not have done so for some considerable time prior to consultation.

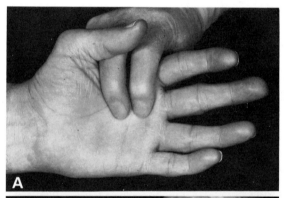
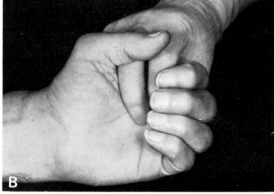

Fig. 4.34 (A) Testing a patient for the presence of trigger finger. The examiner's fingers are placed over the region of the proximal pulley at the palmar crease and, (B) the patient is invited to flex the fingers over those of the examiner. This may be impossible. If flexion can be achieved the examiner may feel a small nodule passing beneath his fingers and the patient will complain of concomitant pain.

Examination

Tenderness is almost always present over the proximal pulley region. If the patient then flexes the finger over that of the examiner a *nodule* within the tendon may be palpable (Fig. 4.34).

In some patients flexion has become impossible and the examiner must eliminate other possible causes:

absent or ruptured tendon — this can usually be excluded by asking the patient to attempt flexion during palpation, when an intact tendon can be felt to become tense;

fixed joints — a detailed history of onset and the absence of previous injury usually provide the diagnosis. X-ray examination excludes any articular cause of immobility.

Laboratory studies of a simple nature should be undertaken in all cases of trigger finger on account of the recognized higher incidence in rheumatoid and diabetic patients. Initially, a sedimentation rate and a two-hour postprandial blood sugar estimation are sufficient, any abnormality so detected being investigated further.

Surgery is indicated if steroid injection does not provide lasting relief. A simple release of the proximal pulley will be successful in all cases — but should not be done in rheumatoid patients (p. 283). A synovectomy where the synovium appears overabundant or inflamed will probably reduce the amount of subsequent tenderness.

FLEXOR CARPI RADIALIS TENDINITIS[123]

Although a distinct clinical entity this condition is not widely recognized and is difficult to treat with permanent success. The patient complains of discomfort in the wrist, particularly after strenuous exercise. Diagnosis is simple, there being acute localized tenderness over the flexor carpi radialis just proximal to the scaphoid tubercle (Fig. 4.35).

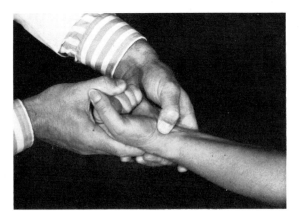

Fig. 4.35 Palpation over flexor carpi radialis just proximal to the ridge of the trapezium may well reveal acute tenderness when compared with the normal side. This is diagnostic of flexor carpi radialis tendinitis.

Once again comparison should be made with the normal wrist to confirm that the tenderness on pressure is greater than normal. *A modified Finkelstein test* has proved useful in making this diagnosis. The relaxed wrist is abruptly deviated as in the Finkelstein, but in a true dorsal direction. Acute pain results in the presence of tendinitis. The scaphotrapezial joint should be studied on appropriate X-rays for it is immediately deep to the tendon and disease there may mimic or cause flexor carpi radialis tendinitis[124]. Surgery is rarely performed for this condition, which is treated conservatively with steroid injection and splintage.

LATERAL EPICONDYLITIS — TENNIS ELBOW

The pathogenesis of this common condition is multiple and often a matter of conjecture. Postulated causes include chronic periostitis of the lateral condyle with spur formation[125], partial tears of the common extensor origin[126,127] or granulation tissue therein[128] traumatic capsulitis of the radiohumeral joint, chondromalacia of the radial head[129,130], radioulnar bursitis, cervical spine disease[131] and radial tunnel syndrome, which is dealt with elsewhere (p. 215).

The condition is characteristic of a chronic inflammatory disorder as it usually occurs on the first occasion as an acute attack of differing intensity, often following on a period of vigorous extensor activity. Treatment or simply rest causes the acute attack to abate, but less severe trouble persists with increasingly frequent attacks of an acute nature, often initiated by the original causative activity. The patient either ceases engaging in that activity, which may alone eliminate the problem, or he consults his physician.

Symptoms

Despite the name which it is commonly given, the majority of cases occur in the fourth decade in patients who never play tennis. In one series, less than 5% of those afflicted played any sport.

The patient complains of pain centered at the elbow but radiating both proximally and distally, mainly the latter, along the extensor muscles. In the acute phase, extension of the arm and flexion of the wrist are avoided as they exacerbate the pain.

Examination

Tenderness is sought at three anatomical points which are in line proximal to distal over the lateral aspect of the elbow (Fig. 4.36)

lateral epicondyle — periostitis, partial tears
radial head (while rotating the forearm) — synovitis, capsulitis
neck of the radius — posterior interosseous nerve

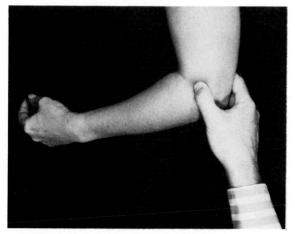

Fig. 4.36 The tenderness in tennis elbow is localized over the anterior aspect of the lateral condyle of the humerus.

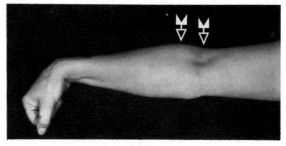

Fig. 4.37 Full flexion of all fingers and the wrist produces discomfort in the patient with tennis elbow more severe than that produced by the middle finger test (p. 00). This contrasts with the findings in a patient with radial tunnel syndrome.

The patient is asked which of the three elicits the most discomfort, remembering that multiple pathology is possible, indeed likely, in this condition. In this examination it is particularly important to compare the affected with the normal side, for pressure at these points normally produces fairly marked discomfort.

Postural discomfort is produced by flexing the wrist and fingers passively, while the patient holds the arm in extension (Fig. 4.37). Pain referred to the epicondyle will frequently cause the patient to ask the examiner to desist before the fingers and wrist have been fully flexed.

The middle finger test should be performed (p. 216). If epicondylitis is the primary problem, pressure on the extended middle finger should cause little more pain than pressure on any of the others. It certainly should not produce as much discomfort as the postural test described above. If this is not so, then radial nerve compression must be considered, especially if the patient has not responded to conservative therapy.

X-ray examination of the elbow should always be undertaken, which may reveal disorders of the humerus or radial head.

Indications

Surgery is indicated when severe symptoms persist despite rest and repeated injections with steroid. Some authors recount that they almost always find a tear, resection and suture providing a cure. Other have designed a number of procedures including removal of calcifications, release of the extensor origin and excision of a portion of the annular ligament. The very multiplicity of techniques indicates that universal success has been achieved with none.

REFERENCES

1. Kanavel A B 1925 Infections of the hand. Lea and Fibiger, Philadelphia
2. Shrewsbury M, Johnson R K 1975 The fascia of the distal phalanx. The Journal of Bone and Joint Surgery 57A: 784–788
3. Hueston J T 1952 Pathology of the inter-digital pilonidal sinus. Australian and New Zealand Journal of Surgery 21: 226–229
4. Mandel M 1978 Immune competence and diabetes mellitus: Pyogenic human hand infections. Journal of Hand Surgery 3: 458–461
5. Mann R J, Peacock J M 1977 Hand infections in patients with diabetes mellitus. Journal of Trauma 17: 376–380
6. Sneddon J 1970 The care of hand infections. Williams and Wilkins, Baltimore
7. Sneddon J 1969-70 Sepsis in hand injuries. The Hand 1-2: 58–62
8. Barlow A, Chattaway F, Holgate M, Aldersley T 1970 Chronic paronychia. British Journal of Dermatology 82: 448–453
9. Howard J B, Highgenboten C L, Nelson J D 1976 Residual effects of septic arthritis in infancy and childhood. Journal of The American Medical Association 236: 932–935
10. Berkowitz R L, Hentz V R 1977 Herpetic whitlow — A non-surgical infection of the hand. Plastic and Reconstructive Surgery 60: 125–127
11. Larossa D, Hamilton R 1971 Herpes simplex infections of the digits. Archives of Surgery 102: 600–603
12. Louis D S, Silva J Jr 1979 Herpetic whitlow: Herpetic infections of the digits. Journal of Hand Surgery 4: 90–94
13. Ogiela D M, Peimer C A 1981 Acute gonococcal flexor tenosynovitis. Case report and literature review. Journal of Hand Surgery 6: 470–472
14. Rosenfeld N, Kurzer A 1978 Acute flexor tenosynovitis caused by gonococcal infection. A case report. The Hand 10: 213–214
15. Thompson S E, Jacobs N F, Zacarias F, Rein M F, Shulman J A 1980 Gonococcal tenosynovitis — dermatitis and septic arthritis. Intravenous penicillin vs oral erythromycin. Journal of The American Medical Association 244: 1101–1102

16. Carithers H A, Carithers C M, Edwards R O 1969 Cat scratch disease: Its natural history. Journal of The American Medical Association 207: 312–316

17. Margileth A M 1968 Cat scratch disease. Pediatrics 42: 803–818

18. Chuinard R G, D'Ambrosia R D 1977 Human bite infections of the hand. Journal of Bone and Joint Surgery 59A: 416–418

19. Farmer C, Mann R 1966 Human bite infections of the hand. Southern Medical Journal 59: 515–518

20. Hooper G 1978 Tooth fragment in a metacarpophalangeal joint. The Hand 10: 215–216

21. Malinowski R W, Strate R G, Perry J F, Fischer R 1979 The management of human bite injuries of the hand. Journal of Trauma 19: 655–659

22. Peeples E, Boswick J A, Scott F A 1980 Wounds of the hand contaminated by human or animal saliva. Journal of Trauma 20: 383–389

23. Zook E G, Miller M, VanBeek A L, Wavek P 1980 Successful treatment protocol for canine fang injuries. Journal of Trauma 20: 243–247

24. Mann R J, Hoffeld T A, Farmer C B 1977 Human bites of the hand: Twenty years of experience. Journal of Hand Surgery 2: 97–104

25. Goldstein E, Miller T, Citron D, Finegold S 1978 Infections following clenched-fist injury: A new perspective. Journal of Hand Surgery 3: 455–457

26. McDonald I 1979 Eikenella corrodens infection of the hand. The Hand 11: 224–227

27. Arons M S, Fernando L, Polayes I M 1982 Pasteurella multocida — the major cause of hand infections following domestic animal bites. The Journal of Hand Surgery 7: 47–52

28. Lucas G L, Bartlett D H 1981 Pasteurella multocida infection in the hand. Plastic and Reconstructive Surgery 67: 49–53

29. Lee B 1960 Dog bites and local infection with pasteurella septica. British Medical Journal I: 1969–1976

30. Veitch J M, Omer G E 1979 Case report: Treatment of catbite injuries of the hand. Journal of Trauma 19: 201–203

31. Goldstein E, Miller T, Citron D, Wield B, Finegold S 1979 Clenched-fist injuries: Infection and empiric antibiotic selection. Contemporary Orthopaedics 1: 30–33

32. Whitaker L A 1973 Management of hand infections in the narcotic addict. Plastic and Reconstructive Surgery 52: 384–389

33. Ross G N, Baraff L J, Quismorio F P 1975 Serratia arthritis in heroin users. The Journal of Bone and Joint Surgery 57A: 1158–1160

34. Gifford D B, Patzakis M, Ivler D, Swezey L 1975 Septic arthritis due to pseudomonas in heroin addicts. The Journal of Bone and Joint Surgery 57A: 631–635

35. Carter S, Mersheimer W 1970 Infections of the hand. Orthopaedic Clinics of North America 1-2: 455–466

36. Neviaser R 1978 Closed tendon sheath irrigation for pyogenic flexor tenosynovitis. Journal of Hand Surgery 3: 462–466

37. Linschieod R, Dobyns J 1975 Common and uncommon infections of the hand. Orthopaedic Clinics of North America 6: 1063–1103

38. Gunther S F, Elliott R C, Brand R L, Adams J P 1977 Experience with atypical mycobacterial infection in the deep structures of the hand. Journal of Hand Surgery 2: 90–96

39. Herndon J H. Lanoue A M 1972 Mycobacterium fortuitum infections involving the extremities. Journal of Bone and Joint Surgery 54A: 1279–1282

40. Gunther S F, Elliott R C 1976 Mycobacterium kansasii infection in the deep structures of the hand. Report of two cases. Journal of Bone and Joint Surgery 58A: 140–142

41. Zvetina J R, Foster J, Reves C V 1979 Mycobacterium kansasii infection of the elbow joint. Journal of Bone and Joint Surgery 61A: 1099–1102

42. Parker M D, Irwin R S 1975 Mycobacterium kansasii tendinitis and fasciitis. The Journal of Bone and Joint Surgery 57A: 557–559

43. Dixon J H 1981 Non-tuberculous mycobacterial infection of the tendon sheaths in the hand. Journal of Bone and Joint Surgery 4: 542–544

44. Williams C S, Riordan D C 1973 Mycobacterium marinum (atypical acid-fast bacillus) infections of the hand. The Journal of Bone and Joint Surgery 55A: 1042–1050

45. Perlman R, Jubelirer R A, Schwarz J 1972 Histoplasmosis of the common palmar tendon sheath. Journal of Bone and Joint Surgery 54A: 676–678

46. Winter W G, Larson R K, Honeggar M H, Jacobesen D, Pappagianis D M, Huntington R W 1975 Coccidioidal arthritis and its treatment — 1975. The Journal of Bone and Joint Surgery 57A: 1152–1157

47. Iverson R E, Vistnes L M 1973 Coccidioidomycosis tenosynovitis in the hand. Journal of Bone and Joint Surgery 55A: 413–417

48. Liseki E J, Curl W W, Markey K L 1980 Hand and forearm infections caused by aeromonas hydrophila. Journal of Hand Surgery 5: 605

49. Hanson P G, Standridge J, Jarrett F, Maki D 1977 Freshwater wound infections due to Aeromonas hydrophila Journal of American Medical Association 238: 1053–1054

50. Childers J C 1980 Pyogenic arthritis due to bacteroides fragilis infection. Orthopedics 3: 319–320

51. Korn J A, Gilbert M S, Siffert R S, Jacobson J H 1975 Clostridium welchii arthritis. The Journal of Bone and Joint Surgery 57A: 555–557

52. Fee N F, Dobranski A, Bisla R S 1977 Gas gangrene complicating open forearm fractures. Report of five cases. Journal of Bone and Joint Surgery 59A: 135–138

53. VanBeek A, Zook E, Yaw P, Gardner R, Smith R, Glover J 1974 Nonclostridial gas-forming infections. Archives of Surgery 108: 552–557

54. Bessman A N, Wagner W 1975 Nonclostridial gas gangrene. Journal of The American Medical Association 233: 958–963

55. Scott F A, German C, Boswick J A 1981 Hemophilus influenzae cellulitis of the hand. Journal of Hand Surgery 6: 506–509

56. Borgsmiller W K, Whiteside L A 1980 Tuberculous tenosynovitis of the hand ('Compound palmar ganglion'): Literature review and case report. Orthopedics 3: 1093–1096

57. Ekerot L, Eiken O 1981 Tuberculosis of the hand. Scand Journal of Plastic and Reconstructive Surgery 15: 77–79

58. Leung P 1978 Tuberculosis of the hand. The Hand 10: 285–291

59. Pinstein M L, Scott R L, Sebes J I 1981 Tuberculous arthritis of the wrist: Differential diagnosis and case report. Orthopaedics 4: 1016–1018

60. Donovan T L, Chapman M W, Harrington K D, Nagel D A 1976 Serratia arthritis. Report of seven cases. The Journal of Bone and Joint Surgery 58A: 1009–1011

61. Southwick G, Lister G D 1979 Actinomycosis of the hand: A case report. Journal of Hand Surgery 4: 360–362

62. Robinson R A 1945 Actinomycosis of the subcutaneous tissue of the forearm secondary to a human bite. Journal of American Medical Association 142: 1049–1051

63. Eastridge C E 1972 Actinomycosis: A 24 year experience. Southern Medical Journal 65: 839–843
64. Goldberg B, Eversmann W W, Eitzen E M 1982 Invasive aspergillosis of the hand. Journal of Hand Surgery 7: 38–42
65. Monroe P W, Floyd W E 1981 Chromohyphomycosis of the hand due to Exophiala jeanselmei (Phialophora jeanselmei, Phialophora gougerotii) — Case report and review. Journal of Hand Surgery 6: 370–373
66. Lichtman D, Johnson D, Mack G, Lack E 1978 Maduromycosis (Allescheria boydii) infection of the hand: A case report. Journal of Bone and Joint Surgery 60A: 546–548
67. Hennessy M J, Mosher T F 1981 Mucormycosis infection of an upper extremity. Journal of Hand Surgery 6: 249–252
68. Smith J, Ruby L K 1977 Nocardia asteroides thenar space infection: A case report. Journal of Hand Surgery 2: 109–110
69. Petersen D P, Wong L B 1981 Nocardia infection of the hand. Case report. Journal of Hand Surgery 6: 502–505
70. Nahas L F, Bennett J E 1981 Case reports: Nocardiosis of the upper limb. Plastic and Reconstructive Surgery 68: 593–595
71. DeHaven K E, Wilde A H, O'Duffy J D 1972 Sporotrichosis arthritis and tenosynovitis. Report of a case cured by synovectomy and Amphotericin B. Journal of Bone and Joint Surgery 54A: 874–877
72. Holcomb H S III, Behrens F, Winn W C Jr, Hughes J M, McCue F C III 1981 Prototheca wickerhamii — An alga infecting the hand. Journal of Hand Surgery 6: 595–599
73. Ahbel D E, Alexander A H, Lichtman D M 1980 Protothecal olecranon bursitis. Journal of Bone and Joint Surgery 62A: 835–836
74. Belsole R, Fenske N 1980 Cutaneous larva migrans in the upper extremity. Journal of Hand Surgery 5: 178–180
75. Simmons E H, Peteghem K V, Tramell T R 1980 Onchocerciasis of the flexor compartment of the forearm: A case report. Journal of Hand Surgery 5: 502–504
76. Carroll R E, Sinton W, Garcia A 1955 Acute calcium deposits in the hand. Journal of American Medical Association 157: 422–426
77. Pagalidis T, Kuczynski K, Lamb D W 1981 Ligamentous stability of the base of the thumb. The Hand 13: 29–35
78. Kuczynski K 1975 The thumb and the saddle. The Hand 7: 120–122
79. Eaton R G, Littler J W 1973 Ligament reconstruction for the painful thumb carpometacarpal joint. Journal of Bone and Joint Surgery 55A: 1655–1666
80. Swanson A B 1972 Disabling arthritis at the base of the thumb. Journal of Bone and Joint Surgery 54A: 456–471
81. Carroll R E, Hill N A 1973 Arthrodesis of the carpometacarpal joint of the thumb. Journal of Bone and Joint Surgery 55B: 292–294
82. Stark H H, Moore J F, Ashworth C R, Boyes J H 1977 Fusion of the first metacarpotrapezial joint for degenerative arthritis. Journal of Bone and Joint Surgery 59A: 22–26
83. Kessler I 1973 Silicone arthroplasty of the trapezio-metacarpal joint. Journal of Bone and Joint Surgery 55B: 285–291
84. Dell P C, Brushart T M, Smith R J 1978 Treatment of trapeziometacarpal arthritis: Results of resection arthroplasty. Journal of Hand Surgery 3: 243–249
85. Gervis W H 1973 A review of excision of the trapezium for osteoarthritis of the trapezio-metacarpal joint after 25 years. Journal of Bone and Joint Surgery 55B: 56
86. Menon J, Schoene H, Hohl J 1981 Trapeziometacarpal arthritis — Results of tendon interpositional arthroplasty. Journal of Hand Surgery 6: 442–446
87. Wilson J H 1972 Arthroplasty of the trapezio-metacarpal joint. Plastic and Reconstructive Surgery 49: 143–148
88. Eaton R G 1979 Replacement of the trapezium for arthritis of the basal articulations. A new technique with stabilization by tenodesis. Journal of Bone and Joint Surgery 61A: 76–83
89. Ferlic D C, Busbee G A, Clayton M L 1977 Degenerative arthritis of the carpometacarpal joint of the thumb: A clinical follow-up of eleven Niebauer prostheses. Journal of Hand Surgery 2: 212–215
90. Lister G D, Kleinert H E, Kutz J E, Atasoy E 1977 Arthritis of the trapezial articulations treated by prosthesic replacement. The Hand 9: 117–129
91. Poppen N, Niebauer J 1978 'Tie-in' trapezium prosthesis: Long-term results. Journal of Hand Surgery 3: 445–450
92. Swanson A B, Swanson G, Watermeier J J 1981 Trapezium implant arthroplasty — Long term evaluation of 150 cases. Journal of Hand Surgery 6: 125–141
93. Crosby E B, Linscheid R L, Dobyns J H 1978 Scaphotrapezial trapezoidal arthrosis. Journal of Hand Surgery 3: 223–234
94. Eiken O 1979 Implant arthroplasty of the scapho-trapezial joint. Scand Journal of Plastic and Reconstructive Surgery 13: 461–468
95. Green W L, Kilgore E S 1981 Treatment of fifth digit carpometacarpal arthritis with silastic prosthesis. Journal of Hand Surgery 6: 510–514
96. Green D P 1979 Pisotriquetral arthritis: A case report. Journal of Hand Surgery 4: 465–467
97. Helal B 1978 Racquet player's pisiform. Hand 10: 87–90
98. Kienbock R 1910 Uber traumatische malacie des mondbeins und ihre folgezustande; entartungsformen und kompressionfrakturen. Fortschr Geb Rontgenstrahlen 16: 78
99. Kienbock R 1980 Concerning traumatic malacia of the lunate and its consequences: Degeneration and compression fractures. Reprinted in Clinical Orthopedics and Related Research 149: 4–8
100. Gelberman R H, Bauman T, Menon J, Akeson W 1980 The vascularity of the lunate bone and Kienbock's disease. Journal of Hand Surgery 5: 272–278
101. Lee M L H 1963 The intraosseous arterial pattern of the carpal lunate bone and its relation to avascular necrosis. Acta Orth Scand 33: 43–55
102. Gelberman R H, Salamon P B, Jurist J M, Posch J L 1975 Ulnar variance in Kienbock's disease. The Journal of Bone and Joint Surgery 57A: 674–676
103. Eiken O, Niechajev I 1980 Radius shortening in malacia of the lunate. Scand Journal of Plastic and Reconstructive Surgery 14: 191–196
104. Ovesen J 1981 Shortening of the radius in the treatment of lunatomalacia. Journal of Bone and Joint Surgery 63B: 231–232
105. Lichtman D M, Mack G R, MacDonald R I, Gunther S F, Wilson J N 1977 Kienbock's disease: The role of silicone replacement arthroplasty. Journal of Bone and Joint Surgery 59A: 899–907
106. Roca J, Beltran J E, Alvarez A 1976 Treatment of Kienbock's disease using a silicone rubber implant. Journal of Bone and Joint Surgery 58A: 373–376
107. Ekerot L, Eiken O 1981 Idiopathic avascular necrosis of the scaphoid. Scand Journal of Plastic and Reconstructive Surgery 15: 69–72
108. Match R M 1980 Nonspecific avascular necrosis of the pisiform bone: A case report. Journal of Hand Surgery 5: 341–342
109. Eiken O, Jonsson K 1980 Carpal bone cysts. A clinical and radiographic study. Scandinavian Journal of Plastic and Reconstructive Surgery 14: 285–290
110. Heberden W 1802 Commentaries on history and cure of disease. T Payne, London

111. Bouchard C 1891 Semaine Med (Paris). 11: 387
112. Kleinert H E, Kutz J E, Fishman J H, McCraw L H 1972 Etiology and treatment of the so-called mucous cyst of the finger. The Journal of Bone and Joint Surgery 54A: 1455–1458
113. Eaton R G, Dobranski A I, Littler J W 1973 Marginal osteophyte excision in treatment of mucous cysts. Journal of Bone and Joint Surgery 55A: 570–574
114. Straub L R, Smith J W, Carpenter G K, Dietz G H 1961 The surgery of gout in the upper extremity. The Journal of Bone and Joint Surgery 43A: 731
115. Williams J G P 1977 Surgical management of traumatic non-effective tenosynovitis of the wrist extensors. Journal of Bone and Joint Surgery 59B: 408–410
116. Brooker A F 1978 Extensor carpi radialis tenosynovitis. An occupational affliction. Orthopaedic Review 6: 99–100
117. Mogensen B A, Mattsson H S 1980 Stenosing tendovaginitis of the third compartment of the hand. Scand Journal of Plastic and Reconstructive Surgery 14: 127–128
118. Hooper G, McMaster M J 1979 Stenosing tenovaginitis affecting the tendon of extensor digiti minimi at the wrist. The Hand 11: 299–301
119. De Quervain F 1895 Ueber eine form von chronischer tendovaginitis. Correspondenz-Blatt F Schweizer Aerzte 25: 389–394
120. Finkelstein H 1930 Stenosing tendovaginitis at the radial styloid process. The Journal of Bone and Joint Surgery 12: 509–540

121. Wood M B, Linscheid R L 1973 Abductor pollicis longus bursitis. Clinical Orthopedics and Related Research 93: 293–296
122. Dinham J M, Meggitt B F 1974 Trigger thumbs in children. Journal of Bone and Joint Surgery 56B: 153–155
123. Weeks P 1978 A cause of wrist pain: Non-specific tenosynovitis involving the flexor carpi radialis. Plastic and Reconstructive Surgery 62: 263–266
124. Fisson J M, Shea F W, Goldin W 1968 Lesions of the flexor carpi radialis tendon and sheath causing pain at the wrist. Journal of Bone and Joint Surgery 50B: 359
125. Begg R E 1980 Epicondylitis or tennis elbow. Orthopaedic Review 9: 33–42
126. Coonrad R W, Hooper W R 1973 Tennis elbow: Its source, natural history, conservative and surgical management. Journal of Bone and Joint Surgery 55A: 1177–1182
127. Garden R S 1961 Tennis elbow. Journal of Bone and Joint Surgery 43B: 100–106
128. Nirschl R P, Pettrone F A 1979 Tennis elbow. Journal of Bone and Joint Surgery 61A: 823–839
129. Bosworth D M 1965 Surgical treatment of tennis elbow. Journal of Bone and Joint Surgery 47A: 1533–1536
130. Newman J H, Goodfellow J W 1975 Fibrillation of head of radius as one cause of tennis elbow. British Medical Journal 1: 328–330
131. Gunn C, Milbrandt W E 1976 Tennis elbow and the cervical spine. Canadian Medical Association Journal 114: 803–809

FURTHER READING

Aghasi M, Rzetelni V, Axer A 1981 Osteochondritis dissecans of the carpal scaphoid. Journal of Hand Surgery 6: 351–352
Ashworth C, Blatt G, Chuinard R, Stark H 1977 Silicone rubber interposition arthroplasty of the carpometacarpal joint of the thumb. Journal of Hand Surgery 2: 345–357
Beckenbaugh R D, Steffee A D 1981 Total joint arthroplasty for the metacarpophalangeal joint of the thumb — A preliminary report 4: 294–298
Bell M S 1976 The changing pattern of pyogenic infections of the hand. The Hand 8: 298–302
Beltran J E, Barjau R, Moreta D 1976 A complication of distal interphalangeal joint arthrodesis. The Hand 8: 36–38
Berger R A, Blair W F, Crowninshield R D, Flatt A E 1982 The scapholunate ligament. Journal of Hand Surgery 7: 87–91
Bilos J, Eskestrand T, Shivaram M 1979 Deep fasciitis of the biceps region. Journal of Hand Surgery 4: 378–381
Bolhofner B, Belsole R J 1981 Kienbock's disease: Current concepts in diagnosis and management. Contemporary Orthopaedics 3: 713–721
de la Caffiniere J Y, Aucouturier P 1979 Trapezio-metacarpal arthroplasty by total prosthesis. The Hand 11: 41–47
Carstam M, Eiken O, Amdren L 1968 Osteoarthritis in the trapezio scaphoid joint. Acta Orthopedic Scandinavica 39: 354–358
Crawford G P 1980 Ligament augmentation with replacement arthroplasty of the carpometacarpal joint of the thumb. The Hand 12: 91–96
Dryer R F, Buckwalter J A 1980 Isolated scaphotrapezial trapezoidal arthrosis. Orthopedics 3: 213–215
Eaton R G, Littler J W 1969 A study of the basal joint of the thumb. Journal of Bone and Joint Surgery 51A: 661–668

Edstrom L E, Robson M C 1978 Destructive DIP joint arthropathy, four unusual case presentations. Orthopaedic Review 7: 61–65
Ehrlich G 1975 Osteoarthritis beginning with inflammation. Definitions and correlations. Journal of the American Medical Association 232: 157–159
Eiken O 1971 Prosthetic replacement of the trapezium. Scand. Journal of Plastic and Reconstructive Surgery 5: 131–135
Engel J, Tsur H, Farin I 1977 A comparison between K-wire and compression screw fixation after arthodesis of the distal interphalangeal joint 60: 611–614
Fisher J R, Conway M J, Takeshita R T, Sandoval M R 1979 Necrotizing fasciitis. Importance of roentgenographic studies for soft-tissue gas. Journal of the American Medical Association 8: 803–806
Fitzgerald R H, Cooney W P, III, Washington J A, Van Scoy R E, Linscheid R L, Dobyns J H 1977 Bacterial colonization of mutilating hand injuries and its treatment. Journal of Hand Surgery 2: 85–89
Grossman J A I, Adams J P, Kunec J 1981 Prophylactic antibiotics in simple hand lacerations. Journal of the American Medical Association 245: 1055–1056
Hall T D 1981 Loose body in the pisotriquetral joint. Report of two cases. Journal of Bone and Joint Surgery 63A: 498–500
Harrison S H 1976 The by-pass operation for arthritis at the first carpometacarpal joint. The Hand 8: 145–149
Hartz C, Beckenbaugh R D 1979 Long-term results of resection of the distal ulna for post-traumatic conditions. Journal of Trauma 19: 219–226
Hergenroeder P T, Penix A R 1981 Bilateral scapholunate dissociation with degenerative arthritis. Journal of Hand Surgery 6: 620–622

Iyer K M 1981 The results of excision of the trapezium. The Hand 13: 246–250

Jackson I T, St Onge R A 1977 The use of palmaris longus tendon to stabilise trapezium implants. The Hand 9: 42–44

Kessler I, Axer A 1971 Arthroplasty of the first carpometacarpal joint with a silicone implant. Plastic and Reconstructive Surgery 47: 252–257

Leach R E, Bolton P E 1968 Arthritis of the carpo-metacarpal joint of the thumb. Journal of Bone and Joint Surgery 50A: 1171–1177

Muller G M 1949 Arthrodesis of the trapezio-metacarpal joint for osteoarthritis. Journal of Bone and Joint Surgery 31B: 540–542

Nylen S, Carlsson B 1980 Time factor, infection frequency and quantitative microbiology in hand injuries. Scand Journal of Plastic and Reconstructive Surgery 14: 185–189

Pierce R O 1980 Tears of the intra-articular cartilage at the wrist joint. Orthopaedic Review 9: 57–61

Pieron A P 1973 The mechanism of the first carpometacarpal joint. An anatomical and mechanical analysis. Acta Orthopedica Scandinavica Supp 148

Pollen A 1974 Acute infection of the tendon sheaths. The Hand 6: 21–25

Roberts A H N, Teddy P J 1977 A prospective trial of prophylactic antibiotics in hand lacerations. British Journal of Surgery 64: 394–000

Schecter W, Meyer A, Schecter G, Giuliano A, Newmeyer W, Kilgore E 1982 Necrotizing fasciitis of the upper extremity. Journal of Hand Surgery 7: 15–19

Smith S, Kuczynski K 1978 Observations on the joints of the hand. The Hand 10: 226–231

Stone N, Hursch H, Humphrey C, Boswick J 1969 Empirical selection of antibiotics for hand infections. The Journal of Bone and Joint Surgery 51A: 899–903

Wavak P 1981 The use of antibiotics in acute hand injuries. Orthopaedic Review 10: 141–143

Weilby A Surgical treatment of osteoarthritis of the carpometacarpal joint of the thumb. Scand Journal of Plastic and Reconstructive Surgery 5: 136–141

Weilby A, Melone C 1978 Results following removal of silicone trapezium metacarpal implants. Journal of Hand Surgery 3: 154–156

5

Rheumatoid

In the hands rheumatoid disease affects primarily the synovium which is found in all of the joints and around the flexor and extensor tendons. Tendons are covered with synovium wherever they pass beneath pulleys. They pass beneath pulleys wherever they run across the concavity of a joint or series of joints. Thus, synovium is present around both flexor and extensor tendons at the wrist beneath their respective retinacula, and also around the flexor tendons in the fibrous sheaths along the fingers. These sheaths commence over the metacarpophalangeal joints, that is, beneath the proximal palmar crease on the radial side of the palm of the hand and beneath the distal palmar crease on the ulnar side. There are three stages in rheumatoid disease:

1. *Proliferative,* characterized by synovial swelling which produces pain on motion, limitation of movements and nerve compression;
2. *Destructive,* in which synovial erosion causes irreversible changes — tendon rupture, capsular weakness and disruption, bone erosion and joint subluxation and deformity;
3. *Reparative.* Synovial activity has now 'burnt out' and fibrosis replaces chronic inflammation, causing tendon adhesions, fibrous ankylosis and finally fixed deformity.

These three stages produce differing and characteristic problems for the patient. Examination is directed at identifying these and determining the appropriate management.

HISTORY

Time of onset and pattern of disease
The duration of the disease process should be ascertained. The patient should be questioned regarding exacerbations and remissions of his symptoms, from which the pattern of his disease will be appreciated. Three general patterns are recognised:

Monocyclic — only one attack followed by permanent remission; 10% of rheumatoid patients,

Polycyclic — attacks of varying duration of differing severity occurring at unpredictable intervals; 45%,
Progressive — an unremitting, inexorable course; 45% (Fig. 5.1).

Major problems
The patient should be asked to identify those aspects of his disease which give him most trouble. These may well not be those most apparent on inspection of the upper limb. Nonetheless *these* problems should receive particular attention in the treatment plan, even at the expense of temporarily disregarding more obvious and challenging deformities. Although terribly disabled, the patient is often *functionally* very competent (Fig. 5.2).

Other problem areas
A brief summary should be made of the regions other than the hand and arm which are troublesome. The name of the physician or surgeon treating those problems should be noted so that early cooperative management can be established. If the patient is receiving no medical help with other disabilities then referral should be offered. Surgery previously performed should be recorded. Future plans for other regions should be discussed and, at a later stage, priorities determined.

Functional grading
The patient should be asked to explain his or her difficulties in both occupation and domestic life. This can often best be achieved by asking a series of questions regarding everyday acts which cover all functions of the hand. Alternatively these acts can be used as tests performed by the patient at the examination or during a preliminary assessment by a physical or occupational therapist.

A simple grading of ability to fulfil everyday needs of locomotion and manipulation can now be made according to the following scale

1 no incapacity
2 manages all but the heaviest tasks
3 manages none but the lightest duties
4 chair or bed bound

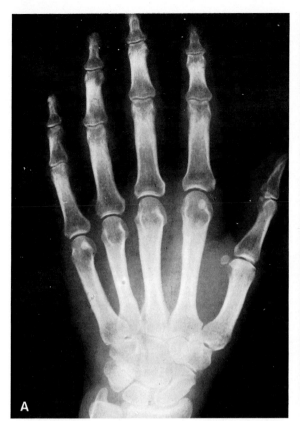 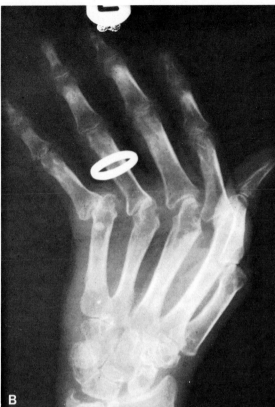

Fig. 5.1A & B. The progression of rheumatoid disease is illustrated by these two X-rays of a young woman in her twenties taken at an interval of four years. At the time of her first X-ray, she had been diagnosed as having sero-positive rheumatoid disease but little evidence of deformity was present. Four years later, rheumatoid disease is all too evident in the radial shift at the wrist and the ulnar deviation of the fingers with metacarpophalangeal joint destruction.

SPECIFIC COMPLAINTS

The patient should now be questioned systematically to determine the presence and duration of symptoms known to be associated with rheumatoid arthritis in the hands.

Pain

The pain of rheumatoid disease is characteristically most severe during the proliferative and early destructive stages of the disease. A recent increase in pain should make the surgeon suspect that a 'flare-up' in the disease is commencing. Except during such exacerbations, the pain is usually not present at rest but is provoked by movement. The patient should be asked to demonstrate the movement which causes pain to aid in localization of the most active synovitis. It may be useful for later assessment of disease progression to grade the pain according to a scale: 0 — no pain; 1 — slight; 2 — moderate; 3 — severe.

Stiffness

It is necessary to distinguish between stiffness and limitation of active joint movements. The latter is a relatively constant feature throughout the day and can be measured. The former is difficulty in movement which cannot be measured and which varies during the course of the day. Attempts have been made to place a value on stiffness by asking the patient how long it takes him to loosen up after getting out of bed in the morning — the time at which stiffness is characteristically present. This has been named the 'limber-up time' (LUT).

Numbness and paraesthesia

Compression, especially of the median nerve, is more common in rheumatoid patients than in the general population due to the increase in the volume of synovium in the rigid confines of the nerve tunnels. The symptoms and signs are the same as those described in the chapter on compression. Very often the rheumatoid patient will not volunteer the symptoms of compression, their presence only being revealed by direct questioning.

Generalized neuropathy, common in the lower limbs of rheumatoid patients, is unusual in the upper.

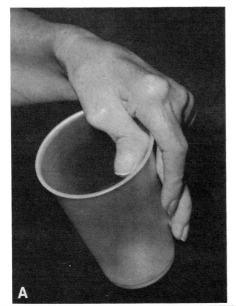

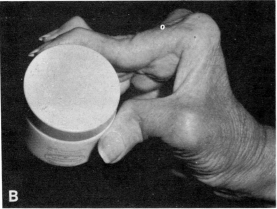

Fig. 5.2 Despite severe disability, rheumatoid patients contrive to perform everyday functions, (A). Not only is compensation due to trick movements but also to the development of additional deformities as seen in (B). Palmar subluxation of the metacarpophalangeal joints and a boutonniere deformity in the thumb has been compensated to some extent by the development of a swan neck deformity in the fingers and of radial instability at the interphalangeal joint of the thumb, giving an otherwise unobtainable grasp on a small jar.

Weakness
Weakness is often generalized and is believed to be part of the systemic disturbance of rheumatoid disease. Some evidence suggests that it is directly related to lack of use either through pain or deformity. Less commonly, weakness of grasp may be due to nerve compression. Rarely, polymyositis masquerading as muscular dystrophy may complicate longstanding rheumatoid disease.[1]

Appearance
On occasion the patient's main complaint is of the ugliness of the deformity. To some the deformed hands are an understandable social embarrassment, to others a disability which prevents them following their occupation.

THERAPY AND ITS EFFECT
It is necessary to know what treatment the patient has previously received and what he is currently taking. The duration of adequate treatment is of significance to the surgeon in timing any planned intervention. For example, synovectomy during the proliferative stage should probably be withheld until a three to six months trial of therapy has been shown to be ineffective in giving relief. This general rule applies unless damage threatens function which it would be difficult to restore, as in gross peritendinous synovitis or marked dorsal subluxation of the ulnar head which may at any stage proceed to tendon rupture.

Steroid intake should be recorded, especially its duration, since therapy for more than 3 years has been shown to delay wound healing[2].

The surgeon should be aware of other effects of rheumatoid disease, that *rheumatoid variants* (p. 284) exist and that rheumatoid disease may be only one aspect of several syndromes. He should examine the patient with this in mind. According to whether or not rheumatoid factor is present in the serum of such patients they are referred to as *sero-positive* or *sero-negative.*

NON-ARTICULAR EFFECTS OF RHEUMATOID DISEASE
Iritis or *uveitis* occurs in 3 to 5% of the patients.
Scleromalacia perforans is rupture of the globe due to necrosis in a rheumatoid nodule.
Anaemia and apparent lack of nutrition are frequently present. 25% show a normocytic normochromic anaemia typical of chronic infection.
Polyneuropathy — as stated above this is mainly confined to the lower limbs.
Lung changes may[3] be any one of the following:

'rheumatoid lung' has a characteristic honeycombed appearance on X-ray due to multiple rheumatoid nodules;
Caplan's syndrome[4] is found in patients with concomitant pneumoconiosis and produces massive pulmonary fibrosis;
idopathic pulmonary fibrosis.

Cardiac manifestations include pericarditis, myocarditis and valvular disease;
Arteritis is uncommon but may rarely be of a fulminating variety.

RHEUMATOID SYNDROMES

Felty's syndrome[5]
  Classical rheumatoid polyarthritis
  Lymphadenopathy
  Splenomegaly   →   granulocytopenia
                    →   anaemia
Rheumatoid sero-positive, these patient's haematological problems can be relieved by steroids and cured by splenectomy, which has no effect, however, on the arthritis.

Sjogren's syndrome[6]
  Classical rheumatoid polyarthritis ⎱
  Keratoconjunctivitis sicca   ⎰   any 2 out of 3
  Xerostomia
Sero-positive for rheumatoid factor, these patients also show several other tissue antibodies. Confirmation of the diagnosis is made by estimating the tear production using the *Schirmer test* or by labial salivary gland biopsy. No cure for the fibrosis of the lacrimal and salivary glands is available.

Social history
At the juncture at which the examiner feels he is beginning to establish rapport with the patient, a picture should be obtained of the patient's social background. Rheumatoid arthritis is economically as well as physically crippling and the number of dependents whom the victim supports may have a great influence upon the time he can devote to surgery. The attitude of employers varies greatly and this must be known to the surgeon for he may be able to influence that attitude to the patient's benefit simply by an explanatory letter or telephone call. In later stages of disease, the availability, health and attitude of relatives is of great importance in helping the patient to conduct a normal daily life.

Allied to the functional assessment already made, knowledge of the home circumstances will clarify the way in which the patient can best be helped by social and welfare services, often by the provision of simple mechanical aids or the management of more elaborate structural alterations to assist the patient in dressing, toilet, cooking and moving about his home.

EXAMINATION

While due attention is paid to sensory loss and motor weakness, skin cover and joint ranges, examination of the rheumatoid hand is conducted more by region than by system. Further, the rheumatoid hand is characterized by certain deformities which would be complex to describe anatomically and then difficult to comprehend even for the well-trained reader. These characteristic deformities have consequently been standardized by the use of generally accepted terms, such as 'ulnar drift', 'swan neck', and 'boutonniere'.

The author personally organises this complexity, and often multiplicity, by summarising all information on one sheet of paper. Down the left hand side are written all the areas of potential involvement — neck, shoulders, elbows, radial head, ulnar head, wrist, extensors, thumb, MP joints, PIP joints, DIP joints, flexors, and nerve compression — in the order in which they are examined. The remainder of the sheet is divided into two columns, the left hand one headed RIGHT, the right hand one LEFT, because the surgeon is facing the patient. On this sheet all the problems can be marked in shorthand giving an overall view from which a quick recollection of the patient can be gained and on which a rational surgical agenda can be planned.

One feature of rheumatoid disease is its *symmetrical distribution*. As a result, the examiner frequently finds the same joints involved in both hands and the same apparently spared. Progression often differs, the dominant hand usually being more advanced in disease than the other.

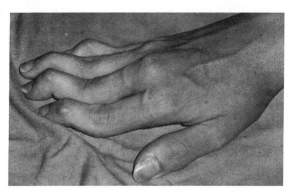

Fig. 5.3 Swan neck deformity of the fingers with hyperextension of the proximal interphalangeal joints and flexion of the distal interphalangeal joints of all fingers.

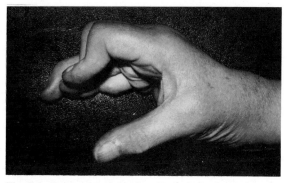

Fig. 5.4 Boutonniere deformity with flexion deformity of the proximal interphalangeal joints and compensatory hyperextension of the distal interphalangeal joints.

Table 5.1

		PIP joint effect			
PIP synovitis	⟶	palmar plate laxity ⎫	⟶	PIP hyperextension ⎱	Swan
Intrinsic tightness	⟶	extensor PLUS ⎬		↓	neck
FDS synovitis	⟶	flexor MINUS ⎭		DIP(MP) flexion ⎰	(Fig. 5.3)
PIP synovitis					
→ central slip* attrition	⟶	extensor MINUS ⎫	⟶	PIP flexion ⎱	
→ lateral band*	⟶	extensor MINUS ⎬		↓	Boutonniere
palmar subluxation		flexor PLUS ⎭		DIP(MP) hyperextension ⎰	(Fig. 5.4)

*Read *'extensor pollicis brevis'* for 'central slip' and extensor hood for 'lateral band' and the mechanism of boutonniere in the *thumb* is explained (Fig. 5.5).

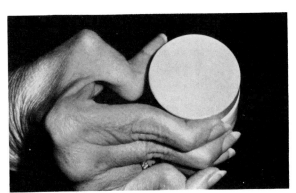

Fig. 5.5 Boutonniere deformity of the thumb with palmar subluxation of the metacarpophalangeal joint and hyperextension of the interphalangeal joint. This is the same patient as seen in Fig. 5.1.

General inspection
An early indication of the patient's main problems may be obtained by inspection of the upper extremity.

DEFORMITY
Several deformities may be evident:
  Posterior subluxation of the elbow
  Volar subluxation of the wrist
  Radial shift of the wrist
  Ulnar drift of the fingers
  Palmar subluxation of the metacarpophalangeal joints
  'Swan neck' ⎱ deformities of the fingers
  'Boutonniere' ⎰
  Z-deformity of the thumb, either into 'swan neck' or 'boutonniere'
  Lateral dislocation of any of the interphalangeal joints
  Misalignment of digits suggestive of tendon rupture.

The Z mechanism
This phenomenon underlies the development of many of the characteristic deformities of the rheumatoid hand. It can be defined: when a joint, for whatever reason, persistently adopts an angulation in one direction, the joints on either side of it will tend to go in the opposite direction, provided other local conditions in those joints permit it. The mechanism is due to the changes in relative mechanical advantage of the tendons acting on a series of joints and to an increase in the extraneous loads borne by joints adjacent to one primarily deformed. It is seen in the hand in several instances (Table 5.1). The pathogenesis of the swan neck and boutonniere deformities of the thumb can best be understood if the metacarpophalangeal joint of the thumb is considered rather as being the proximal interphalangeal joint (which indeed it is in some respects cf. the location of the epiphyses).

Gross instability; arthritis mutilans[7]; 'opera-glass hands'[8] (Fig. 5.6)
This degree of instability results when the bone ends are excessively eroded. In later stages the diaphyses become tapered. This results in totally flail joints with marked digital shortening. Grasp of almost any object becomes impossible. The excess of skin falls into folds which telescope out as the digit is restored to its original length by traction — hence the term 'opera-glass hands' or *'la main en lorgnette'*. Occasionally ankylosis of a joint arrests the shortening, so that one digit may be disproportionately long. This effect is the aim of surgery, which should be performed relatively early and consists of arthrodesis of all effected interphalangeal joints, adding bone grafts for length wherever appropriate. Only the carpo-metacarpal joint of the thumb and the metacarpophalangeal joints of the fingers can be kept mobile in the most advanced cases.

Swellings
Rheumatoid nodules. These subcutaneous swellings may be found at any site over the hands and arms, but are by far most commonly located over the subcutaneous ulnar border (Fig. 5.7) just distal to the elbow. They may be present in conjunction with a swollen olecranon bursa from which they should be distinguished. Rheumatoid nodules are firm and rubbery, not fluctuant as is a swollen olecranon bursa. The presence of rheumatoid nodules has been shown to be a poor prognostic factor in rheumatoid disease. Nodules are uncomfortable and may ulcerate.

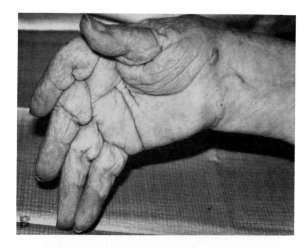

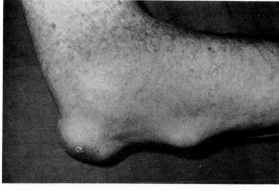

Fig. 5.7 Rheumatoid nodules are most commonly found over the subcutaneous border of the ulna.

Redness is only seen in the presence of very severe, active synovitis. On the dorsum of the wrist the extent of the synovial swelling indicates whether the extensor tendon synovial sheaths are involved or the wrist joint alone. In the former case, the swelling extends well on to the dorsum of the hand distally and on to the forearm proximally (Fig. 5.8). It is also a much more clearly delineated swelling than that in the wrist joint proper where swelling is difficult to see and may only be detected on palpating and moving the

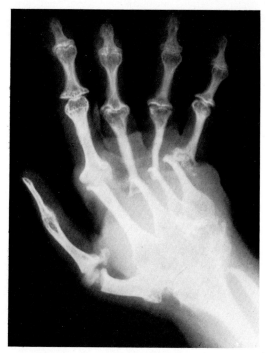

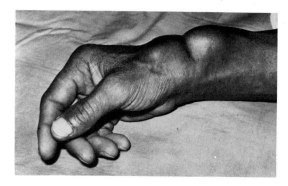

Fig. 5.8 Synovial swelling associated with extensor compartment disease is often prominent and extends over the wrist proximally and the dorsum of the hand distally.

Fig. 5.6 (A) Gross destruction of the metacarpophalangeal and interphalangeal joints particularly on the right hand in this patient has resulted in the collapse of the skeleton with consequent excess of skin. Traction on the digits produces marked telescoping, hence the term 'opera-glass hands'. (B) *Arthritis mutilans* (see text).

They should be excised and this is usually undertaken in conjunction with other procedures on the hand.

Pseudo rheumatoid nodules, identical histologically, but without other stigmata of rheumatoid disease, have been reported.[9]

Prominent ulna head — see p. 264

Synovial swelling. Markedly swollen joints can be detected on inspection, as can any associated inflammation.

joint. Undue fullness on the palmar aspect over the proximal phalanx, in the palm (Fig. 5.9), and above the wrist (Fig. 5.10) suggests flexor synovitis.

SKIN

The skin of the rheumatoid patient is typically thin and papery, especially susceptible to trauma. This is particularly so in the patient who has been treated for some time with steroids. As a result, the skin frequently shows *bruising, petechiae* and *finger tip haemorrhages and infarcts,*

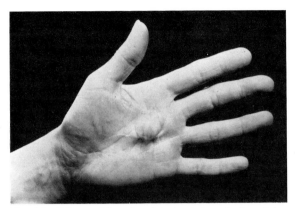

Fig. 5.9 Fullness of the palm of the hand along the line of the middle finger is most evident just proximal to the fibrous tendon sheath. This is indicative of flexor tendon synovitis.

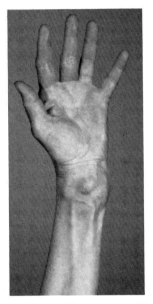

Fig. 5.10 An accumulation of flexor tenosynovitis can be seen in the wrist proximal to the carpal tunnel.

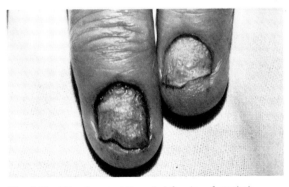

Fig. 5.11 The characteristic nail deformity of psoriasis.

especially at the nail folds. Other causes should be sought, for example, petechiae may be evidence of the thrombocytopenia of Felty's spenomegaly.

Psoriasis — the characteristic skin lesion should be sought and is most commonly found around the elbow. Deformity of the nails may also help in establishing the diagnosis (Fig. 5.11). If the patient proves to be sero-negative then one is dealing with psoriatic rather than rheumatoid arthritis and surgery should be approached more guardedly as the outcome is often less satisfactory (p. 285).

Palmar erythema — not associated with hepatic dysfunction, this is seen in many rheumatoid patients, mainly over the thenar and hypothenar eminences.

Intertrigo — this is often encountered in the grossly deformed hand and is due to the accumulation of moisture, most often between the fingers and in the palm in the presence of severe metacarpophalangeal joint disease. Every effort, including splinting, regular cleansing and drying and the application of appropriate local medication, should be made to heal the skin before surgery.

MUSCLE WASTING

A common general feature in rheumatoid disease, excessive wasting of the thenar or hypothenar eminences should suggest possible median or ulnar nerve compression respectively. The first dorsal interosseous commonly shows marked atrophy evidenced by the deep concavity on the dorsal aspect of the first web space (Fig. 5.12), masked only by the equally common adduction deformity of the thumb. This wasting results in unusual prominence of the second matacarpal head and allows ulnar drift (p. 273).

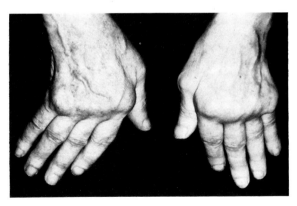

Fig. 5.12 The wasting of the first dorsal interosseous especially evident in the right hand was due to rheumatoid atrophy, ulnar nerve function being intact.

SYSTEMATIC REGIONAL ASSESSMENT

The surgeon should now proceed to assess the upper extremity joint by joint, tendon by tendon, nerve by nerve.

In assessing joints, certain facts are determined in almost all of them. These are

Pain
Synovial swelling
Tenderness
Range of motion — active
                   — passive
                   — associated pain
Stability
Crepitus

Although the patient was asked generally about pain while his history was being taken, this question should be asked specifically at the start of examination of each joint and during passive range of motion. If pain is experienced equally throughout the range and worsened by applying some longitudinal compression during motion, the cause is probably articular erosion. If the pain is mainly at the extremes of the range and indeed arrests passive motion, the cause is more likely to be synovial inflammation (Fig. 5.13).

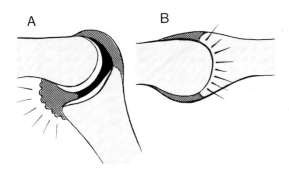

Fig. 5.13 This diagramatically shows how (*left*) in the presence of inflamed synovium, compression of the synovium and stretching on the opposite aspect of the joint produce pain, whereas (*right*) where the cartilaginous surface has been completely worn down, the pain is due to rubbing of one bone end on another.

Neck

Rheumatoid involvement of the joints in the cervical spine is common. Three deformities occur as a result:

atlanto - axial subluxation
superior migration of the odontoid process into the
   foramen magnum
subaxial subluxation of the vertebral bodies.

These may result in *pain* of varying degree, *instability* of the cervical spine and *neurological disturbance* which at worst can result in fatal cord transection. This may well occur during general anaesthesia and full assessment of the neck before anaesthesia of any rheumatoid patient is therefore mandatory.

Examination should include:
Passive range of movement. In most patients with cervical spine disease this will be limited and in about three-quarters of them will produce pain characteristically in the distribution of the greater occipital nerve[10]. Audible and palpable crepitation may be present. Stressing the neck at extremes may produce pain but must be hazardous and *should not be attempted.*

Trigeminal nerve testing. Due to involvement of the descending tract of the fifth cranial nerve, about 20 per cent of the patients with narrowing of the canal will show suppressed sensation in the area of the ophthalmic division of the trigeminal nerve.

Lower limb reflexes. Patients may show reduced reflexes due to peripheral neuropathy but in canal narrowing *hyperreflexia* occurs in about one-third of the patients due to involvement of the pyramidal tracts.

If any of these tests suggests the presence of atlanto-axial subluxation full neurological assessment should be undertaken and the patient fitted immediately with a soft cervical collar pending more detailed evaluation.

At the Hospital for Special Surgery in New York[11] they classify neural deficit as follows:

I — nil
II — subjective weakness, hyperreflexia, dysaesthesia
IIIa — objective long tract signs
IIIb — quadriparesis

All patients with rheumatoid disease should have anteroposterior and lateral X-rays in extension and flexion performed (Fig. 5.14).

The following relationships should be studied

(i) the gap between the dens and the arch — this
    should not exceed 3 mm in any position[12]
(ii) McGregor's line — from the upper surface of the
    hard palate to a point most caudal on the curve
    of the occiput — the distance by which the dens
    is above that line should not exceed 4.5mm[13].
(iii) the C_2 – C_3 relationship.

Changes progress with time[14]. Only 1% of patients come to posterior fusion, which is indicated for intractable pain, significant instability and Grade II or certainly IIIa neural deficit.

Shoulder

The shoulder is the hub around which the hand moves and disease will indirectly but seriously limit hand function. The range of motion in the shoulder can quickly be tested by inviting the patient to touch the interscapular region in three ways with the hand being examined

over the ipsilateral shoulder — abduction, external
   rotation
over the contralateral shoulder — flexion, adduction
beneath the ipsilateral axilla — extension, internal
   rotation.

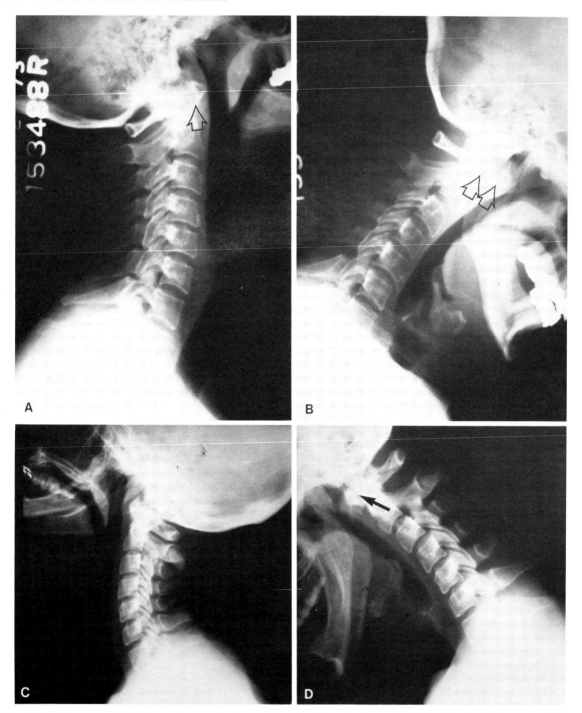

Fig. 5.14 The contrast in the distance between the dens and the arch of the atlas in extension (A) and flexion (B) is very marked in this patient being some 11 mm when measured on a true lateral view. The dens was not the seat of erosion on a transoral film and this very hazardous subluxation was therefore due to laxity of the transverse ligament of the atlas. (C) and (D) show that the space in a non-rheumatoid patient does not alter with flexion.

Difficulty in performing any of these movements should be followed by more detailed clinical and radiological assessment, which falls within the province of the orthopaedic rather than the hand surgeon.

Elbow

Subcutaneous rheumatoid nodules are most commonly found about the elbow joint, usually situated over the subcutaneous border of the ulna about 5 cm from the olecranon. They may, however, be in the wall of an olecranon bursa and if this is the seat of effusion a double swelling of differing pathology may present.

Synovium

In extension of the normal elbow, there is a depression just above the radial head. This depression overlies the joint space between the radial head and the capitulum of the humerus and is largely obliterated by swelling in the presence of active synovitis of the joint. With the elbow flexed to 90 degrees, it is also possible to feel synovial swelling to the medial side of the olecranon. Fluid if present can be felt to fluctuate from the lateral to the medial aspect.

Range of motion: pain

The elbow should now be moved through a full range of active and passive movements, recording the results obtained. The normal range is 0°-145° extension to flexion. The passive movement here, as in all joints, must be produced slowly and gently. Pain is much more severe if produced by rapid movement, and the recorded range therefore less.

Active synovitis is suggested by pain towards the extremes of the range, increasing as they are reached and indeed often being itself the limiting factor. These patients tend to have less range of active than passive movement. Synovectomy has been shown to be effective in relieving pain and improving the range of motion. The approach appears to make little difference — bilateral incisions[15], transolecranon[16] or by excising the radial head[17] — provided all synovium is removed from both humero-radial and humero-ulnar compartments[18].

Pain experienced throughout the range, especially if associated with crepitus and worsened by longitudinal compression, indicates probable erosion of articular cartilage (Fig. 5.15). Provided the joint is relatively stable, such patients may be considerably relieved by synovectomy with insertion of a 2 millimetre thick sheet of silastic between the humerus and ulna — a silastic sheet interpositional arthroplasty. Reduction in range of motion due to joint destruction may be very pronounced, even to the point of spontaneous ankylosis. Where neither hand can be used to feed the patient or to perform toilet activities, total elbow joint replacement can restore function in a large proportion of patients[19-21], although the

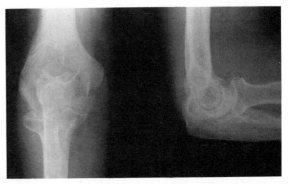

Fig. 5.15 This AP and lateral X-ray of the elbow reveals loss of joint space and was associated with pain experienced throughout the range of flexion and extension of the elbow joint.

procedure is attended by a high rate of complications[22, 23] and reoperation[24].

Crepitus

If the elbow joint is cupped in the palm of one hand and the joint is then slowly moved passively through a short arc, creaking or grinding may be felt by the supporting hand. This may be due to marked synovitis or more frequently to advanced erosion of the articular surfaces.

Stability

Dislocation of the elbow is relatively rare in rheumatoid disease since it requires not only disruption of the ligaments of the joint and weakening of the muscles but also considerable erosion of the humerus and ulna. If it does occur the clinical picture is similar to that of trauma in that posterior dislocation of the olecranon is the common displacement and can be detected by increase in the distance from olecranon to either epicondyle when compared with the interepicondylar distance. It differs from traumatic dislocation in that any of these bony landmarks may be destroyed by erosion and in the fact that the dislocation in the rheumatoid is usually remarkably painless.

The much less severe instability of the subluxed joint can be detected by grasping both upper and forearms with the elbow joint at 90 degrees and attempting to displace the ulnar first backwards and then forwards in relation to the trochlea of the humerus. Being a perfect hinge joint, the normal elbow cannot be subluxed at all by this manoeuvre (Fig. 5.16).

Gross instability of one or other collateral ligament should be assessed by holding the arm in full extension and supination, placing the palm of one hand over the opposite side of the joint as a fulcrum and then stressing the collateral ligament with force applied laterally with the other hand just above the wrist, using the forearm as a lever. Instability is a contraindication to silastic sheet interpositional arthroplasty. The one compensation for

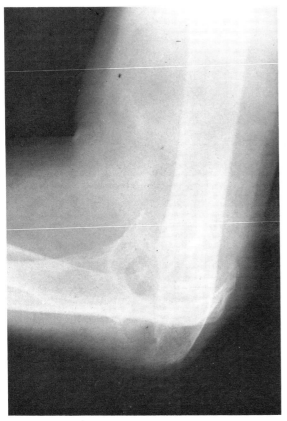

Fig. 5.16 This X-ray shows almost total destruction of the elbow joint associated with gross instability on clinical examination.

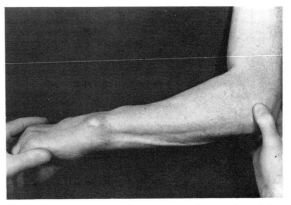

Fig. 5.17 With the elbow flexed some 90 degrees, the radial head is sought with the examiner's thumb while the arm is carried into pronation and supination with the other hand.

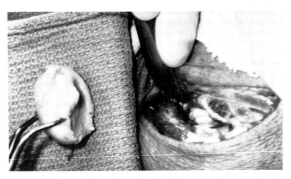

Fig. 5.18 At excision, the radial head is seen to be the site of erosive arthritis.

instability is that it is usually accompanied by a functional range of motion.

RADIAL HEAD

With the patient's arm abducted somewhat and the forearm flexed to 90 degrees, the arm should be supported beneath the elbow with the palm of the hand while the radial head is sought with the thumb of that hand (Fig. 5.17). Its identification can be greatly facilitated by passively pronating and supinating the forearm with the other hand causing the radial head to rotate.

Crepitus

During this movement crepitus may be detected and this may be accompanied by discomfort. This is due to loss of articular cartilage in the superior radioulnar joint and will clearly not be helped by the interpositional arthroplasty recommended for this painful crepitus in the humeroulnar joint. Rather is excision of the radial head indicated (Fig. 5.18). This procedure relieves pain and increases the range of motion in the majority of patients.[25] Replacement of the head with a silastic prosthesis appears to give inferior

results and is associated with a significant incidence of prosthesis fracture.[26-28]

Range of motion

Supporting the elbow with the palm of the hand, the patient's hand should be held and the forearm carried into full pronation and supination, and the passive and then active ranges recorded. These ranges are measured taking 0° to be with the plane of hand vertical. The average normal range is pronation 70°, supination 85°. Care should be taken to immobilize the elbow during this test for the apparent ranges can be greatly increased by movement of the shoulder and trunk. This is particularly common in supination and becomes an unconscious everyday movement of the patient, adducting the shoulder and laterally flexing the trunk in order to place the palm of the hand in a flat, receptive position.

Pain

With the elbow stabilized, passive pronation and supination of the forearm are very commonly accompanied by pain, especially on extreme supination (Fig. 5.19). This

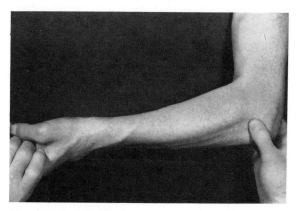

Fig. 5.19 When the forearm is carried into extreme supination, the patient very commonly complains of pain, usually at the ulnar head.

should be accurately localized by the patient. The pain may be experienced at the elbow which suggests superior radioulnar joint disease, but much more commonly is very accurately referred to the ulnar head (see below).

Wrist

As already indicated, inspection of the wrist frequently reveals significant disease in the form of synovial swelling. This is most often observed in two sites:

(a) the *dorsum of the wrist*. Swelling here is often encountered but is often not in the wrist joint proper, but in the extensor synovial compartment.

(b) *ulnar aspect*. The collection may be overlooked for it is partially hidden beneath the overhanging ulnar head.

Postural change

The changes in resting posture vary from mild deviation to frank and gross subluxation of the joint. In either event they invariably occur in one or other of two directions. Each has distinct significance distal to the wrist joint.

1. *flexion*. This deformity arises with synovitis of both wrist and midcarpal joints and may progress even as far as total anterior dislocation of the carpus on the radius (Fig. 5.20). The functional effect is highly significant, for full power of the long finger flexors can only be achieved with the wrist in dorsiflexion.
2. *radial deviation*. This comes about for two reasons

   (a) loss of articular cartilage in the radiocarpal joint,
   (b) accumulation of synovium around the ulnar head.

Cradling the wrist in one hand the examiner should proceed to feel and then to move the wrist joint.

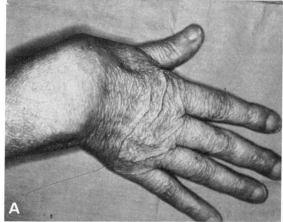

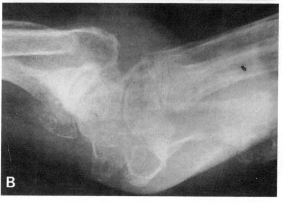

Fig. 5.20 (A) Total anterior dislocation of the wrist joint is evident even on clinical examination, the radius and ulna being abnormally prominent on the dorsum of the wrist. In less marked anterior dislocation radiological examination, (B) may reveal its presence.

Synovium

The synovium on the dorsum of the wrist and ulnar aspect should be palpated using the three finger test for fluctuation to confirm its relatively fluid nature (Fig. 5.21). By firm pressure or by placing the wrist in flexion, the boundaries of the synovial swelling are made more apparent. In the case of dorsal swelling, the exact location of the diseased synovium can often be deduced by the wider and obviously superficial extent of that around the extensor tendons compared with that in the radiocarpal joint. Very occasionally the examiner may be led to this conclusion erroneously by an unusually large amount of synovium in the midcarpal joint — not a common finding.

Range of motion

The wrist joint should be carried into maximum flexion, extension, radial deviation and ulnar deviation, both actively and passively. The average normal range is flexion 75°, extension 70°, ulnar deviation 35°, radial deviation 20°.

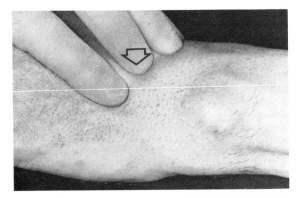

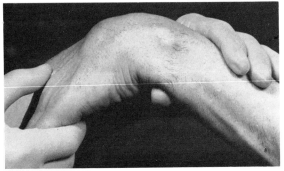

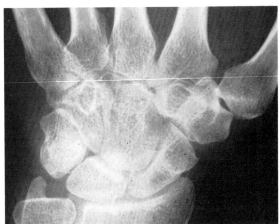

Fig. 5.21 (A) The presence of synovium in the wrist joint and the extensor compartment can be palpated by fixing the swelling with two fingers of one hand and palpating it with a finger of the examiner's other hand, thereby eliciting fluctuation (B) By carrying the wrist into palmar flexion the precise boundaries of the synovium swelling can be made more apparent.

Pain

If pain is experienced in the more extreme arcs of the range and is accompanied by joint swelling synovitis of the composite radiocarpal and midcarpal joint is the most likely cause (Fig. 5.22). To distinguish between the two components of the joint is difficult.

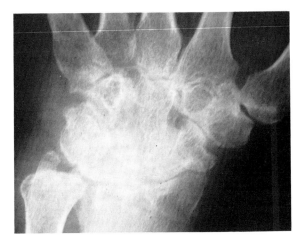

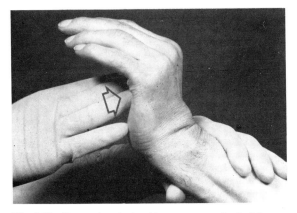

Fig. 5.22 By carrying the hand into extremes of wrist joint motion the presence of pain most marked at either end of the arc is suggestive of synovitis.

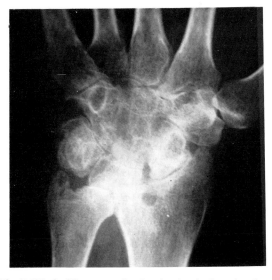

Fig. 5.23A-C The progressive deterioration in the wrist of a patient in her 30's is seen in these X-rays taken at two year intervals.

If on the other hand, pain is experienced throughout a limited arc with little or no swelling present, then loss of articular cartilage is the more likely cause. This is supported by the detection of crepitus.

Crepitus

As with the elbow crepitus can best be detected by cradling the joint in the palm of one hand while gently flexing and extending the joint. Pain with crepitus can be helped appreciably by silastic sheet interpositional arthroplasty,[29] provided the joint is stable (Fig. 5.23).

Instability

Minor degrees of subluxation may not be detectable on inspection, being masked by dorsal synovitis. The lower forearm should be grasped firmly in one hand and the hand and carpus in the other. Alternate dorsal and palmar movement of one hand relative to the other in a shearing manner will reveal instability (Fig. 5.24). In the normal wrist little or no movement can be achieved by this manoeuvre.

Significant instability of the wrist severely impairs hand function. Were the disease unilateral, arthrodesis would be a simple and effective solution. However, the disease is not and the examiner must be aware of the distinct possibility that surgery will be required on the opposite wrist in the future. For this reason attempts should be made to restore stability while retaining some motion. If motion is retained in the subluxed joint, then relocation of the joint with temporary Kirschner wire fixation and dorsal stabilisation[30] by reefing the capsule and buttressing it with the extensor retinaculum[31], will relieve pain and retain a degree of stable mobility in the majority[32]. If the joint is fixed in subluxation but the wrist extensors are still functional[33] — usually revealed on exploration — then wrist joint replacement with a silastic spacer gives good results with increased strength[34]. Finally, if the wrist extensors have been destroyed, arthrodesis is indicated. This may be done formally in the presence of good bone stock[35], but where

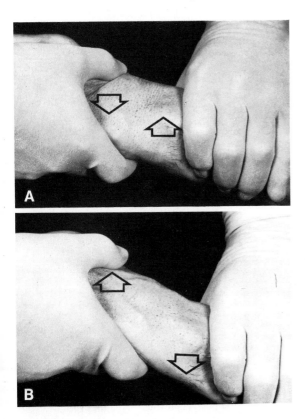

Fig. 5.24A & B By grasping the forearm and hand and attempting to produce a shearing action at the wrist joint which in normal patients is stable, the early stages of subluxation can be demonstrated.

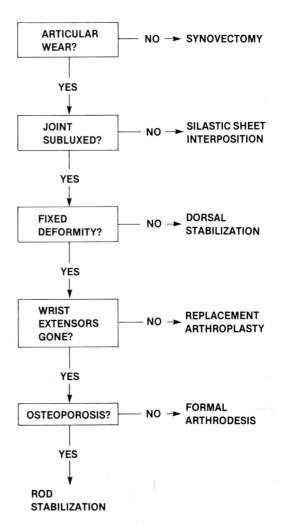

Fig. 5.25 This flow chart illustrates the method of selecting the appropriate procedure in rheumatoid disease of the wrist (see text).

that is osteoporotic, transfixion of the joint with a Rush nail[36] or Steinman pin[37] is swift and invariably successful. Where arthrodesis is necessary, the surgeon must be mindful that personal toilet and hygiene can only be performed with some wrist flexion so one of the two wrists must have either mobility or be flexed in 20° of flexion. The process of selecting the correct operative procedure for the wrist is outlined in Figure 5.25.

ULNAR HEAD

With either the thumb of the supporting hand or the index finger of the other, the surgeon should firmly depress the prominent ulnar head. It may be stable in which event the patient simply has a naturally large ulnar head. In rheumatoid patients, however, the prominence can be depressed by 5 mm or more, usually with accompanying pain (Fig. 5.26). This movement has been described as the *'piano key'* sign for, like a piano key, when the bone is released it springs back into its original position.

Depression of the ulnar head often has two effects apart from producing pain.

1. recurrence of radial deviation of the wrist. As the ulnar head is depressed the carpus can often be felt to rotate radially with a grinding sensation. This radial deviation was probably present before disruption of the triangular radioulnar articular disc allowed the ulnar head to sublux dorsalwards.

2. increased prominence of synovial swelling on the ulnar border of the wrist.

Ulnar head subluxation, especially with pain on supination and depression, is an indication for excision of the ulnar head, one of the most effective operations in surgery of the rheumatoid hand not only because it relieves pain, restores motion and gives increased grip strength[38,39], but also because it removes a major threat to the extensor tendons.

Extensor tendons

Synovium

The distinguishing features of synovitis around the extensor tendons at the wrist have already been stated:

discrete, well-demarcated, often prominent swelling,
  extension of the swelling on to the dorsum of the hand, thumb and forearm,
 absence of pain, even on passive movement of the wrist,
 bogginess to palpation,
 crepitus on palpation during finger motion.

Significant synovitis requires synovectomy as it is a major factor in producing tendon rupture (Fig. 5.27).

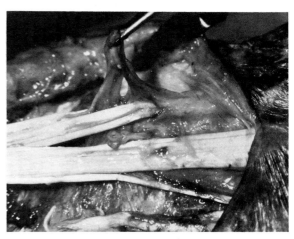

Fig. 5.27 Diseased synovium is here shown being dissected off the extensor tendons during exploration of the tendon rupture.

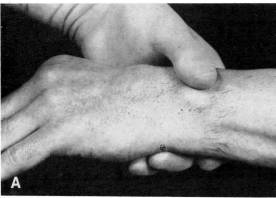

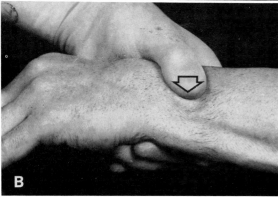

Fig. 5.26A & B *The piano key sign.* Pressure exerted over the ulnar head will cause distinct motion in the presence of dislocation and surrounding synovitis. On release the ulnar head jumps back into its original position.

TENDON RUPTURE[40]

The most apparent cause of rupture of tendons, namely attrition against rough or prominent bone (Fig. 5.28) has been refuted by some who emphasize the importance of synovitis within the tendon and interference with its blood supply. Certainly tendon disruptions in rheumatoid disease only occur where the tendon lies within a synovial sheath. Nonetheless, the most common sites for rupture are related to bony prominences:

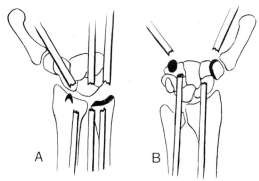

Fig. 5.28   This diagram highlights the bony points at which tendinous rupture is likely to occur. On the left dorsally, the radial tubercle and the dislocated ulnar head, and on the right anteriorly, the ridge on the trapezium and the hook of the hamate.

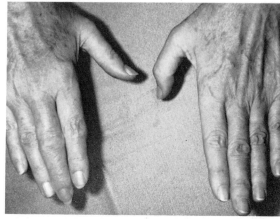

Fig. 5.30   *Extensor pollicis longus rupture* is revealed by the posture of the metacarpophalangeal and interphalangeal joints on the right.

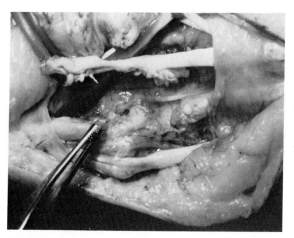

Fig. 5.29   The erosion produced in this tendon by the ulnar head which has here been removed can clearly be seen to conform to the hemispherical shape of that head.

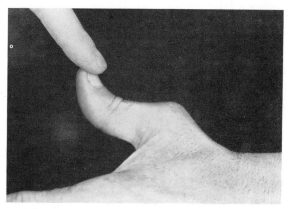

Fig. 5.31   This patient with rheumatoid disease is able to perform extension against resistance indicating a normal extensor pollicis longus, which is palpable over the metacarpal of the thumb.

extensor pollicis longus at the tubercle on the radius, extensor digiti minimi and extensor digitorum of small and ring fingers over the dorsally subluxed ulna head (Fig. 5.29).

These ruptures are usually evident on inspection but may require active testing.

Extensor pollicis longus rupture

Posture: Flexion of both metacarpophalangeal and interphalangeal joints of the thumb (Fig. 5.30).

Active test: Resisted extension of the interphalangeal joint of the thumb (Fig. 5.31). Partial rupture may be present with little effect on the normal posture. However, active testing reveals weakness and often pain over the site of partial rupture.

Extensor digiti minimi rupture
Extensor digitorum rupture

Posture: drooping of the affected fingers at the metacarpophalangeal joint (Fig. 5.32). This becomes increasingly apparent as the patient actively attempts to straighten the fingers, for this results in unbalanced action of the intrinsic muscles which extend the interphalangeal joint but flex the metacarpophalangeal joint.

Active test: resisted extension of the metacarpophalangeal joint (Fig. 5.33).

A mistaken diagnosis of extensor tendon rupture may be made for any one of three reasons:

1. *Subluxation of the metacarpophalangeal joint* with intrinsic contracture and palmar plate shortening may make the joint incapable of extension. This possibility

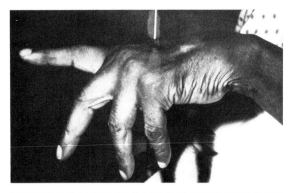

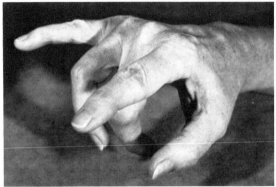

Fig. 5.32 The most common order of rupture of the extensor tendons has occurred in this patient with progressive loss of extension in the small, ring, and middle fingers. It should be noted that some extension remains in the middle finger and this may be evidence of an intertendinous connection from the intact extensor to the index.

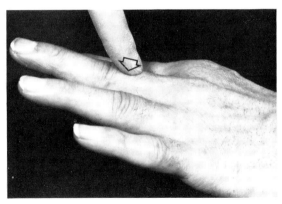

Fig. 5.33 The metacarpophalangeal joint is extended by the long extrinsic extensor and this should be tested in each finger.

can be eliminated by testing passive extension of the metacarpophalangeal joints (Fig. 5.34).

2. *Ulnar displacement of the extensor tendons* (Fig. 5.35) at the metacarpophalangeal joints may be so marked that they fall below the axis of that joint losing all power to extend it. In extreme cases they become weak flexors. This is more difficult to detect but should be suspected if the tendons can be felt to tighten on attempted extension and if their line passes towards the ulnar aspect of the relevant metacarpophalangeal joint. In early stages of this extensor tendon dislocation, the patient cannot initiate finger extension but can maintain it if the fingers are first placed in that position.

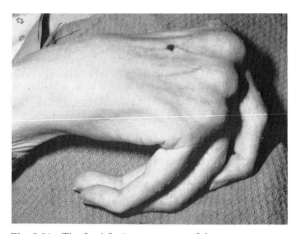

Fig. 5.34 The fixed flexion contracture of these metacarpophalangeal joints is due to severe palmar subluxation of the proximal phalanges.

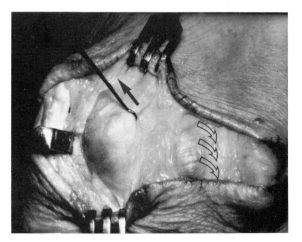

Fig. 5.35 In this patient about to undergo metacarpophalangeal replacement, the ulnar displacement of the extensor tendon to the middle finger is clearly shown. The tendon has fallen into the space between the metacarpophalangeal joints and here is being pulled up into its normal position using a skin hook.

3. *Posterior interosseous nerve palsy*[41] resulting from compression of that nerve by synovitis of the radiohumeral joint may mimic extensor tendon rupture (see Chapter 3).

Ruptured extensor tendons require early surgical reconstruction lest joint flexion contractures ensue. In those cases in which too much tendon length has been destroyed to allow direct repair, early intervention *may* allow reconstruction using a tendon graft while power remains in the motor unit. Tendon transfers are usually required and the integrity of appropriate tendons should be determined during examination — extensor indicis, extensor carpi ulnaris, flexor digitorum superficialis and others. The transfers commonly employed are:

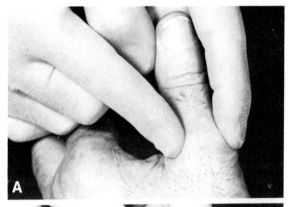

for EPL — EI or EDM or EPB

    EDM — EI

    1 ED — link to an adjacent intact tendon

    2 ED — EI + adjacent

    3 or 4 ED — FDS[43] or ECU or FCU

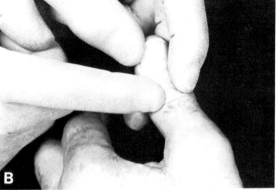

Thumb

At each joint — trapeziometacarpal, metacarpophalangeal and interphalangeal — the presence of pain and of the signs of rheumatoid disease should be noted.

Synovium

In all the small joints of the hand active synovitis can be felt as a 'boggy' swelling between the finger and thumb of the examining hand or perhaps more precisely, between the two index fingers of the examiner (Fig. 5.36). The synovium may be made more evident and obviously fluctuant by gently flexing the joint under examination. Because of the relative resistance of the palmar plate all joint synovitis in the hand is more pronounced dorsally.

Tenderness

Should be recorded during palpation.

Range of motion

Should be recorded both actively and passively. The normal range of motion in the joints of the thumb varies very widely from a combined range in normal metacarpophalangeal and interphalangeal joints of 120 degrees to over 300 degrees. The average accepted by the American Academy of Orthopaedic Surgeons is

	CM	MP	IP
extension	20°	10°	15°
flexion	15°	55°	80°
abduction	60°	—	—

Of greater significance than recording the active and passive ranges is careful observation of specific points

    pain: throughout range, emphasized by compression — articular loss; at extremes of range — synovitis;

Fig. 5.36A & B Synovial swelling in the metacarpophalangeal and interphalangeal joints of the thumb can best be palpated by using two fingers. Its presence is evidenced by a 'boggy' fluctuance between the two digits.

    passive range: the examiner must be able to correct passively any deformity of the thumb joints, if soft tissue reconstruction is to prove effective;

    instability.

Stability

Collapse of the skeleton of the thumb in rheumatoid disease is very common. The resultant deformity tends to conform to one of four patterns, which have been classified and described by Nalebuff[44].

TYPE I = 'BOUTONNIERE' (Fig. 5.37)

Disease commences at the metacarpophalangeal joint. Synovial expansion of the dorsal capsule produces attrition of extensor pollicis brevis and ulnar displacement of extensor pollicis longus. Thus the thumb becomes 'extrinsic-minus' and progressive metacarpophalangeal flexion results. The consequent palmar subluxation of the base of the proximal phalanx in addition to the dorsal synovial expansion causes distal and palmar displacement of the intrinsics — abductor pollicis brevis and adductor

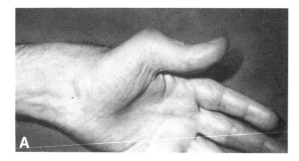

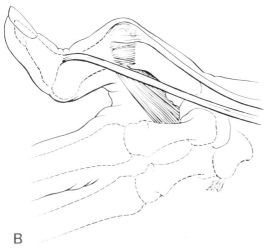

Fig. 5.37(A) Here an early boutonniere deformity of the thumb is demonstrated with palmar subluxation of the metacarpophalangeal joint and the commencement of hyperextension of the interphalangeal joint.

(B) The mechanism is here diagrammatically illustrated. The synovial swelling in the metacarpophalangeal joint results in attenuation of the extensor pollicis brevis with resultant loss of extension of that joint. It also causes distal shift of the intrinsic tendons going to the extensor expansion. Contrasting with their normal neutral function, the intrinsics become flexors of the metacarpophalangeal joint.

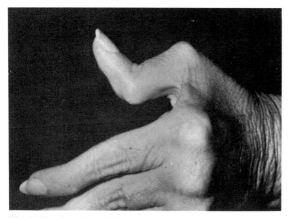

Fig. 5.38 An advanced boutonniere deformity of the thumb known also as an intrinsic plus or '90-90' thumb.

pollicis — which further increases the metacarpophalangeal flexion and hyperextends the interphalangeal joint (Fig. 5.38).

Indications in type I [45]
if (i) joints can be reduced passively,
  (ii) joints are stable laterally in the reduced position,
 (iii) articular surfaces are adequate on X-ray
   → synovectomy + insertion of extensor pollicis longus into the base of the proximal phalanx

if any of the above not present
   → stabilization of the metacarpophalangeal joint by arthrodesis or peg [46] or replacement arthroplasty [47]

TYPE II – uncommon
Type II is identical to Type I but is consequent upon disease in the trapeziometacarpal joint with adduction of the first metacarpal.

TYPE III = 'SWAN-NECK' (Fig. 5.39)
Disease commences at the trapeziometacarpal joint resulting in adduction and flexion of the first metacarpal. In the presence of concomitant disease in the metacarpophalangeal joint, the Z-mechanism (p. 254) produces hyperextension of that joint and hyperflexion of the interphalangeal joint.

Indications in Type III
1. correct adduction of first metacarpal [48] by release of adductor pollicis, or first dorsal interosseous or the overlying fascia or all three;
2. maintain correction by attending to the trapeziometacarpal disease. (See Chapter 4). It is highly desirable to maintain motion at this joint in rheumatoid disease, therefore fusion is rarely performed.

if (i) articular surfaces adequate on X-ray
 (ii) no evident disease in other trapezial joints
  then, synovectomy
   + ligament reconstruction with FCR or ECRL
if (iii) articular surfaces not adequate
  add, silastic interposition [49]

if (iv) other trapezial articulations diseased
  then, trapezial excision
   + silastic replacement
   or + tendon interposition

It is essential to ensure adequate function in the thenar muscles if the abducted position is to be maintained.
3. Once the adduction contracture has been overcome, the metacarpophalangeal and interphalangeal joint deformities can be corrected —

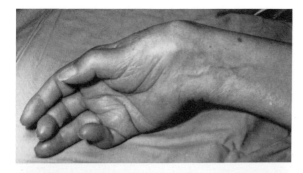

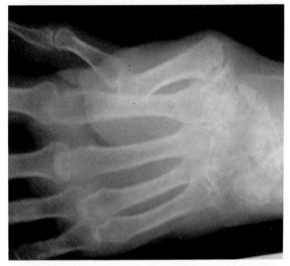

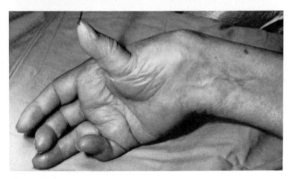

Fig. 5.39 (A) *Swan-neck deformity of the thumb* seen on X-ray (B) to be due to basal joint disease followed by adduction contracture and hyperextension deformity. The deformity is fixed as is shown in (C) resulting in severe loss of first web space span.

if (i) joints reducible passively
 (ii) joints stable laterally in the reduced position
 (iii) articular surfaces adequate on X-ray
    → synovectomy and soft tissue stabilization by palmar capsulodesis or tenodesis[50]
 if any of (i), (ii) or (iii) not present
    → stabilization or replacement arthroplasty.

TYPE IV (Fig. 5.40)
Disease again commences at the trapeziometacarpal joint, resulting in adduction of the first metacarpal. However in this instance collateral ligament laxity at the metacarpophalangeal and/or interphalangeal joint produces radial deviation at either or both of these articulations (Fig. 5.41).

Indications in Type IV
1. correct adduction and basal joint disease as in type III
2. manage the metacarpophalangeal and/or interphalangeal joints as follows:

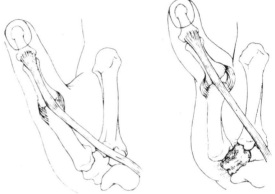

Fig. 5.40 The mechanism of a Type IV deformity of the thumb is here illustrated diagrammatically. Disease at the trapeziometacarpal joint results in adduction deformity of the first metacarpal towards the second. This is compensated for by stretching of the collateral ligaments of either the metacarpophalangeal joint as illustrated here or of the interphalangeal joint. The normal relationships are demonstrated in the diagram on the left.

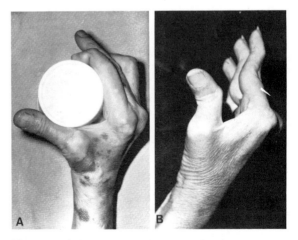

Fig. 5.41 (A) Radial deviation has occurred at the metacarpophalangeal joint following adduction deformity in a Type IV rheumatoid thumb.
 (B) The radial deviation has here occurred at the interphalangeal joint.

if articular surfaces adequate on X-ray (uncommon)
  → synovectomy
    + collateral ligament reconstruction
if articular surfaces poor (common)
  → stabilization or replacement arthroplasty of the
    metacarpophalangeal joint
    + stabilization of the interphalangeal joint.

As has been emphasized previously the pathogenesis of
Type I and Type III can be understood in the terms of the
pathological anatomy of the rheumatoid finger if the
metacarpophalangeal joint of the thumb is equated to the
proximal interphalangeal joint of the finger. The following
substitutions would then be made

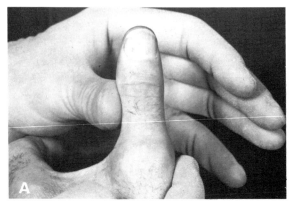

Thumb	*Finger*
metacarpophalangeal joint	proximal inter- phalangeal joint
abductor pollicis brevis and adductor pollicis	intrinsic lateral bands
extensor pollicis brevis	central slip of extensor digitorum
interphalangeal joint	distal inter- phalangeal joint

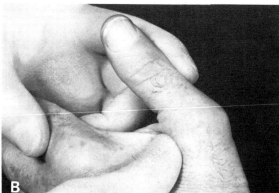

In those cases in which a full-blown deformity of Types
I–IV has not occurred, stability should be assessed at each
joint in turn.

Trapeziometacarpal — as subluxation develops, the base
of the first metacarpal moves radially and anterior relative
to the trapezium (these directions are referred to the plane
of the palm of the hand). Such subluxation can be detected
by the examiner placing his thumb over the metacarpal
base and his index finger on the flexor aspect of the
patient's thumb. Pressing with both digits will reduce any
subluxation usually with accompanying pain. No
movement is present in the normal joint with this
manoeuvre.

Metacarpophalangeal and interphalangeal joints — each
collateral ligament should be stressed in turn with the joint
held in maximum extension (Fig. 5.42). In the normal hand
this produces only a few degrees of pain-free movement.
The palmar plate should be stressed by firm extension. The
normal hyperextension in these joints of the thumb is very
variable.

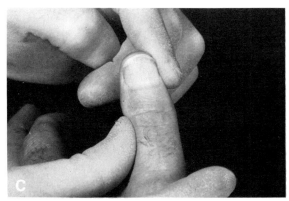

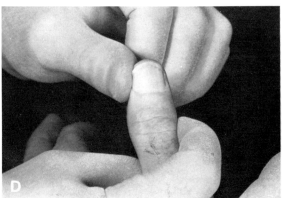

Fig. 5.42A-D The integrity of the collateral ligaments of the
metacarpophalangeal and interphalangeal joints of the thumb
should be tested by laterally stressing these when held in
maximum extension. (B) shows that there is some laxity of the
radial collateral ligament of the metacarpophalangeal joint.

Crepitus

If the whole thumb is grasped in one hand and the wrist in the other with the examiner's thumb over the trapeziometacarpal joint and the joint rotated while applying some force along the axis of the thumb, crepitus can be detected. This is evidence of loss of articular cartilage, especially if the movement is accompanied by pain. It should be treated as indicated above (Type III; 2 (iii) or (iv)).

Metacarpophalangeal joints

Synovium

As in all other digital joints, the capsule of the metacarpophalangeal joint is most substantial on its palmar and lateral aspects, where it is thickened into the palmar plate, accessory collateral and collateral ligaments. These structures allow motion while providing strong stability. Synovitis is therefore best detected on the dorsal aspect where swelling can be felt as fluctuation between two of the examiner's digits with the joints held in gentle flexion of some 40 to 50 degrees (Fig. 5.43).

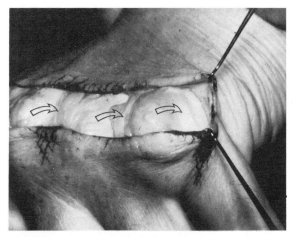

Fig. 5.44 The extreme ulnar subluxation of the extensor tendons is seen here prior to metacarpophalangeal joint replacement. The extensor digiti minimi can be seen on the ulnar aspect of the neck of the metacarpal.

radial movement is replaced by ulnar dislocation of the extensor tendons. In late stages, the extensor tendons fall between the metacarpal heads (Fig. 5.44). In this position they are unable to extend the fingers and a mistaken diagnosis of tendon rupture may be made.

In periods of active synovitis, palpation of the synovium will produce marked *tenderness*.

Indications

Synovectomy of the metacarpophalangeal joints is indicated in the following situations:

1. persistent painful swelling despite adequate medical therapy;
2. early erosions evident on radiological examination; these are most likely to be seen on Brewerton views (p. 283) (Fig. 5.45);

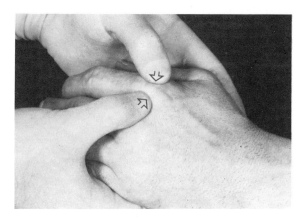

Fig. 5.43 Synovitis in the metacarpophalangeal and interphalangeal joints of the digits can be detected by the two thumbs of the examiner with the joint held in gentle flexion. Its presence is revealed by a 'boggy' fluctuance between the two examining digits.

In time the synovium erodes through the capsule and comes to bear on the extensor expansion. The expansion is significantly thinner on the radial aspect than on the ulnar, especially in the index finger. Stretching of the expansion results in ulnar dislocation of the tendons. This displacement should be noted for it is one of the factors responsible for the production of ulnar drift. In the normal hand, the extensor tendons are held over the metacarpophalangeal joints by the dorsal hood. Indeed, in power grasp they can be seen to shift radially as full force is applied. As the dorsal hood is weakened and stretched this

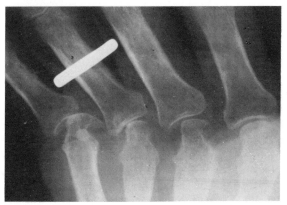

Fig. 5.45 A Brewerton view of the metacarpophalangeal joints demonstrates very clearly the erosions of the metacarpal heads particularly beneath the radial collateral ligaments of these joints. This occurs at an area of bare bone within the capsule of the joint.

3. displacement of the extensor tendons in the presence of synovitis. The radial extensor hood can be reefed following synovectomy, but care must be taken not to limit flexion. Release of the ulnar hood and intrinsic is often necessary to achieve recentralization[51].

In one review, synovectomy was effective in relieving pain in about half of the patients while almost all lost motion, with an average reduction of 20°[52].

All patients being prepared for synovectomy should be warned of the possible need for joint replacement, since the condition of the bone ends cannot be fully assessed clinically or by X-ray (Fig. 5.46). Only 18% of patients in one series were seen to have erosions on X-ray, whereas they were found to be present on exploration in 81%.[53]

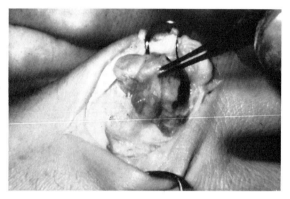

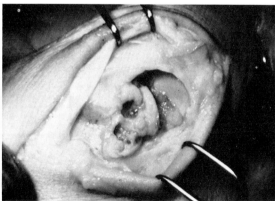

Fig. 5.46A & B   Synovium frequently obscures large erosions in the underlying metacarpal head.

Range of motion

The range of both active and passive motion in each metacarpophalangeal joint should be recorded with the goniometer, taking note of whether or not motion is limited by pain.

Stability[54]

While the normal metacarpophalangeal joint shows a wide range of motion both in flexion and extension and, when the fingers are extended, in a lateral direction, their stability is essential for normal hand function. In the extended position, where stability is required for strong lateral pinch, it is provided mainly by the interosseous muscles and that primarily by the powerful first dorsal interosseous. When the joints are flexed, and stability is necessary for power grasp, the normal metacarpophalangeal joint is locked in lateral immobility by its collateral ligaments. This laxity in extension and immobility in flexion is provided by virtue of the eccentric attachment of the ligament to the cam-shaped metacarpal head. The metacarpal head is also wider on its palmar aspect than dorsally and this also serves to tighten the collateral ligaments.

Instability in rheumatoid disease results from

weakness of the first dorsal interosseous which should therefore be tested in all cases to detect early loss of stability (Fig. 5.47);

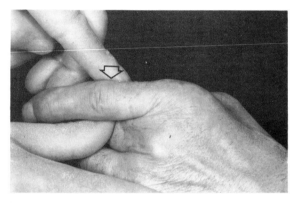

Fig. 5.47   The first dorsal interosseous is tested by asking the patient to abduct the index finger against pressure exerted by the examiner.

disruption of the collateral ligaments. [55] This results from synovial erosion of the only area of bare bone within the joint capsule, namely that beneath the proximal attachment of the collateral ligament. A deep erosion is commonly detected in this situation, both radiologically (Fig. 5.48) and during synovectomy (Fig. 5.49). This eventually causes detachment of the collateral ligament from its insertion with significant loss of stability. This can be detected by flexing the index finger at the metacarpophalangeal joint and exerting lateral pressure. In the normal hand no motion results. In the advanced rheumatoid there is considerable movement, while in the incipient case the patient complains of pain on this manoeuvre.

When these two stabilizing factors have been eliminated or significantly weakened, other forces, mechanical and pathological, produce the characteristic deformities of the rheumatoid metacarpophalangeal joints, *ulnar drift* and *palmar subluxation.*

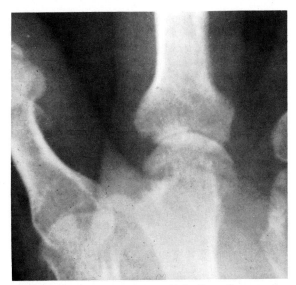

Fig. 5.48 This metacarpophalangeal joint X-ray illustrates the erosion on the radial aspect of the metacarpal head of the index finger. It results in disruption of the collateral ligament attachment on that side which permits the development of ulnar drift.

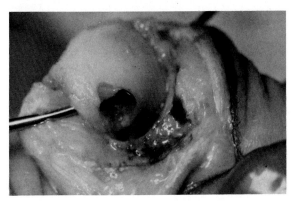

Fig. 5.49 Significant erosions may only be detected at the time of synovectomy.

increased by a slip of tendon from extensor digiti minimi which becomes increasingly powerful as the extensor becomes dislocated in an ulnar direction.

These forces produce the *ulnar deviation* seen in the normal hand in extension and which increases in power grasp.

The pathological forces which produce *ulnar drift* once stability has been lost should be sought at the appropriate stage in the examination.

Radial deviation of the wrist which by the Z-mechanism induces ulnar drift of the metacarpophalangeal joints[58]

> *ulnar shift of the extensor tendons;*
> *ulnar applied force of the flexor tendons* (Fig. 5.50);[59]
> *intrinsic tightness.* (p. 275)

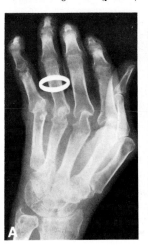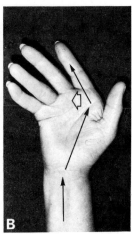

Fig. 5.50A & B As was emphasized in the section on Surface Anatomy, the flexor tendons cross the wrist joint to the ulnar side of the midline. With radial deviation of the wrist the angle of incidence of these tendons to the index finger in particular is increasingly from an ulnar direction. As laxity in the flexor tendon sheath develops so the force of the flexor tendons on the metacarpophalangeal joint is applied further out on the proximal phalanx and becomes progressively more and more powerful in its ulnar moment.

ULNAR DRIFT[56]

Flatt describes ulnar drift as having two components[57].

Ulnar deviation, an ulnar rotation of the phalanx around the metacarpal head, is present in the normal hand and only pathological when uncorrectable. *Ulnar shift,* an ulnar translocation of the base of the phalanx on the metacarpal head, is always abnormal.

The normal usage and structure of the hand impose pressures on the metacarpophalangeal joints which displace them into ulnar deviation.

Thumb pressures in all pinch grips;
the ulnar inclination of the head of the metacarpal bone;
the action of abductor digiti minimi which is a strong ulnar deviator of the small finger proximal phalanx. Its action is

All of these abnormal ulnar deviating forces are self-perpetuating. That is, in each instance, once ulnar drift has arisen as a result of removal of the radial stabilizing factors and application of the ulnar deviating forces, the mechanical advantage of those forces to further produce ulnar drift is enhanced (Fig. 5.51).

PALMAR SUBLUXATION

This displacement can only occur when the collateral ligaments have been stretched or their attachments disrupted. It is further encouraged by the stretching of the dorsal expansion of the extensor mechanism with dislocation of the extrinsic extensor tendons to lie between the metacarpal heads. These changes remove the dorsal structures which normally resist palmar subluxation and

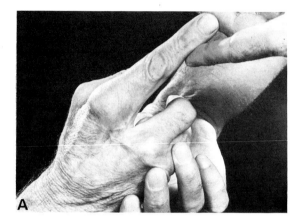

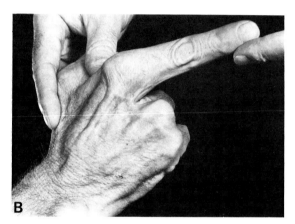

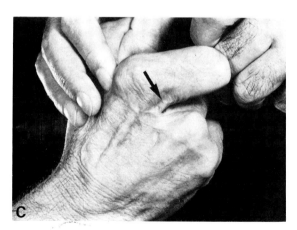

Fig. 5.51 This patient who does not suffer from rheumatoid disease but has been subjected to a ray resection of the middle finger with subsequent scarring illustrates well two of the factors which play a part in producing ulnar drift of the fingers. In (A) the finger is held extended without any active effort by the patient. In (B) active extension shows that the extensor tendon is lying to the ulnar aspect of the metacarpophalangeal joint and that active extension results in ulnar deviation of the finger.

(C) Here the intrinsic test is being applied and it can be seen how the patient's finger swings into ulnar drift on account of tightness of the intrinsic on the ulnar aspect of his index finger.

often create a flexion deformity of the metacarpophalangeal joints. The forces which then produce the subluxation are *intrinsic tightness* and the powerful palmar moment of the *extrinsic flexor tendons*.

Palmar subluxation is commonly evident on inspection, the metacarpal heads being prominent dorsally to a marked extent (Fig. 5.52). In less apparent cases, usually where florid synovitis still persists, the presence of subluxation can be demonstrated by stabilizing the metacarpal with one hand, gripping the proximal phalanx with the other and

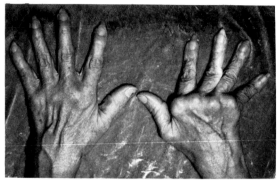

Fig. 5.52 Palmar subluxation of the metacarpophalangeal joints is clearly evident in the right hand of this patient, the metacarpal heads being evident as a ridge across the dorsum of the hand.

testing the motion of one on the other in a palmar-dorsal direction (Fig. 5.53). In the normal hand, little or no motion is possible. In the extreme case of palmar subluxation, the joint cannot be reduced (Fig. 5.54). Proximal-distal motion of the proximal phalanx may then be present and, when extreme, is referred to as *telescoping*.

Indications
The various agents producing ulnar drift should be dealt with as detailed in their respective sections. However, ulnar drift can only arise once the stabilizing influences have been removed. No satisfactory means of soft tissue reconstruction of the disrupted collateral ligament has been described. Attempts to correct ulnar drift by crossed intrinsic transfer into the adjacent proximal phalanx have showed a recurrence rate of 20% with an average loss of metacarpophalangeal motion of 27°.[60] Established ulnar drift and palmar subluxation are usually associated with pronounced destruction of cartilage and bone. For these reasons instability of the metacarpophalangeal joints is usually treated by arthroplasty. This may be excisional with or without tendon interposition as described by Vainio, Tupper and Fowler. More commonly replacement is performed using any of the several joints which have been described.[61] These are not without problems[62] but

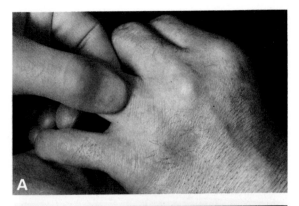

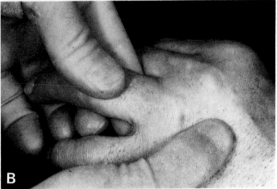

Fig. 5.53A & B. By gripping the hand and proximal phalanx of the digit under examination, subluxation of the phalanx on the metacarpal head can be detected by moving the proximal phalanx alternately dorsally and palmarwards on the metacarpal head.

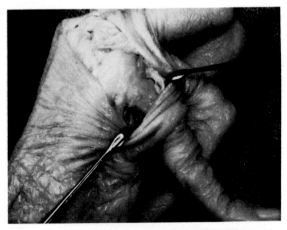

Fig. 5.54 At operation the relationship of the head of the metacarpal to the base of the proximal phalanx can be seen. Stress being applied to the tip of the small finger (Bottom left) is placing this metacarpophalangeal joint in maximum *extension*.

provide the best solution with good alignment and relief of pain and fair range of motion and grip strength.

Intrinsic muscles

Tightness of the intrinsic muscles of the hand contributes to several of the major problems of the rheumatoid patient:

    weakness of power grasp, (Fig. 5.55)

    ulnar drift,

    palmar subluxation of the metacarpophalangeal joints,

    swan neck deformity of the fingers.

The muscles primarily involved are the interossei and the lumbricals. The pathogenesis of intrinsic tightness has not been clearly established, but spasm provoked by the inflamed metacarpophalangeal joints is the probable cause.

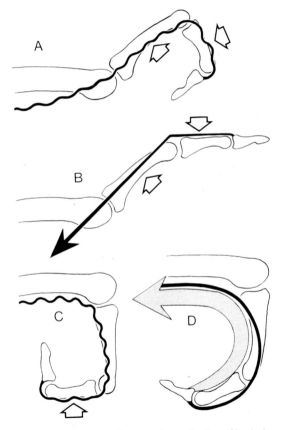

Fig. 5.55 This diagram illustrates the mechanism of intrinsic tightness. (A) In the normal finger the intrinsics are sufficiently loose to permit flexion of the proximal interphalangeal joint when the metacarpophalangeal joint is fully extended. (B) In intrinsic tightness the proximal interphalangeal joint cannot be flexed with the metacarpophalangeal in that position. (C) In relaxed flexion the intrinsics are loose in both the normal circumstance and also in the presence of intrinsic tightness. (D) In intrinsic tightness powerful flexion draws the flexor digitorum profundus proximally and therefore translocates the origin of the lumbrical. The intrinsic tightness then serves to paradoxically extend the interphalangeal joints, thereby resisting the power of flexion and resulting in weakness of grip.

Secondary fibrosis results in the fixed intrinsic contracture. In testing for intrinsic tightness, the examiner should firstly assess the range of passive joint motion and the extent to which that is impaired by joint disease or tendon adhesions.

The intrinsics flex the metacarpophalangeal joints and extend the interphalangeal joints. Therefore the test for tightness should be performed as follows:

1. Hold the metacarpophalangeal joint in full passive extension (Fig. 5.56).
2. Gently flex the proximal interphalangeal joint with the other hand. In the normal hand, full proximal interphalangeal joint flexion will be possible.

By contrast, in the presence of intrinsic tightness, firm, rather resilient, resistance will be encountered. The angle of the proximal interphalangeal joint at which this is met should be recorded (p. 139).

3. The metacarpophalangeal joint should now be allowed to fall progressively into flexion while keeping pressure applied to the middle phalanx. The proximal interphalangeal joint will flex further as the metacarpophalangeal joint is lowered from extension.

In pure intrinsic tightness, the proximal interphalangeal joint will flex fully once the metacarpophalangeal joint has been allowed to pass into flexion. The extent by which it fails to achieve full flexion is a measure of proximal interphalangeal joint disease or extrinsic tendon adhesion.

The test should then be repeated while deviating the finger both radially and ulnarwards. This will reveal whether the tightness in the initial test is primarily of the ulnar or radial intrinsics

ulnar — when more tightness is encountered with the finger deviated radially,
radial — when there is greater tightness in ulnar deviation.

Commonly, the ulnar intrinsics are significantly tighter than the radial.

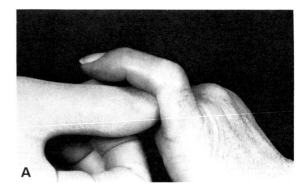

A

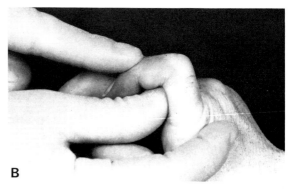

B

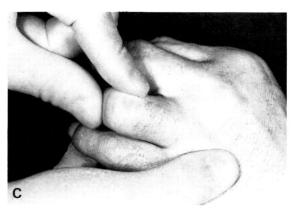

C

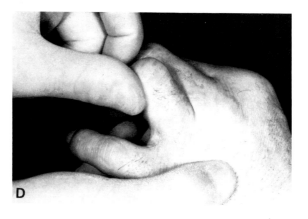

D

Fig. 5.56 Testing for intrinsic tightness. (A) The metacarpophalangeal joint is held in full extension. (B) The proximal interphalangeal joint is then fully flexed and resistance to this movement suggests tightness of the intrinsics. Differentiation between tightness in the radial and ulnar intrinsics can be achieved by deviating the digit into both radial and ulnar directions while in this intrinsic minus position (C and D).

Indications

Intrinsic release is possibly one of the swiftest and most effective procedures in surgical practice. Complete excision of the wing tendon (Fig. 5.57) as advocated by Littler should be employed, as its removal eliminates not only the lateral band tightness which causes the weakness of grasp and contributes to the swan neck deformity, but also that of the dorsal digital expansion which passes over the extrinsic extensor to form an extensor hood. Tightness of this expansion, together with the palmar moment of the flexor tendons, are the subluxing forces which dislocate the unstable metacarpophalangeal joint.

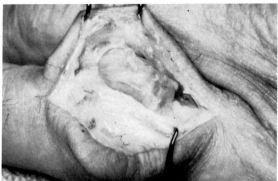

Fig. 5.58 The mass of diseased synovium is seen here being dissected from beneath the extensor apparatus at the proximal interphalangeal joint. The tip of the finger is to the left of the picture and the lateral bands and central slip are being supported by a retractor. The synovial mass has been dissected out entirely and is being gripped by the forceps in the lower part of the illustration.

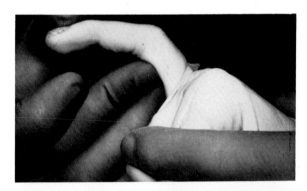

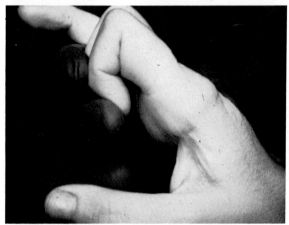

Fig. 5.57 The effect of intrinsic release. In (A) an unreleased finger is being stressed into flexion at the proximal interphalangeal joint with the metacarpophalangeal extended. In (B) two digits previously equally tight are being placed in the same position. The improvement in range is apparent.

medial and deep fibres of the lateral bands of the extensor tendon insert into the base of the middle phalanx. This firm tendinous insertion drives the bulging synovium proximally along the dorsum of the proximal phalanx. This has been called descriptively 'the synovial snail' (Fig. 5.58). The presence of synovium can be detected as in other joints, by fluctuation beneath the examiner's thumbs with the joint held in gentle flexion to some 45 degrees (Fig. 5.59).

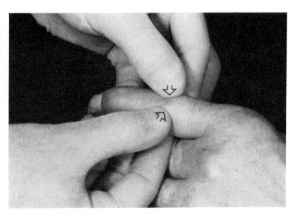

Fig. 5.59 Synovium is detected in the interphalangeal joint as a fluctuant swelling between the examiner's thumb.

Proximal interphalangeal joints

Synovium

The proximal interphalangeal joint of the rheumatoid patient is one of the earliest and most commonly afflicted. The synovium is driven dorsally by intra-articular pressures during flexion, where, as in other joints, it encounters less resistance. The central slip and the more

The destructive effect of synovitis on the soft tissues around the proximal interphalangeal joint depends on other forces acting on the joint and may take one of several forms

boutonniere deformity (Fig. 5.60)
swan neck deformity
joint destruction
lateral instability.

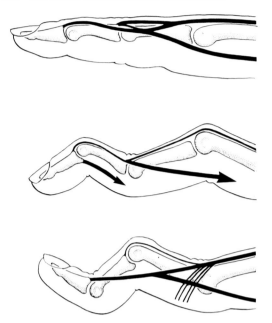

fibrous flexor tendon sheath. In resisted finger flexion, this cruciate portion moves away from the skeleton, as can be palpated quite distinctly in the normal hand, and this serves to stabilize the extensor apparatus and, by its embracing nature, the entire joint structure. In rheumatoid disease the 'synovial snail' stretches and often herniates through the weakest portion of the expansion which is that on either side of the central slip, between it and the lateral bands (Fig. 5.62). As this weakness increases, the lateral bands are pulled further anteriorly with each finger flexion by the transverse retinacular ligament. Flexor tenosynovitis, by stretching the flexor sheath, allows the flexor tendon to move further away from the skeleton, increasing the subluxing force applied to the lateral bands. The synovial erosion continues dorsally and, as in the

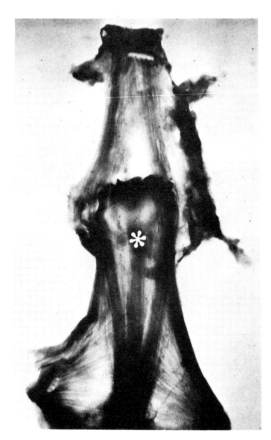

Fig. 5.60 The mechanism of development of swan neck and boutonniere deformities is shown here in diagrammatic form. In the upper figure the extrinsic and intrinsic tendons, the central slip and lateral bands bear their normal relationship to the finger joints. In the centre illustration, tightness of the intrinsics associated with disease in the proximal interphalangeal joint has resulted in hyperextension of the proximal interphalangeal joint with compensatory flexion at the distal interphalangeal joint. In the lowermost diagram, disease in the proximal interphalangeal joint has caused weakness in the central slip and disruption of the aponeurosis between the central slip and lateral bands which have consequently fallen below the axis of the joint and become flexors rather than extensors. As a result the proximal interphalangeal joint has gone into flexion and the distal interphalangeal joint assumed compensatory hyperextension.

BOUTONNIERE DEFORMITY[63] (Fig. 5.61)

The extensor apparatus of the proximal interphalangeal joint is braced against the joint by the transverse retinacular ligament. This thin but distinct structure overlies the collateral and accessory collateral ligaments laterally. Dorsally it blends with the surface of the extensor components and ventrally with the cruciate part of the

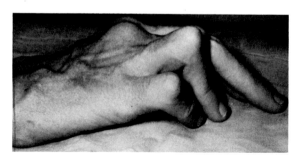

Fig. 5.61 Boutonniere deformity.

Fig. 5.62 This specimen of the entire extensor apparatus shows the central slip marked with an asterisk. Distal to the asterisks, towards the upper part of the photograph there is a weak point evident in the central slip. On either side of that the connection between the central slip and lateral bands can also be seen to be somewhat thinner than the other parts of the extensor apparatus. These thin areas are those which are eroded by synovium in the proximal interphalangeal joint allowing the lateral bands to slip palmarwards. Attached to the lateral bands are the transverse retinacular ligaments which connect the bands to the cruciate part of the fibrous flexor tendon sheath (dissection by Dr D. C. Riordan).

metacarpophalangeal joint of the thumb, causes weakening and eventually complete disruption of the central slip. This results in loss of extensor power.

Imbalance in favour of flexion at the proximal interphalangeal joint results in a flexion deformity and the Z-mechanism produces compensatory hyperextension at the metacarpophalangeal and distal interphalangeal joints. This deformity is initially *mobile*, that is, the joint shows a normal passive range of motion but later becomes *fixed*.[64]. Only the former is amenable to soft-tissue reconstruction.

SWAN NECK DEFORMITY (Fig. 5.63)[65]

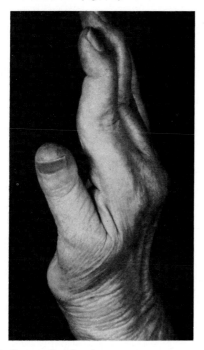

Fig. 5.63 Swan neck deformity.

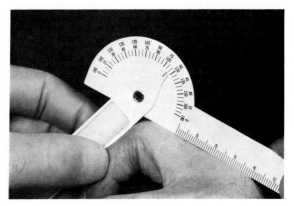

Fig. 5.64 The range of motion in the interphalangeal joints should be recorded using a goniometer.

in each joint in turn. Hyperextension is recorded as a negative value. This may be misleading if the negative sign is misunderstood or overlooked. This problem can be overcome by illustrating the measurement with a small stick diagram.

Instability
The proximal interphalangeal joint is often unstable in

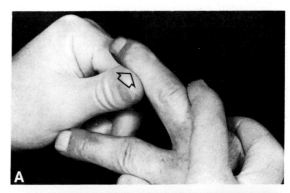

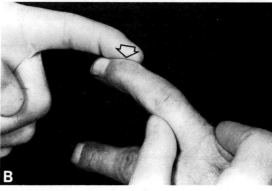

Fig. 5.65A & B Lateral stress should be applied in a three point fashion to test the collateral ligaments on both the ulnar and radial aspects of all interphalangeal joints in maximum extension.

This deformity also has its basis in weakening of the periarticular structures of the proximal interphalangeal joint by active synovitis. The abnormal force applied to the joint is tightness of the intrinsic muscles. Some believe that swan neck will develop only with decreased flexor power, this resulting from synovitis around the flexor digitorum superficialis. The resultant hyperextension of the joint is initially added to a normal range of motion. However, joint disease allied to the inability of the weakened flexors to pull the middle phalanx around the head of the proximal phalanx from the increasingly hyperextended position results in a decreased range of motion. The Z-mechanism causes flexion in both distal interphalangeal and metacarpophalangeal joints.

Range of motion (Fig. 5.64)
The range of motion should be recorded with a goniometer

swan neck deformity as described above. Lateral instability should be tested by applying three point stress with the finger in extension (Fig. 5.65). If the joint cannot be fully extended, too much importance should not be laid on minor degrees of apparent lateral instability (p. 142).

Indications

Early *swan neck* deformity, that is before irreversible changes occur in the articular surface, can be corrected by
1. intrinsic release to eliminate the deforming force,
2. flexor synovectomy when synovitis is present,
3. correction of the hyperextension, which may be achieved by capsulodesis or by tenodesis.

Early, mobile *boutonniere* deformity may be improved by synovectomy and reconstruction of the extensor apparatus. This is an operation in which it is difficult to achieve improvement as is attested to by the large number of described procedures[66-75].

Advanced proximal interphalangeal deformities are amongst the most difficult to correct. Thus, the indications for synovectomy and intrinsic release are applied at an early juncture. Those for synovectomy are
1. Persistent intractable painful synovitis;
2. Early erosions seen on radiological examination;
    These are best seen on true anteroposterior and lateral views using a dental plate (Fig. 5.66);

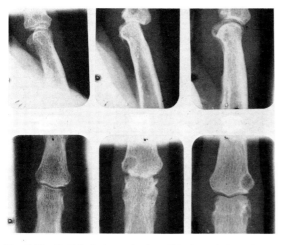

Fig. 5.66 Radiological examination of the interphalangeal joints in the rheumatoid patient is best performed using dental films which allow true anteroposterior and lateral films to be obtained.

3. Incipient boutonniere deformity as evidenced by synovitis associated with some lag to proximal interphalangeal joint extension.

Synovectomy of the proximal interphalangeal joint has been shown to result in significant relief of pain and improvement of grip strength in 60% of patients five years after surgery[76] and even to result in the healing of small erosions[77]. Flexor tendon disease has great significance in limiting motion of the proximal interphalangeal joint (p. 283).

Advanced swan neck or boutonniere with articular changes, lateral instability or joint destruction precludes soft tissue reconstruction. The choice lies between

stabilization — by formal arthrodesis or by peg stabilization[78], and
replacement arthroplasty.

The choice is made according to the extent of disease in other parts of the hand, especially in the metacarpophalangeal joints and in the tendons acting on the proximal interphalangeal joint, the age and occupation of the patient and the digit which requires treatment. The index finger most requires stability for pinch manoeuvres and stabilization is there more often indicated than in the ulnar digits where a range of motion is required for power grasp. In those digits therefore the poorer the range of motion in the metacarpophalangeal joint, the more replacement arthroplasty is indicated.

Distal interphalangeal joint

Rheumatoid synovitis is uncommon in the distal interphalangeal joint when compared with its incidence in other joints of the hand. Indeed, the presence of synovitis in the distal joint should arouse the examiner's suspicion that the patient is suffering not from rheumatoid disease but from *psoriasis* which is especially likely to cause distal joint disease.

The distal joint is certainly affected by classical rheumatoid but mainly in a secondary manner consequent upon proximal interphalangeal joint deformities. Deformity of the distal joint in both swan neck and boutonniere deformities of the proximal interphalangeal joint is initially mobile, but later fixed. In the boutonniere especially, correction of a fixed contracture of the proximal interphalangeal joint must often be accompanied by attention to the distal interphalangeal joint. In almost all instances arthrodesis or peg stabilization is the procedure most likely to aid function. The angle at which fusion is performed increases from radial to ulnar across the four digits.

Flexor tendons

Synovium

A smoothly contoured swelling proximal to the wrist creases is evidence of increase in the volume of synovium beneath the flexor retinaculum. This swelling can be seen to move a little proximally as the fingers are flexed. The presence of synovium in the digital sheaths is suggested if the skin over the proximal phalanges especially is unnaturally tense and shiny.

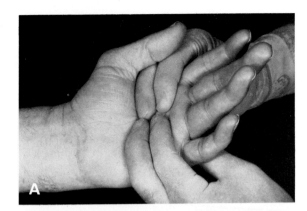

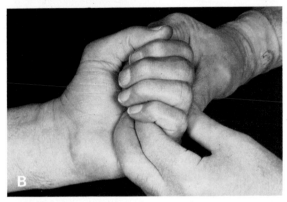

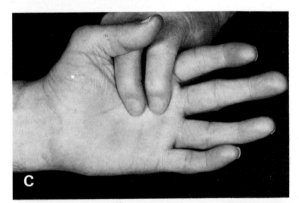

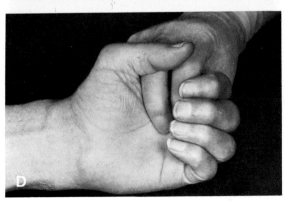

Fig. 5.67 A. The index and middle fingers of both hands of the examiner are placed across the palm of the patient and the patient is then asked to flex the fingers strongly, B. Crepitation can be detected in those synovial sheaths in which synovitis is present. This can be further localized by palpating the sheaths individually as in C and D, while the patient repeats the manoeuvre.

By supporting the supinated hand with his thumbs and placing the index and middle fingers of both hands across the palm so that the middle fingers are in contact with one another at the level of the palmar creases, the examiner is able to palpate the region of the flexor tendons as they emerge from the digital sheaths (Fig. 5.67). If the patient is then asked to slowly close all the fingers down over those of the examiner, the crepitus created by increased, diseased synovium can be detected. By adjusting the finger tips to lie over each sheath in turn, the examiner can localise which tendons are involved. Not uncommonly, one or two fingers are involved and the others not. Further evidence of this selective involvement is gained by then asking the patient to open and close the hand repetitively as rapidly as possible. This may reveal that there is a 'slow finger' which flexes out of phase with the others, indicating active flexor synovitis even to the extent of causing a 'trigger finger'.

Trigger finger in rheumatoid disease may be due to locking at the proximal pulley as in non-rheumatoid patients. However, it may equally be caused by a nodule of synovium in the tendon, catching in the bifurcation of the flexor digitorum superficialis (Fig. 5.68).

A 'slow finger' can also be caused by a swan neck deformity, flexion of the proximal interphalangeal joint being delayed until sufficient force has been generated by the flexor tendon to pull the middle phalanx around the head of the proximal phalanx (Fig. 5.69).

Palpation of the wrist in similar manner to that described above during finger flexion will detect crepitations due to diseased synovium.

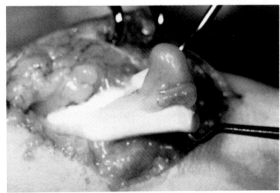

Fig. 5.68 This intratendinous nodule on the flexor digitorum profundus produced locking of the finger by blocking on the bifurcation of the flexor digitorum superficialis.

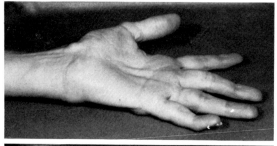

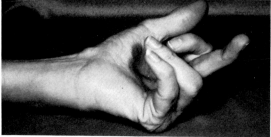

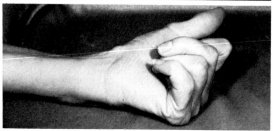

Fig. 5.69 A 'slow' finger. As this hand is closed so the swan-neck deformity of the middle finger causes it to delay, (B) until increasing force of the flexor tendons pulls it suddenly and painfully around the head of the proximal phalanx into flexion (C).

NERVE COMPRESSION

Significant increase in the volume of synovium around the flexor tendons in the carpal tunnel may cause compression of the median nerve with typical symptoms of carpal tunnel syndrome (p. 194) — numbness and paraesthesia in the median nerve distribution and weakness and atrophy of the thenar muscles. More rarely, the sensory and motor loss will be in the distribution of the ulnar nerve indicating compression in Guyon's canal (p. 204).

The radial nerve may also be compressed by synovitis around the radial head, resulting in a posterior interosseous syndrome (p. 217).

It is important to seek these pathognomonic symptoms and signs in the rheumatoid patient who will frequently fail to volunteer them, either because they have been masked by his many other problems or because he or she believes that they are of little consequence by comparison.

TENDON RUPTURE

Rupture of tendons occurs as a result of interference with their blood supply and also of intratendinous infiltration of

synovium. At surgery, smooth, relatively firm nodules of visceral synovium are found penetrating deeply between the tendon fibres. Individual testing of each flexor tendon should therefore be performed as described elsewhere. Weakness and pain on resisted flexion have less significance than in the injured tendon, since it is not possible to determine to what extent they are due to the synovitis itself or to impending rupture. Frequently tendon adhesions coexist with ruptures and incomplete tendon erosions. Thus the surgeon undertaking flexor syno-vectomy must prepare the patient for possible tendon graft and distal interphalangeal joint fusion and prepare himself for an often perplexing encounter.

Indications
Release of the carpal tunnel with complete flexor

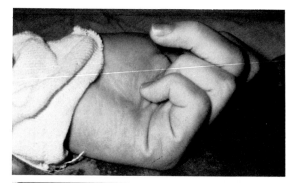

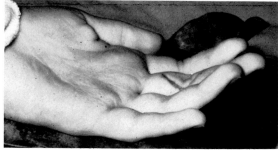

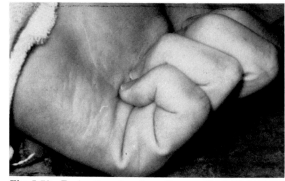

Fig. 5.70 Exploration of a trigger finger under local anaesthesia (A) The patient is unable to form a full fist. (B) A nodule could be palpated over the proximal interphalangeal joint (figure 5.68). Excision resulted in full flexion (C).

synovectomy is indicated in the presence of median nerve compression. Trigger fingers should be treated by synovectomy where indicated, particular attention being paid to the presence of intratendinous nodules of synovium which may be the primary cause of the triggering. Wherever possible, the A₁ pulley should be preserved for its excision will increase the force of the ulnar moment of the flexor on the metacarpophalangeal joint. Where meticulous synovectomy does not eliminate triggering, one slip of the superficialis should be excised rather than incur that risk[79]. When triggering alone is being treated, surgery should be done under wrist block to ensure full active function after treatment (Fig. 5.70). The efficacy of flexor tenosynovectomy is considerable in improving motion in the proximal interphalangeal joint — in one series the range increased by from 40° – 84°[80].

Synovectomy is indicated whenever a significant bulk of synovium is detected around the flexor tendons (Fig. 5.71).

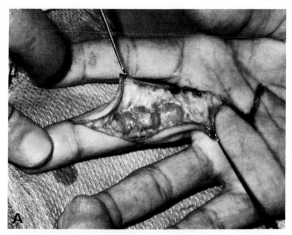
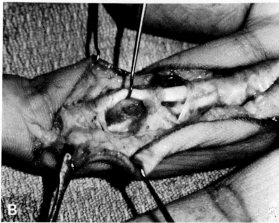

Fig. 5.71 Through a Bruner incision the flexor tendon sheath has been displayed in this patient with rheumatoid flexor synovitis. (A) The bulging, particularly of the cruciate part of the tendon sheath, is clearly to be seen. (B) When the tendon sheath is opened the extensive nature of the diseased synovium can be appreciated.

Delay in this situation is not justified, largely because it is not possible to determine clinically to what extent tendon erosion has progressed and also because the results of tendon graft in the rheumatoid patient are too poor to justify the risk of delay. When rupture is encountered, it should be managed as follows:

flexor pollicis longus — graft
flexor digitorum profundus — fuse distal interphalangeal joint
both FDS and FDP — transfer adjacent FDS to FDP.

Radiological assessment

All patients complaining of rheumatoid disease in the upper limb should undergo radiological examination of

neck — especially requesting lateral views taken in extension and flexion,
elbow
wrist and hands, including Brewerton views of the metacarpophalangeal joints.

As emphasized above, all rheumatoid patients are in danger of cervical cord compression and transection (p. 257).

The *Brewerton view*[81] of the metacarpophalangeal joints is taken with the fingers flat on the plate, the metacarpals at

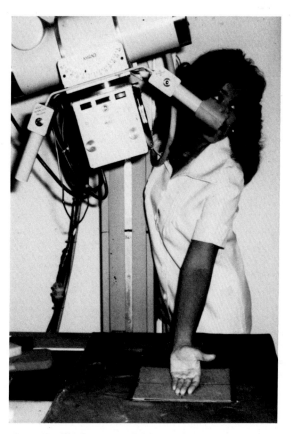

Fig. 5.72 *The Brewerton view* (see text).

65 degrees inclination to them and the tube at 15 degrees from the ulnar side of the hand (Fig. 5.72). In early rheumatoid disease, when the standard anteroposterior view of the hand shows little change, the Brewerton view may show a surprising amount of bony erosion beneath the collateral ligaments of the metacarpophalangeal joints.

Apart from these standard views, X-rays should be taken of any other joints of which the patient specifically complains. In the severely diseased hand, the standard views do not always demonstrate the proximal interphalangeal joints clearly, in which case true individual anteroposterior and lateral views should be taken of each proximal interphalangeal joint.

In all joints involved by rheumatoid disease, the changes are similar on X-ray examination, in order of appearance.

> *loss of joint space* — due to loss of articular surface, this may be seen relatively early in the patient's clinical course, but is evidence of fairly advanced disease;
> *bony erosions* — bony erosion is always evidence of advanced rheumatoid disease;
> *subluxation;*
> *ankylosis.*

'Egg-cup' deformity is encountered on occasion in the metacarpophalangeal joint (Fig. 5.73). This nomenclature is used when the erosion in that joint is into the base of the proximal phalanx, the head of the metacarpal being bluntly conical. No subluxation or ulnar drift of significance accompanies this deformity, and the patient usually has a good range of motion with little pain. No surgical intervention is indicated.

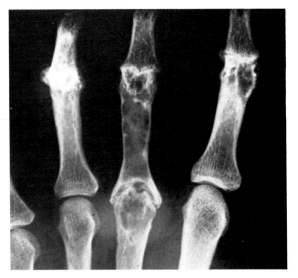

Fig. 5.73 This X-ray demonstrates an 'egg cup deformity' of the metacarpophalangeal joint of the middle finger. In this no subluxation or deviation has occurred and the erosion in the metacarpophalangeal joint is at the base of the proximal phalanx. This commonly results in a painfree joint having an excellent range of motion. No surgical intervention is indicated.

Giant bone cysts may occur in conjunction with rheumatoid disease, most commonly in the ulnar head[82].

As several authors have emphasized, the assessment of rheumatoid disease is made clinically, not radiologically. Quite frequently, patients with severe clinical disease show little X-ray change. Less often the converse is true.

RHEUMATOID VARIANTS

Certain patients, while having polyarthritis apparently indistinguishable from rheumatoid arthritis, show certain features which set them in a different category.

Juvenile rheumatoid arthritis (JRA)[83]
This presents in three different clinical forms

1. *systemic onset type JRA* (Still's disease[84]) is characterised by polyarthritis associated with systemic manifestations such as *uveitis, pericarditis, splenomegaly, hepatomegaly,* and *fever.*
2. *polyarticular JRA* is very similar to the adult form of the disease by distribution, although having different effects as outlined below. This is the most likely form to continue unabated into adult rheumatoid disease.
3. *mono-articular or pauci-articular JRA* affects four or less joints. In one series[85], 32% progressed to involve other joints at a later stage. Eye problems were common.

The great majority of children with JRA are sero-negative. The deformities in the upper extremity are often quite different from the adult form —

> shortening of the ulna
> flexion and *ulnar* deviation of the wrist, often progressing to ankylosis
> *radial* deviation and loss of flexion of the metacarpophalangeal joints (Fig. 5.74)
> boutonniere common (swan-neck rare)

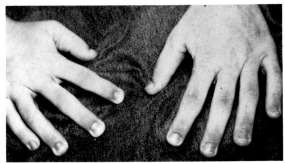

Fig. 5.74 *Juvenile rheumatoid arthritis.* The ulnar deviation at the wrist with radial drift of the fingers commonly encountered in juvenile rheumatoid disease.

Knowing the dynamics of the hand one can see how the deformities might develop progressively from polyarthritis and destruction of the ulnar epiphysis. Similarly it can be seen that the key to management is splintage of the wrist in good position at virtually all times. Regular therapy to maintain finger motion during the day allied to night resting splints will help to prevent deformity. Surgery has little part to play although, contrary to general belief, synovectomy has been shown in one series to cause no harm[86].

Ankylosing spondylitis

This condition usually commences at the sacroiliac joints and involves the spine. Clinically, the diagnosis can be made on the basis of five specific historic features[87]

> back pain of insidious onset
> patient under 40 (M/F = 10/1)
> present for more than 3 months
> morning stiffness which
> improves with exercise.

20% show peripheral arthritis indistinguishable from rheumatoid disease, although there is a much greater tendency to ankylosis of joints than to their destruction. Less than ten percent show positive tests for rheumatoid factor. The HLA type B27[88] is present in the serum of well over 90% of patients with ankylosing spondylitis as compared with 4% of the general population.

Systemic lupus erythematosus[89] (S.L.E.)

S.L.E. causes painful, swollen, but rarely destroyed, joints. If deformity does occur it is due to ligamentous laxity and takes the form of subluxation, with *little evidence of X-ray changes*. Swan-neck deformities and hyperextension of the interphalangeal joint of the thumb are common but the first is not accompanied by intrinsic tightness nor the latter by a flexion contracture of the metacarpophalangeal joint. In the rare cases in whom destruction and X-ray changes do occur then some 'overlap' of rheumatoid and systemic lupus erythematosus is probable.

Raynaud's phenomenon is found in some 50% of these patients (p. 184) and may be responsible for the major part of the symptoms in the hand.

Where ligamentous laxity becomes extreme to the point of impairing hand function, resection of a subluxed ulnar head and stabilisation of the basal joint of the thumb are of value. Other, soft tissue, procedures are not generally successful and in severe deformities, arthroplasty of the wrist or metacarpophalangeal joints may be necessary[90].

Systemic sclerosis

Scleroderma shows polyarthritis but the joint deformities result from fibrous contractures of skin and muscle rather than from erosive synovitis. However, when it presents as a polyarthritis without any of its other features, it may not be possible to distinguish it from rheumatoid, especially since 20 to 40% will be sero-positive. Other manifestations should therefore be sought in patients presenting with joint deformity, muscle wasting but little bony change. *Calcinosis circumscripta* can occur independently but in the majority of cases is associated with scleroderma[91] (Fig. 5.75).

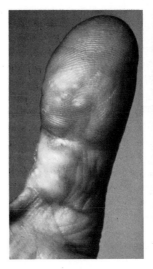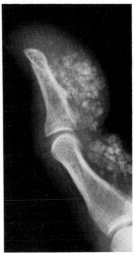

Fig. 5.75 *Calcinosis circumscripta* in a patient with systemic sclerosis. Excision of the calcific nodular deposits may relieve the discomfort they cause, but caution is required since healing in scleroderma is not normal.

In scleroderma the hand surgeon can only be of assistance by

1. prescribing careful splintage and active and passive exercise to prevent contracture,
2. urgently treating early infections which will otherwise progress to extensive ulceration.

Mixed connective tissue disease (MCTD)[92]

This disorder has features in common with both lupus and scleroderma; the majority of patients show Raynaud's phenomenon and also decreased oesophageal motility. Serology can distinguish between the three disorders, of which MCTD appears most responsive to steroid therapy.

The striking feature in the hands of patients with MCTD is *tightness of the long flexors*, resulting in a significant decrease in finger extension, which progressively worsens with wrist extension. Less common manifestations are intrinsic tightness and boutonniere deformity of the thumb.

Psoriatic arthritis

Psoriatic arthritis[93] may resemble rheumatoid very closely.

However, it is distinguished by several features

    sero-negative rheumatoid factor
    absence of rheumatoid nodules
    presence of a typical skin rash
    involvement of the distal interphalangeal joints

and radiologically,

    osteolysis of the distal phalanges
    cortical erosions of the phalangeal shafts
    periosteal new bone formation near the joints.

Usually the deformity shows much less destruction of articular cartilage and deformities are due more to contracture than collapse, although a small minority may show *arthritis mutilans* (p. 254). Surgery is undertaken later than in rheumatoid disease and is designed to overcome deformity, for example of the metacarpophalangeal joints by metacarpal osteotomy[94].

Ulcerative colitis; Regional enteritis (Crohn's)

Patients with colitis or enteritis often show transient arthritis of the peripheral joints. Only 10% of these progress to classical rheumatoid-like changes. Sero-negative, if these patients are cured of their visceral disorder, their arthritis invariably shows marked improvement.

Behcet's syndrome (= mucocutaneous ocular syndrome)

This condition, probably a cell-mediated immunological response, has many varied manifestations, major amongst which are recurrent oral and genital ulceration and relapsing iritis.

Arthritis is common, usually occurring long after the onset, and resembling the arthropathy of ulcerative colitis. It usually effects the elbow and wrist and is not associated with permanent changes. The sedimentation rate is increased and the patients are sero-negative for rheumatoid factor.

Reiter's syndrome

    Polyarthritis
    Non-gonococcal urethritis
    Conjunctivitis

Mucocutaneous papules, vesicles or pustules are often encountered on the glans penis, the soles and palms and in the mouth. Sero-negative, their joint changes are usually transitory but may show recurrent exacerbations. Diagnosis then rests on the other manifestations. As with ankylosing spondylitis, the incidence of B27-positive cases is very high.

Other forms of so-called *reactive arthritis* have been described in association with infections by *Salmonella, Yersimia, Brucella,* and *Gonococcus.*

Surgical planning

Choosing the time at which to operate on the rheumatoid patient depends upon the stage of their disease, the degree of their disability, priority with respect to other parts of the body and convenience in their normal work and social schedule. This latter consideration is of more importance in the rheumatoid than in others, for several surgical assaults can be anticipated over the years. Urgency exists with respect to nerve compression and tendon rupture or the threat of it, most commonly by extensor synovitis and a dislocated ulnar head. Synovectomy is prophylactic in protecting tendons at the dorsal wrist and in the proximal interphalangeal joint. It appears to improve function and may have some protective value in the elbow joint and in the flexor tendons. Its merits in other areas are unproven. Soft tissue reconstruction is of benefit in the presence of good articular cartilage in deformities of the thumb and in mobile boutonniere or swan-neck deformities.

Once joints are irrevocably deformed or destroyed, the surgeon must be aware of the functional needs in each joint. Stability is required in the wrist, the metacarpophalangeal and interphalangeal joints of the thumb and the distal interphalangeal joints of the fingers. Mobility is required in *one* elbow, the basal joint of the thumb and the metacarpophalangeal joints of the fingers. Hence, ankylosis in the first group and instability in the second is not nearly as disabling as if the situation were reversed. It follows further that arthrodesis of the first group and arthroplasty of the second are the required procedures, modified only by such considerations as the need for one flexed or flexible wrist to reach the perineum. Only the proximal interphalangeal joints remain in limbo: they do well with arthrodesis in the index finger and in the others if the metacarpophalangeal joints show a good range; they require arthroplasty if those joints do not show motion and cannot be made to do so. The minimal aims in treating the rheumatoid finger is to achieve coordinate motion of all fingers at one of the joints at least, with the non-mobile joints in a functional position and the whole finger complex showing good lateral stability.

Consulting the summary sheet and remembering the need for compatibility of simultaneous operations during postoperative care and therapy, the surgeon should construct a surgical programme with the patient. If to do so would not ignore priorities imposed by specific patient problems, the programme should work from proximal to distal. It should combine procedures which are complementary and serve to remove at the same operation mutually deforming disorders. For example, the correction of radial deviation of the wrist with metacarpophalangeal joint replacement is logical[95]. Finally, the necessary work under tourniquet control should be limited to one inflation time, that is, a maximum of two hours. Second inflation greatly increases oedema, with resultant difficulty in skin closure and in early postoperative mobilization. It is also likely that the rheumatoid patient, resourceful and uncomplaining though he undoubtedly is, suffers untold discomfort in other parts from prolonged periods on the operating table. Further, recovery, rehabilitation and therefore return for other necessary surgery are all speeded by so limiting our endeavours.

REFERENCES

1. Labbate V A, Ehrlich E E 1976 Rheumatoid arthritis with unusual myositis resembling muscular dystrophy. Journal of Bone and Joint Surgery 58A: 571–572

2. Garner R W, Mowat A G, Hazleman B L 1973 Wound healing after operations on patients with rheumatoid arthritis. Journal of Bone and Joint Surgery 55B: 134–144

3. Cervantes-Perez Col P, Toro-Perez Col A H, Rodriguez-Jurado P 1980 Pulmonary involvement in rheumatoid arthritis. Journal of The American Medical Association 243: 1715–1719

4. Caplan A 1953 Certain unusual appearances in the chest of coal miners suffering from rheumatoid arthritis. Thorax 8: 29–37

5. Felty A R 1924 Chronic arthritis in the adult associated with splenomegaly and leukopenia. Bulletin of John Hopkins Hospital 35: 16–20

6. Sjogren H 1933 A new conception of kerato conjunctivitis sicca. Acta Ophthal Kbh Supp. 2: 1

7. Froimson A I 1971 Hand reconstruction in arthritis mutilans. Journal of Bone and Joint Surgery 53A: 1377–1382

8. Nalebuff E A, Garrett J 1976 Opera-glass hand in rheumatoid arthritis. The Journal of Hand Surgery 1: 210–220

9. Williams H J, Biddulph E C, Coleman S S, Ward J R 1977 Isolated subcutaneous nodules (Pseudorheumatoid). Journal of Bone and Joint Surgery 59A: 73–76

10. Sadeghpour E, Noer H R, Mahinpour S 1981 Skull-C2 fusion in rheumatoid patients with atlanto-axial subluxation. Orthopedics 4: 1369–1374

11. Ranawat C S, O'Leary P, Pellicci P, Tsairis P, Marchisello P, Dorr L 1979 Cervical spine fusion in rheumatoid arthritis. Journal of Bone and Joint Surgery 61A: 1003–1010

12. Rana N A, Hancock D O, Taylor A R, Hill A G S 1973 Atlanto-axial subluxation in rheumatoid arthritis. Journal of Bone and Joint Surgery 55B: 458–470

13. Rana N A, Hancock D O, Taylor A R, Hill A G S 1973 Upward translocation of the dens in rheumatoid arthritis. Journal of Bone and Joint Surgery 55B: 471–477

14. Pellicci P M, Ranawat C S, Tsairis P, Bryan W J 1981 A prospective study of the progression of rheumatoid arthritis of the cervical spine. Journal of Bone and Joint Surgery 63A: 342–350

15. Copeland S A, Taylor J G 1979 Synovectomy of the elbow in rheumatoid arthritis. Journal of Bone and Joint Surgery 61B: 69–74

16. Inglis A E, Ranawat C S, Straub L R 1971 Synovectomy and debridement of the elbow in rheumatoid arthritis. Journal of Bone and Joint Surgery 53A: 652–662

17. Marmor L 1972 Surgery of the rheumatoid elbow. Follow-up study on synovectomy combined with radial head excision. Journal of Bone and Joint Surgery 54A: 573–578

18. Wilson D W 1973 Synovectomy of the elbow in rheumatoid arthritis. Journal of Bone and Joint Surgery 55B 106–111

19. Pritchard R 1979 Semiconstrained elbow prosthesis. A clinical review of five years of experience. Orthopaedic Review 8: 33–43

20. Kudo H, Iwano K, Watanabe S 1980 Total replacement of the rheumatoid elbow with a hingeless prosthesis. Journal of Bone and Joint Surgery 62A: 277–285

21. Pritchard R W 1981 Long-term follow-up study: Semi-constrained elbow prosthesis. Orthopedics 4: 151–155

22. Ewald F C, Scheinberg R D, Poss R, Thomas W H, Scott R D, Sledge C B 1980 Capitellocondylar total elbow arthroplasty. Journal of Bone and Joint Surgery 62A: 1259–1263

23. Morrey B F, Bryan R S, Dobyns J H, Linscheid R L 1981 Total elbow arthroplasty. A five year experience at the Mayo Clinic 63A: 1050–1063

24. Inglis A E, Pellicci P M 1980 Total elbow replacement. Journal of Bone and Joint Surgery 62A: 1252–1258

25. Taylor A R, Mukerjea S K, Rana N A 1976 Excision of the head of the radius in rheumatoid arthritis. Journal of Bone and Joint Surgery 58B: 485–487

26. Mayhall W S T, Tiley F T, Paluska D J 1981 Fracture of silastic radial-head prosthesis. Case report. Journal of Bone and Joint Surgery 63A: 459–460

27. Morrey B F, Askew L , Chao E T 1981 Silastic prosthetic replacement for the radial head. Journal of Bone and Joint Surgery 63A: 454–458

28. Bohl W R, Brightman E 1981 Fracture of a silastic radial-head prosthesis: diagnosis and localization of fragments by xerography. The Journal of Bone and Joint Surgery 63A: 1482–1483

29. Jackson I T, Simpson R G 1979 Interpositional arthroplasty of the wrist in rheumatoid arthritis. The Hand 11: 169–175

30. Straub L R, Ranawat C S 1969 The wrist in rheumatoid arthritis. The Journal of Bone and Joint Surgery 51A: 1–20

31. Clayton M L 1965 Surgical treatment at the wrist in rheumatoid arthritis. Journal of Bone and Joint Surgery 47A: 741–750

32. Kulick R G, DeFiore J C, Straub L R, Ranawat C S 1981 Long-term results of dorsal stabilization in the rheumatoid wrist. Journal of Hand Surgery 6: 272–280

33. Lamberta F J, Ferlic D C, Clayton M L 1980 Volz total wrist arthroplasty in rheumatoid arthritis: A preliminary report. Journal of Hand Surgery 5: 245–252

34. Goodman M J, Millender L H, Nalebuff E A, Philips C A 1980 Arthroplasty of the rheumatoid wrist with silicone rubber: An early evaluation. The Journal of Bone and Joint Surgery 5: 114–121

35. Haddad R J, Riordan D C 1967 Arthrodesis of the wrist. Journal of Bone and Joint Surgery 49A: 950–954

36. Mikkelsen O T 1980 Arthrodesis of the wrist joint in rheumatoid arthritis. The Hand 12: 149–153

37. Millender L H, Nalebuff E A 1973 Arthrodesis of the rheumatoid wrist. Journal of Bone and Joint Surgery 55A: 1026–1234

38. Rana N A, Taylor A R 1973 Excision of the distal end of the ulna in rheumatoid arthritis. Journal of Bone and Joint Surgery 55B: 96–105

39. Ansell B M, Harrison S H 1974 The results of ulna styloidectomy in rheumatoid arthritis. Scandinavian Journal of Rheumatology 3: 67

40. Straub L R, Wilson E H 1956 Spontaneous rupture of extensor tendons in the hand associated with rheumatoid arthritis. Journal of Bone and Joint Surgery 38A: 1208–1217

41. Millender L H, Nalebuff E A, Holdsworth D E 1973 Posterior interosseous nerve syndrome secondary to rheumatoid synovitis. Journal of Bone and Joint Surgery 55A: 753–757

42. Nalebuff E A 1969 Surgical treatment of tendon rupture in the rheumatoid hand. Surgical Clinics of North America 49: 811–822

43. Nalebuff E A, Patel M R 1973 Flexor digitorum superficialis transfer for multiple extensor tendon ruptures in rheumatoid arthritis. Plastic and Reconstructive Surgery 52: 530–533

44. Nalebuff E A 1968 Diagnosis classification and management of rheumatoid thumb deformities. Bulletin of Hospital Joint Diseases 29: 119–137

45. Inglis A E, Hamlin C, Sengelmann R P 1972 Reconstruction of the metacarpophalangeal joint of the thumb in rheumatoid arthritis Journal of Bone and Joint Surgery 54A: 704–712

46. Harrison S, Smith P, Maxwell D 1977 Stabilization of the first metacarpophalangeal and terminal joints of the thumb. The Hand 9: 242–249

47. Swanson A B, Herndon J H 1977 Flexible (silicone) implant arthroplasty of the metacarpophalangeal joint of the thumb. Journal of Bone and Joint Surgery 59A: 362–368

48. Kessler R 1973 Aetiology and management of adduction contracture of the thumb in rheumatoid arthritis. The Hand 5: 170–174

49. Millender L, Nalebuff E, Amadio P, Philips C 1978 Interpositional arthroplasty for rheumatoid carpometacarpal joint disease. Journal of Hand Surgery 3: 533

50. Kessler I 1979 A simplified technique to correct hyperextension deformity of the metacarpophalangeal joint of the thumb. Journal of Bone and Joint Surgery 61A: 903–905

51. Zancolli E 1970 Arthritic ulnar drift. An operation for metacarpophalangeal dislocation before cartilage destruction. Journal of Bone and Joint Surgery 52A: 1067

52. Ellison M R, Kelly K J, Flatt A E 1971 The results of surgical synovectomy of the digital joints in rheumatoid disease. Journal of Bone and Joint Surgery 53A: 1041–1060

53. McMaster M 1972 The natural history of the rheumatoid metacarpophalangeal joint. Journal of Bone and Joint Surgery 54B: 687–697

54. Smith R J, Kaplan E B 1967 Rheumatoid deformities at the metacarpophalangeal joints of the fingers. The Journal of Bone and Joint Surgery 49A: 31–47

55. Hakstian R W, Tubiana R 1968 Ulnar deviation of the fingers. The Journal of Bone and Joint Surgery 49A: 299–316

56. Backhouse K M 1968 Mechanics of normal digital control in the hand and an analysis of ulnar drift of the rheumatoid hand. Annals of Royal College of Surgeons of England 43: 154–173

57. Flatt A E The care of the rheumatoid hand, 2nd edn. C V Mosby, St Louis. In press

58. Pahle J.A., Raunio P. 1969 Influence of wrist position on finger deviation in rheumatoid arthritis. The Journal of Bone and Joint Surgery 51B: 664–676

59. Wise K S 1975 The anatomy of the metacarpo-phalangeal joints, with observations of the aetiology of ulnar drift. The Journal of Bone and Joint Surgery 57B: 485–490

60. Ellison M R, Flatt A E, Kelly K J 1974 Ulnar drift of the finger in rheumatoid disease. Journal of Bone and Joint Disease 53A: 1061–1082

61. Swanson A B 1973 Flexible implant arthroplasty in the hand and extremities. C V Mosby, St Louis

62. Beckenbaugh R D, Dobyns J H, Linscheid R L, Bryan R S 1976 Review and analysis of silicone-rubber metacarpophalangeal implants. Journal of Bone and Joint Surgery 58A: 483–487

63. Nalebuff E A, Millender L H 1975 Surgical treatment of the boutonniere deformity in rheumatoid arthritis. Orthopedic Clinics of North America 6: 753–763

64. Heywood A W B 1969 Correction of the rheumatoid boutonniere deformity. Journal of Bone and Joint Surgery 51A: 1309–1314

65. Nalebuff E A, Millender L H 1975 Surgical treatment of the swan-neck deformity in rheumatoid arthritis. Orthopedic Clinics of North America 6: 733–752

66. Dolphin J A 1965 Extensor tenotomy for chronic boutonniere deformity of the finger. Journal of Bone and Joint Surgery 47A: 161–164

67. Harris C, Rutledge G L 1972 The functional anatomy of the extensor mechanism of the finger. Journal of Bone and Joint Surgery 54A: 713–726

68. Kilgore E S, Graham W P 1968 Operative treatment of boutonniere deformity. Surgery 64: 999–1000

69. Littler J W, Eaton R G 1967 Redistribution of forces in the correction of the boutonniere deformity. Journal of Bone and Joint Surgery 49A: 1267–1274

70. Matev I 1964 Transposition of the lateral slips of the aponeurosis of long-standing boutonniere deformity of the fingers. British Journal of Plastic Surgery 17: 281–286

71. Salvi V 1969 Technique for the bottonhole deformity. The Hand 1: 96–97

72. Snow J W 1976 A method for reconstruction of the central slip of the extensor tendon of a finger. Plastic and Reconstructive Surgery 57: 455–459

73. Souter W A 1974 The problem of boutonniere deformity. Clinical Orthopaedics 104: 116–133

74. Urbaniak J R, Hayes M G 1981 Chronic boutonniere deformity — An anatomic reconstruction. Journal of Hand Surgery 6: 379–383

75. Weeks P M 1967 The chronic boutonniere deformity: A method of repair. Plastic and Reconstructive Surgery 40: 248–251

76. Ansell B, Harrison S 1975 A five year follow-up of synovectomy of the proximal interphalangeal joint in rheumatoid arthritis. The Hand 7: 34–36

77. Ansell B M, Harrison S H, Little H, Thouas B 1970 Synovectomy of proximal interphalangeal joints. British Journal of Plastic Surgery 23: 380–385

78. Harrison S H 1974 The Harrison Nicolle intramedullary peg. Follow-up study of 100 cases. The Hand 6: 304–307

79. Ferlic D, Clayton M 1978 Flexor tenosynovectomy in the rheumatoid finger. Journal of Hand Surgery 3: 364–367

80. Mills M B, Millender L H, Nalebuff E A 1976 Stiffness of the proximal interphalangeal joints in rheumatoid arthritis. The role of flexor tenosynovitis. Journal of Bone and Joint Surgery 58A: 801–805

81. Brewerton D A 1967 A tangential radiographic projection for demonstrating involvement of metacarpal heads in rheumatoid arthritis. British Journal of Radiology 40: 233–234

82. Magyar E, Talerman A, Feher M, Wouters H W 1974 Giant bone cyst in rheumatoid arthritis. Journal of Bone and Joint Surgery 56B: 121–129

83. Granberry W M, Mangum G L 1980 The hand in the child with juvenile rheumatoid arthritis. The Journal of Hand Surgery 5: 105–113

84. Still G F 1897 On a form of chronic joint disease in children. Med Chir Trans 80: 47–59

85. Blockey N J, Gibson A A M, Goel K M 1980 Monarticular juvenile rheumatoid arthritis. Journal of Bone and Joint Surgery 62B: 368–371

86. Eyring E J, Longert A, Bass J C 1971 Synovectomy in juvenile rheumatoid arthritis. Journal of Bone and Joint Surgery 53A: 638–651

87. Calin A, Porta J, Fries J F, Schurman D J 1977 Clinical history as a screening test for ankylosing spondylitis. Journal of The American Medical Association 237: 2613–2614

88. Constantz R, Bluestone R 1980 Diagnosis of the seronegative spondyloarthropathies: HL-A B27 testing as an aid to diagnosis Contemporary Orthopaedics 2: 141–147

89. Bleifeld C J, Inglis A E 1974 The hand in systemic lupus erythematosis. The Journal of Bone and Joint Surgery 56A: 1207–1215

90. Dray G J, Millender L H, Nalebuff E A, Philips C 1981 The surgical treatment of hand deformities in systemic lupus erythematosis. Journal of Hand Surgery 6: 339–345

91. Schlenker J D, Clark D D, Weckesser E C 1973 Calcinosis circumscripta of the hand in scleroderma. Journal of Bone and Joint Surgery 55A: 1051–1056

92. Lewis R A, Adams J P, Gerber N L, Decker J L, Parsons D B 1978 The hand in mixed connective tissue disease. Journal of Hand Surgery 3: 217–222

93. Loebl D, Kirby S, Stephenson R, Cook E, Mealing H, Bailey J 1979 Psoriatic arthritis. Journal of The American Medical Association 242: 2447–2451

94. Stern H S, Lloyd G J 1978 Metacarpal shortening. The Hand 10: 202–204

95. Millender L H, Philips C 1978 Combined wrist arthrodesis and metacarpophalangeal joint arthroplasty in rheumatoid arthritis. Orthopedics 1: 43–48

FURTHER READING

Arden G P, Harrison S H, Ansell B M 1970 Surgical treatment in rheumatoid arthritis. British Medical Journal 4: 604–609

Beckenbaugh R D, Linscheid R L 1977 Total wrist arthroplasty: A preliminary report. Journal of Hand Surgery 2: 337–344

Bucholz R W, Burkhead W Z 1979 The pathological anatomy of fatal atlanto-occipital dislocations. Journal of Bone and Joint Surgery 61A: 248–251

Conaty J P, Mongan E S 1981 Cervical fusion in rheumatoid arthritis. Journal of Bone and Joint Surgery 63A: 1218–1227

Cummings J K, Taleisnik J 1971 Peripheral gangrene as a complication of rheumatoid arthritis. Journal of Bone and Joint Surgery 53A: 1001–1006

Davidson C D, Horn J R, Herndon J, Grin O D 1977 Brain-stem compression in rheumatoid arthritis. Journal of the American Medical Association 238: 2633–2634

Ferlic D C, Clayton M L, Leidholt J D, Gamble W E 1975 Surgical treatment of the symptomatic unstable cervical spine in rheumatoid arthritis. The Journal of Bone and Joint Surgery 57A: 349–354

Fielding J W, Hawkins R J, Ratzan S A 1976 Spine fusion for atlanto-axial instability. Journal of Bone and Joint Surgery 58A: 400–407

Gama C 1979 Results of the Matev operation for correction of boutonniere deformity. Plastic and Reconstructive Surgery 64: 319–324

Gottlieb N L, Riskin W G 1980 Complications of local corticosteroid injections. Journal of the American Medical Association 243: 1547–1548

Hakstian R W 1967 Ulnar deviation of the fingers. Journal of Bone and Joint Surgery 49A: 299–316

Harris R W 1981 The pathophysiology of rheumatoid hand deformities. Orthopaedic Review 10: 33–46

Harrison S H 1979 The surgical management of the arthritic hand. Annals of the Royal College of Surgeons of England 61: 17–28

Hart F D, Huskisson E C 1972 Measurement in rheumatoid arthritis. Lancet 1: 28–30

Holt P J L 1969 Assessment of suitability for joint replacement. The physician's viewpoint. Annals of Rheumatoid Disease 28: 69–73

Kemble J V H 1977 Functional disability in the rheumatoid hand. The Hand 9: 234–241

Moore J R, Weiland A J 1980 Bilateral attritional rupture of the ulnar nerve at the elbow. Journal of Hand Surgery 5: 358–360

Nakamo K K 1975 The entrapment neuropathies of rheumatoid arthritis. Orthopaedic Clinics of North America 6: 837–860

Nalebuff E A 1969 Hand surgery and the rheumatoid patient. Surgical Clinics of North America 49: 787–797

Pulkki T, Vainio K 1962 Compression of the ulnar nerve due to rheumatoid arthritis of the elbow. Ann Chir Gyn Fenniae 51: 327–330

Ropes M W, Bennett G A, Cobb S, Jacox R, Jessar R A 1959 Revision of diagnostic criteria for rheumatoid arthritis. Arthritis and Rheumatism 2: 16–20

Savage O 1966 Measurements in rheumatoid arthritis. Proc R Soc Med 59: Supp 85–88

Souter W A 1979 Planning treatment of the rheumatoid hand. The Hand 11: 3–17

Stark D, Miller R 1978 Anesthesia for patients with rheumatoid arthritis. Orthopaedic Review 7: 21–30

Steinbrocker O, Traeger C H, Batterman R C 1949 Therapeutic criteria in rheumatoid arthritis. Journal of the American Medical Association 140: 659–662

Swanson A B 1972 Flexible implant arthroplasty for arthritic finger joints. The Journal of Bone and Joint Surgery 54A: 435–455

Swanson A B, Mays J D, Yamauchi Y 1969 A rheumatoid arthritis evaluation record for the upper extremity. Surgical Clinics of North America 48: 1003–1013

Swezey R L, Bjarhason D, Austin E S 1973 Nerve conduction studies in resorptive arthropathies. Journal of Bone and Joint Surgery 55A: 1680–1684

Trevhaft P S 1971 A rapid method for evaluating the structure and function of the rheumatoid hand. Arthritis and Rheumatism 14: 75–86

Upton A R M, Darracott J, Bianchi F A 1978 Ulnar neuropathies in rheumatoid arthritis. The Hand 10: 77–81

6

Swelling

Swellings may arise from any tissue in the hand — skin, subcutaneous tissue, fascia, nerve, artery, tendon, synovium, muscle, cartilage or bone. Some are very common and are recognized at a glance. Others are rare requiring histological examination and even consultation amongst pathologists for their identification. To consider them all would involve producing a pathological catalogue which has no place in a text on diagnosis and indications. (A guide to the hand surgery literature is given in the bibliography at the end of this chapter. It is broken down for ease of reference into tissues and tumours.)

This brief chapter is confined to a consideration of an approach to hand swellings common to them all with short notes on the few for which more detail seems necessary. With regard to surgical indications, these are simple. All swellings of the hand, with very few exceptions, require excision. The margin of normal tissue taken in the course of the excision varies with the anticipated malignancy of the lesion. Where doubt exists whether or not a lesion is one which would require wide, ablative resection, such as melanoma or an osteosarcoma, biopsy is acceptable since, contrary to previous opinion, it appears to have no influence on the eventual outcome.

HISTORY

The facts sought in the course of taking a history are those required in diagnosing a swelling in any part of the body.

Duration
Presence since birth, increasing in size with the patient, suggests a *hamartoma*.

Swift growth indicates inflammation or high-grade malignancy.

Bursts of growth at puberty and during pregnancy are characteristic of *cavernous haemangioma* but growth in previously quiescent lesions should be viewed with suspicion. For example, a plexiform neurofibroma may develop a *malignant Schwannoma*, evidenced by sudden enlargement in one area.

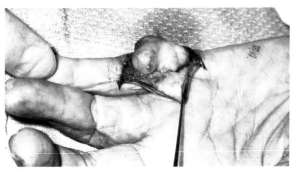

Fig. 6.1 This lesion which had developed over the course of two to three years at the proximal digital crease was attached to the skin and was an *epidermoid* or *implantation cyst*.

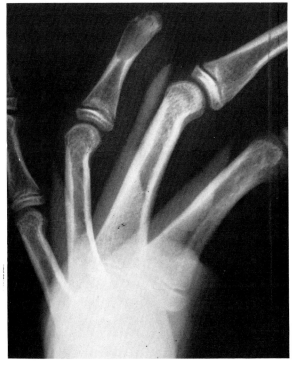

Fig. 6.2 The space occupying lesion in the distal half of the middle phalanx of this digit following amputation was an *epidermoid cyst*.

Nature of onset
If sudden and related to injury, vascular involvement is probable, in the form of a traumatic aneurysm.

Previous trauma to the area
    Epidermoid cysts follow minor trauma to the skin (Fig. 6.1). In a series of rare cases which involved bone — always the distal phalanx — the majority of patients surprisingly remembered the incident even though the delay was long, averaging eight and a half years (Fig. 6.2).
    Foreign body granulomas likewise follow minor injury.

Previous similar swellings
Recurrence after adequate previous excision should always arouse concern. The original histological sections should be reviewed before further surgery.

Similar swellings elsewhere
    Neurofibromatosis invariably produces multiple swellings in the skin.
    Lesions associated with *systemic disorders* may be multiple, such as xanthomata in patients with hyperlipidaemia.

Variation in size
This is characteristically a feature of *ganglion cysts* which develop to significant size, disperse often as a result of a forgotten blow only to recur at a later date.

Associated symptoms
    Pain with a swelling in the hand is rarely severe and when it is so is diagnostic of an inflammatory lesion, either infective or due to gout or calcific deposits (Chapter 4). Severe pain with no swelling, provided neuropathic and inflammatory causes have been excluded, should make the examiner suspect a *glomus tumour* (p. 00) or an *osteoid osteoma* as being the cause.
    Numbness or weakness in a specific distribution indicates that the lesion, if appropriately situated, is producing nerve compression (Chapter 3).

Symptoms related to other systems
Metastatic tumours in the hand are rare but they do occur and the examiner should seek evidence of the primary focus (Fig. 6.3).

EXAMINATION

A system for examination of swellings should be adopted from which the examiner never strays. The mnemonic ascribed to Learmonth is useful.

$S^3 C^2 M$ site   colour   mobility
              size   consistency
              shape

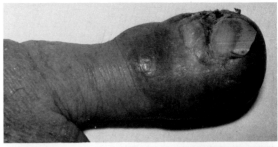
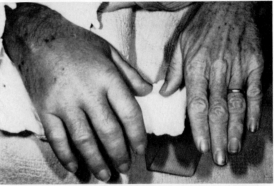
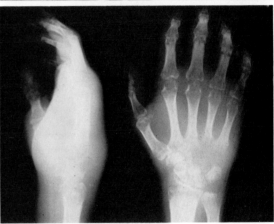

Fig. 6.3 *Metastatic tumours.*(A) Consequent upon renal carcinoma. (B) & (C) Consequent upon bronchogenic carcinoma.

SITE
The situation of a swelling may be virtually diagnostic. For example, a swelling located over the distal phalanx in the region of the nailbed, especially if grooving of the nail is apparent, can only be a ganglion of the distal interphalangeal joint, the so-called 'mucous cyst' (pp. 241, 298). A firm swelling on the palmar aspect of the proximal phalanx of the thumb of the dominant hand which is mobile transversely but not longitudinally, is a neuroma on the digital nerve — a 'bowler's thumb' (p. 158). A firm, small, immobile swelling beneath the proximal digital crease of the finger is almost always a ganglion of the tendon sheath (p. 298).

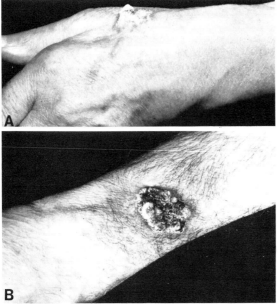

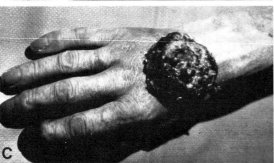

Fig. 6.4 *Squamous cell carcinoma* on the hand may be encountered at a very early hyperkeratotic stage (A), in a more florid but excrescent form with little involvement of the underlying tissues (B), or quite commonly in an advanced stage with some involvement of the underlying tissue, usually with superadded infection (C). In this last case, quite marked lymphadenopathy was present. This was observed for a period of six weeks after excision of the primary tumour and disappeared completely. This phenomenon is often encountered with squamous cell carcinoma and is due to secondary infection.

Skin lesions on the dorsum of the hand or forearm, especially of those who have worked a lifetime in the sun, are likely to be squamous cell carcinomata (Fig. 6.4). However far progressed this may be, a good prognosis can be given to the patient for actinic lesions of this type are relatively benign. For this reason, while a full centimetre clearance should be given on the skin and care taken to excise through normal tissue on the deep aspect of the tumour, extensive resection is not commonly necessary.

Determining the site also requires the examiner to attempt to localize the swelling to a particular tissue. This is considered further under mobility.

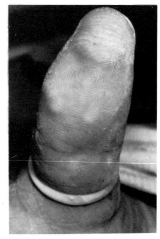

Fig. 6.5 This patient presented with the nodular lesion beneath the thumb pulp with multiple seed nodules further proximal. Biopsy showed this to be *Bowen's disease* which was thereafter observed, and showed no progression.

SIZE

The size of a lesion should be recorded. In the unusual case where the decision is made not to excise the lesion — as for example in Bowen's disease affecting an important structure (Fig. 6.5) — then the record will be of value in ensuring that no active growth is occurring between visits. Large lesions, as a general rule, are benign, provided they have not ulcerated the skin or produced associated symptoms.

SHAPE

To determine the shape of a swelling, the surgeon must be able to define its margins. If with a soft tissue lesion this is not possible because the margins appear to merge into surrounding tissues, the possibility of malignancy must be entertained. Some swellings may appear to be multilocular and some indeed are. However, the many rigid structures in the hand, especially tendons and fascia, may mould a benign lesion growing beneath them into an irregular form (Fig. 6.6).

COLOUR

Any pigmented lesion, especially beneath the nail or on the palms of the hand should be considered as dangerous (Fig. 6.7). Mitotic activity in a malignant melanoma is classically indicated by any of the following: alteration in colour, increase in size, elevation of a previously flat lesion, bleeding and itching (Fig. 6.8). In short, any change in a pigmented lesion should be treated as *prima facie* evidence of malignancy. The subungual *melanoma* may be a relatively slow-growing tumour, the patient often giving a lengthy history only of an increasing dark spot beneath the nail. Radical excision of the distal phalanx and the distal half of the adjacent phalanx with soft tissue to the base of the digit is indicated.

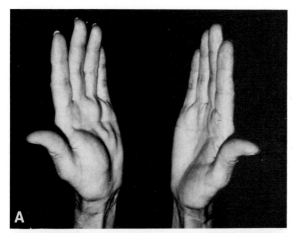

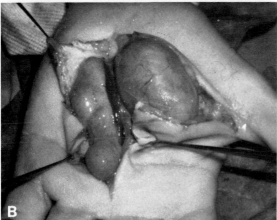

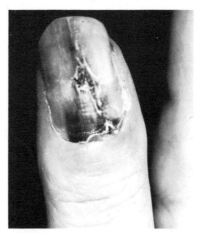

Fig. 6.7   This patient presented with a history of a dark lesion deep to the nail of the thumb present for some twelve months. Histological examination following radical excision showed this to be a *malignant melanoma*.

Fig. 6.6   (A) This patient presented with a history of a gradually developing mutilocular lesion in the palm of the left hand. While it appeared clinically that this was composed of several lesions it was appreciated at surgery, (B) that because this *lipoma* arose beneath the tendons and nerves of the palm of the hand, it had been distorted by them from its basic unilocular form.

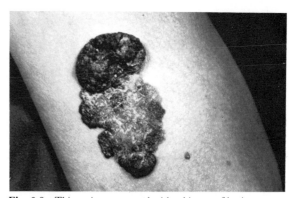

Fig. 6.8   This patient presented with a history of having a previously flat pigmented lesion on the inner aspect of the upper arm. This subsequently underwent an increase in size, the development of an excrescent area in the upper part of the lesion, changes in colour, persistent irritation, and recent bleeding on contact with clothing. As anticipated, it proved to be a *malignant melanoma*.

All *naevi* of the palm of the hand are *junctional* in location and therefore excision should be recommended in all cases.

The typical appearance of a *'strawberry naevus'* in the newborn is well-known — raised and pinkish-red. The main significance to the examiner is that he should know to always leave such lesions completely alone to follow their natural course.

CONSISTENCY

To determine whether the swelling is *fluctuant*, the consistency should be assessed with two fingers fixing the lesion and a third exerting intermittent pressure (Fig. 6.9). At body temperature in the relatively unyielding surroundings of the hand, a *lipoma* is a fluctuant swelling.

When the consistency is yielding and apparently fluid, steady pressure should be applied to it. If this serves to empty the swelling which then *refills*, it is clearly a *vascular*

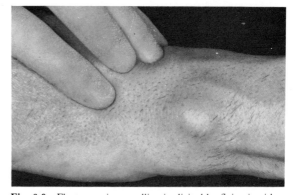

Fig. 6.9   Fluctuance in a swelling is elicited by fixing it with two fingers of one hand and exerting pressure with a third digit. Although usually evidence of free fluid, fluctuance is encountered in lipomata at body temperature.

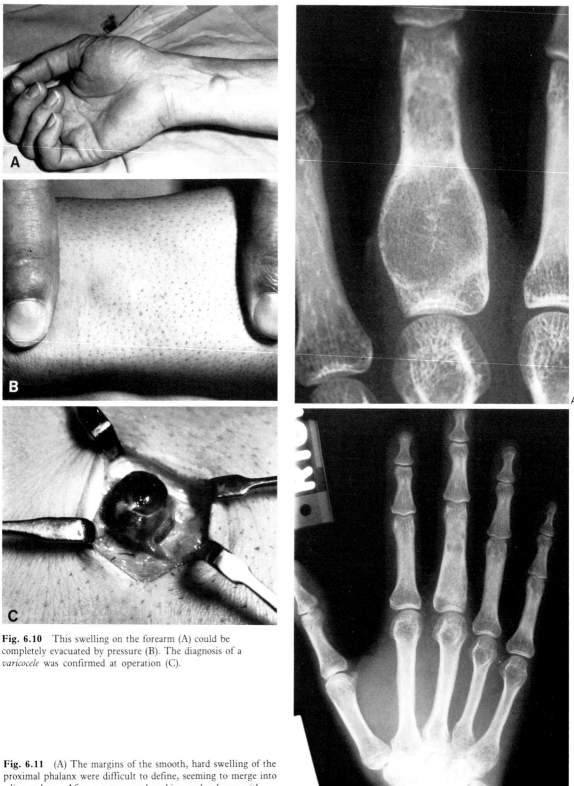

Fig. 6.10 This swelling on the forearm (A) could be completely evacuated by pressure (B). The diagnosis of a *varicocele* was confirmed at operation (C).

Fig. 6.11 (A) The margins of the smooth, hard swelling of the proximal phalanx were difficult to define, seeming to merge into adjacent bone. After curettage and packing *enchondroma* with cancellous bone remodelling occurred as seen two years later (B).

lesion of which a cavernous *haemangioma, aneurysm* or *varicocele* are the most likely (Fig. 6.10). If hard and unyielding, a swelling is probably arising from bone, although *gouty tophi* and the calcium deposits of *calcinosis* are of similar consistency. However, they are both craggy, irregular and usually show some mobility. Lesions of bone often present as a smooth hard lump, totally immobile, the margins of which are difficult to define in both benign and malignant lesions (Fig. 6.11). The one common exception is a *Heberden's node* (p. 239), the margins of which can be clearly palpated.

MOBILITY

The tissues to which the swelling is attached can often be determined by checking its mobility with respect to skin, bone and tendon. The skin overlying the lesion should be lifted and the fingers rolled to detect whether or not the swelling moves with the skin inseparably. Certain lesions which do not involve the skin surface are nonetheless always attached to it — *epidermoid cyst, Dupuytren's disease* (p. 137) and *juvenile dermatofibroma* (Fig. 6.12) are the most common.

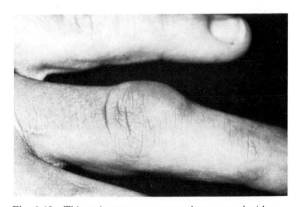

Fig. 6.12 This patient was a teenager who presented with a history of a swelling which had developed over the proximal interphalangeal joint of his left ring finger. This was firmly attached to skin and proved to be a juvenile dermato-fibroma..

If fully developed to contracture Dupuytren's offers no diagnostic difficulties. However, a patient may complain of a tender palmar nodule with no evidence of contracture. Examination will reveal a smooth rounded mass firmly attached to the skin in most instances in the line of the ring finger between the proximal and distal palmar creases. Provided the possibility occurs to the examiner no doubt will exist regarding the diagnosis. Excision is not indicated unless the patient finds the tender nodule interferes with power grasp. Often he is content with reassurance regarding the nature of the condition.

Garrod's knuckle pads, fibrous thickening over the dorsum of the proximal interphalangeal joints appear to be related to Dupuytren's disease and to have the same familial tendency.

If the swelling is not attached to the skin, it may appear to be attached to bone, being firmly immobile in all directions. If such a lesion is well-defined it is unlikely to arise from the bone itself but rather from the tendon sheath, a *ganglion* or *giant cell tumour* being most likely.

Some swellings may be mobile in one direction and not in another implying that they arise from, or are attached to, a longitudinally running structure. This is the case, for example, with a *neurilemmoma* of a digital nerve, a fusiform swelling which moves freely from side to side but very little along the axis of the finger. Excision of a neurilemmoma does not require resection of normal fascicles, especially since this lesion never becomes malignant. Using magnification the lesion can be dissected cleanly out of the nerve (Fig. 6.13). Other lesions may move as the patient

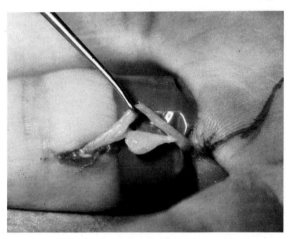

Fig. 6.13 This patient came with a somewhat tender, small nodular swelling over the proximal phalanx of her middle finger. This was freely mobile in the transverse direction but not at all in the longitudinal and could therefore be adjudged to be attached to either nerve or artery. At operation it appeared to be intimately involved in the structure of the digital nerve but careful dissection under the microscope showed that it could be completely separated from the fasicles of the nerve. It was a *neurilemmoma.*

moves the hand, a feature which is pathognomonic of a *ganglion on the extensor tendon,* most commonly seen in children (Fig. 6.14).

If the swelling has ulcerated, certain features of the *ulcer* should be examined. An ulcer arising in the nailbed will declare itself only by the presence of discharge from beneath the nail. Should such a discharge persist for more than three weeks biopsy must be performed and may reveal an unsuspected *squamous cell carcinoma.*

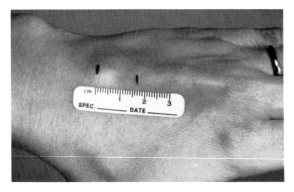

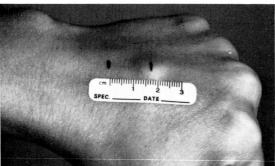

Fig. 6.14A & B   The movement of this small, hard mass through a distance of $1\frac{1}{2}$ cm is characteristic of a *ganglion* of the extensor tendon.

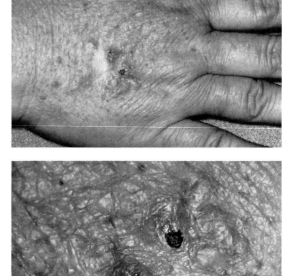

Fig. 6.16A & B   *Basal cell carcinoma* of the 'self-healing, cicatrizing, or field fire' variety.

Ulcers

Edge

The characteristically heaped-up margins of a *squamous carcinoma* contrast with the flat, normal skin which surrounds a *pyogenic granuloma* (Fig. 6.15). *Basal cell carcinoma* is rarely encountered in the hand and the 'pearly edge' with which it is credited is not always apparent. If the surgeon places the skin on stretch, however, and inspects the edge of the ulcer, preferably with magnification, the typical pearly appearance becomes more evident, the whiteness being interrupted by fine telangiectatic vessels coursing across the margin (Fig. 6.16).

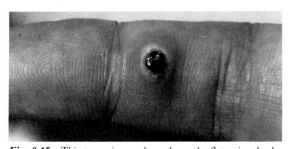

Fig. 6.15   This *pyogenic granuloma* shows the flat uninvolved surrounding skin and exuberant granulation which is characteristic.

Floor

The floor of an ulcer is that portion which the examiner can inspect. A red, overgrown granulating floor which overflows the edge of the ulcer is found most frequently in a *pyogenic granuloma*. The surgeon must be aware, however, that the relatively rare totally *amelanotic melanoma* (Fig. 6.17) may have a very similar appearance. Once he has encountered such a melanoma he will take care to explain the remote possibility to subsequent patients, thereafter undertaking early surgery.

The floor of an ulcer is often crusted over. If it can be done without pain, this crust should be removed. Should this produce brisk bleeding and there be no evidence of attempts at marginal re-epithelialization, *squamous carcinoma* is likely (Fig. 6.18).

Keratocanthoma with a characteristic circular plug of keratin should be excised for it may rarely be a swiftly growing carcinoma (Fig. 6.19).

Base

The base of an ulcer is that part underlying it which the examiner can palpate. If the base is thickened and indurated and especially if it is fixed to underlying tissues, the possibility of malignancy is considerable.

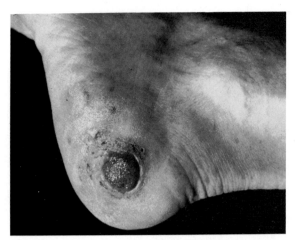

Fig. 6.17 This lesion on the heel was totally without pigment even after careful examination under magnification. Suspicions were entertained regarding its nature and wide excision performed. It was indeed an *amelanotic melanoma*.

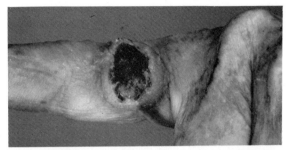

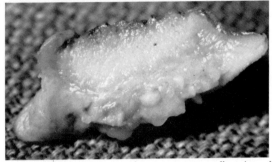

Fig. 6.19A & B *Kerato-acanthoma or squamous cell carcinoma?* This lesion proved on biopsy to be a squamous cell carcinoma of the index finger.

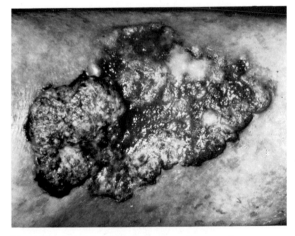

Fig. 6.18 This ulcer had been present for some sixteen years and showed change in that the edges began to become heaped up in appearance. A crust formed over the ulcer which on removal produced brisk bleeding. Subsequent histological examination showed this to be *squamous cell carcinoma*.

Calcification in the soft tissues is seen in acute calcific tendinitis (p. 233), calcinosis circumscripta, and quite frequently in haemangioma, juvenile aponeurotic fibroma, synovial sarcoma, lipoma and liposarcoma.

Calcinosis circumscripta presents as tender calcific deposits which quite commonly afflict the finger pads, in which position they are troublesome to the patient. They give no diagnostic difficulties, but are mentioned here because of the high incidence of *scleroderma* in patients with this condition (p. 285).

Angiography is required to determine the location and extent of vascular lesions and the nature of feeding vessels and run-off. It may also define the location and extent of certain bony tumours.

Bone scan may be employed to locate symptomatic but undetectable lesions such as an osteoid osteoma.

Indications

Complete excision of any benign swelling presenting in the hand proves curative. Difficulties arise only when the lesion is believed to be malignant or when doubt exists as to the nature of any deep tumour.

Squamous cell carcinoma in the hand is relatively benign. Excision of the lesion with a 1 cm margin is indicated: the deep margin is at the plane in which dissection is free — this can best be determined by preliminary injection of fluid beneath the tumour. When no such plane can be demonstrated, indicating involvement of bone or tendon, appropriate amputation is required. This is most likely to occur in the 'danger area' of the interdigital clefts, so

Regional nodes

These should always be examined, taking care not to omit the supratrochlear node.

X-rays

Radiological examination may reveal

1. the presence of lesions arising primarily from bone,
2. any effects produced on the bone by soft tissue swellings,
3. the presence of calcification in the soft tissues.

described by Rayner. Squamous cell carcinoma of the nailbed requires ablation of the distal phalanx. Carcinomata of the hand are frequently infected and this may result in reactive lymphadenopathy. For this reason the presence of enlarged nodes should not lead to gloom or even immediate node dissection. Rather should the nodes be left for six weeks after excision of the primary, at which stage dissection should be undertaken in the rare cases in which they are still enlarged.

Many factors have been cited as influencing the prognosis, and therefore the appropriate surgical treatment, of malignant melanoma — age, sex, size, ulceration, presence of satellites, absence of melanin and nodularity. Certainly, if a suspected lesion is ulcerated or nodular, the prognosis is poorer and the excision should be wider. However, more accurate guidance can be obtained by histological examination: Breslow has shown that the incidence of metastases is directly related to the maximal thickness of the tumour; for example, those less than 1 mm thick rarely, if ever, metastasise. Where deemed desirable incisional biopsy for staging followed by later wide resection has been shown to carry no added stigma, contrary to previous teaching. Where nodes are involved, dissection is indicated and may be effective, in inverse proportion to the number of nodes found to be involved.

The close liaison between surgeon and pathologist necessary for management of melanoma is also essential for the appropriate treatment of suspicious soft tissue or bony swellings. Together they must plan the evaluation and determine the staging of the lesion. The hazards and technique of biopsy of such lesions have been clearly stated in three articles in the October 1982 issue of the *Journal of Bone and Joint Surgery*. Once the stage has been determined on the basis of pathological grading, accurate location of the anatomical site and detection of metastases by X-ray and scan, adequate excision of the malignant primary as part of the planned treatment requires ablation of the anatomical compartment containing it. This may be achieved only by amputation.

SPECIFIC LESIONS

GANGLION

Ganglion is the most common swelling encountered in the hand. It may arise virtually anywhere in the limb and be significant more for its effects than its mere presence as in Guyon's canal or the cubital tunnel where it produces nerve compression (see Chapter 3). It is most commonly found in one of four sites.

Distal phalanx (Fig. 6.20) — overlying the nailbed, this ganglion from the distal interphalangeal joint, formerly considered to be a mucous cyst, invariably produces a groove or even a split in the nail. Not infrequently this ganglion erodes the overlying skin or is incised. It is then often the seat of chronic or recurrent infection. A local flap may be required to cover the defect created by excision.

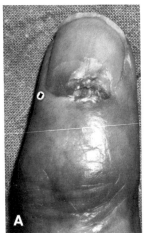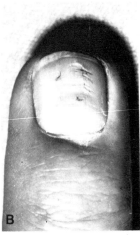

Fig. 6.20 (A) A *ganglion* over the distal phalanx arising from the distal interphalangeal joint in the presence of osteoarthritis commonly produces distortions of the nail which grow out after excision (B) This is the so-called 'mucous cyst'.

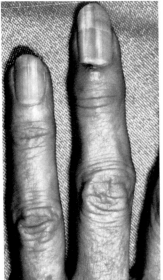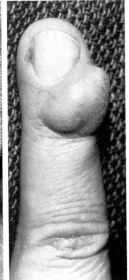

Fig. 6.20 (C & D) Two other presentations of a *ganglion* of the distl interphalangeal joint.

Proximal digital crease — the ganglion here emerges from the tendon sheath just distal to the proximal pulley. It presents as a small, very firm, immobile and often tender mass palpable to one or other side of the midline (Fig. 6.21). It is most commonly encountered in the middle finger and in one series more than 25 per cent of the patients were full-time typists.

Anterior aspect of the wrist (Fig. 6.22) — ganglia in this site are almost always found just lateral to the flexor carpi radialis tendon, in close proximity to the radial artery

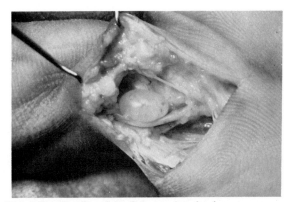

Fig. 6.21 *Ganglion* of the flexor tendon sheath.

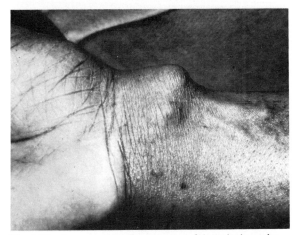

Fig. 6.22 A common site for a *ganglion* of the wrist is on the radial side of the anterior aspect. Some of these ganglia arise from the intercarpal joints and pass along the tendon of flexor carpi radialis in its tunnel under the ridge of the trapezium before emerging on the wrist. This should be carefully pursued at the time of surgery if recurrence is to be avoided.

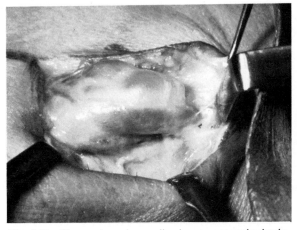

Fig. 6.23 The anterior wrist ganglion is very commonly closely adherent to the radial artery. In these instances, the integrity of the ganglion should be sacrificed if any danger exists of entering the wall of the radial artery.

which they have been reported to occlude (Fig. 6.23). Although in most instances they arise from the radiocarpal or inferior radioulnar joint, they may have their origin in the carpus and pass along the tunnel of flexor carpi radialis in the trapezium. The surgeon must be aware of this fact so that he may pursue it and thereby reduce the chances of recurrence.

Dorsal aspect of the wrist (Fig. 6.24) — all the ganglia so far considered are cystic, well-defined masses. The dorsal ganglion may also be so, but not uncommonly is a more sessile, ill-defined swelling sometimes causing the surgeon to doubt its very existence. Commonly arising from the scapholunate or midcarpal joints, this ganglion is intimately involved in the dorsal capsule and probably as a result is often associated with complaints of pain and weakness of the wrist.

Because of similar aching, its position and its sessile character, an anomalous *extensor digitorum brevis manus* (p. 219) is often misdiagnosed as a dorsal ganglion. A *carpometacarpal boss* also presents in a similar site, being an excess of bone at the base of the second or less commonly third metacarpal. However, its consistency and X-ray appearance (Fig. 6.25) distinguish it from a ganglion.

X-ray of the appropriate area should always be performed. The distal interphalangeal joint is often the seat of osteoarthritis. Any pathology of the carpus must be excluded before surgery, since excision involves dissection amongst the ligaments of the wrist.

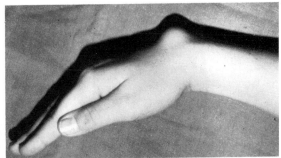

Fig. 6.24 A dorsal swelling not attached to the skin characteristic of a cystic *ganglion*.

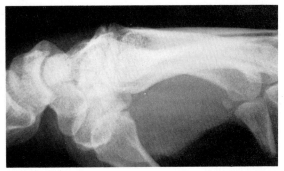

Fig. 6.25 *Carpometacarpal boss.*

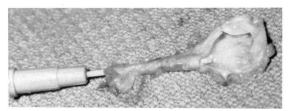

Fig. 6.26 The neck to a ganglion is frequently longer than the width of the ganglion itself.

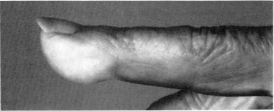

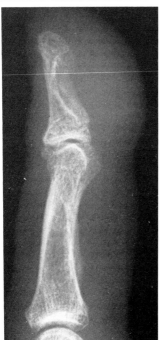

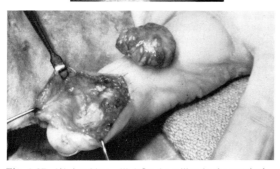

Fig. 6.27 (A) A rubbery, ill-defined swelling in the terminal pulp produced (B) scalloping of the distal phalanx. The lesion proved to be a well-localized *giant cell tumor.* (C)

Recurrence of a ganglion after excision is not uncommon. The best safeguard against this embarrassment is to pursue the neck of the ganglion to its very source, often a lengthy chase (Fig. 6.26). It is possible, of course, that the recurrence may be a second, new lesion.

GIANT CELL TUMOUR (= pigmented villonodular synovitis)
This is the second most common swelling encountered in the hand following ganglion cyst. The aetiology is not clear, but it is always found in the presence of synovial tissue, most commonly arising from the flexor tendon sheath or interphalangeal joints. It presents therefore on the finger, somewhat more often on the palmar than on the dorsal surface. Because it is usually symptomless, the

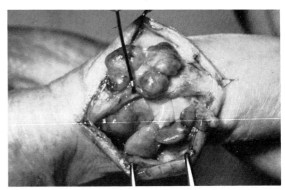

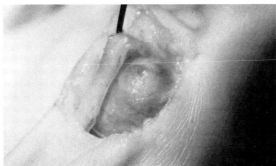

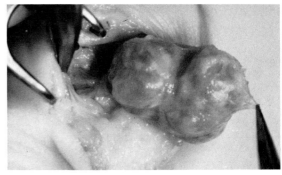

Fig. 6.28A *Giant cell tumor.* The tumor passes through the interstices in the extensor tendon, and can be seen emerging from various aspects of the proximal interphalangeal joint. (B) & (C) The giant cell tumor characteristically envelops normal structures, here the digital nerve, which has grooved the tumor.

patient may present late, by which time there may be a visible, irregular swelling. On palpation, it has the consistency of soft rubber and it may be difficult to define its boundaries.

On occasion it produces X-ray changes by pressure (Fig. 6.27), by eroding the osteochondral juction like rheumatoid pannus, or by migrating along the foramina of bony vessels. Exploration reveals the very characteristic yellow and brown mottled tumour which surrounds normal structures rather than displacing them (Fig. 6.28).

Excision cures the condition only if the lesion is pursued throughout its often tortuous path which may be circumferential and also involve the entire flexor tendon sheath. Otherwise recurrence is common.

ARTERIOVENOUS FISTULA (Fig. 6.29)

A fistula presents as a collection of varicose veins on the upper extremity. The patient may consult the physician because of a recent wound which has failed to heal. This is because of a 'steal' phenomenon whereby the flow through the fistula is so high that no blood reaches the more distal circulation to the digits. Examination reveals obvious varicosities in a limb which may or may not be hypertrophied. The skin temperature is elevated. The varicosities can be emptied by firm pressure but quickly refill. A thrill should be sought with the palpating hand and auscultation performed to detect a bruit. Blood flow through such fistulae has been recorded as being as much as forty times normal. When the arteriovenous shunt is that severe, the pulse pressure is greatly increased and the patient is in danger of developing high-output cardiac failure. Occlusion of the main artery to the limb therefore often results in *bradycardia* (the *Branham reaction*). Studies

of the oxygen saturation of the venous blood should be performed. In the presence of an arteriovenous fistula the saturation will exceed that of central venous samples.

Radiological signs (Fig. 6.30) in arteriovenous fistula are

1. dilatation of arteries leading to the fistula,
2. absence of normal filling distal to the fistula,
3. pooling of the medium in the fistula, referred to as 'snowflakes',
4. the presence of contrast medium in the veins on the first film in the angiographic series.

Such arteriovenous fistulae may arise as a result of trauma (Fig. 6.31) — commonly a penetrating wound —, or iatrogenically. Iatrogenic fistulae may of course be intentional for the purposes of dialysis or arise as a complication of cardiac catheterisation (p. 40). The dialysis patient with 'shunt steal' problems has a swollen, blue, cold hand with ulceration on one or more fingertips. Surprisingly on examination, bounding pulses can be felt throughout the hand, especially marked in the dilated,

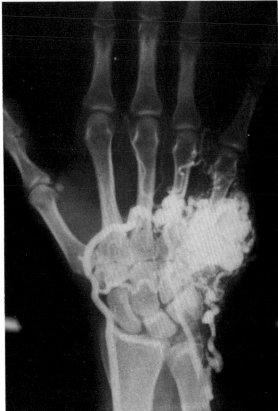

Fig. 6.30 All of the features of arteriovenous fistulae are shown in this radiographic examination, with dilatation of the arteries, absence of normal filling distal to the fistula, 'snowflake' pooling of the medium in the fistula and the presence of contrast in the veins in this early film in the angiographic series.

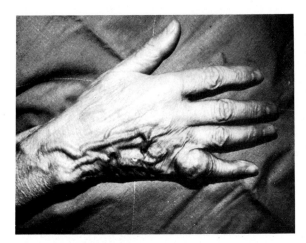

Fig. 6.29 *Arteriovenous fistula.* The swelling at the base of the small finger was pulsatile and the temperature of the overlying skin was significantly higher than that of the adjacent normal fingers. The grossly varicose veins on the ulnar aspect of the dorsum of the hand made the diagnosis virtually certain.

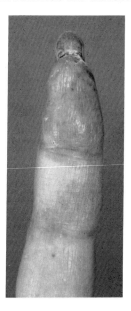

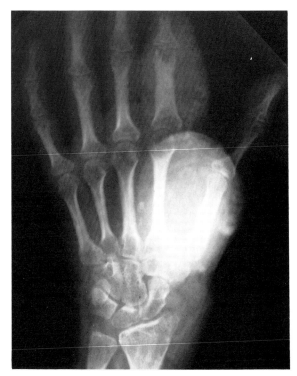

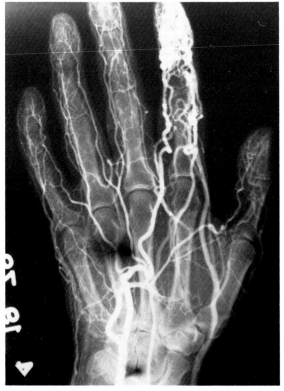

Fig. 6.31 This patient presented with cold intolerance and incipient necrosis of the tip of the finger. (A) Examination revealed that the finger was pulsatile, and arteriography (B) showed a traumatic arteriovenous fistula.

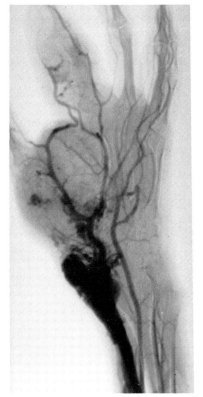

Fig. 6.32 *Congenital arteriovenous fistula.* (A) Shows the mass in the first web space with scalloping of the bone indicative of its involvement. (B) Angiography reveals the extent of the lesion.

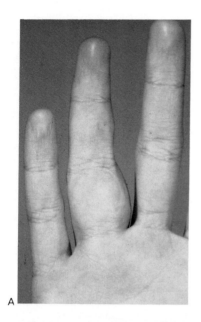

A

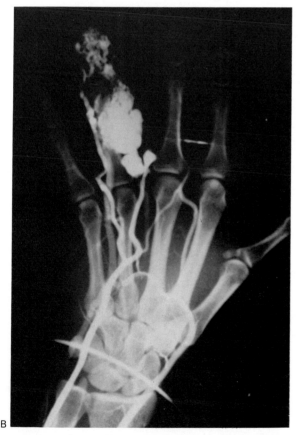

B

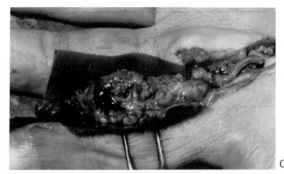

C

Fig. 6.33 (A) This patient had a pulsatile mass which could be evacuated on the base of the ring finger. (B) Arteriography revealed that this was well-localized to the radial digital artery. (C) Excision was therefore performed.

tortuous veins. Revision of the shunt resolves the situation. Congenital lesions rarely show a single discrete arteriovenous communication but rather present as diffuse *cavernous haemangiomata*, the extent of which is only apparent on angiography, and often involving bone (Fig. 6.32). Excision should be undertaken only on very localised lesions and even then warning should be given of potential recurrence (Fig. 6.33). . Larger lesions or recurrences should be managed with protective, compressive garments (Fig. 6.34). Microembolisation may offer some relief for these patients in the future, for they are often troubled by pain and fatigue, quite apart from the potential cardiac effects.

GLOMUS TUMOUR

Glomus tumour may present as a swelling and Riddell and Martin reported one of unusual size. However, more commonly the patient presents with no swelling but only *pain* of spasmodic and excruciating nature. Sometimes triggered by trauma or mere contact, it is more often entirely spontaneous, radiating from the site of the tumour in a lancinating manner. It is characteristically precipitated by exposure to cold and relieved by warmth, although it may be sensitive to any temperature change.

Examination, if the tumour can be located — for its most common situation is beneath the nail — reveals an unimpressive, small, purplish patch in the skin (Fig. 6.35).

Tenderness is extreme and very well localized. This is best demonstrated by *Love's pin test*, in which the head of a pin is pressed around the area, finally coming on the tumour. Only then is pain elicited.

ANEURYSM

Three types of aneurysm are encountered

mycotic — which is rare;
atherosclerotic — uncommon, usually dorsal;
traumatic — most common, invariably palmar.

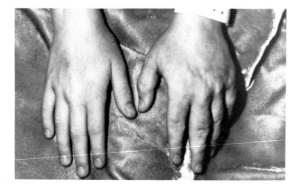

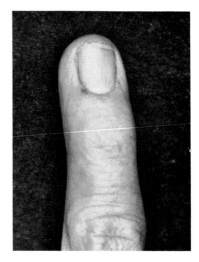

Fig. 6.35 *Glomus tumour.* This patient complained of excruciating pain in the right small finger. Examination revealed a small and insignificant purple patch on the eponychial fold which was however extremely tender.

The *traumatic aneurysm* (Fig. 6.36), which is *not* the result of a penetrating injury (p. 37) comes about as a result of repeated blows to the hand and has a similar aetiology to the ulnar artery thrombosis encountered in the 'hypothenar hammer syndrome' (p. 183). In the latter the injury is to the intima, while aneurysm formation follows disruption of the media. The most common sites for such aneurysmal formation are

the ulnar artery where it is exposed between Guyon's canal and the palmar fascia and overlies the hook of the hamate (Fig. 6.37).

the superficial branch of the radial artery as it enters the thenar eminence over the tubercle of the scaphoid.

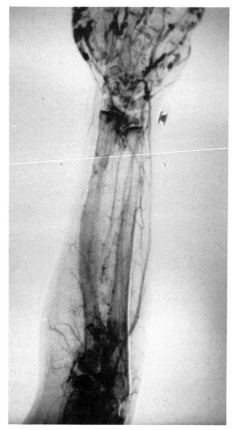

Fig. 6.34 (A) Multiple congenital arteriovenous fistulae produced irregular swellings and discoloration of the left hand which is painful on dependency. (B) Angiography reveals the extent of the disorder. This is currently controlled by compression garments.

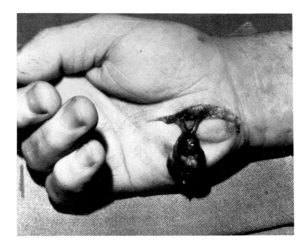

Fig. 6.36 *Traumatic aneurysm.* This patient gave a history of having struck his hand very forcibly over the ulnar aspect some two weeks previously and presented with a painful, pulsatile swelling.

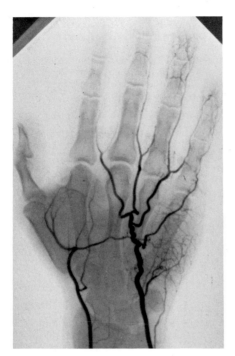
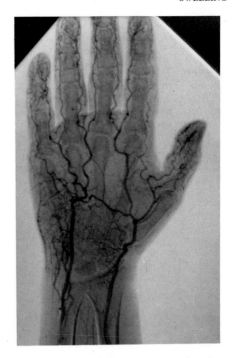

Fig. 6.37 Tortuous *aneurysm* formation is seen over the line of the ulnar artery just at and distal to the hypothenar region.

The aneurysm may be true or false.

The diagnosis is suggested when the patient complains of the development of a painful swelling after sustaining a blow to the hand. He may also complain of coolness in his fingers, most commonly the ring and cold intolerance may progress as far as ulceration of the digital pulp. Rarely he may give symptoms indicative of ulnar nerve compression (p. 202).

The presence of a pulsatile mass is pathognomonic. When no pulsation is detectable, a positive Allen test (p. 181) will confirm the diagnosis. Angiography will provide further evidence but is not required in the presence of the stated symptoms and signs.

Excision is indicated and if circumstances allow, a reversed vein graft should be inserted. Rarely, multiple small venous aneurysms may present, usually in middle-aged women (Fig. 6.38). There is no treatment possible or necessary.

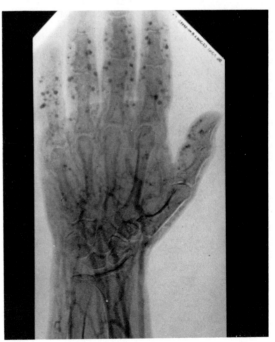

Fig. 6.38 *Venous aneurysms.* During the arterial phase (A) these lesions are not evident, but once the angiogram enters the venous phase, the multiple small venous aneurysms can be seen. (Angiograms by courtesy of Dr C. S. Wheeler)

REFERENCES

Survey

1. Butler E D, Hamill J P, Seipel R S, DeLorimier A A 1960 Tumors of the hand. A ten-year survey and report of 437 cases. American Journal of Surgery 100: 293–302
2. Gaisford J C 1960 Tumors of the hand. Surgical Clinics of North America 40: 549
3. Haber M H, Alter A H, Wheelock M C 1965 Tumors of the hand. Surgery, Gynecology and Obstetrics 121: 1073–1080
4. Mason M L 1937 Tumors of the hand. Surgery, Gynecology and Obstetrics 64: 129
5. Posch J L 1956 Tumors of the hand. Journal of Bone and Joint Surgery 38A: 517–540
6. Stack H G 1964 Tumours of the hand. Postgraduate Medical Journal 40: 290–298

Skin

Basal cell carcinoma
7. Enna C 1978 Adenoid basal cell epithelioma involving a finger. The Hand 10: 309–311
Bowen's disease
8. Bowen J T 1912 Precancerous dermatoses: Study of two cases of chronic atypical epithelial proliferation. Journal of Cancerous Diseases 30: 241–255
9. Defiebre B K 1978 Bowen's disease of the nail bed: A case representation and review of the literature. Journal of Hand Surgery 3: 184–186
10. Stilwell J H, Maisels D O 1981 Subungual Bowen's disease. The Hand 13: 287–290
Dermatofibrosarcoma protuberans
11. Schvarcz L W 1977 Congenital dermatofibrosarcoma protuberans of the hand. The Hand 9: 182–185
12. Wirman J A, Sherman S, Sullivan M R 1981 Dermatofibrosarcoma protuberans arising on the hand. The Hand 13: 187–190
Epidermoid cyst
13. Carroll R E 1953 Epidermoid (epithelial) cyst of the hand. American Journal of Surgery 85: 327–334
14. St Onge R A, Jackson I T 1977 An uncommon sequel to thumb trauma: epidermoid cyst. The Hand 9: 52–56
15. Sieracki J C, Kelly A P 1959 Traumatic epidermoid cysts involving digital bones: Epidermoid cysts of the distal phalanx. Archives of Surgery 78: 597–703
16. Zadek I, Cohen H G 1953 Epidermoid cyst of the terminal phalanx of a finger with a review of literature 85: 771
Juvenile aponeurotic fibroma
17. Booher R J, McPeak C J 1959 Juvenile aponeurotic fibromatosis. Surgery 46: 924–931
18. Specht E E, Konkin L A 1975 Juvenile aponeurotic fibroma. The cartilage analogue of fibromatosis. Journal of American Medical Association 236: 626–628
19. Specht E E, Staheli L T 1977 Juvenile aponeurotic fibroma. Journal of Hand Surgery 2: 258–260
20. Zeide M S, Wiessel S, Terry R Juvenile aponeurotic fibroma. Plastic and Reconstructive Surgery 61: 922–923
Keratoacanthoma
21. Lamp J C, Graham J H, Urbach F, Burgoon C F 1964 Keratoacanthoma of the subungual region. A clinicopathological and therapeutic study. The Journal of Bone and Joint Surgery 46A: 1721–1731, and 1752
Melanoma
22. Banzet P, Glicenstein J, Dufourmentel C 1975 Melanotic tumors of the hand. The Hand 7: 183–184

23. Breslow A, Macht S D 1978 Evaluation of prognosis in Stage I cutaneous melanoma. Plastic and Reconstructive Surgery 61: 342–346
24. Rushfort G F 1971 Two cases of subungual malignant melanoma. British Journal of Surgery 58: 451
25. Ware J W 1977 Subungual malignant melanoma presenting as sub-acute paronychia following trauma. The Hand 9: 49–51
Poroma
26. Mamoun S M, Shaw D T, Li C S, Richey D G 1972 Eccrine poroma of the hand. Plastic and Reconstructive Surgery 50: 295–298
Squamous cell carcinoma
27. Bunkis J, Mehrhof A I, Stayman J W 1981 Radiation-induced carcinoma of the hand. Journal of Hand Surgery 6: 384–387
28. Fitzgerald R H, Brewer N S, Dahlin D C 1976 Squamous-cell carcinoma complicating chronic osteomyelitis. Journal of Bone and Joint Surgery 58A: 1146–1148
29. Forsythe R L, Bajaj P, Engeron O, Shadid E A 1978 The treatment of squamous cell carcinoma of the hand. The Hand 10: 104–108
30. Rayner C R W 1981 The results of treatment of two hundred and seventy-three carcinomas of the hand. The Hand 13: 183–186
31. Silverman I 1935 Epithelioma following chronic paronychia. American Journal of Surgery 19: 141–142, 151
— *subungual*
32. Attiyeh F F, Shah J, Booher R J, Knapper W H 1979 Subungual squamous cell carcinoma. Journal of the American Medical Association 241: 262–263
33. Canipe T L, Howell J A, Howell C M 1964 Subungual carcinoma. Plastic and Reconstructive Surgery 33: 263–265
34. Carroll R E 1976 Squamous cell carcinoma of the nail bed. The Journal of Hand Surgery 1: 92–97
35. Eichenholtz S N, Deangelis C 1965 Squamous cell carcinoma of nail bed. Journal of the American Medical Association 191: 102–104
36. Long P I, Espiniella J L 1978 Squamous cell carcinoma of the nail bed 239: 2154–2155
37. Onukak E E 1980 Squamous cell carcinoma of the nail bed: a diagnostic and therapeutic problem 67: 893–894
38. Shneidman D W, Barr R J, Graham J H 1979 Chronic cutaneous herpes simplex. Journal of the American Medical Association 241: 592–594

Subcutaneous and soft tissue

Epithelioid sarcoma
39. Boyes J, Marroum M 1978 Epithelioid sarcoma of hand and forearm. The Hand 10: 302–305
40. Bryan R S, Soule E H, Dobyns J H, Pritchard D J, Linscheid R L 1974 Primary epithelioid sarcoma of the hand. Journal of Bone and Joint Surgery 56: 458
41. Button M 1979 Epithelioid sarcoma: A case report. Journal of Hand Surgery 4: 368–371
42. Enzinger F M 1970 Epithelioid sarcoma. Cancer 26: 1029–1040
43. Peimer C A, Smith R J, Sirota R L, Cohen B E 1977 Epithelioid sarcoma of the hand and wrist: Patterns of extension. Journal of Hand Surgery 2: 275–282
44. Serciou S P, Reid D A C 1980 Epithelioid sarcoma — two case reports. The Hand 12: 304–307
Fibroma
45. Poppen N K, Niebauer J J 1977 Recurring digital fibrous tumor of childhood. Journal of Hand Surgery 2: 256–257
46. Schenkar D L, Kleinert H E 1977 Desmoplastic fibroma of the hand. Plastic and Reconstructive Surgery 59: 128–133

47. Sugiura I 1976 Desmoplastic fibroma. Case report and review of the literature. Journal of Bone and Joint Surgery 58A: 126–130

Fibrosarcoma
48. Akbarnia B A, Wirth C R, Colman N 1976 Fibrosarcoma arising from chronic osteomyelitis. Case report and review of the literature. Journal of Bone and Joint Surgery 58A: 123–125
49. Rasi H B, Mascardo T, Jinkdrak K 1980 Congenital fibrosarcoma of hand. Orthopaedic Review 9: 49–54

Histiocytoma
50. Hubbard L F, Burton R I 1977 Malignant fibrous histiocytoma of the forearm. Report of a case and review of the literature. Journal of Hand Surgery 2: 292–296
51. Karev A 1979 Malignant histiocytoma of the arm in a four year old boy. The Hand 11: 106–108
52. McDowell C L, Hencreoth W D 1977 Malignant fibrous histiocytoma of the hand. A case report 2: 297–298
53. Spector D, Miller J, Viloria J 1979 Malignant fibrous histiocytoma. Journal of Bone and Joint Surgery 61B: 190–193

Lipoma
54. Booher R J 1965 Lipoblastic tumors of the hands and feet. Review of the literature and report of thirty-three cases. The Journal of Bone and Joint Surgery 47A: 727–740
55. Hart J A L 1973 Intraosseus lipoma. Journal of Bone and Joint Surgery 55B: 624–632
56. Leffert R D 1972 Lipomas of the upper extremity. Journal of Bone and Joint 54A: 1262–1266
57. Schmitz R L, Keeley J L 1957 Lipomas of the hand. Surgery 42: 696–700
58. Strauss A 1922 Lipoma of the tendon sheaths: With report of a case and review of the literature. Surgery, Gynecology and Obstetrics 35: 161
59. Sullivan C R, Dahlin D C, Bryan R S 1956 Lipoma of the tendon sheath. Journal of Bone and Joint Surgery 38A: 1275–1280

Sarcoma
60. Tyler G, Wirman J, Neale H W 1980 Melanin containing clear cell sarcoma in a fingertip: case report and review of the literature. The Hand 12: 308–315

Synovium
Ganglion
61. Andren L, Eiken O 1971 Arthrographic studies of wrist ganglions. Journal of Bone and Joint Surgery 53A: 299–302
62. Angelides A C, Wallace P F 1976 The dorsal ganglion of the wrist: Its pathogenesis, gross and microscopic anatomy, and surgical treatment. The Journal of Hand Surgery 1: 228–235
63. Barnes W E, Larsen R D, Posch J L 1964 Review of ganglia of the hand and wrist with analysis of surgical treatment. Plastic and Reconstructive Surgery 34: 570–578
64. Janzon L, Niechajev I A 1981 Wrist ganglia. Scandinavian Journal of Plastic and Reconstructive Surgery 15: 53–56
65. McEvedy B V 1962 Simple ganglion. British Journal of Surgery 49: 585–594
66. Nelson C L, Sawmiller S, Phalen G S 1972 Ganglions of the wrist and hand. Journal of Bone and Joint Surgery 54A: 1459–1464
67. Orsay R H, Mecray P M, Ferguson L K 1937 Pathology and treatment of ganglion. American Journal of Surgery 36: 313–319

— children
68. MacCollum M S 1977 Dorsal wrist ganglions in children. Journal of Hand Surgery 2: 325

— flexor sheath
69. Matthews P 1973 Ganglia of the flexor tendon sheaths in the hand. Journal of Bone and Joint Surgery 55B: 612–617
70. Sarpyener M A, Ozcurumez O, Seyhan F 1968 Multiple ganglions of tendon sheaths. The Journal of Bone and Joint Surgery 50A: 985–990

— intraosseous
71. Bowers H, Hurst L 1979 An intra-articular intraosseous carpal ganglion. Journal of Hand Surgery 4: 375–377
72. Brown I, Huffstadt A J C 1981 Intraosseous ganglia. The Hand 13: 51–54
73. Grange W J 1978 Subperiosteal ganglion: A case report. Journal of Bone and Joint Surgery 60B: 124–125
74. Helal B, Vernon-Roberts B 1976 Intraosseous ganglion of the pisiform bone. The Hand 8: 150–154
75. Kambolis C, Bullough P G, Jaffe H I 1973 Ganglionic cystic defects of bone. Journal of Bone and Joint Surgery 55A: 496–505
76. Mogan J V, Newberg A H, Davis P H 1981 Intraosseous ganglion of the lunate. Journal of Hand Surgery 6: 61–63
77. Schauowicz F, Sainz M C, Slulitell J A 1979 Juxta-articular bone cysts (Intra-osseous ganglia). Journal of Bone and Joint Surgery 61B: 107–117

— radial artery
78. Crowley J G 1980 Cystic adventitial arterial disease. Journal of the Royal College of Surgeons of Edinburgh 25: 194–197
79. Kelly G L 1973 Radial artery occlusion by a carpal ganglion. Plastic and Reconstructive Surgery 52: 191–193
80. Lister G D, Smith R R 1978 Ideas and innovations. Protection of the radial artery in the resection of adherent ganglions of the wrist. Plastic and Reconstructive Surgery 61: 127–129

Giant cell tumour
81. Crawford G P, Offerman R J 1980 Pigmented villonodular synovitis in the hand. The Hand 12: 282–287
82. Fletcher A G, Horn R C 1951 Giant cell tumors of tendon sheath origin. A consideration of bone involvement and report of two cases with extensive bone destruction. Annals of Surgery 133: 374–385
83. Fyfe I S, MacFarlane A 1980 Pigmented villonodular synovitis of the hand. The Hand 12: 179–188
84. Galloway J D B, Borders A C, Ghormely R K 1940 Xanthomas of tendon sheath and synovial membranes: A clinical and pathological study. Archives of Surgery 40: 485–538
85. Hamilton W C, Ramsey P L, Hanson S M, Schiff D C 1975 Osseous xanthoma and multiple hand tumors as a complication of hyperlipidemia. The Journal of Bone and Joint Surgery 57A: 551–553
86. Hoehn J 1978 Multiple fibrous xanthomas of tendon sheath. The Hand 10: 306–308
87. Matthews R E, Gould J S, Kashlan M B 1981 Diffuse pigmented vollonodular tenosynovitis of the ulnar bursa — a case report. Journal of Bone and Joint Surgery 6: 64–69
88. Phalen G S, McCormack L J, Gazale W J 1959 Giant cell tumor of tendon sheath (benign synovioma) in the hand. Evaluation of 56 cases. Clinical Orthopedics 15: 140–151
89. Zook E G 1977 Extensive giant cell tumor of the finger. A case history. Orthopedics 2: 267–268

Synovial cell sarcoma
90. Kazayeri M, Gallo G 1979 Synovial sarcoma: A case report. Orthopedics 2: 496–498

Nerve
Review
91. Strickland J W, Steichen J B 1977 Nerve tumors of the hand and forearm. Journal of Hald Surgery 2: 285–291

Neurilemmoma

92. Blair W F 1980 Granular cell schwannoma of the hand. Journal of Hand Surgery 5: 51-52
93. Lewis R C, Nannini L H, Cocke W M 1981 Multifocal neurilemmomas of median and ulnar nerves of the same extremity — Case report. Journal of Hand Surgery 6: 406-408
94. Robb J 1978 Trigger finger due to neurilemmoma in the carpal tunnel. The Hand 10: 229-301

Neurofibromatosis

95. Bloem J J A M, Van Der Meulen J C 1978 Neurofibromatosis in plastic surgery. British Journal of Plastic Surgery 31: 50-53, 1978
96. Monballiu G 1981 Plexiform neurofibroma of the median nerve. Chirurgia Plastica 6: 141-145
97. Shereff M J, Posner M A, Gordon M H 1980 Upper extremity hypertrophy secondary to neurofibromatosis: A case report. Journal of Hand Surgery 5: 355-357

— malignant change

98. Sands M J, McDonough M T, Cohen A M, Rutenberg H L, Elsner J W 1975 Fatal malignant degeneration in multiple neurofibromatosis. Journal of the American Medical Association 233: 1381-1382

Tumours within nerve

99. Abu Jamra F N, Rebeiz J J 1979 Lipofibroma of the median nerve. Journal of Hand Surgery 4: 160-164
100. Mikhail I K 1964 Median nerve lipoma in the hand. The Journal of Bone and Joint Surgery 46B: 726
101. Morely G H 1964 Intraneural lipoma of the median nerve in the carpal tunnel. Report of a case. The Journal of Bone and Joint Surgery 46B: 734-735
102. Paletta F X, Senay L C 1981 Lipofibromatous haematoma of median nerve and ulnar nerve: surgical treatment. Plastic and Reconstructive Surgery 68: 915-926
103. Patel M, Silver J, Lipton D, Pearlman H 1979 Lipofibroma of the median nerve in the palm and digits of the hand. Journal of Bone and Joint Surgery 61A: 393-397
104. Peled I, Iosipovich Z, Rousso M, Wexler M R 1980 Hemangioma of the median nerve. Journal of Hand Surgery 5: 363-365
105. Pulvertaft R G 1964 Unusual tumours of the median nerve. Report of two cases. The Journal of Bone and Joint Surgery 46B: 731-733
106. Rowland S A 1977 Case report: Ten year follow-up of lipofibroma of the median nerve in the palm. Journal of Hand Surgery 2: 316-317
107. Rusko R A, Larsen R D 1981 Intraneural lipoma of the median nerve — case report and literature review. Journal of Hand Surgery 6: 388-391
108. Terzis J K, Daniel R K, Williams H B, Spencer P S 1978 Benign fatty tumors of the peripheral nerves. Annals of Plastic Surgery 1: 193-216
109. Watson-Jones R 1964 Encapsulated lipoma of the median nerve at the wrist. The Journal of Bone and Joint Surgery 46B: 736
110. Yeoman P M 1964 Fatty infiltration of the median nerve. The Journal of Bone and Joint Surgery 46B: 737-739

Vessel

Review

111. Booher R J 1961 Tumors arising from blood vessels in the hands and feet. Clinical Orthopedics 19: 71-98

Aneurysm

112. Baxt S, Mori K, Hoffman S 1975 Aneurysm of the hand secondary to Kaposi's sarcoma. Case report. Journal of Bone and Joint Surgery 57A: 995-997

113. Carneiro R D S 1974 Aneurysm of the wrist. Plastic and Reconstructive Surgery 54: 483-489
114. Dormandy J A, Barkley H 1979 Bilateral axillary artery aneurysms in a child. British Journal of Surgery 66: 650
115. Jenkins A McL, Macpherson A I S, Nolan B, Housely E 1976 Peripheral aneurysms in Behcet's disease. British Journal of Surgery 63: 199-202
116. Kleinert H E, Burget G C, Morgan J A, Kutz J E, Atasoy E 1973 Aneurysms of the hand. Archives of Surgery 106: 554-557
117. Malt S 1978 An arteriosclerotic aneurysm of the hand. Archives of Surgery 113: 762-763
118. Thorrens S, Trippel O H, Bergan J J 1966 Arteriosclerotic aneurysms of the hand. Archives of Surgery 92: 937-939

Angiomyoma

119. Neviaser R J, Newman W 1977 Dermal angiomyoma of the upper extremity. Journal of Hand Surgery 2: 271-274

Arteriovenous fistula

120. Leb D E, Sharma J K 1978 Clubbing secondary to an arteriovenous fistula used for hemodialysis. Journal of the American Medical Association 240: 142-143

— congenital

121. Bogumill G P 1977 Clinico-pathological correlation in a case of congenital arterio-venous fistula. The Hand 9: 60-64
122. Curtis R M 1953 Congenital arteriovenous fistulae of the hand. The Journal of Bone and Joint Surgery 35A: 917-928
123. Gelberman R, Goldner J L 1978 Congenital arteriovenous fistulas of the hand. Journal of Hand Surgery 3: 451-454
124. Griffin J M, Vasconez L O, Schatten W E 1978 Congenital arteriovenous malformations of the upper extremity. Plastic and Reconstructive Surgery 62: 49-58
125. Veal J R, McCord W M 1936 Congenital abnormal arteriovenous anastomoses of the extremities with special reference to diagnosis by arteriography and by the oxygen saturation test. Archives of Surgery 33: 848-866

Glomus

126. Carroll R E, Berman A T 1972 Glomus tumors of the hand. Review of the literature and report of 28 cases. Journal of Bone and Joint Surgery 54A: 691-703
127. Chan C W 1981 Intraosseous glomus tumor — Case report. Journal of Hand Surgery 6: 368-369
128. Cornell S J 1981 Multiple glomus tumors in one digit. The Hand 13: 301-302
129. Davis T S, Graham W P, Blomain E W 1981 A ten year experience with glomus tumors. Annals of Plastic Surgery 6: 297-299
130. Love J G 1944 Glomus tumors: Diagnosis and treatment. Mayo Clinic Proceedings 19: 113-116
131. Maley E D, McDonald C J 1975 Bilateral subungual glomus tumors. Plastic and Reconstructive Surgery 55: 488-489
132. Maxwell G P, Curtis R, Wilgis F 1979 Multiple digital glomus tumors. Journal of Hand Surgery 4: 363-367
133. Mullis W F, Rosato E F, Butler C J, Mayer L J 1972 The glomus tumor. Surgery, Gynecology and Obstetrics 135: 705-707
134. Rettig A C, Strickland J W 1977 Glomus tumor of the digits. Journal of Hand Surgery 2: 261-265
135. Riddell D H, Martin R S 1951 Glomus tumor to unusual size. Annals of Surgery 133: 401-403
136. Riveros M, Pack G T 1951 The glomus tumor. Report of 20 cases. Annals of Surgery 133: 401-403
137. Sugiura I 1976 Intra-osseous glomus tumor. The Journal of Bone and Joint Surgery 58B: 245-247
138. Varian J P, Cleak D K 1980 Glomus tumors in the hand. The Hand 12: 293-299

Haemangioma

139. Ekerot L, Jonsson K, Eiken O, Cederholm C 1981 Hemangioma of the lunate (Klippel-Trenaunay syndrome) Scandinavian Journal of Plastic and Reconstructive Surgery 15: 153–156

140. Frazier C H 1980 Hemangioma of the fingertip. Orthopedics 3: 1211

141. Geister J H, Eversmann W W 1978 Closed system venography in the evaluation of upper extremity hemangiomas. Journal of Hand Surgery 3: 173–178

142. Pezehski C, Daneshbod K, Faghihi E 1980 Multiple hemangiomas of bone of upper extremity. Orthopaedic Review 9: 67–69

143. Tunon J B, Gonzalez F P 1977 Angiomatosis of the metacarpal skeleton. The Hand 9: 88–91

Haemangioendotheliomas

144. Acharya G, Merritt W H, Theogaraj S D 1980 Hemangioendotheliomas of the hand. Case reports. The Journal of Hand Surgery 5: 181–182

145. Ekerot L, Eiken O, Jonsson K, Lindstrom C 1981 Malignant hemangioendothelioma of metacarpal bones. Scandinavian Journal of Plastic and Reconstructive Surgery 15: 73–76

146. Finsterbush A, Husseini N, Rousso M 1981 Multifocal hemangioendothelioma of bones in the hand — a case report. Journal of Hand Surgery 6: 353–356

147. Larsson S E, Lorentzon R, Boquist L 1975 Malignant haemangioendothelioma of bone. Journal of Bone and Joint Surgery 57A: 84–89

148. Moss L D, Stueber K, Hafiz M A 1982 Congenital hemangioendothelioma of the hand — case report. Journal of Hand Surgery 7: 53–56

149. Patel M, Srinivason K, Pearlman H 1978 Malignant hemangioendothelioma in the hand. Journal of Hand Surgery 3: 585

Hemangiopericytoma

150. Ratna S 1976 Case reports: Hemangiopericytoma of the hand. Plastic and Reconstructive Surgery 57: 746–748

Leiomyoma

151. Hauswald K R, Kasdan M L, Weis D L 1975 Vascular leiomyoma of the hand. Plastic and Reconstructive Surgery 55: 89–91, 1975

Muscle

Myoblastoma

152. Bielejeski T R 1973 Granular cell tumor (myoblastoma) of the hand. Journal of Bone and Joint Surgery 55A: 841–843, 1973

Rhabdomyosarcoma

153. Mutz S B, Curl W 1977 Alveolar cell rhabdomyosarcoma of the hand. Case report with four year survival and no evidence of recurrence. Journal of Hand Surgery 2: 283–284

154. Potenza A D, Winslow D J 1961 Rhabdomyosarcoma of the hand. Journal of Bone and Joint Surgery 43A: 700–708

Cartilage

Chondroblastoma

155. Neviaser R J, Wilson J N 1972 Benign chondroblastoma in the finger. Journal of Bone and Joint Surgery 54A1: 389–392

Chondroma

156. Dellon A L, Weiss S W, Mitch W E 1978 Bilateral extraosseous chondromas of the hand in a patient with chronic renal failure. Journal of Hand Surgery 3: 139–141

157. Takigawa K 1971 Chondroma of the bones of the hand. Journal of Bone and Joint Surgery 53A: 1591–1600

158. Takigawa K 1971 Carpal chondroma. Journal of Bone and Joint Surgery 53A: 1601–1604

Chondromatosis, synovial

159. Constant E, Harebottle N H, Davis D G 1974 Synovial chondromatosis of the hand. Plastic and Reconstructive Surgery 54: 353–358

160. DeBennedetti M J, Schwinn P 1979 Tenosynovial chondromatosis in the hand. Journal of Bone and Joint Surgery 898–902

161. Heiple K G, Elmer R M 1972 Chondromatous hamartomas arising from the volar digital plates. The Journal of Bone and Joint Surgery 54A: 393–398

162. Lynn M D, Lee J 1972 Periarticular tenosynovial chondrometaplasia. Repoct of a case at the wrist. Journal of Bone and Joint Surgery 54A: 650–652

163. Sim F H, Dahlin D C, Ivins J C 1977 Extra-articular synovial chondromatosis. Journal of Bone and Joint Surgery 59A: 492–495

164. Strong M L 1975 Chondromas of the tendon sheath of the hand. Report of a case and review of the literature. The Journal of Bone and Joint Surgery 57A: 1164–1165

Chondrosarcoma

165. Block R S, Burton R I 1977 Multiple chondrosarcomas in a hand. A case report. Journal of Hand Surgery 2: 310–313

166. Gottschalk R G, Smith R T 1963 Chondrosarcoma of the hand. The Journal of Bone and Joint Surgery 45A: 141–150

167. Granberry W M, Bryan W 1978 Chondrosarcoma of the trapezium: A case report. Journal of Hand Surgery 3: 277–279

168. Jokl P, Albright J A, Goodman A H 1971 Juxtacortical chondrosarcoma of the hand. Journal of Bone and Joint Surgery 53A: 1370–1376

169. Patel M R, Pearlman H S, Engler J, Wollowick B S 1977 Chondrosarcoma of the proximal phalanx of the finger. Review of the literature and report of a case. Journal of Bone and Joint Surgery 59A: 401–403

170. Roberts P H, Price C H G 1977 Chondrosarcoma of the bones of the hand. Journal of Bone and Joint Surgery 59B: 213–221

171. Wu K K, Collon D J, Guise E R 1980 Extraosseous chondrosarcoma. Report of five cases and review of the literature. Journal of Bone and Joint Surgery 62A: 189–194

172. Wu K K, Kelly A P 1977 Periosteal (juxta-cortical) chondrosarcoma. Report of a case occurrilg in the hand. Journal of Hand Surgery 2: 314–315

Enchondroma

173. Jewusiak E M, Spence K, Sell K 1971 Solitary benign enchondroma of the long bones of the hand. Journal of Bone and Joint Surgery 53A: 1587–1590

174. Mosher J F 1976 Multiple enchondromatosis of the hand. A case report. Journal of Bone and Joint Surgery 58A: 717–719

Bone

Aneurysmal bone cyst

175. Burkhalter W, Schroeder F, Eversmann W 1978 Aneurysmal bone cysts occurring in the metacarpals. Journal of Hand Surgery 3: 579

176. Chalmers J 1981 Aneurysmal bone cysts of the phalanges. The Hand 13: 296–300

177. Fuhs S E, Herndon J H 1979 Aneurysmal bone cysts involving the hand: A review and report of two cases. Journal of Hand Surgery 4: 160–164

Carpometacarpal boss

178. Artz T D, Posch J L 1973 The carpometacarpal boss. The Journal of Bone and Joint Surgery 55A: 747–752

179. Cuono C B, Watson H K 1979 The carpal boss: surgical treatment and etiological considerations. Plastic and Reconstructive Surgery 63: 88–94

Ectopic ossification
180. Altner P C, Singh S K 1981 An unusual case of ectopic ossification in a finger. Journal of Hand Surgery 6: 142–145
181. Johnson M K, Lawrence J F 1975 Metaplastic bone formation (myositis ossificans) in the soft tissue of the hand. Case report 57A: 999–1000
182. Ogilvie-Harris D J, Fornasier V L 1980 Pseudomalignant myositis ossificans: Heterotopic new bone formation without a history of trauma. Journal of Bone and Joint Surgery 62A: 0274–1283
183. Schecter W P, Wong D, Kilgore E S, Newmeyer W L, Howes E L, Clark G 1982 Peripartum pseudomalignant myositis ossificans of the finger. Journal of Hand Surgery 7: 44–46
184. Wissiner H A, McClain E J, Boyes J H 1966 Turret exostosis. Ossifying hematoma of the phalanges. The Journal of Bone and Joint surplus 48A: 105

Ewings
185. Dreyfuss U Y, Auslander L, Bialik V, Fishman J 1980 Ewing's sarcoma of the hand following recurrent trauma. A case report. The Hand 12: 300–303
186. Dryer R, Buckwalter J, Flatt A, Bonfiglio M 1979 Ewing's sarcoma of the hand. Journal of Hand Surgery 4: 372–374

Giant cell tumour, osteoclastoma
187. Averill R M, Smith R J, Campbell C J 1980 Giant cell tumors of the bones of the hand. Journal of Hand Surgery 5: 39–50
188. Crawford J, Akbarnia M D 1975 Giant cell tumor of the radius treated by massive resection and tibial-bone graft. Journal of Bone and Joint Surgery 57A: 982–990
189. Fitzpatrick D J, Bullough P G 1977 Giant cell tumor of the lunate bone: A case report. Journal of Hand Surgery 2: 269–270
190. Gutpa S, Kumar A, Gupta I 1980 Giant cell tumor of the first metacarpal bone. The Hand 12: 288–292
191. Larsson S E, Lorentzon R, Boquist L 1975 Giant cell tumor of bone. Journal of Bone and Joint Surgery 57A: 167–173
192. Peimer C A, Schiller A L, Mankin H J, Smith R J 1980 Multicentric giant cell tumor of bone. Journal of Bone and Joint Surgery 62A: 652–656
193. Smith J A, Millender L H 1979 Treatment of recurrent giant cell tumor of the digit by phalangeal excision and toe phalanx transplant. A case report. Journal of Hand Surgery 4: 164–168
194. Smith R J, Mankin H J 1977 Allograft replacement of distl radius for giant cell tumor. The Journal of Hand Surgery 2: 299–309

Osteoblastoma
19. Mosher J, Peckham A 1978 Osteoblastoma of the metacarpal: A case report. Journal of Hand Surgery 3: 358–360

Osteochondroma
196. Callan J E, Wood V E 1975 Spontaneous resolution of an osteochondroma. Journal of Bone and Joint Surgery 57A: 723
197. Ganzhorn R W, Bahri G, Horowitz M 1981 Osteochondroma of the distal phalanx. Journal of Hand Surgery 6: 625–626
198. Ishizuki M, Isobe Y, Arai T, Nagatsuka Y, Tanabe K, Okumura S 1977 Osteochondromatosis of the finger joints. The Hand 9: 198–200

199. Medlar R C, Sprague H H 1979 Osteochondroma of the carpal scaphoid. Journal of Hand Surgery 4: 150–152
200. Murphy A F, Wilson J N 1958 Tenosynovial osteochondroma in the hand. Journal of Bone and Joint Surgery 40A: 1236

Osteoid osteoma
201. Aulicino P L, Dupuy T E, Moriarity R P 1981 Osteoid osteoma of the terminal phalanx of finger. Orthopaedic Review 10: 59–63
202. Carroll R E 1953 Osteoid osteoma in the hand. Journal of Bone and Joint Surgery 35A: 888–893
203. Ghiam G F, Bora F W 1978 Osteoid osteoma of the carpal bones. Journal of Hand Surgery 3: 280–283
204. Giannakis A, Papachristou G, Tiniakos G, Chrysafidis G, Hartofilakidis-Garofalidis G 1977 Osteoid osteoma of the terminal phalanges. The Hand 9: 295–300
205. Grundberg A B 1977 Osteoid osteoma of the thumb. Report of a case. Journal of Hand Surgery 2: 266
206. Jensen E G 1979 Osteoid osteoma of the capitate bone. The Hand 11: 102–105
207. Lamb D W, Castillo F D 1981 Phalangeal osteoid osteoma in the hand. The Hand 13: 291–295
208. Murray J A, Thaggard A, Wallace S, Benmenachem G 1979 Arteriography of osteoid osteoma: An aid in differentation and management. Orthopedics 2: 359–365
209. O'Hara J P, Tegtmeyer C, Sweet D E, McCue F C 1975 Angiography in the diagnosis of osteoid osteoma of the hand. Journal of Bone and Joint Surgery 57A: 163–166
210. Rosenfeld K, Bora F W, Lane J M 1973 Osteoid osteoma of the hamate. Journal of Bone and Joint Surgery 55A: 1085–1087
211. Sim F H, Dahlin D C, Beabout J W 1975 Osteoid osteoma: diagnostic problems. Journal of Bone and Joint Surgery 57A: 154–159

Osteosarcoma
212. Brostrom L, Harris M, Simon M, Cooperman D, Nilsonne U 1979 The effect of biopsy on survival of patients with osteosarcoma. The Journal of Bone and Joint Surgery 61B: 209–212
213. Campanacci M, Bacci G, Pagani P, Giunti A 1980 Multiple drug chemotherapy for the primary treatment of osteosarcoma of the extremities. The Journal of Bone and Joint Surgery 62B: 93–101
214. Fleegler E J, Marks K E, Sebek B A, Groppe C W, Belhobek G 1980 Osteosarcoma of the hand. The Hand 12: 316–322
215. Stark H H, Jones F E, Jernstrom P 1971 Parosteal osteogenic sarcoma of a metacarpal bone. The Journal of Bone and Joint Surgery 53A: 147–153

Metastatic
216. Aggarwal N D, Mittal R L, Bhalla B 1972 Delayed solitary metastasis to the radius of renal-cell carcinoma. Journal of Bone and Joint Surgery 54A: 1314–1316
217. Bevan D A, Ehrlich G E, Gupta V P 1977 Metastatic carcinoma simulating gout. Journal of the American Medical Association 237: 2746–2747
218. Kent K W, Guise E R 1978 Metastatic tumors of the hand: A report of six cases. Journal of Hand Surgery 3: 271–276
219. Kerin R 1958 Metastatic tumors of the hand. The Journal of Bone and Joint Surgery 40A: 263
220. Marmor L, Horner R L 1959 Metastasis to a phalanx simulating infection in a finger. American Journal of Surgery 97: 236

221. Prystowsky S D, Herndon J H, Freeman R G 1975 Bronchogenic carcinoma metastatic to the hand. Cutis 16: 678–681

222. Uriburu I J F, Morchio F J, Marin J C 1976 Metastases of carcinoma of the larynx and thyroid gland to the phalanges of the hand. Report of two cases. Journal of Bone and Joint Surgery 58A: 134–136

223. Wu K K, Winkelman N Z, Guise E R 1980 Metastatic bronchogenic carcinoma to the finger simulating acute osteomyelitis. Orthopedics 3: 25–28

Treatment — general

224. Clifford R H, Kelly A P 1959 Diagnosis and treatment of tumors of the hand. Clinical Orthopaedics 13: 204–212

225. Pearson D 1980 Radiotherapy and chemotherapy of limb tumours. Annals of the Royal College of Surgeons of England 62: 99–102

226. Smith R J 1977 Tumors of the hand. Who is best qualified to treat tumors of the hand? Journal of Hand Surgery 2: 251–255

Congenital

The classification indicated above by Roman numerals is that adopted by the International Federation of Hand Societies and by the International Society for Prosthetics and Orthotics.[1] Those conditions presented in italics are considered in this chapter. This is not a complete list of congenital deformities. It does, however, represent 89.1% of one large series of affected hands[2] the balance being made up of conditions with which the author has no experience — such as arthrogryposis and ulnar club hand — or for which no treatment is available or required — brachydactyly and Madelung's deformity.[3] Greek and Latin 'unpronouncables' are avoided where possible for it seems unfair to copy them from another book into this. Should the reader encounter them or be invited by a learned geneticist to see a patient with a multi-eponymous syndrome, then he is referred to the Glossary and the Index of Syndromes in Adrian Flatt's excellent book, *The Care of Congenital Hand Anomalies*[2].

And so to the task in hand. It is different, challenging and rewarding. Firstly, before becoming preoccupied with the deformity of the hand, the examiner should inquire about other associated anomalies[4] and ensure that they are being properly handled. If a full examination has not been undertaken it should be performed or arranged. Consultation and planning may be necessary with other treating physicians.

Secondly, diagnosis is made more difficult by the total lack of active participation of the patient. The history must be taken from the parents who may seem surprisingly uncertain about the manual capabilities and limitations of their child. This is because they are of course untrained in clinical observation. Where the information is required, they must be trained to look for particular features, such as use of a part or its active motion. No facts can be obtained where active participation is required, for example, two point discrimination, active motion and the Allen test. Thus much more weight comes to rest on *inspection*; on *palpation* and *passive motion*; on *X-ray evaluation*. Clinical examination should be appropriately prolonged to permit observation, supplemented and stimulated by the provision of two-handed toys if the child is old enough. An occupational therapist can greatly expedite this assessment. Some tricks may help — *active motion* is indicated by the presence of normal skin creases; its absence by their absence. Active motion can be revealed sometimes by holding the digit or limb at the extremes of the range for some moments and then releasing it. Thus, holding the fingers in full flexion may cause the child to keep them there momentarily after release, or, holding them in full extension may induce reflex flexion when freed. Clearly only positive observations are valid. In the few situations where sensation is in doubt — for example, in constriction ring syndrome — tactile adhesion and wrinkling tests (pp. 154, 158) can be used. X-ray evaluation is made more difficult, sometimes worthless, by the fact that much of the infant hand is present only in cartilage. Ossification centres appear at different ages (Table 7.1)[5]. These ages vary considerably in the normal individual, but knowledge of them — as of other radiological variables[6] — is of value, both in routine reading of films and also because there are specific causes of *advanced, retarded* and *dysharmonic maturation* which are outwith the scope of this text. For the above and other reasons — changes with growth, establishment of rapport — it is often desirable to see the

Table 7.1 Age of appearance of ossification centres. (Figures are for the 50th percentile in girls; centres appear later in boys by a multiplication factor of 1.55 ± 0.14 SD)

Carpus	
Capitate and hamate	2 months
Triquetral	1.7 years
Lunate	2.6 years
Scaphoid, trapezium, trapezoid	4.1 years
Metacarpus and Phalanges	
Metacarpophalangeal joints	
of the fingers (both centres) all by	1.5 years
Metacarpal of thumb	1.6 years
Proximal phalanx of thumb	1.7 years
Middle phalanges	all by 2.0 years
Distal phalanges	all by 2.5 years

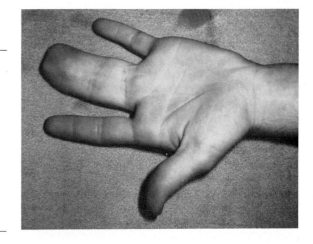

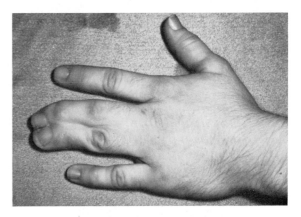

child on two or more occasions before making surgical plans.

Finally, the surgeon should remember that while he examines and operates upon the baby, he is treating the parents. For the infant is sublimely unaware that he has any problem and he certainly does not present with a complaint. The parents by contrast are distraught to a degree that may seem out of all proportion. But it is not, for their concern is heightened by the potential of personal guilt, by the disappointment of having other than the expected perfect child, by the fear of anaesthesia and surgery at an age they believe to be so delicate, by the possibility of further abnormal children. They must therefore be informed with clarity and precision, reassured with honesty and compassion. From an early stage in the relationship, they must be told, with tact and sympathy, of the limitations of surgical endeavour. They must be brought as far as possible to view function as beauty, regardless of uncorrectable deviations from the norm. They should not be given false hopes, either by too glowing or inadequate a prognosis. Restoration, manufacture rather, of a normal hand is possible in only the most simple of defects. In rare and complex cases there is much to be said for a second opinion arranged by the surgeon. It gives support and often information to the doctor, and reassurance to the parents with invariably a perceptible increase in their confidence about their first choice of physician.

The surgeon may do much less surgery to the child with more informed consent than he could to the parents themselves. This is only right and proper for such protectiveness is an expression of their biological function. Having performed that surgery he must maintain the information link: speaking to the parents immediately on completion of their child's operation; telling them at what time rounds are made so that they may be there; inviting them if concerned to the office or clinic at any time in the post-operative period; sharing plans for future

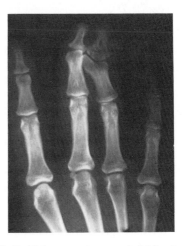

Fig. 7.1 (A–C) *Adult presentation congenital deformity.* This patient with a complete simple syndactyly and concealed distal central polydactyly of the left middle and ring fingers presented at the age of 28. Some months following correction the patient became sufficiently disturbed psychiatrically as to require prolonged hospital admission. Psychiatric opinion at the time indicated that the patient subconsciously associated her unwed status with the syndactyly (see also Fig. 7.29).

management. Only in these ways will the surgeon gain that which he needs in addition to knowledge and technical skill in dealing with congenital deformity — the trust of the family.

Congenital anomalies in adults

The adult who presents with a congenital defect uncorrected requires evaluation of an entirely different kind. Evidently, they have functioned efficiently to that stage. Why then do they now come forward seeking surgical correction? The possibility of underlying psychiatric disturbance must never be overlooked. The evident symbolism of the unseparated complete syndactyly of the left middle and ring fingers in an unmarried 28 year old woman is very clear (Fig. 7.1). The subconscious reliance that another patient may be placing on surgical correction may be less evident, but nonetheless devastating when it fails to yield the desired social result. Psychiatric consultation should always be suggested — the patient who readily assents in order to have surgery is well balanced and does not need the consultation! (see Fig. 7.29).

FAILURE OF FORMATION OF PARTS

Transverse absence — upper third of forearm

This is the most common transverse absence in the upper limb and is almost entirely a problem for the prosthetist. The length of forearm below the normal elbow joint is 5 to 7 cm at birth, but growth is relatively decreased and the adult length rarely exceeds 10 cm.[7] The child should be fitted with a simple prosthesis at six months which aids considerably in crawling and climbing.[8] More sophisticated devices are provided at 12 to 18 months and even myoelectric prostheses are now being fitted in some centres at the age of three. The infant and child does well with prostheses[9], even bilateral, but renewed counselling is required at adolescence when social pressures may cause him to reject it.

Transverse absence — carpus, metacarpus, phalanges

The absence of digits may present as a result of several congenital anomalies, the most common being:

(i) true transverse absence
(ii) cleft hand (p. 321)
(iii) amputations from constriction ring syndrome (p. 346)
(iv) symbrachydactyly

While the carpus is rarely complete, these children have a normal wrist joint and may also have vestigial digits (Fig. 7.2). If left alone, they will become remarkably adroit at crude grasp and release by the age of two to three, using the flexed wrist against the torso. The back of the carpus is also used and when they present at an older age, both the palmar and dorsal two point discrimination are more acute than normal.

Initially, the infant should be fitted with a palmar plate prosthesis which, by motion of the wrist, permits grasp of smaller objects than otherwise.[7] Management can continue with prostheses, by conversion to a split hook with simple hinge control by the wrist joint.

However, there are some limited possibilities employing surgery, particularly where some metacarpal remnants are present. These include any or all of the following:

distraction manoplasty
free phalangeal transfer
ulnar post construction
microvascular toe to hand transfer

Examination and counselling should be directed at determining whether these are indicated or desired.

EXAMINATION
Skeletal parts should be palpated, paying particular attention to *wrist motion* and *vestigial metacarpus*. The former is important for prosthesis design and for possible tendon transfers, both because they will probably be of wrist motors and because a full active range of wrist motion will add excursion to such transfers through the tenodesis effect. Good vestigial metacarpals at the thumb position and at the fifth or fourth ray are especially valuable. If any of the thumb metacarpal is present, the thenar area should be examined for passive range of the basal joint and observed for intrinsic muscle function, revealed both by contour and by voluntary active motion.

When vestigial digits are present they are simply nubbins of tissue often bearing a minute nail. Some authorities state that the presence of nails and a hypoplastic skeleton indicates a symbrachydactyly rather than a true transverse absence (Fig. 7.3). These vestigial digits are retracted into the pad of the transverse absence by the action of rudimentary long extrinsic tendons. These nubbins should be grasped gently and distracted, both to assess the presence and to some degree the strength of these extrinsics and also to evaluate the size of the skin envelope of the distal remnant. X-rays are of limited value at the probable age of first presentation.

INDICATIONS
Armed with the information regarding skeleton, skin, passive and active motion gleaned from examination, the surgical possibilities can be discussed with the parents.

Fingers
[Transverse absence of the *thumb* at metacarpal level is considered with *partial aplasia of the thumb* (p. 347).]

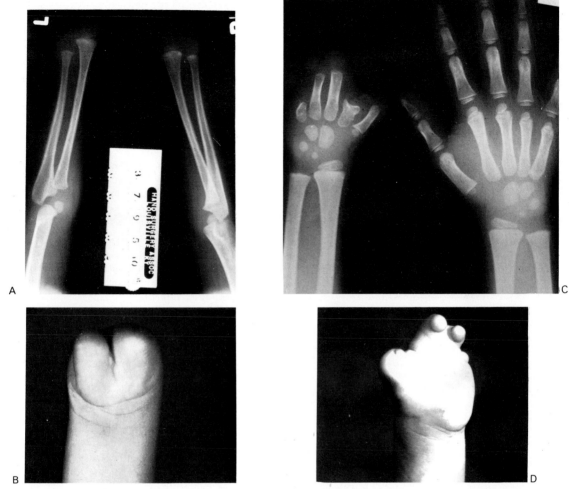

Fig. 7.2 (A) This child presented with bilateral transverse absence, on X-ray apparently at the level of the wrist. (B) It was evident on clinical examination, however, that there were mobile vestigial metacarpals at the thumb and ring or small finger positions. For this reason, he is scheduled for toe to hand transfer. (C) This somewhat older child clearly has metacarpals and (D) demonstrates crude grasp between them. The proposed management here is for second toe transfer to the first metacarpal, ablation of the vestigial second metacarpal, and subsequent second and third toe transfer from the opposite foot to the middle and ring metacarpals.

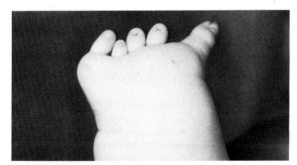

Fig. 7.3 *Symbrachydactyly or transverse absence with vestigial digits.* This child showed a stable skeleton in the rudimentary thumb, but only rudimentary cartilaginous fragments in the vestigial digits. There were extrinsic tendons evidenced by the retraction of the nubbins when they were drawn distally.

Distraction manoplasty has been said to lengthen the skin envelope of the vestigial digits.[10] Done by transfixing the pulps with wire and applying steady traction over some weeks, it is more effective if there are cartilaginous elements in the pulp for they reduce the chance of the wire cutting out and the speed with which it does so. After distraction has been applied for four to six weeks, *phalangeal transfer* should be undertaken, with Z-plasty lengthening if necessary of the annular ring constriction which is often present at the base of the vestigial digit. The reports of success with phalangeal transfer vary very widely from highly reputable and experienced authors: Carroll reports no growth in 159 transferred phalanges in 79 cases[11], Watson 90% of expected growth in 20 of 27 cases[12]. Other experience suggests that free bone grafts survive

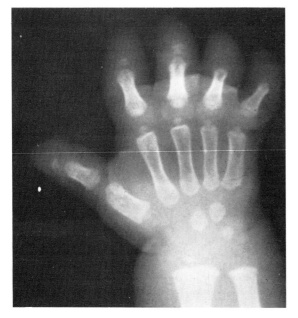

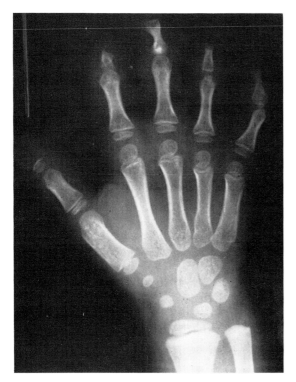

Fig. 7.4 (A) This hand demonstrates uniform transverse absence of the fingers possibly due to constriction ring syndrome since there are no nails and that skeleton which is present is normal. After a period of distraction, phalangeal transfers were undertaken to all four fingers from the second and third toes of both feet. It can be seen four years later (B) that the phalanges in the middle, ring, and small have survived but with no clear evidence of a growth centre while that placed in the index finger has not.

more certainly and are integrated well when they are employed as an interposition rather than a cantilever graft and when they are fixed, cancellous bone to cancellous[13,14]. Carroll's pessimism would more closely fit this contention, since the phalanges are placed in the skin envelope with no local bone distally and usually no bone to bone contact (Fig. 7.4).

If fourth (or fifth) metacarpal remnants are present on examination, these can be put to good use. The ulnar remnant can be lengthened by interposition cancellous bone grafting, the skin envelope being enlarged by peroperative distraction or — rarely necessary[14] — by advancing the thenar cone and applying a full-thickness graft to the base — somewhat akin to a Gillies 'cocked-hat' procedure[15]. An alternative to bone-grafting is the microsurgical transfer of one or two toes, a procedure still under evaluation (p. 122). While it is technically possible to achieve survival, the acquisition of function is even more difficult in congenital absence than following traumatic loss of fingers[16], because of the vestigial nature of all structures in the hand (Fig. 7.5):

— tendons are rudimentary, often represented by a sheet of fascia; transfer of wrist motors are often required
— the median and ulnar nerves, having nowhere to go, are underdeveloped; digital nerves have to be joined to cutaneous branches such as the terminal radial, the dorsal sensory branch of the ulnar nerve and the palmar cutaneous branch of the median nerve.

All of these surgical procedures may be tried and are not incompatible. Distraction manoplasty at six months with phalangeal transfer thereafter, using the proximal phalanges of the third and fourth toes, can be followed by a two year observation period during which phalangeal survival, epiphyseal development and overall growth can be assessed. If no grasp is so restored, ulnar post construction and toe-to-hand transfer can be performed knowing that all less complex avenues have been explored.

This plan potentially exposes the child to several surgical procedures at an early age, which must be made clear to the parents when discussing the choice between prosthesis and surgery.

Longitudinal absence — distal radial — radial club hand[17]

As a diagnosis, the term 'radial club hand' emphasises the main feature of the disorder, namely the hypoplasia or absence of the radius with resultant radial deviation of the hand on the forearm (Fig. 7.6). The condition is commonly associated with other anomalies and these should not be overlooked during examination (see below). There is no clearly understood aetiology, either genetic or environmental. Both extremities are affected in 50–72% of cases, depending on the series.

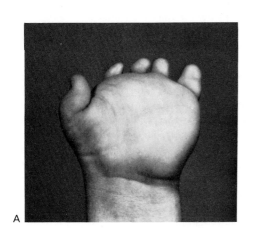

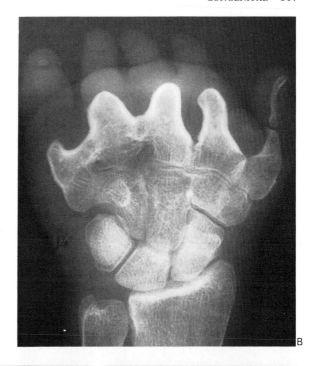

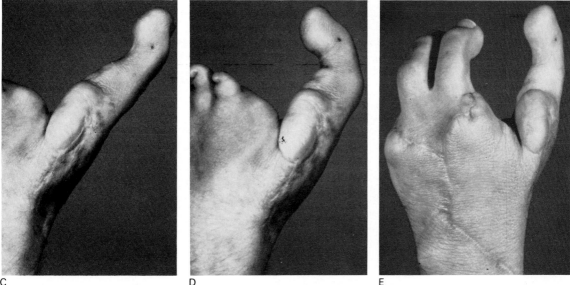

Fig. 7.5 (A & B) This eighteen year old presented for reconstruction of symbrachydactyly of all digits. (C & D) This was achieved successfully with respect to thumb reconstruction, but (E) transfer of two toes to the middle and ring finger positions has thus far been unsuccessful with regards to motion and sensation. This is largely due to the rudimentary nature of the flexor and extensor tendons and to the fact that both median and ulnar nerves were vestigial. The digital nerves to the thumb were joined to the radial cutaneous and palmar cutaneous branch of the median nerves while those to the fingers were attached to the dorsal sensory branch of the ulnar nerve.

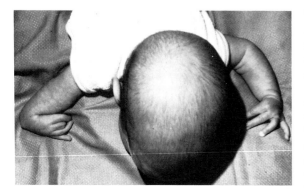

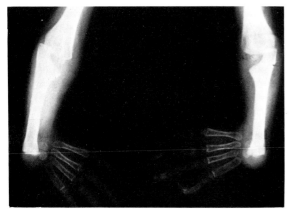

Fig. 7.6 *Bilateral radial club hand.* (A) Note that the right hand is more severely affected, and the absence of wrinkles on the extensor surface of the fingers indicates the lack of digital motion. The elbow as seen here is in full extension, and passive flexion was markedly limited at birth. With manipulation this improved to the point where centralisation could be performed. (B) The radius is totally absent. The ulna is short and wide, though in this case not curved.

EXAMINATION

The wrist is radially deviated to a variable degree. Passive motion reveals a significant reduction in the range of motion available, when compared with normal, both in palmar and dorsiflexion of the wrist and in ulnar deviation. The degree to which the radial deviation can be corrected is important, as it may indicate the power of deviating forces which will work against any surgical correction and certainly determines the need for manipulation with or without splintage before surgery. When fully deviated ulnarward, skin webbing on the radial aspect and redundancy on the ulnar will be noted. The former may contain a tight band which may be the fibrous anlage of the radius, which must be excised, or, more importantly, the median nerve — this is frequently the most radial structure and in one fourth of cases is duplicated, one branch serving radial and the other median territory.

The thumb may be normal, hypoplastic, rudimentary or absent, the incidence varying widely in different series.

The *rudimentary* thumb is present, but has no function, being distally located and having neither normal articulations or motors — a 'pouce flottant'. The *hypoplastic* has function which is impaired to a varying degree (p. 340).

The elbow of the child with radial club hand is held in the extended posture and attempts at passive motion will reveal that this is a fixed extension in many of the cases seen early. The passive motion improves with age and this should be encouraged by manipulation and splintage of both elbow and wrist. Certainly, the wrist should *not* be centralised where lack of elbow flexion would prevent the corrected hand from reaching the head.

Motion in the *finger joints* is most impaired in the radial digits. Thus the passive range of motion is more significantly reduced in the index than in the small finger. The metacarpophalangeal joint, while lacking flexion, usually shows normal or increased hyperextension (Fig.

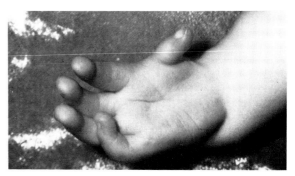

Fig. 7.7 *Radial club hand.* Following centralisation and prior to pollicisation, the relative lack of flexion in the index finger when compared with the small can be detected by the relative absence of flexion skin creases.

7.7). The proximal interphalangeal joints in one series[17] showed average active ranges of motion as follows:

> index 24°
> middle 35°
> ring 57°
> small 78°

Despite this reduced motion, true symphalangism (p. 324) rarely occurs. It is not known to what extent the reduced motion is due to primary changes in the joint and what to anomalies of the motors, but muscle inadequacies certainly occur. On the extensor aspect, the extensor digitorum may be fused to the wrist extensors. The long flexors, especially the superficial, may be incomplete, atrophic or fused. Here again the degree of involvement is greatest in the index finger.

The *absence of muscles* or their anomalies may be detected in some small part by *loss of contour*, of *flexion creases*, or of *passive range* and *lack of voluntary motion* when the child is

confirmed only at surgery or at a much later age when the child can co-operate in active testing. While almost all upper extremity muscles may be affected (Table 7.2)[18] those most commonly so are

pectoralis major
biceps[19]
brachioradialis
supinator
extensor carpi radialis
flexor carpi radialis
the muscles of the thumb

The nerves and arteries of the radial club hand are also usually abnormal but this cannot be determined on examination of the infant nor need it affect the surgical

observed for some time. However, the deficiency may be correction provided the surgeon exercises appropriate caution.

X-ray, depending upon the age of the child, will reveal to a varying degree the following anomalies:

radius — completely absent = total aplasia
— present proximally = partial aplasia
— complete but short = hypoplasia
ulna curved, thickened and, on average, only 60% of normal length (Fig. 7.8)
humerus also shorter than normal
carpal bone fusions and absence, the latter especially of the trapezium and scaphoid — other carpal bones may be absent, but are more likely to show fusion or delayed ossification
thumb absence or hypoplasia (p. 340)

Table 7.2 Muscle anomalies in radial club hand (after Skerik and Flatt[17])

*MM	ABSENT ⩾ 50%	ABERRANT		FUSION with
		ORIGIN	INSERTION	
PM	sterno-costal head		///////////////	
D				
BB	long head	///////////////	///////////////	coraco-brachialis, PT
T				
BR	///////////////		///////////////	ECRL
PT				BB, PL, FCR
PQ	///////////////			
S	///////////////		///////////////	
FCR	///////////////	///////////////	///////////////	PT
FCU			///////////////	ECU
PL	///////////////		///////////////	FDS, PT
FDS	index	radial head		FDP, PL
FDP	index		///////////////	FDS
FPL	///////////////		///////////////	
FPB	///////////////	///////////////	///////////////	
APB	///////////////	///////////////	///////////////	
AP	///////////////	///////////////	///////////////	
ADM				FDM
FDM				ADM
IO	1st DORSAL			
EPL	///////////////		///////////////	
EPB	///////////////		///////////////	
APL	///////////////		///////////////	
EI	///////////////		///////////////	
EDM				ED or ECU
ED				ECRL or EDM or ECU
ECU		///////////////	///////////////	ED or FCU or EDM
ECRL	///////////////			ECRB, ED, BR
ECRB	///////////////			ECRL

*Abbreviations for muscles are those given in the Appendix (pp. 352–364)

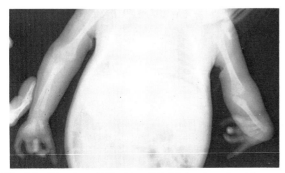

Fig. 7.8   Here in a child with radial club hand on the right and polydactyly with a triphalangeal thumb on the left the relatively shorter and thicker ulna of the radial club hand can be seen.

Associated anomalies must also be sought either by the surgeon himself or by referral to a pediatrician. These may affect the decision to undertake surgery and its timing. *Cardiac defects* occur in 10–13% of patients with radial club hand.[2] *Blood dyscrasias* are also common.

INDICATIONS

Manipulation should be taught to the parents to be undertaken twice daily, emphasising both ulnar deviation of the wrist and flexion of the elbow. Splintage is difficult to apply and of doubtful value provided manipulation is being faithfully administered.

If elbow flexion has been achieved, centralisation of the carpus on the ulna should be undertaken at six to twelve months of age[20]. This is achieved by appropriate carpal excision and accompanied by transfer of radial wrist motors to ulnar motors and, where necessary, by angulation closing wedge osteotomy of the curved ulna[14]. Centralisation should aim to preserve the distal ulnar epiphysis,

although premature fusion is a recognised complication[2]. The limb is however always shorter than normal and the loss of length is more than balanced by the improvement in appearance and, to a lesser degree, function[21,22].

Where required, pollicisation is performed six months after centralisation. It is always required in absent or rudimentary thumbs while the indications in hypoplasia are discussed below (p. 340).

While some will centralise and pollicise only in bilateral cases and then on only one side, current practice increasingly favors surgical treatment of all cases with good elbow motion and no other complicating anomalies.

Longitudinal absence — distal central — cleft hand[23]

Typical[24]: bilateral: familial: absent metacarpus: usually middle ray absence, sometimes index, rarely ring; V-shaped defect: foot often involved.

Atypical: unilateral: non-genetic: metacarpus present: several rays absent: U-shaped defect; no foot involvement (Fig. 7.9).*

The typical cleft hand can vary in severity:

simple cleft between middle and ring fingers, no absence
→   absent middle
→   progressive hypoplasia of radial digits (Fig. 7.10)
→   syndactyly of remaining digits (Fig. 7.11)

Early forms of radial hypoplasia show a degree of adduction contracture of the thumb with varying hypoplasia of the intrinsic muscles of the thumb. A reduced range of motion, with or without flexion contracture, may limit the function of any of the proximal interphalangeal joints. Transverse bones may be present, usually in the metacarpus.

In the extreme forms of either typical or atypical cleft hand there may be only two border digits, either of which may have arisen from fusion — the 'lobster claw' hand[25].

EXAMINATION

Observation should be directed at assessing the function in the border digits and in the wrist.

Border digits:

grasp — this may be achieved by the cleft or by the usual mechanism of the thumb-index web space

pinch may be easily performed by two residual border digits, for example, in the atypical, U-shaped cleft

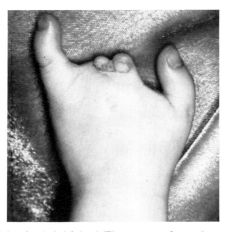

Fig. 7.9   *Atypical cleft hand.* The presence of normal metacarpals in the cleft is characteristic. (Some authorities would classify this as a symbrachydactyly for the reasons given in the footnote.)

*The distinction between atypical cleft hand, transverse finger defects, constriction ring syndrome and symbrachydactyly is difficult. The last named demonstrates nails and a rudimentary skeleton. The others have no finger nails and what bones are present are normal[14].

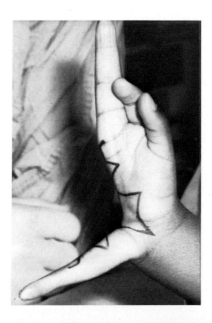

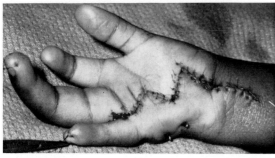

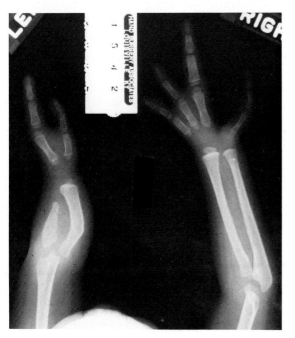

hand or may be prevented by a number of different factors, namely,

inadequate rotation, the ulnar digit being too pronated or the radial digit too supinated or both

blocking by the remaining metacarpus of the missing digits in the atypical cleft

impaired digital motion which may be due to poor joint range, to the point of symphalangism, or to anomalous or absent motors — the digit may be flail.

The wrist motion is usually normal and its motors may be required for tendon transfers.

Palpation will assess the *passive range of motion,* both normal and abnormal, in the joints, *contracture,* especially of the first web space, and the presence of normal and abnormal *skeleton.* The latter is confirmed by *X-ray* evaluation.

INDICATIONS

Since the syndactyly, when it exists, is between digits of unequal length in the first and the fourth web space early correction is required to prevent further deformity of the longer digit. This should be performed at six months of age and both ulnar and radial components can be separated simultaneously.

Reconstruction of the thumb may require simple deepening of the first web space, tendon transfers, rotational osteotomy or even full pollicisation. The skin from the cleft can be transferred as a palmar based flap into the first web such as described by Snow and Littler[26,27] thus combining the two procedures of *cleft closure* and *first space widening. Rotational osteotomy* of border digits, the radial into pronation and the ulnar into supination, is performed at the metacarpal level and is designed to bring the tips into pinch contact. It is important that the osteotomies be so positioned that active flexion of the digits carries them beyond, and not just into contact with, one another, otherwise no power can be exerted in pinch activities. Full *pollicisation* is required where the radialmost digit is triphalangeal and supinated into the plane of the fingers (Fig. 7.11). This invariably occurs in association with syndactyly. Caution must be exercised in this circumstance for frequently the blood supply comes from as few as two common digital arteries, one to the radial and one to the ulnar component of the cleft. Prudence dictates that correction be achieved in two stages, first syndactyly separation, second cleft closure and pollicisation. The

Fig. 7.10 (A & B) The typical cleft hand shown here at the time of cleft closure demonstrates the relative hypoplasia of the radial digits with adduction contracture of the thumb. (C) the X-ray shows the hand seen in (A) and (B) on the right; the radial hypoplasia and deep cleft is evident. The left hand shows an even more severe cleft, with only two digits and ulnar hypoplasia. (This case is also shown in Fig. 7.45C & D.)

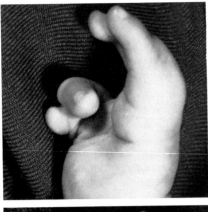

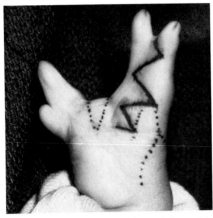

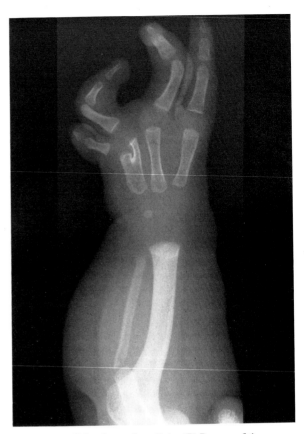

Fig. 7.11 *Cleft hand.* (A) This is an advanced form with syndactyly of the two radial and two ulnar digits. (B) Because of the probability that each set of syndactylised digits had only one artery between them — a fact which subsequently proved to be true — separation of the syndactylised digits was undertaken before pollicisation. The dotted lines indicate the incisions for pollicisation and Snow-Littler web space reconstruction to be performed at a later stage. (C) The X-ray illustrates the curvature which ensued in the second finger after syndactyly release. The radial digit, to be pollicised, is triphalangeal.

parents must be warned of the potential for vascular compromise.

Where a digit is flail, *tendon transfers* employing wrist motors extended by a tendon graft may restore active function. However, this will not restore more than the pre-existing passive motion and that passive motion can rarely be increased by joint release procedures. Further, where normal tendons are absent, so also is both the pulley mechanism on the flexor surface and the complex extensor apparatus.

By comparison with the anomalies which may occur in the border digits, *closure* of the typical cleft itself is relatively simple. It is important to employ zig-zag incisions, to design a distally based flap to restore the web and to reconstitute the deep transverse metacarpal ligament.

Rather than closure, the atypical cleft hand may require *deepening* to facilitate grasp by the border digits. This is achieved by excision of the intervening metacarpus.

The function of cleft hands if often remarkably good (Fig. 7.12) the patient being capable of all manipulative activities, provided of course that all five digits are not required. However, the appearance of the hand is socially unacceptable and may cause great distress to the parents and later to the child. The surgeon must nonetheless be aware of the severe limitations, indeed the sometimes meddlesome nature, of surgical correction. Here as much as in any other congenital anomaly, emphasis must be laid on support and counselling, stressing that the unscarred, functioning, supple hand, however deformed, is much more acceptable aesthetically than a scarred, clumsy and stiff extremity — still deformed.

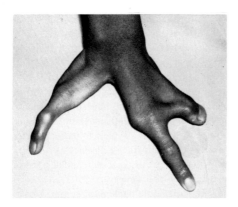

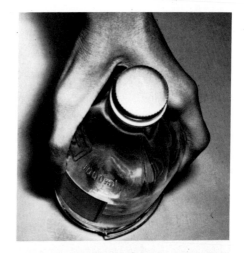

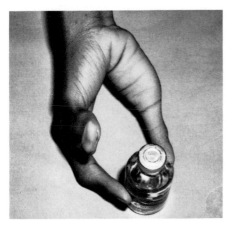

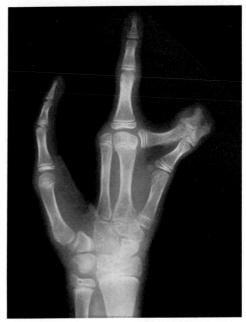

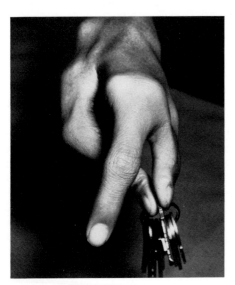

Fig. 7.12 *Typical cleft hand.* (A) This boy presented for evaluation at the age of 18. (B to D) It can be seen he has full prehensile function using the different digits in unique fashion. Such function would only be impaired at this late age by surgical intervention. (E) The X-ray reveals a typical cleft with symphalangism and complex syndactyly of the index and thumb and resultant deviation.

FAILURE OF DIFFERENTIATION OF PARTS

Radio-ulnar synostosis

This condition occurs at the proximal forearm in the large majority and is bilateral in 60% of cases. There are two types described — *primary* in which the radial head is absent and the synostosis is more extensive than in the *secondary* form, in which the radial head is normal, although often dislocated.

Examination reveals a fixed pronation deformity which exceeds 50° in about 50%. Some compensation for this limitation is provided by hypermobility of the wrist which permits up to 50° of rotation.

X-ray evaluation confirms the diagnosis and shows the radius to be heavy and bowed, the ulna to be straight and narrow (Fig. 7.13).

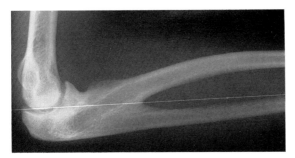

Fig. 7.13 *Primary radioulnar synostosis.* The radial head is absent. The synostosis is extensive. The radius is heavy and bowed, and the ulna is straight and narrow.

Indications. Attempts to restore active rotation by a variety of methods have proved unsuccessful. Therefore, where a case is unilateral and minor, no treatment is indicated. In severe cases, a rotational osteotomy through the synostosis should be performed at age 5. In unilateral cases the limb is placed at 10–20° of pronation, in bilateral the dominant is fixed at 30–45° pronation, the non-dominant at 20–35° supination[28].

Symphalangism[29]

While strictly defined by Cushing[30] as hereditary stiffness of the proximal interphalangeal joints symphalangism has come to mean congenital stiffness of a finger at any joint, genetically transmitted or not. Nonetheless, the condition does affect mainly the proximal interphalangeal joint and is commonly associated with varying degrees of shortness of the middle phalanx.

Hereditary symphalangism is transmitted as a dominant trait: it may affect one digit but usually more: it is more common in ulnar than in radial digits. Where the digit is of normal length, the distal interphalangeal joint commonly shows an increased, compensatory range of motion. More frequently the middle phalanx is short — *symbrachydactyly*

— and then the distal joint may also show some stiffness. In either case the patient cannot make a fist.

Non-heriditary symphalangism occurs in association with syndactyly, Apert's syndrome (see Fig. 7.23) Poland's syndrome and anomalies of the feet — in that order of incidence.

Examination shows that the fingers are commonly short and always atrophic, the skin being shiny and unmarked by creases on either dorsal or palmar surface. Attempts at *passive motion* will confirm the absence of motion, usually at the proximal interphalangeal joint and also the relatively slender nature of the bones. *X-ray evaluation* may be confusing for the middle phalangeal epiphysis may appear to be a joint space.

Indications for surgery in infancy do not exist. Attempts to restore motion by release or replacement arthroplasty will fail, in part due to the lack of normal motors, both flexor and extensor. Surgery also carries the risk of damaging the epiphysis, further shortening an already short finger. Both function and appearance can be improved only by an angulation osteotomy in late adolescence, once the epiphysis has fused. The angles chosen should be those recommended for proximal interphalangeal joint arthrodesis — index 20°, middle 30°, ring 40°, small 50°.

Camptodactyly[31,32]

This is a congenital flexion deformity of the digit, usually at the proximal interphalangeal joint and by far most commonly encountered in the small finger (Fig. 7.14A). It can occur, with rapidly decreasing frequency, in the ring, middle and very rarely the index fingers, usually in association with camptodactyly of the small. It is commonly bilateral and may be transmitted by an autosomal dominant trait or occur sporadically.

Debate exists over this simple condition, both with respect to the anatomical cause and also as to whether or not there are two distinct types of camptodactyly. The balance would appear to favour there being two types, one which appears in infancy and affects the sexes equally and one which usually first presents in girls in their early adolescence. Both types of deformity may become much more marked during the teenage growth spurt. Function is rarely if ever affected and therefore it is usually appearance which prompts the patient to present. This, allied with the growth spurt deterioration, probably accounts for the fact that the majority of cases are seen during the second decade of life.

As to the anatomical cause, most structures around the proximal phalanx have been implicated at one time or another. Cases seen by the author have all been due to one of two anomalies:

abnormal insertion of the lumbrical (7.14B and D)
abnormal origin and/or insertion of the superficialis

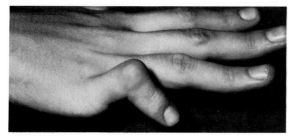

Fig. 7.14 (A)   Camptodactyly affecting here, as is most common, the small finger alone.

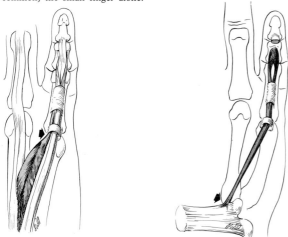

Fig. 7.14(B and C)   Two more common causes of camptodactyly.
B. The fourth lumbrical inserting with the superficialis.
C. Superficialis arising from the retinaculum or palmar fascia.

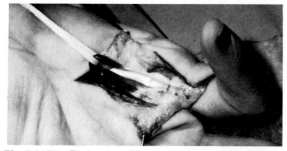

Fig. 7.14(D)   Exploration of this camptodactyly revealed that the lumbrical tendon inserted into the superficialis producing flexion of proximal interphalangeal joint as demonstrated here, rather than its usual function of extending the proximal interphalangeal joint.

Where these cases have been established for some years, secondary changes occur in the proximal interphalangeal joint.

Examination should first be directed at determining the number of fingers involved and then measuring the *extension deficit*, both active and passive

(a) with the metacarpophalangeal joint extended
(b) with the metacarpophalangeal joint held in flexion[31].

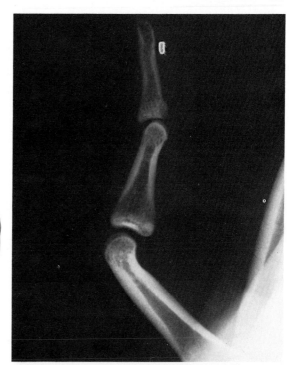

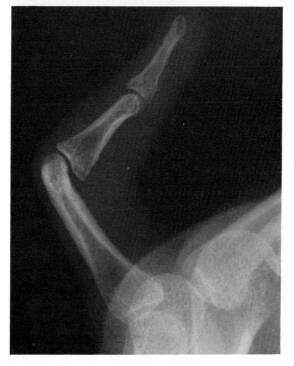

Fig. 7.15   *Camptodactyly.* (A) The neck of the proximal phalanx shows an indentation corresponding to the anterior lip of the base of the middle phalanx. (B) The base of the middle phalanx is wider than normal and also shows an indentation. The head of the proximal phalanx lacks the anterior portions of both condyles. These X-ray changes indicate that a soft tissue release alone will be unsuccessful.

The distal interphalangeal joint is never involved. If it shows fixed hyperextension, a traumatic boutonniere is the likely cause of the flexion contracture of the proximal interphalangeal joint.

X-ray evaluation should be undertaken on a *true lateral* of the involved proximal interphalangeal joint. Particularly in those cases in which full passive extension could not be attained, characteristic changes are seen (Fig. 7.15).

    (i)   the neck of the proximal phalanx may show an indentation corresponding to the anterior lip of the base of the middle phalanx when in full flexion

   (ii)   the base of the middle phalanx which is wider than normal in an antero-posterior direction may also show an indentation of its articular surface, impairing the normal smooth arc of that feature.

  (iii)   the head of the proximal phalanx, rather than being a full, smooth arc of a circle matching other heads and congruous with the base of the middle phalanx, has a blunt-pointed configuration such as would be produced by grinding off the palmar surface of the head

Indications for surgical correction depend very largely on these X-ray findings[31]. When they are well-established, soft tissue procedures are unlikely to restore full extension. Where the deformity is pronounced and troublesome, a dorsal angulation osteotomy of the neck of the proximal phalanx can be proposed. It must be made clear to the patient, however, that the procedure only changes the arc of motion of the joint and that for every degree of extension gained, one of flexion and therefore of grasp must be sacrificed.

When the X-ray reveals a normal joint, the palmar aspect of the digit should be explored, seeking in particular anomalies of the lumbrical and/or superficialis. Where flexion of the metacarpophalangeal joint produced full active proximal interphalangeal joint extension only *release* of the abnormal tendon is necessary. Where only passive extension was achieved a tendon transfer to the radial lateral band is needed in addition. This can be of:

    (i)   an anomalous lumbrical if superficialis is normal

   (ii)   an anomalous superficialis provided it is normal proximally as demonstrated by normal excursion on traction

  (iii)   the normal superficialis of the adjacent finger if the superficialis of the affected digit is abnormal proximally as well as distally.

Clinodactyly[33]

This is curvature of a digit in a radio-ulnar plane. It is most commonly seen in the small finger and next frequently in the triphalangeal thumb (p. 336). In most instances the resultant curvature turns the tip of the digit towards the mid-line of the hand and is due to a deformity of the middle phalanx. As emphasised in the assessment of malunited fractures, the two articular surfaces of the phalanx should be parallel. In clinodactyly, they are not. There are three different forms of clinodactyly encountered in the small finger:

    (i)   minor angulation — normal length — very common

   (ii)   minor angulation — short phalanx — present in 25% of mongoloid children, only 3% of normal

  (iii)   marked angulation — delta phalanx

The *delta phalanx*[34,35] comes about as a result of an abnormal epiphysis, which extends from one end of the normal proximal epiphysis around and along the short side — a 'J-shaped epiphysis', sometimes continuing to form an abnormal distal epiphysis to the bone, thus creating a 'C-shaped epiphysis' or *longitudinally bracketed diaphysis*[36] (Fig. 7.16).

Examination should measure the degree of angulation and confirm that all other functions of the digit are normal.

X-ray evaluation should determine whether the phalanx is short as well as angled and whether or not it is a delta phalanx. During the first 18 months to 2 years of life this is suggested by the location of the diaphyseal portion of the

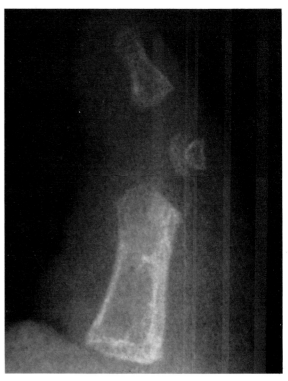

Fig. 7.16 *Delta phalanx.* The middle phalanx of this small finger demonstrates a 'C-shaped epiphysis' or longitudinally bracketed diaphysis.

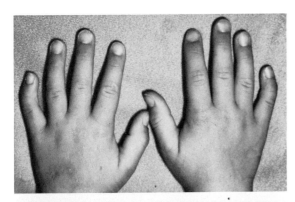

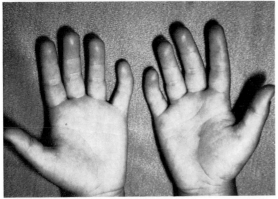

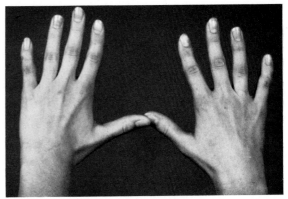

Fig. 7.17 *Clinodactyly.* (A–C) The clinodactyly of each small finger is due to an angulated short middle phalanx. (D) An opening wedge osteotomy of the middle phalanx with interposition of a small bone graft taken from the distal radius has resulted in normal growth and reasonable correction of the clinodactyly.

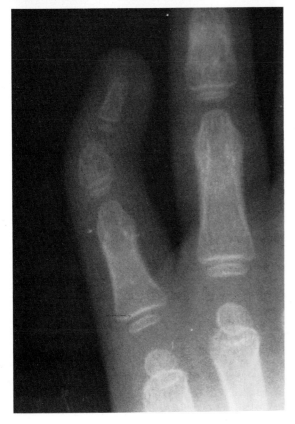

phalanx displaced towards the convex side of the curve. The abnormal epiphysis ossifies thereafter.

Indications. Minor clinodactyly is only of aesthetic importance and surgery should be discouraged. Where the patient, usually an adolescent, is clearly distressed by the deformity, *closing wedge osteotomy* should be performed where the phalanx is of normal length, *opening wedge* where the phalanx is short the necessary cortico-cancellous bone graft being taken from the distal radius (Fig. 7.17). The delta phalanx usually creates much more severe clinodactyly and therefore presents in infancy. When the digit is too long, especially where the phalanx is an additional one, as in triphalangeal thumb, then early excision should be performed (Fig. 7.18). The ligaments

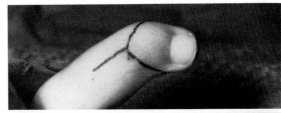

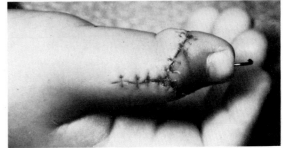

Fig. 7.18 *Delta phalanx in a triphalangeal thumb.* (A) The marked angulation present in this triphalangeal thumb of a nine month old was corrected by total excision and reconstruction of the collateral ligaments (B).

should be preserved and repaired and, where possible, the extensor tendon should be shortened appropriately. When the delta phalanx replaces a normal constituent of a consequently short finger, opening wedge osteotomy should be performed. This not only straightens and lengthens the digit — it also breaks the continuity of the abnormal epiphysis. In all instances the possibilities of residual deformity, non-union and tendon adhesions must be made clear to both patient and parents.

Flexed thumb

The infant's thumb is normally flexed and for this reason abnormal fixed flexion may not be noticed until some months after birth. The two main causes are *trigger thumb* and *clasped thumb*, distinguished by the fact that the fixed flexion in the first is of the interphalangeal joint alone while in the latter the metacarpophalangeal joint is affected also.

Weckesser[37] and others have classified clasped thumb as follows:

Group I	— deficient extension alone	70%
Group II	— + flexion contracture	24%
Group III	— + thumb hypoplasia	} 5%
Group IV	— miscellaneous	

Examination will reveal the persistently flexed posture of the thumb. Such persistence, associated with adduction, showing no spontaneous active extension at 3 months after birth, is diagnostic of clasped thumb. *Passive motion* will show

trigger thumb	—	flexed interphalangeal joint, which *may* extend suddenly with a click
	—	hyperextension of the metacarpophalangeal joint
clasped thumb	—	in the majority Group I cases, easy full passive extension will be achieved.

X-ray evaluation is not required for the skeleton is not affected in either condition, with the exception of the hypoplasia associated with the rare Group III clasped thumb.

Indications

Trigger thumbs present at birth can be left for one year, for 30% will resolve spontaneously in that time, and joint contracture has not been reported in any child operated on before the age of four. Surgical release of the A_1 pulley at the metacarpophalangeal joint will cure all residual cases (Fig. 7.19).

Group I clasped thumb diagnosed in infancy should be splinted for 3 months in extension. If, after that treatment, extension is present but weak it should be continued for a further three months. Recurrence does not occur if the response to primary conservative treatment has been good.

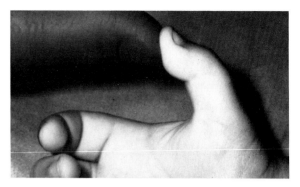

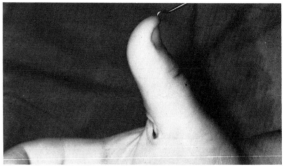

Fig. 7.19 *Congenital trigger thumb.* This persistent trigger thumb (A) was corrected by release of the A_1 pulley at an age of eighteen months. (B).

Older cases of Group I progressively develop flexion contracture, thereby becoming Group II. Cases which are Group II from birth are probably arthrogrypotic in nature. *Tendon transfers* to the deficient extensors with or without release of the flexion contracture are therefore required in Group II and late Group I.

Syndactyly[38]

Complete:	the involved digits are united as far as the distal phalanx
Incomplete:	united further than the mid-point of the proximal phalanx but short of the distal phalanx
Complex:	bony union exists between the involved digits
Simple:	no such bony union exists
Acrosyndactyly[39]:	fusion between the more distal portions of the digits; always some proximal fenestration from dorsal to palmar surfaces (Fig. 7.20).

While in the simple, incomplete syndactyly, the union of the involved digits is a web, which may provide sufficient local skin for correction, it is preferable to view the digits as ones which have failed to separate rather than ones which are webbed for a true web is rarely present. By this approach, the need for additional skin in the form of full

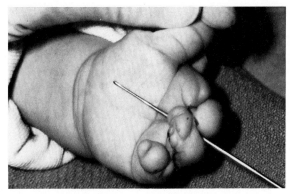

Fig. 7.20 *Acrosyndactyly.* The index, middle, and ring fingers are here fused at the tips producing the so-called 'rosebud' hand. The proximal fenestration which is always present from dorsal to palmar surfaces is here demonstrated with a probe.

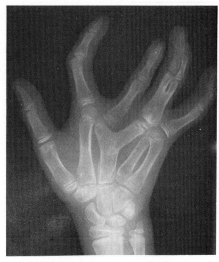

Fig. 7.21 *Syndactylised concealed central polydactyly.* This hand shows a bifid third metacarpal, an anomalous forth metacarpal, and an additional digit forming part of a syndactylised duplication of the ring finger.

thickness grafts in the surgical separation of the great majority of cases is readily appreciated by all.

Syndactyly is the most common congenital deformity, both in its pure form and more so still when one includes its presentation as one feature of syndromes such as Poland's and Apert's (see below). When syndactyly presents alone — endogenous — it is transmitted by a dominant gene, but with reduced penetrance and variable expression, so that a family history is present in from 10 to 40% of patients, depending on the series. Fifty per cent of such cases are bilaterally symmetrical.

The incidence of ray involvement also varies according to the source and can best be recalled by the mnemonic 5.15.50.30

Thumb — index	5%
Index — middle	15%
Middle — ring	50%
Ring — small	30%

Accessory phalanges may be present between the skeletons of syndactylised digits either in an organised form — concealed central polydactyly — or in an apparent jumble of bones, lying transversely and obliquely as well as longitudinally (Fig. 7.21, see also Fig. 7.1).

Anomalies of tendons, nerves and vessels occur with increasing frequency the more complete a syndactyly. Even in the most simple complete syndactyly the bifurcations of both nerve and artery lie distal to the normal location. As the condition becomes more complex, the bifurcation of the common vessel becomes progressively more distal and, as shown in a recent study of infantile angiograms, the arteries on the outer aspect become progressively more rudimentary. The implications of vascular compromise at the time of division are self-evident.

Acrosyndactyly is commonly associated with constriction ring syndrome (p. 346) and has been classified by Walsh.[40]

moderate	—	two phalanges and one interphalangeal joint in each digit
severe	—	one phalanx (Fig. 7.22)

The deviation, distortion and 'jumbling' of the involved digits increases with the severity.

Poland's syndrome[41] is a rare, non-genetic disorder characterised by four features[42]

(i) unilateral shortening of the digits, mainly the index, long and ring, due largely to shortness or absence of the middle phalanx
(ii) syndactyly of the shortened digits, usually of a simple, complete type
(iii) hypoplasia of the hand, and, to a lesser degree, of the forearm

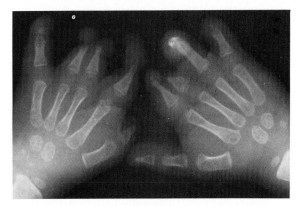

Fig. 7.22 *Acrosyndactyly.* These digits demonstrate both moderate and severe acrosyndactyly as defined by Walsh, there being some digits with two phalanges and an interphalangeal joint and other digits with only one.

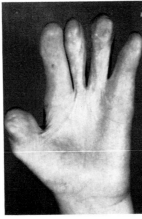

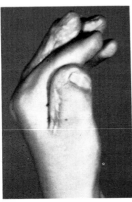

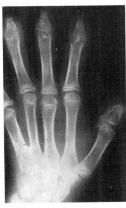
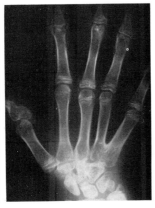

Fig. 7.23 *Apert's syndrome.* This child shows the total complex syndactyly with a common nail for the thumb and index, so typical of Apert's syndrome. (B, C, D) An adolescent patient who had undergone syndactyly release at an early age presented for improvement of grasp. Maximum flexion is shown in (C). (D) The X-rays demonstrate the symphalangism of all fingers, the delta middle phalanx of the thumb which has been fused at a previous surgical procedure, and the flattening of the metacarpal head. Grasp was improved by angulation osteotomy of the long proximal phalanx in each finger.

(iv) absence of the sternocostal head of the pectoralis major muscle on the same side, associated in a decreasing proportion[43] with
  (a) absence of the pectoralis minor
  (b) hypoplasia of the breast and nipple (33% of affected females[44])
  (c) contraction of the anterior axillary fold
  (d) absence of serratus anterior, latissimus dorsi and deltoid
  (e) rib deficiencies, thoracic scoliosis and dextrocardia

Apert's syndrome[45] occurs initially by mutation, but is thereafter a strongly dominant gene, a fact of increasing significance as craniofocial surgery improves the mental and aesthetic status of these patients. The features are

(i) acrocephaly with hypertelorism
(ii) bilateral complex syndactyly with symphalangism (Fig. 7.23)

The index, middle and ring fingers frequently share a common nail. The thumb is involved in the syndactyly in one-third of cases; it often demonstrates a delta proximal phalanx with resultant radial deviation. Vascular and tendinous anomalies are the rule.

EXAMINATION

Examination in syndactyly should determine the rays involved and how complete the involvement. The *nails* should be examined for they are commonly united especially in complex, complete cases. Any *deformity* in the involved digits should be noted. The *length* of the digits compared with normal may reveal *brachysyndactyly*. *Passive motion* should be undertaken on all joints for *symphalangism* may co-exist. The presence of these latter two conditions — brachydactyly or symphalangism — in conjunction with syndactyly suggests that more than the hand may be involved and a full physical examination is required.

X-ray evaluation should reveal the number of digits, the number of metacarpals, the number of phalanges, the presence and situation of complex cross-union, delta phalanges and, in later cases the configuration of joint surfaces.

INDICATIONS
Early separation, between six and twelve months of age, is indicated in certain situations.

1. *Acrosyndactyly*
2. *Syndactyly between rays of unequal length*
  If this is not done the longer ray will develop rotation and flexion deformities which may not be corrected even with additional later surgery. The urgency is increased the greater the discrepancy between the digits, thus the rare thumb-index syndactyly should be

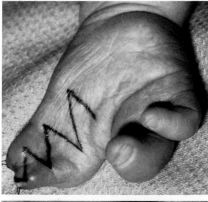

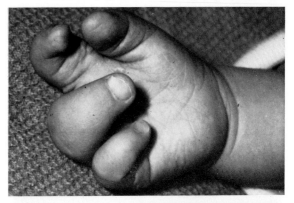

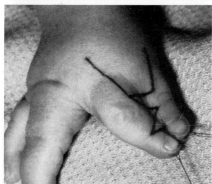

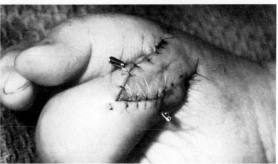

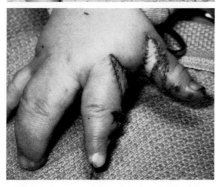

Fig. 7.25 *Complex complete syndactyly — nail union.* (A) The union of the nails of the syndactylised middle and ring fingers is separated in a preliminary procedure with application of a thenar flap, (B) providing extra tissue to resurface the contiguous surfaces of the distal phalanges at later division. The Kirschner wires maintain the distal phalangeal separation in order to avoid circulatory embarrassment of the thenar flap. The pronation of the index finger referred to in Figure 7.24 is seen here more clearly.

Fig. 7.24 *Simple complete syndactyly.* (A & B) The simple complete syndactyly between the thumb and index finger in this child is here being separated at the age of seven months. Despite this the rotation and angulation of the index finger can be detected in C (see same patient in Fig. 7.25).

separated when first seen. (Fig. 7.24) It follows that involved border digits in Poland's and Apert's syndrome require early release[45].

While technique is outwith the range of this text, certain points are worthy of emphasis since they involve planning based on examination:

— where two digits have a common nail, syndactyly separation should be preceded by nail division with introduction of additional skin using a thenar flap[46] (Fig. 7.25)

— the sinus fenestration present in acrosyndactyly is always too far distal to form the new web space, and must always be excised during division

— syndactyly release should not be performed simultaneously on adjacent webs, that is, on both sides of one digit

— the shorter the digit, the more proximal should be the new web, the limit being the level of the metacarpophalangeal joint

— the new web must always be constructed of local skin (Fig. 7.26)

— skin grafts will always be required, except in the least of incomplete cases

— when the thumb is involved, as in Apert's syndrome, simultaneous rotation and angulation osteotomy is required where all metacarpals are in the same plane and there is absence of the thenar musculature[14]

— bilateral syndactyly should be operated upon by two teams at the same operation in order to reduce the number of procedures.

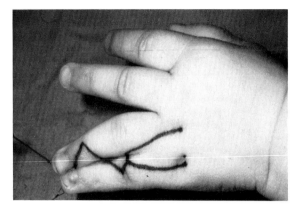

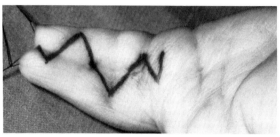

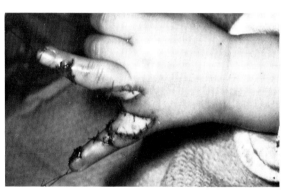

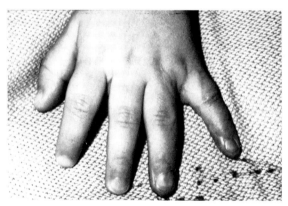

Patients, and their parents, must be made aware that the limbs in Poland's and Apert's syndrome will always be smaller than normal and the fingers stiff. Where symphalangism exists, angulation osteotomy in adolescence is indicated. Delta phalanges should be dealt with by excision or wedge osteotomy as discussed under triphalangeal thumb (below) and clinodactyly (above).

DUPLICATION

Polydactyly is a common congenital disorder, vying with syndactyly for first place. Duplication of the small finger, in strong contrast to that of the thumb, is usually the result of an autosomal recessive trait and is often part of a syndrome. Its presence therefore dictates the need for a full physical examination. The radial aspect of the hand is involved a little more than the ulnar and both are much more common than central polydactyly. The latter is almost always associated with syndactyly and often shows disorganisation of the skeleton, such as transverse orientation of the additional metacarpal. The varying manifestations of duplication have been classified by Stelling[47]

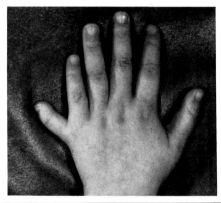

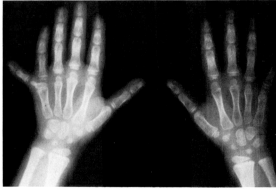

Fig. 7.26 *Complete simple syndactyly.* (A–C) The general principles of release are here illustrated. The new web is constructed entirely of local skin. A number of full thickness grafts taken from the groin are required. The resultant separation shown in D is pleasing — and permanent.

Fig. 7.27 (A & B) *Ulnar duplication — Stelling type II.* The additional digit shown here articulates with a relatively normal metacarpal although the epiphysis and metaphysis are somewhat widened. Reconstruction of the ulnar collateral ligament was necessary at the time of excision.

Type I: soft tissue mass containing no skeletal structure; rare in the thumb

Type II: a digit or part thereof, containing all normal components and articulating with a normal or bifid metacarpal or phalanx (Fig. 7.27)

Type III: a digit, complete with metacarpal; rare (see Wassel VI below)

Radial duplication

Duplication of the thumb can occur at any level and clarity has been given by the introduction of the following classification by Wassel[48]

Type I —	*Bifid* distal phalanx	2%
II —	distal phalanx *duplicated*	15%
III —	*Bifid* proximal phalanx	6%
IV —	proximal phalanx *duplicated*	43%
V —	*Bifid* metacarpal	10%
VI —	metacarpal *duplicated*	4%
VII —	Triphalangia, in either or both of the thumbs and at any level II–VI	20%

It can be seen that confusion may arise between the Stelling and Wassel classifications. In practice, this does not occur since the Wassel classification is used exclusively when describing thumb duplications. By contrast with ulnar polydactyly, thumb duplication is usually unilateral and sporadic, except for Type VII triphalangia which results from a dominant gene.

EXAMINATION

Examination should initially place the duplication in the appropriate Wassel category and then, with the exception of the majority of Types I and II (see below), should be directed at determining which of the two thumbs should be retained on the basis of the following criteria.

Size (Fig. 7.28) — while most duplications are of similar size and that smaller than the normal, unaffected thumb, one of the two may be rudimentary — this is most common in Type VI, the radial being small and functionless.

Deviation may be present both at the point of duplication and at joints distal to that point[49]. Where a digit is markedly deviated at its base frequently it deviates in the opposite direction at more distal joints under the influence of anomalous tendon insertions and of the Z-ing phenomenon similar to that seen in rheumatoids (Fig. 7.29).

Function may differ markedly in two thumbs of similar size and this may only be revealed by repeated, quite prolonged observation. Frequently functions may be shared, extension being good in one, flexion in the other. Even in the youngest infant, complete loss of motion will be revealed by absence of the matching skin creases. The tendon insertions are often anomalous, both flexor and extensor attaching more on the facing aspects of the phalanges in a manner which encourages deviation of the distal phalanges of the two thumbs towards one another. On occasion the flexor may insert into the extensor as in pollex abductus (see below) serving then solely as a deviating force.

Passive mobility, both normal and abnormal, should be assessed in all joints. The *first web space* is contracted in certain cases of thumb duplication and this should not be overlooked.

X-ray evaluation will confirm the classification of the duplication and in triphalangeal thumb should determine the nature of the extra phalanx (see below).

INDICATIONS

In Types I and II where the thumb are usually of equal size, the Bilhaut-Cloquet sharing procedure should be performed.[50] Since the thumbs are usually small, a little more than half should be taken from each. The difficulties associated with this procedure are residual nail deformity and unintentional epiphyseodesis. If the thumbs are of almost normal size, the first problem can be avoided by taking the entire nail from only one of them, discarding that from the other. The second problem is avoided by accurate matching of the epiphyseal plate, disregarding any incongruity in the joint surface which can be shaved down later in the procedure — the two epiphyses are rarely of equal thickness.

In the more proximal types, *size, deviation, function* or *passive mobility* may make the choice easy. Where, however, the thumbs are equal in all respects, then the choice may await exploration before a final decision is made on the basis of tendon and nerve anatomy. In the bifid Types III and V the surgeon can be entirely unbiased. In the duplicated Types IV and VI — especially the former which is also the most common — he should favour retention of the ulnar thumb thereby avoiding reconstruction of the ulnar collateral ligament so important for thumb stability. In any event certain steps are indicated in Type IV to ensure the best result[51] (Fig. 7.30):

— exploration and appropriate realignment of the insertions of both flexor and extensor tendons

— shaving of the metacarpal head on the side of excision of the duplicate, in order to eliminate an unsightly prominence, whilst ensuring

— preservation of both ligaments — that between the two duplicated proximal phalanges and that between the metacarpal and the discarded phalanx — for reconstruction of the one collateral

— reattachment of the intrinsic muscles.

Where the first web space is contracted, the skin from the duplicated thumb to be discarded should be preserved as a dorsally based flap to be transposed into the defect created by release (Fig. 7.31).

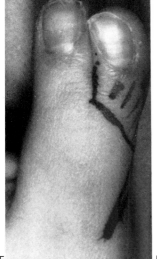

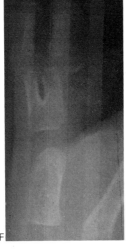

Fig. 7.28 *Radial polydactyly — duplicated thumb.* Selection of the appropriate surgical procedure is illustrated by these cases. (A & B) Case 1. Wassel type II: the digits are relatively equal in size and somewhat smaller than usual. (C & D) Case 2. Wassel type II: the radialmost digit is clearly the smaller and least functional. (E & F) Case 3. Wassel type III: both thumbs are relatively small. In case 1, a Bilhaut-Cloquet procedure was performed. In case 2, the radial of the two digits was excised with good result. In case 3, the radial of the two digits was excised producing an unsatisfactorily small distal thumb. A Bilhaut-Cloquet procedure was not performed in case 3 because of the difficulty anticipated in achieving congruity of the joint surfaces.

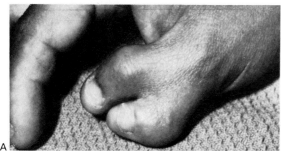

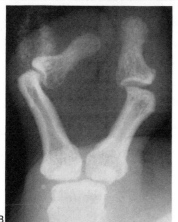

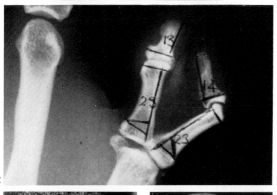

Fig. 7.29 *Duplicated thumb — Wassel type IV.* (A, B) This thumb shows deviation both at the metacarpophalangeal joint and also at the interphalangeal joints distally. This is somewhat similar to the Z-ing phenomenon seen in rheumatoids. (C) A Bilhaut-Cloquet procedure with multiple osteotomies was undertaken with an acceptable result. (D & E) This patient presented at the age of 28. When psychiatric evaluation was suggested, she readily assented. It was therefore not performed. She has had no psychiatric consequences to surgical correction (see also Fig. 7.1).

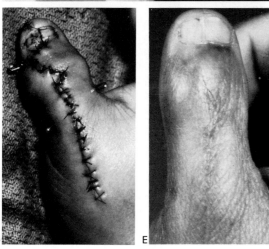

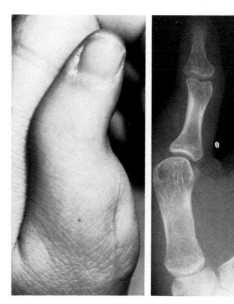

Fig. 7.30 (A & B) This patient previously had a radialmost digit excised from a Wassel type IV. This was clearly performed without shaving of the metacarpal head or reconstruction of the radial collateral ligament. This has resulted in the Z-ing deformity shown here affecting both the metacarpophalangeal and the interphalangeal joint. It was found on exploration that there was a communication between flexor and extensor tendons on the radial aspect of the proximal phalanx (see Fig. 7.42).

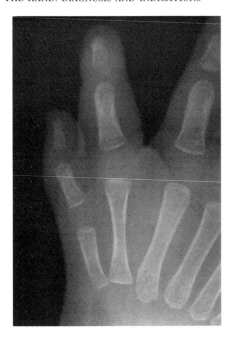

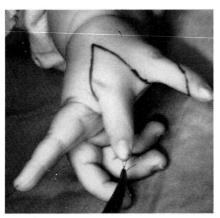

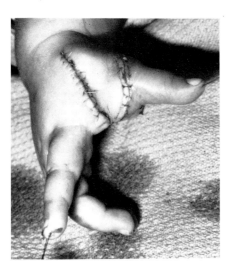

Fig. 7.31 (A) *Duplicated thumb — Wassel type VI.* The radialmost digit here was excised. The first web space was contracted and also showed shortage of skin. This was corrected (B & C) by transposing the skin from the digit to be discarded into the first web space and by translocating the metacarpal which was retained on to the articular surface of the trapezium previously occupied by the excised metacarpal.

TRIPHALANGEAL THUMB

Triphalangeal thumb[52] may present as part of a Type VII duplication (Fig. 7.32) or as an isolated entity. It may be inherited as a dominant trait[53]. The additional phalanx lies between the proximal and distal phalanges and may be any one of three types

— delta phalanx, producing increasing deviation (see also p. 326)
— rectangular phalanx which is short
— rectangular phalanx of normal length

In the latter two types the metacarpal is longer than normal adding even more length to the already lengthened thumb. If in addition, the digit is supinated, the first web space is contracted and the thenar muscles small, then there is little distinction from a five finger hand, a diagnosis which would be confirmed by finding a deep transverse metacarpal ligament.

Indications

A *delta phalanx* should be totally excised as early as possible and the soft tissues reconstructed. If seen late, arthrodesis of one joint with wedge osteotomy is required. A *rectangular phalanx* is treated by resection and arthrodesis of the distal joint, where necessary accompanied by an opponensplasty, widening of the first web space and shortening of the metacarpal. The closer the triphalangeal thumb comes to being a five-fingered hand, the more should formal pollicisation be considered (see below).

Central duplication

This, the least common of the duplications, affects the ring finger in more than half of the cases and the middle and index fingers in about equal number of cases. Stelling Types I and III present little problem requiring simple excision of the supernumerary digit. Type II, which is most common, and is almost invariably associated with syndactyly, thereby producing a '*hidden central poly-dactyly*', is most difficult to treat. This is both because it is intimately involved anatomically with both of the digits between which it lies and because they also are impaired to a differing degree (Fig. 7.33).

Examination may reveal what appears to be a simple complete syndactyly. The presence of an additional digit may be detected clinically only with *palpation*. Both active and *passive motion* may be impaired and should be carefully assessed.

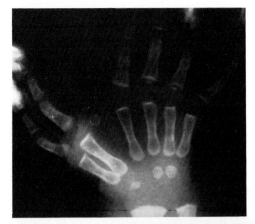

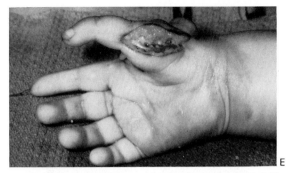

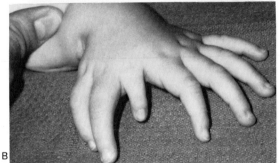

Fig. 7.32 *Radial polydactyly with triphalangeal thumb.* (A & B) The radial polydactyly shown here consists of two triphalangeal thumbs and a Stelling type II additional radial duplication. (This is not a mirror hand since the two forearm bones are of relatively normal nature.) In another Wassel type VII duplication (C & D) following excision of the radialmost of these duplicated digits, (E) the excessive length and additional joint of the triphalangeal remaining thumb is clearly evident.

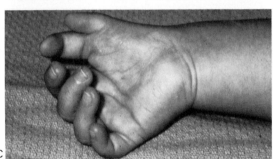

X-ray evaluation should determine the Stelling type of polydactyly, the point of duplication with especial attention to shared epiphyses, and the condition of the 'normal' digits with particular reference to complex syndactyly, symphalangism, deviation and abnormal phalanges.

Indications[54].
Early surgery is indicated since deviation of the digits to be retained only worsens and correction becomes more difficult with time. It is important to emphasise to the parents a number of points:

(i) impairment of motion may be due to the interposed extra digit or to an indeterminable degree of limitation in the apparently normal digits alongside, even to the point of *symphalangism*, the implications of which must be explained

(ii) *tendons and nerves* may be shared between two, or even three, digits in central polydactyly. The flexor, and more so the extensor, tendons may be a conjoined sheet of tissue difficult to separate and even more difficult to impart with function

(iii) *deviation* of the 'normal' digits which may be evident or concealed may require ligament reconstruction with simultaneous or subsequent angulation osteotomy

(iv) Flatt[2] has pointed out that the anomalies existing within an apparently simple complete syndactyly may be so great that only one functional finger can be obtained from the three digital skeletons available.

Ulnar duplication is common especially in black children, is often inherited and is associated with a number of syndromes, demanding full physical examination. The principles outlined above for diagnosis and indications apply.

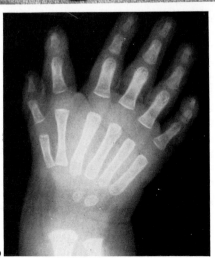

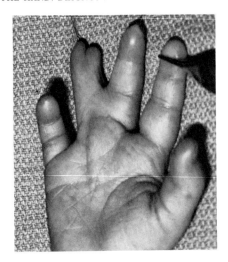

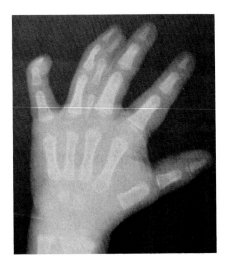

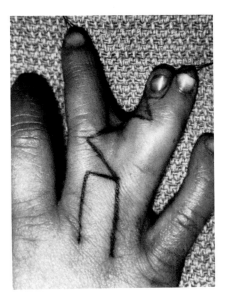

Fig. 7.33 (A & C) *Hidden central polydactyly.* Here the Stelling type II additional ring finger is not entirely concealed. There is however syndactyly between the middle and ring fingers. The X-ray (B) reveals that the main ring finger is somewhat hypoplastic in structure. Indeed, the collateral ligaments had to be reconstructed in this finger which despite that reconstruction, went on to show some rotation and slight deviation.

OVERGROWTH

Macrodactyly

Macrodactyly is a non-hereditary congenital enlargement of a digit. It is unilateral in 90% of cases. In 70% of those afflicted the condition affects more than one digit, those always being adjacent and corresponding to the territory of one or more peripheral nerves[55], most commonly the median (Fig. 7.34). The enlargement is more pronounced distally than proximally — thus phalanges are affected more frequently than metacarpals (Fig. 7.35). All tissues that respond late in development to neurogenic influence are enlarged — nerves, fat, skin appendages and bone. Two facts follow from this:

1. The cause of macrodactyly is neurogenic — probably a form of neurofibromatosis[56], the enlarged nerves being similarly infiltrated with fat and fibrous tissue (Fig. 7.36).
2. Tendons and blood vessels are of normal size — the latter fact results in relatively poor blood supply to all tissues, with a consequently higher incidence of avascular necrosis of skin flaps.

Two types of macrodactyly have been described[57]

static — present at birth, the enlargement keeps pace with growth of the normal digits

progressive — sometimes not apparent until as late as 2 years of age, this form is more aggressive, growing more quickly than adjacent digits and involving the adjacent palm.

Examination yields a swift diagnosis. The involved digit should be watched during manipulation for it may be excluded either because it is clumsy or because of *joint stiffness* which becomes progressively more severe with age and excessive growth. *Deviation* is a common accompaniment, due to uneven overgrowth of the two borders of the digit. *Palpation* will detect any temperature difference suggestive of locally poor circulation and may also reveal significant increase in tension which in part explains both the stiffness and the diminished blood supply. *Passive motion* should be recorded. While sensation is usually normal in the young, in adult patients, compression of the enlarged median nerve may lead to carpal tunnel syndrome[58]. *Ulceration* of the fingertips may be evidence of

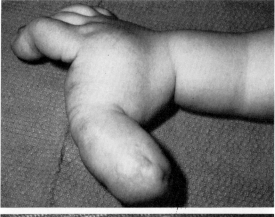

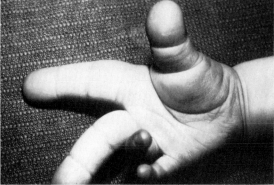

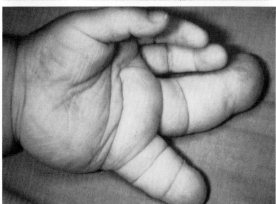

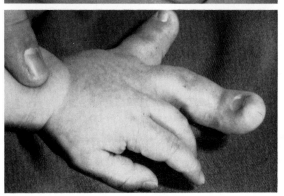

Fig. 7.34 *Macrodactyly.* It can be seen here that the median (A & B) and ulnar nerve (C & D) distributions are primarily affected in these three cases. Case B is that of Mr Gwyn Morgan FRCS.

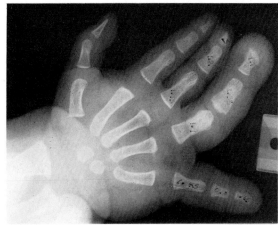

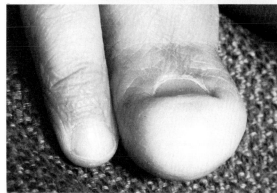

Fig. 7.35 It can be seen from the X-ray (A) that the phalanges are markedly enlarged while the metacarpals are of normal size. (B) illustrates the difference between the ring finger of the normal hand and that of the macrodactylous hand of the same patient.

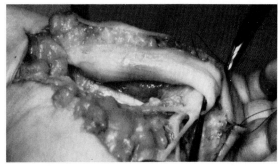

Fig. 7.36 The marked enlargement of the median nerve of the patient shown in Fig. 7.34A.

impaired neurovascular status. The most likely differential diagnosis — cavernous hemangioma — is excluded by the entirely different consistency of the digit and appropriate vascular observations (p. 303)

X-ray evaluation plays a significant role. Comparison should be made between the involved fingers and films taken by identical technique of:

(i)   the same digits on successive visits
(ii) the corresponding digit on
    (a) the opposite uninvolved hand
    (b) the parent of the same sex (Fig. 7.37)

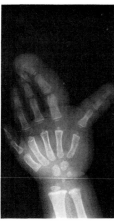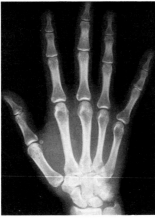

Fig. 7.37   Here on the same X-ray are shown the hands of the patient shown in Figure 7.34C and Figure 7.35 and the mother of that patient. The grossly macrodactylous ring finger of the child is still 1.3 cm shorter than that of the mother. This demonstrates the impracticality in some progressive macrodactyly cases of the recommendation that one should undertake epiphyseal arrest when the digit is equal to that of the same finger in the parent.

Careful measurements should be made and recorded. While of course particular attention should be paid to the involved fingers, adjacent digits should be assessed equally closely for any evidence of incipient macrodactyly.

Indications
Macrodactyly reduces even the giants of hand surgery. The severely affected single digit which has little motion, gross curvature and poor circulation presents only the problem of informing the parents of what they feared — that amputation is the correct treatment. But what of the thumb?[59] And of multiple digits? Reduction is the only answer and that both time-consuming and inadequate — espiphyseal ablation when the bone in question equals parental length; osteotomies both shortening to reduce length and angulatory to correct deviation. Even this is insufficient — further shortening with nail preservation as described by Barsky[57] or Tsuge[60] and longitudinal narrowing osteotomies are required. Nerve stripping

(Tsuge)[60] and extensive defatting to the extent of creating 'flap grafts' (Edgerton)[56] achieve some meagre soft tissue reduction. Many operations are required and each reduces blood and nerve supply and contributes to scarring and stiffness. The whole is an experience frustrating for the surgeon, painful for the child, harrowing for the parents. A test of rapport.

UNDERGROWTH

Hypoplasia and aplasia of the thumb
Hypoplasia of the thumb has been classified by Blauth[61]

Grade I	—	minor hypoplasia, in which all elements are present, the thumb being overall somewhat smaller than normal
Grade II (Fig. 7.38)	—	adduction contracture of the first web space
	—	laxity of the ulnar collateral ligament of the metacarpo-phalangeal joint
	—	hypoplasia of the thenar muscles[62,63]
	—	normal skeleton, with respect to articulations
Grade III (Fig. 7.39)	—	significant hypoplasia, with aplasia of intrinsics, rudimentary extrinsic tendons, if any
	—	skeletal hypoplasia, especially of the carpometacarpal joint which is vestigial
Grade IV (Fig. 7.40)	—	floating thumb = pouce flottant a vestigial, totally uncontrolled digit attached just proximal to the metacarpophalangeal joint of the index finger
Grade V (Fig. 7.41)	—	total absence

Hypoplasia, especially of Grade II, may be associated with:[64]

(i)   duplication of the thumb
(ii) triphalangia, with or without delta phalanx
(iii) anomalies of tendons and muscles
    (a) flexor pollicis longus, which may be absent[65,66], rudimentary or attached to the extensor tendon — the *pollex abductus*[67] (Fig. 7.42)
    (b) eccentric insertion of extrinsic motors on the distal phalanx with resultant deviation of the distal phalanx, early or late
    (c) anomalous extensors[68,63]
    (d) aplasia of the thenar muscles.

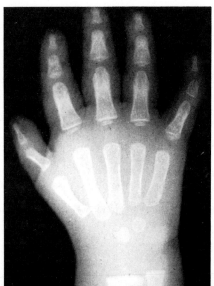

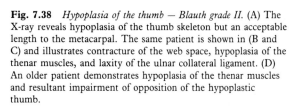

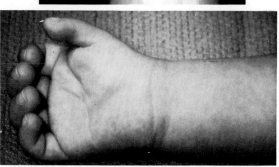

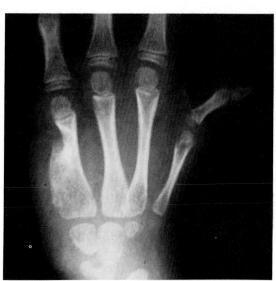

Fig. 7.38 *Hypoplasia of the thumb — Blauth grade II.* (A) The X-ray reveals hypoplasia of the thumb skeleton but an acceptable length to the metacarpal. The same patient is shown in (B and C) and illustrates contracture of the web space, hypoplasia of the thenar muscles, and laxity of the ulnar collateral ligament. (D) An older patient demonstrates hypoplasia of the thenar muscles and resultant impairment of opposition of the hypoplastic thumb.

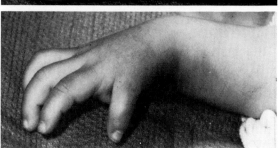

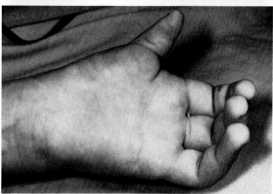

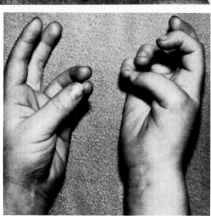

Fig. 7.39 (A & B) *Hypoplasia of the thumb — Blauth grade III.* The skeletal hypoplasia is evident. This thumb would normally be treated by excision and pollicisation, but the absence of the small finger made reconstruction desirable. Despite epiphysiodesis of the metacarpophalangeal joint, deepening of the first web space, reconstruction of the thenar musculature, and tendon transfer to replace the absent flexor pollicis longus, the resultant thumb function was less than optimal.

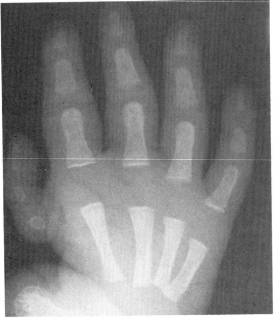

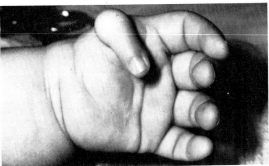

Fig. 7.40   (A & B) *Hypoplasia of the thumb — Blauth grade IV* 'Pouce flottant'.

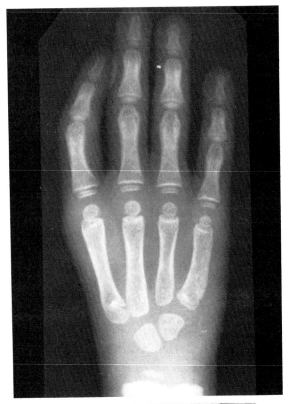

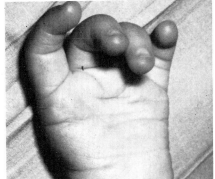

Fig. 7.41   (A & B) *Aplasia of the thumb — Blauth grade V.*

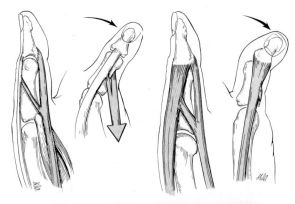

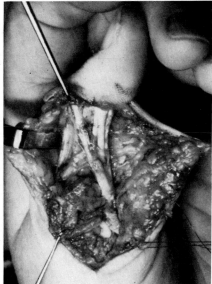

Fig. 7.42 *Pollex abductus.* In this condition the extensor and flexor tendons are conjoined by a band running from the flexor tendon proximally to the extensor tendon distally. Thus, action of the flexor pollicis results in radial deviation of the thumb. This may occur at the level of the metacarpal (A) or the level of the proximal phalanx (B & C). (The patient shown in (C) is that in Fig. 7.30.)

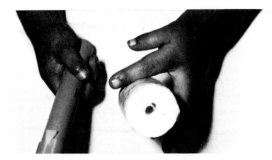

Fig. 7.43 This patient with grade III hypoplasia has undergone pollicisation on the right (by Professor Dieter Buck-Gramcko) while on the left illustrates the use of the 'cigarette grip' between the index and middle fingers.

Examination, once the Grade has been determined, is largely directed at the tendon anomalies which may be associated with Grade II hypoplasia. *Skin creases* should be sought, indicative of active joint motion, which should also be observed. Where flexion creases are absent or rudimentary, abduction at the metacarpophalangeal joint may be seen and the tendon of the absent flexor pollicis longus of a pollex abductus palpated where it crosses the hypoplastic thenar area. *Passive motion* of all joints should be recorded. Laxity of the collateral ligaments of the interphalangeal and, more probably, the metacarpophalangeal joints should be assessed. *X-ray evaluation* should confirm the Grade, seek abnormal phalanges in the thumb and exclude other anomalies.

Indications

    Grade I — no treatment required

    Grade II — see below

    Grades III–V — pollicisation of the index finger[69,70]

Parents, and indeed some surgeons, may express reluctance to sacrifice a hypoplastic thumb, especially of Grade III. However, the deficiencies of basal joint, motors and size can never be restored. If the parents are adamant, the child can be left until grasp movements commence, when he or she will clearly demonstrate that his manipulative potential lies in the index and middle fingers by their use in the so-called 'cigarette grip' for all pick-up manoeuvres (Fig. 7.43). However, where all are agreed, pollicisation of the index should be undertaken within the first year of life[70] (Fig. 7.44).

Grade II hypoplasia requires:

1.   exploration of flexor and extensor tendons and correction of any anomalies[71]
2.   release of the first web space[72]
3.   opponensplasty[73]
4.   stabilisation of the metacarpophalangeal joint

Tendon anomalies are most significant on the flexor surface. Infrequently, an anomalous attachment from flexor to extensor must be divided. Flexor pollicis longus if absent or grossly anomalous, may require to be replaced using immediate or two stage tendon graft[74], employing either the proximal tendon or a superficialis as motor. In such circumstances, and even in some cases where the flexor is adequate, pulley reconstruction will be required at the level of the proximal phalanx, employing extensor retinaculum or fascia.

Release of the web space may be achieved with a two- or four-flap Z-plasty but frequently additional skin is required[75]. In hypoplasia associated with duplication this is available from the discarded digit. In other cases skin is obtained by sliding or transposition flaps from the index finger or the dorsum of the thumb[76] or by rotation flaps

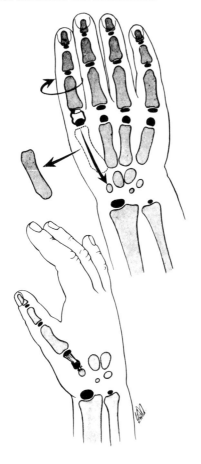

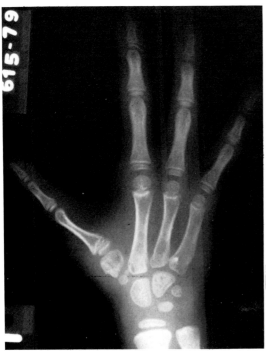

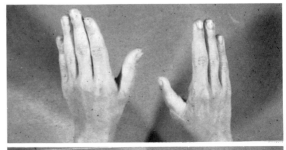

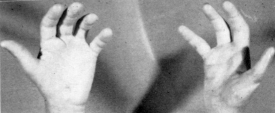

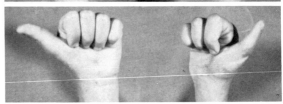

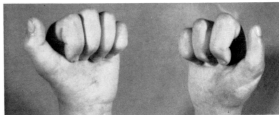

Fig. 7.44   (A) The elements of skeletal adjustment involved in pollicisation are shown diagrammatically. (B) The skeletal appearance three years after pollicisation of the index finger. (C, D, E & F) The appearance and function of the hand shown in B.

from the dorsum of the hand[77] (Fig. 7.45). Distant flaps are *never* necessary[14].

Opponensplasty can be achieved by use of the flexor digitorum superficialis[73] or the abductor digiti minimi[78,79,80]. The author prefers the former both because it is more powerful and also because, by passing it through the metacarpal, the tendon end can serve a second purpose of reconstructing the ulnar collateral ligament.

Stabilisation of the metacarpophalangeal joint is undertaken by one of three techniques (Fig. 7.46)

(i) fusion, taking care to leave the epiphyseal plate undisturbed

(ii) reconstruction using the end of a superficialis opponensplasty, as indicated above

(iii) tendon graft attached to the vestigial ligament or through bone.

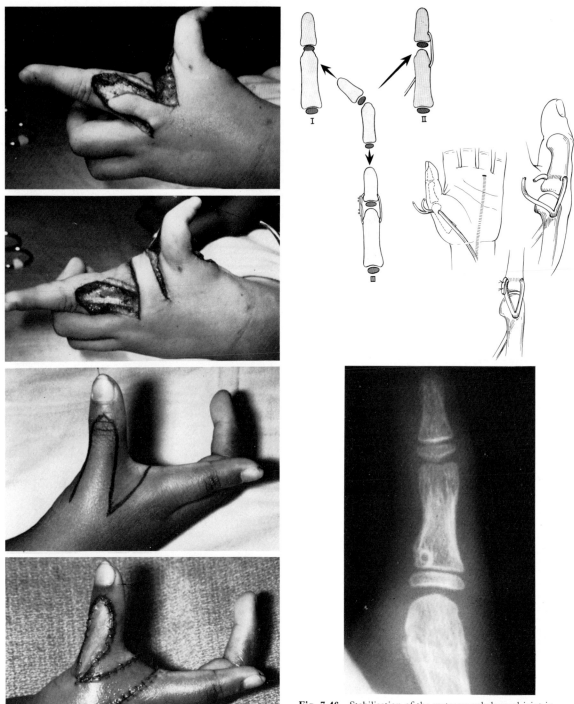

Fig. 7.45 *Transposition flaps to the first web space.* (A & B) From the dorsum of the index finger (after Brand). (C & D) From the dorsum of the thumb (after Strauch). The patients shown are, respectively, in (A & B) the patient in Figure 7.39; in (C & D) the patient shown in Figure 7.10.

Fig. 7.46 Stabilisation of the metacarpophalangeal joint in hypoplastic thumb. (A) The choice lies between (1) fusion, (2) reconstruction employing the end of a superficialis opponensplasty or, (3) tendon graft. (B) The superficialis opponensplasty is passed through the metacarpal to the ulnar aspect where it is used to reconstruct the collateral ligament in a relatively anatomical V-shape. (C) The necessary hole through the metacarpal head and the metaphysis of the proximal phalanx can be seen in this X-ray.

While preservation of joint motion is clearly desirable, stability of this particular joint is even more important. Where this cannot be achieved by either of methods (ii) or (iii), it is appropriate to resort to (i).

Partial aplasia of the thumb, in which the basal structures are normal but the distal portion absent, arises not from undergrowth but from transverse absence or constriction ring amputation. It is considered with the latter.

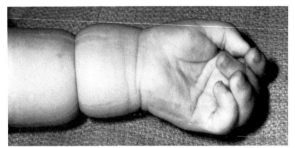

CONSTRICTION RING SYNDROME

This condition occurs sporadically, there being no evidence of heredity. The debate as to cause which commenced with Hippocrates continues[81,82] — but not here! Patterson has classified the cases as follows[83] (Fig. 7.47):

1.   Simple constriction rings
2.   Rings accompanied by distal deformity, with or without lymphoedema
3.   Rings accompanied by distal fusion — acrosyndactyly
4.   Amputations

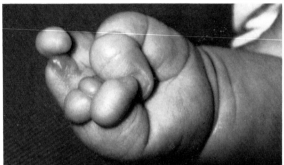

Examination should assess the urgency of the situation. This is usually indicated by severe distal lymphoedema. In the more severe cases even where no emergency exists, both circulation and neurological function will be impaired[84] and these should be assessed as far as possible by measuring temperature gradients, observing for spontaneous movement and assessing sensation by the adherence test (p. 154). The level of amputations should be accurately determined, together with the passive and active motion present in the remaining joints. The presence or absence of intrinsic muscles, especially in the thumb, should be noted from contour, palpation and observation. *X-ray evaluation* will assist in this determination, particular attention being paid in the thumb to the length of metacarpal remaining and the normal function of the basal joint.

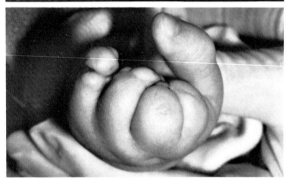

Indications
Early release of constriction rings is required, in the immediate neonatal period where oedema is gross. Contrary to traditional teaching there is no hazard in multiple, circumferential Z-plasties[14] (Fig. 7.48). Amputation fortunately usually occurs in only one or two fingers and good function can be achieved with the remaining digits, which may be enhanced by ray resection of the residual stumps. Amputation of the thumb is another matter entirely and is the major cause of *partial thumb aplasia,* the other being transverse absence.

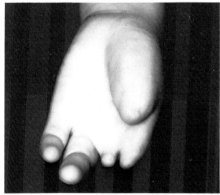

Fig. 7.47 *Constriction ring syndrome.* (A) Simple constriction ring. (B) Rings in the index, ring, and small fingers with distal deformity and lymphodema. (C) Acrosyndactyly. (D) Amputations. (The last case is that of Professor Dieter Buck-Gramcko.)

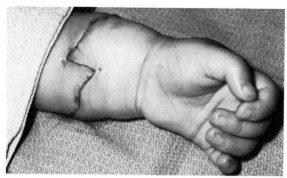

Fig. 7.48 The ring constriction shown in Figure 7.47A was safely released by multiple Z-plasties circumferentially.

Partial aplasia of the thumb is treated by one of the following procedures

1. Phalangisation
2. Metacarpal lengthening[85]
3. Toe to hand transfer[16,86]
4. Digital transfer

The considerations involved in choosing the correct procedure are *existing length, intrinsic function, presence of a basal joint* and the *condition of the other digits,* some of which have been discussed under post-traumatic thumb reconstruction (p. 122). In partial aplasia, as opposed to congenital hypoplasias, the basal joint and proximal metacarpal are sound. Digital transfer therefore is indicated only in those patients in whom the thumb can be lengthened by transfer of another congenitally amputated digit — 'on-top plasty'. Metacarpal lengthening may be stabilised after distraction either without a bone graft,[85] or with an immediate or a secondary bone graft[87].

TIMING OF SURGERY[14]

Some congenital deformities require urgent attention, such as the constriction ring which is causing severe lymphoedema. Some should be treated early although not urgently:

1. Complex syndactyly
2. Syndactyly between digits of differing length
3. Acrosyndactyly
4. Delta phalanges
5. Club hand

Others, like trigger thumb and minor clinodactyly, should be left for they may never require surgical correction. But what of the other, major, proportion of congenital anomalies of the hand? The immunologists advise us to do urgent surgery in the first five weeks while the child retains decreasing amounts of passive immunity derived from the mother, and to delay other procedures until after five months so that active immune mechanisms are sufficiently mature. The child psychologists tell us not to separate mother and child between the second and fifth birthdays, since the infant is fully aware of the trauma of separation but cannot understand its reason or its finite duration.

What are the disadvantages of early surgery? Firstly, the child of that age cannot co-operate in any rehabilitative programme. However, to wait for that co-operation would mean no surgery until age ten or twelve and in any event, the lack of co-operation is far outweighed by the enviable healing properties of infancy. Secondly, the anatomy of the hand is very small and delicate at that early age and the risk of damage must be greater than at a more mature juncture. Here lies a challenge to the surgeon — not the obvious challenge of delicate technique, but the hidden, unrecognised and therefore more potent challenge of self-evaluation. Injuries must be dealt with to the best of our ability for they are emergencies; reconstruction after injury is so influenced by tissue damage as to defy assessment; rheumatoid disease imposes its own influences on our results; release of compression syndromes demands diagnostic and anatomical knowledge more than surgical skill; only in the correction of congenital anomalies do we hand surgeons see so clearly the distinction between the craftsman and the novice. And so each must examine his training, his experience and his inclinations. There is honour, not shame, in delaying surgery or in referring infants after such honest scrutiny. Where, however, the surgeon is competent, the advantages of early surgery aided by magnification heavily outweigh any disadvantages. The results in the child's function and in the parents' contentment attest to this fact.

REFERENCES

1. Swanson A B 1976 A classification for congenital limb malformation. Journal of Hand Surgery 1: 8–22
2. Flatt A E 1977 The care of congenital hand anomalies. C V Mosby, St Louis
3. Nielsen J B 1977 Madelung's deformity: A follow-up study of 26 cases and a review of the literature. Acta Orthopaedica Scandinavica 48: 379–384
4. Miura T 1981 Congenital hand anomalies, and their association with other congenital abnormalities. The Hand 13: 267–270
5. Garn S M, Rohmann C G, Silverman F N 1967 Radiographic standards for postnatal ossification and tooth calcification. Medical Radiography and Photography 43: 45–66
6. Poznanski A K 1974 The hand in radiologic diagnosis. W B Saunders, Philadelphia
7. Lamb D W, Kuczynski K 1981 The practice of hand surgery. Blackwell, Edinburgh
8. MacDonell J A 1968 Age of fitting upper extremity prostheses in children. Journal of Bone and Joint Surgery 40A: 655–662
9. Swanson A B 1968 Restoration of hand function by the use of partial or total prosthetic replacement. Journal of Bone and Joint Surgery 45A: 276–283
10. Cowen N J, Loftus J M 1978 Distraction augmentation manoplasty — technique for lengthening digits of hands. Orthopaedic Review 7: 45–53
11. Carroll R E, Green D P 1975 Reconstruction of the hypoplastic digits. Journal of Bone and Joint Surgery 57A: 727
12. Goldberg N H and Watson H K 1982 Composite toe (phalanx and epiphysis) transfers in the reconstruction of the aphalangic hand. Journal of Hand Surgery 7: 454–459
13. Rank B K 1978 Long-term results in epiphyseal transplants in congenital deformities of the hand. Plastic and Reconstructive Surgery 61: 321–329
14. Buck-Gramcko D 1981 In: Nigst H, Buck-Gramcko D, Millesi H (eds) Handchirurgie. Georg Thieme, Stuttgart English translation 'Atlas of hand surgery' by McGregor A, edited by Lister G D, in press
15. Reid D A C 1980 The Gillies thumb lengthening operation. The Hand 12: 123–129
16. Gilbert A 1982 Toe transfers for congenital hand defects. The Journal of Hand Surgery 7: 118–124
17. Lamb D W 1977 Radial club hand. A continuing study of sixty-eight patients with one hundred and seventeen club hands. Journal of Bone and Joint Surgery 59A: 1–13
18. Skerik S K, Flatt A E 1969 The anatomy of congenital radial dysplasia. Clinical Orthopaedics 66: 125–143
19. Menelaus M B 1976 Radial club hand with absence of the biceps muscle treated by centralisation of the ulna and triceps transfer. Journal of Bone and Joint Surgery 58B: 488–491
20. Riordan D C 1955 and 1963 Congenital absence of the radius. Journal of Bone and Joint Surgery 37A: 1129–1140 and 45A: 1783
21. Bora F W, Nicholson J T, Cheema H M 1970 Radial meromelia. Journal of Bone and Joint Surgery 52A: 966–979
22. Bora F W, Osterman A L, Kaneda R R, Esterhal J 1981 Radial club-hand deformity. Journal of Bone and Joint Surgery 63A: 741–745
23. Nutt J N, Flatt A E 1981 Congenital central hand deficit. Journal of Hand Surgery 6: 48–60
24. Barsky A J 1964 Cleft hand: classification, incidence and treatment. Journal of Bone and Joint Surgery, 46A: 1707–1720
25. Maisels D O 1970 Lobster-claw deformities of the hands and feet. British Journal of Plastic Surgery 23: 269–282
26. Snow J W, Littler J W 1967 Surgical treatment of cleft hand. Transaction of the Fourth International Congress of Plastic and Reconstructive Surgery 888–893
27. Miura T, Komada T 1979 Simple method for reconstruction of the cleft hand with an adducted thumb. Plastic and Reconstructive Surgery 64: 65–67
28. Green W T, Mital M 1979 Congenital radio-ulnar synostosis: Surgical treatment. Journal of Bone and Joint Surgery 61A: 738–743
29. Flatt A E, Wood V E 1975 Rigid digits or symphalangism. The Hand 7: 197–214
30. Cushing H 1916 Hereditary anchylosis of proximal phalangeal joints (symphalangism). Genetics 1: 90–106
31. Smith R J, Kaplan E B 1968 Camptodactyly and similar atraumatic flexion deformities of the PIP joints of the fingers. A study of 31 cases. Journal of Bone and Joint Surgery 50A: 1187–1203
32. Engber W D, Flatt A E 1977 Camptodactyly: An analysis of sixty-six patients and twenty-four operations. Journal of Hand Surgery 2: 216–224
33. Burke F, Flatt A 1979 Clinodactyly — a review of a series of cases. The Hand 11: 269–280
34. Watson H K, Boyes J H 1967 Congenital angular deformity of the digits — delta phalanx. Journal of Bone and Joint Surgery 49A: 333–338
35. Wood V E, Flatt A E 1977 Congenital triangular bones in the hand. Journal of Hand Surgery 2: 179–193
36. Theander G, Carstam N 1974 Longitudinally bracketed diaphysis. Annales de Radiologie 17: 355–360
37. Weckesser E C, Reed J R, Heiple K G 1968 Congenital clasped thumb (congenital flexion-adduction deformity of the thumb). Journal of Bone and Joint Surgery 37A: 1417–1428
38. Entin M A 1976 Syndactyly of upper limb. Clinics in Plastic Surgery 3: 129–140
39. Maisels D O 1962 Acrosyndactyly. British Journal of Plastic Surgery 15: 166–172
40. Walsh R J 1970 Acrosyndactyly: a study of 27 patients. Clinical Orthopaedics 71: 99–111
41. Ravitch M M 1977 Poland's syndrome — a study of an eponym. Plastic and Reconstructive Surgery 59: 508–512
42. Sugiura Y 1976 Poland's syndrome' Clinico-roentgenographic study on 45 cases. Cong. Anom. 16: 17–28
43. Ireland D C R, Takayama N, Flatt A E 1976 Poland's syndrome. A review of forty-three cases. Journal of Bone and Joint Surgery 58A: 52–58
44. Epstein L I, Bennett J E 1970 Syndactyly with ipsilateral chest deformity. Plastic and Reconstructive Surgery 46: 236–240
45. Hoover G H, Flatt A E, Weiss M W 1970 The hand in Apert's syndrome. Journal of Bone and Joint Surgery 52A: 878–895
46. Johannson S H 1982 Nagelwallbildung durch Thenarlappen bei Kompletter Syndaktylie, Handchirurgie 14: 199–203
47. Stelling F 1963 The upper extremity. In: Ferguson A B (ed) Orthopaedic surgery in infancy and childhood, vol 2. Williams and Wilkins, Baltimore, pp 304–308
48. Wassel H D 1969 The results of surgery for polydactyly of the thumb. Clinical Orthopaedics 64: 175–193
49. Marks T W, Bayne L G 1978 Polydactyly of the thumb: Abnormal anatomy and treatment. Journal of Hand Surgery 3: 107–116
50. Hartrampf C R, Vasconez L O, Mathes S 1975 Construction of one good thumb from both parts of a congenitally bifid thumb. Plastic and Reconstructive Surgery 54: 148–152

51. Miura T 1977 An appropriate treatment for post-operative Z-formed deformity of the duplicated thumb. Journal of Hand Surgery 2: 380–386
52. Miura T 1976 Triphalangeal thumb. Plastic and Reconstructive Surgery 58: 587–594
53. Wood V 1978 Polydactyly and the triphalangeal thumb. Journal of Hand Surgery 3: 436–444
54. Wood V E 1971 Treatment of central polydactyly. Clinical Orthopaedics 74: 196–205
55. Frykman G, Wood V 1978 Peripheral nerve hamartoma with macrodactyly in the hand: Report of three cases and review of the literature. Journal of Hand Surgery 3: 307–312
56. Edgerton M T, Tuerk D B 1974 Macrodactyly (digital gigantism): its nature and treatment. In: Littler J W, Cramer L M, Smith J W (eds) Symposium on Reconstructive Hand Surgery. C V Mosby Co, St Louis, pp 157–172
57. Barsky A 1967 Macrodactyly. Journal of Bone and Joint Surgery 49A: 1255–1266
58. Allende B T 1967 Macrodactyly with enlarged median nerve associated with carpal tunnel syndrome. Plastic and Reconstructive Surgery 39: 578–582
59. Rousso M, Katz S, Khodadadi D 1976 Treatment of a case of macrodactyly of the thumb. The Hand 8: 131–133
60. Tsuge K 1967 Treatment of macrodactyly. Plastic and Reconstructive Surgery 39: 590–599
61. Blauth W 1967 Der hypoplastische Daumen. Arch. Orthop. Unfall. Chir. 62: 225–246
62. Fromont: 1895 Anomalies musculaires multiples de la main. Absence due flechisseur propre du pouce. Absence des muscles de l'eminence thenar; lombricaux supplementaires. Bull. Soc. Anat. Paris. 70: 395–401
63. Neviaser R 1979 Congenital hypoplasia of the thumb with absence of the extrinsic extensors, abductor pollicus longus and thenar muscles. Journal of Hand Surgery 4: 301–304
64. Edgerton M T, Snyder C B, Webb W L 1965 Surgical treatment of congenital thumb deformities. Journal of Bone and Joint Surgery 47A: 1453–1474
65. Miura T 1977 Congenital absence of the flexor pollicis longus. The Hand 9: 272–274
66. Tsuchida Y, Kasai S, Kojima T 1976 Congenital absence of flexor pollicis longus and flexor pollicis brevis: A case report. The Hand 8: 294–297
67. Tupper J W 1969 Pollex abductus due to congenital malposition of the flexor pollicis longus. Journal of Bone and Joint Surgery 51A: 1285–1290
68. Kobayashi A, Ohmiya K, Iwakuma T, Mitsuyasu M 1976 Unusual congenital anomalies of the thumb extensors. The Hand 8: 17–21
69. Buck-Gramcko D 1971 Pollicisation of the index finger. Journal of Bone and Joint Surgery 53A: 1605–1617
70. Buck-Gramcko D 1977 Thumb reconstruction by digital transposition. Orthopaedic Clinics of North America 8: 329–342
71. Blair W F, Omer G E 1981 Anomalous insertion of the flexor pollicis longus. Journal of Hand Surgery 6: 241–244
72. Strauch B, Spinner M 1976 Congenital anomaly of the thumb: Absent intrinsics and flexor pollicis longus. Journal of Bone and Joint Surgery 58A: 115–118
73. Su C T, Hoopes J E, Daniel R 1972 Congenital absence of the thenar muscles innervated by the median nerve. Journal of Bone and Joint Surgery 54A: 1087–1090
74. Arminio J A 1979 Congenital anomaly of the thumb: Absent flexor pollicis longus tendon. Journal of Hand Surgery 4: 487–488
75. Lister G D, Milward T M 1975 Skin contracture of the first web space. Transactions Sixth International Congress of Plastic and Reconstructive Surgery 594–604 Paris
76. Strauch B 1975 Dorsal thumb flap for release of adduction contracture of the first web space. Bulletin of the Hospital for Joint Diseases 36: 34–39
77. Flatt A E, Wood V 1970 Multiple dorsal rotation from the hand for thumb web contractures. Plastic and Reconstructive Surgery 45: 258–262
78. Huber E 1921 Hilssoperation bei medianuslahmung. Deutsche Zeitschrift für Chirurgie 162: 271–275
79. Littler J W, Cooley S G E 1963 Opposition of the thumb and its restoration by abductor digiti quinti transfer. Journal of Bone and Joint Surgery 45A: 1389–1396
80. Manske P, McCarroll H 1978 Abductor digiti minimi opponensplasty in congenital radial dysplasia. Journal of Hand Surgery 3: 552–559
81. Field J H, Krag D O 1973 Congenital constricting bands and congenital amputation of the fingers: placental studies. Journal of Bone and Joint Surgery 55A: 1035–1041
82. Yoshitake K 1975 Clinical and experimental studies of the congenital constriction band syndrome, with an emphasis on its etiology. The Journal of Bone and Joint Surgery 57A: 636–642
83. Patterson T J S 1961 Congenital ring-constrictions. British Journal of Plastic Surgery 14: 1–31
84. Moses J M, Flatt A E, Cooper R R 1979 Annular constricting bands. Journal of Bone and Joint Surgery 61A: 562–565
85. Matev J 1979 Thumb reconstruction in children through metacarpal lengthening. Plastic and Reconstructive Surgery 64: 665–669
86. Yoshimura M 1980 Toe-to-hand transfer. Plastic and Reconstructive Surgery 66: 74–83
87. Kessler I, Baruch A, Hecht O Experience with distraction lengthening of digital rays in congenital anomalies. Journal of Hand Surgery 2: 394–401

FURTHER READING

Barsky A J 1951 Congenital anomalies of the hand and their surgical treatment. Journal of Bone and Joint Surgery 33A: 35–64

Boyes J G 1977 Macrodactylism — a review and proposed management. The Hand 9: 172–180

Buck-Gramcko D 1975 Congenital malformations of the hand: Indications, operative treatment and results. Scandinavian Journal of Plastic and Reconstructive Surgery 9: 190–198

Buck-Gramcko D 1981 Hand surgery in congenital malformations. In: Jackson I T (ed) Recent advances in plastic surgery. Churchill Livingstone, Edinburgh

Burman M 1972 Note on duplication of the index finger. Journal of Bone and Joint Surgery 54A: 884

Courtemanche A D 1969 Campylodactyly: etiology and management. Plastic and Reconstructive Surgery 44: 451–454

Dellon A L, Hansen F 1980 Bilateral inability to grasp due to multiple (ten) congenital trigger fingers. The Journal of Hand Surgery 5: 470–472

Engber W D 1981 Cleft hand and pectoral aplasia. Journal of Hand Surgery 6: 574–577

Entin M A 1960 Congenital anomalies of the upper extremity. Surgical Clinics of North America 40: 497

Gonzalez-Crussi F, Lee S C, McKinney M 1977 The pathology of congenital localized giantism. Plastic and Reconstructive Surgery 59: 411–417

Harrison S H 1970 Pollicisation in cases of radial club hand. British Journal of Plastic Surgery 23: 192–200

Huffstadt A J C 1981 Polydactyly — bifid thumb. The Hand 13: 81–84

Jones G B 1964 Delta phalanx. Journal of Bone and Joint Surgery 46B: 226–228

Kelikian H, Doumahian A 1959 Congenital anomalies of the hand. Journal of Bone and Joint Surgery 39A: 1002–1019

Losch G M, Duncker H R 1972 Anatomy and surgical treatment of syndactylism. Plastic and Reconstructive Surgery 50: 167–173

Marumo E, Kojima T, Masuzawa G 1980 Cleft hand and its surgical treatment. Annals of Plastic Surgery 5: 40–50

Miura T 1981 A clinical study of congenital anomalies of the hand. The Hand 13: 59–68

Miura T 1976 Syndactyly and split hand. The Hand 8: 125–130

Miura T 1981 Congenital anomaly of the thumb: Unusual bifurcation of the flexor pollicis longus and its unusual insertion. Journal of Hand Surgery 6: 613–615

Murakami Y, Edashige K 1980 Anomalous flexor pollicis longus muscle. The Hand 12: 82–84

Nathan P A, Keniston R C 1975 Crossed polydactyly: Case report and review of the literature. Journal of Bone and Joint Surgery 57A: 847–848

Opgrande J D 1982 Constriction ring syndrome: Unusual case report. Journal of Hand Surgery 7: 11–12

Palmieri T J 1980 The use of silicone rubber implant arthroplasty in treatment of true symphalangism. Journal of Hand Surgery 5: 242–244

Phillips R S 1971 Congenital split foot (lobster claw) and triphalangeal thumb. Journal of Bone and Joint Surgery 53B: 247–257

Schulstad I, Skoglund K 1979 Surgical treatment of simple syndactyly. Scandinavian Journal of Plastic and Reconstructive Surgery 11: 235–237

Skoog T 1965 Syndactyly: A clinical report on repair. Acta Chirurgica Scandinavica 130: 537–549

Snowdy H A, Omer G E, Sherman F C 1980 Longitudinal growth of a free toe phalanx transplant to a finger. Journal of Hand Surgery 5: 71–73

Tada K, Yonenobu K, Swanson A 1981 Congenital central ray deficiency in the hand. A survey of 59 cases and subclassification. Journal of Hand Surgery 6: 434–441

Thorne F L, Posch J L, Mladick R A 1968 Megalodactyly. Plastic and Reconstructive Surgery 41: 232–239

Tuch B A, Lipp E B, Larsen I J, Gordon L H 1977 A review of supernumerary thumb and its surgical management. Clinical Orthopaedics 125: 159–167

Ueba Y 1981 Plastic surgery for the cleft hand. Journal of Hand Surgery 6: 557–560

Watari S, Tsuge K 1979 A classification of cleft hands, based on clinical findings. Plastic and Reconstructive Surgery 64: 381–389

Appendix: Muscle testing

Figure No.	Muscle	Abbreviation	Action	Nerve	Cord	Root
A.1(a)	Supraspinatus	SS	External rotation of arm fixes shoulder in carrying	Suprascapular (from upper trunk)	—	C5(6)
A.1(b)	Infraspinatus	IS	External rotation of arm	Suprascapular	—	C5 (6)
A.1(c)	Teres major	TMa	Internal rotation of arm adduction, extension	Lower subscapular	Posterior	C6 (7)
A.2	Pectoralis major	PM	Internal rotation of arm	Lateral pectoral Medial pectoral	Lateral Medial	C5 6 C7 8
A.3	Latissimus dorsi	LD	Adduction of arm	Arises from cord	Posterior	C6 7 8
A.4	Deltoid	D	Abduction of arm	Axillary	Posterior	C5 (6)

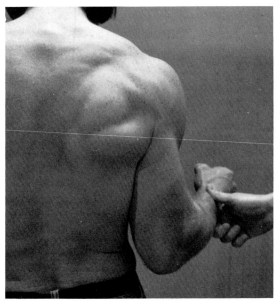
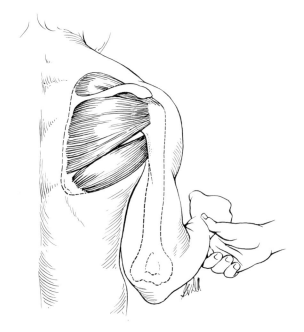

Fig. A.1 a-c

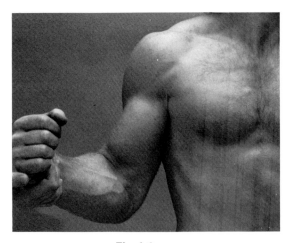
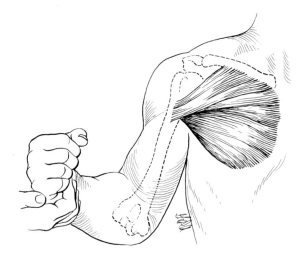

Fig. A.2

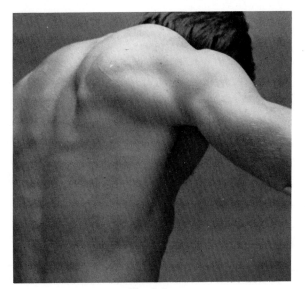
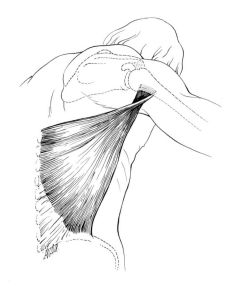

Fig. A.3

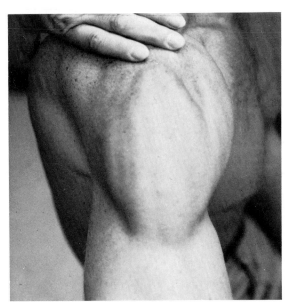
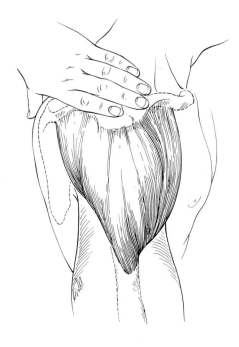

Fig. A.4

Figure No.	Muscle	Abbreviation	Action	Nerve	Cord	Root
A.5	Serratus anterior	SA	Forward rotation of scapula (absence produces 'winging')	Arises directly from roots	—	C5 6 7
A.6	Biceps	BB	Flexion of elbow supination of forearm (flexed)	Musculocutaneous	Lateral	C5 (6)
A.7	Triceps	T	Extension of elbow	Radial	Posterior	C(6) 7
A.8	Brachioradialis	BR	Flexion of elbow	Radial	Posterior	C6
A.9	Pronator teres	PT	Pronation of forearm (extended)	Median	Lateral	C6 7
A.10	Pronator quadratus	PQ	Pronation of forearm (flexed)	Ant. interosseous (median)	Lateral	C7
A.11	Supinator	S	Supination of forearm (extended)	Post. interosseous (radial)	Posterior	C6

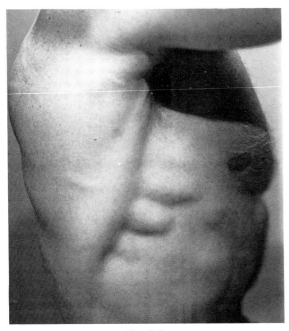
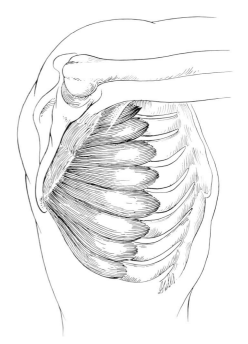

Fig. A.5

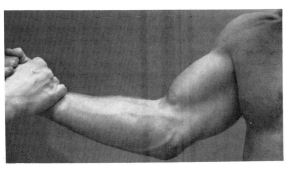
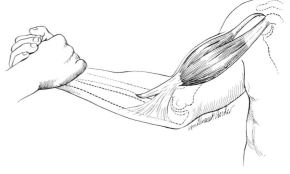

Fig. A.6

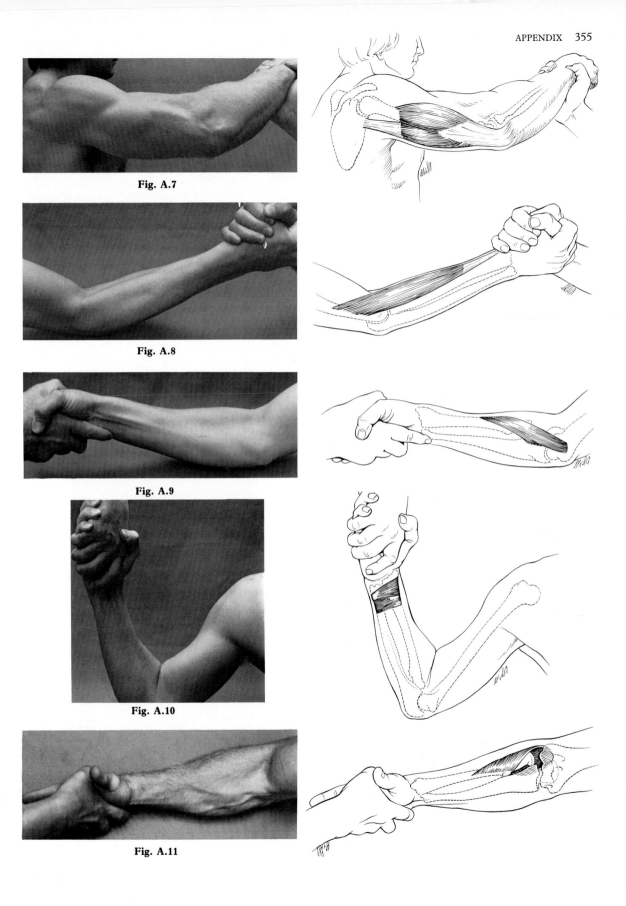

Fig. A.7

Fig. A.8

Fig. A.9

Fig. A.10

Fig. A.11

Figure No.	Muscle	Abbreviation	Action	Nerve	Cord	Root
A.12	Flexor carpi radialis	FCR	Flexion of wrist	Median	Lateral	C6 7
A.13	Flexor carpi ulnaris	FCU	Flexion of wrist Ulnar deviation of wrist	Ulnar	Medial	C8
A.14	Palmaris longus	PL	—	Median	Medial	C8
A.15(a)	Flexor digitorum superficialis	FDS	Flexion of PIP joints	Median	Medial	C7 8
A.15(b)	Flexor digitorum superficialis (index)					
A.16	Flexor digitorum profundus	FDP	Flexion of DIP joints	Anterior interosseous (index and middle) Ulnar (ring and small)	Medial Medial	C8 C8
A.17	Flexor pollicis longus	FPL	Flexion of thumb IP joint	Ant. interosseous	Medial	C8

(see page 29 for explanation of A.15, a and b)

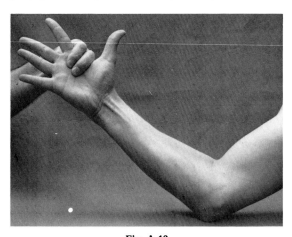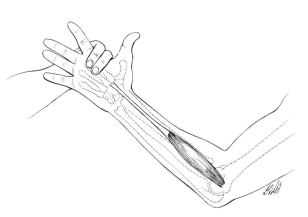

Fig. A.12

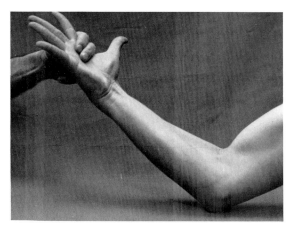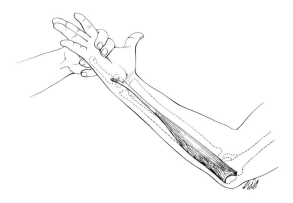

Fig. A.13

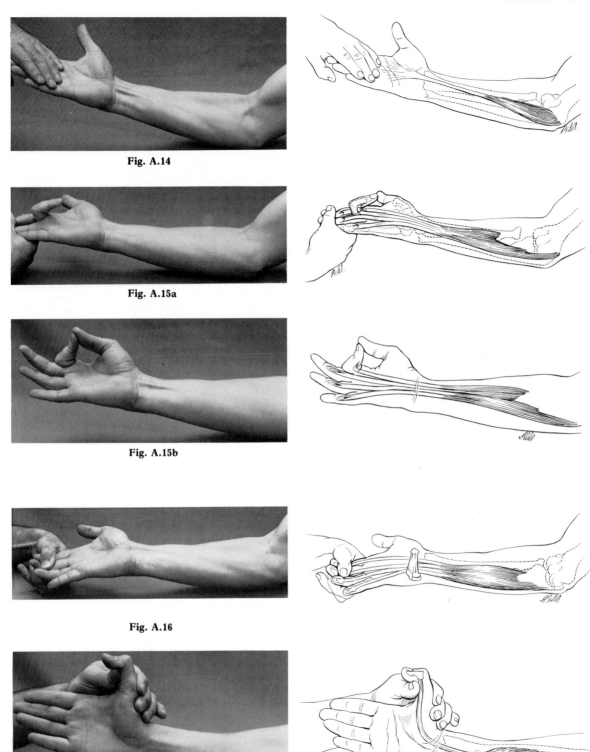

Fig. A.14

Fig. A.15a

Fig. A.15b

Fig. A.16

Fig. A.17

Figure No.	Muscle	Abbreviation	Action	Nerve	Cord	Root
A.18	Flexor pollicis brevis	FPB	Flexion of MP joint of thumb	Median (superficial head) Ulnar (deep head)	Medial	T1
A.19	Abductor pollicis brevis	APB	Abduction of thumb (extension of IP joint)	Median	Medial	T1
A.20	Adductor pollicis	AP	Adduction of thumb (extension of IP joint)	Ulnar	Medial	T1
A.21	Abductor digiti minimi	ADM	Abduction of small finger	Ulnar	Medial	T1
A.22	Flexor digiti minimi	FDM	Flexion of MP joint of small finger	Ulnar	Medial	T1

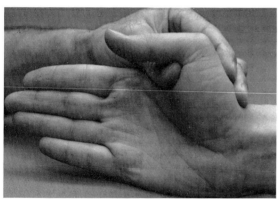
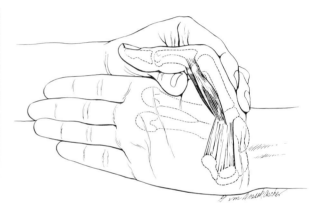

Fig. A.18

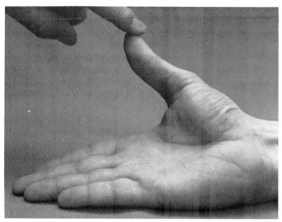
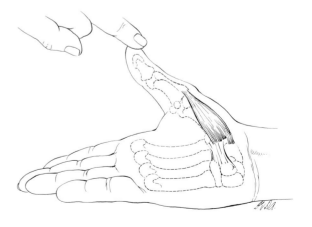

Fig. A.19

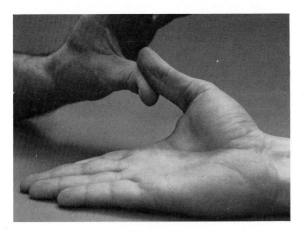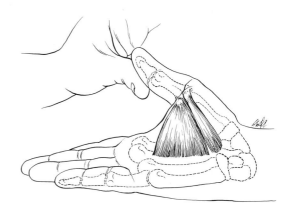

Fig. A.20

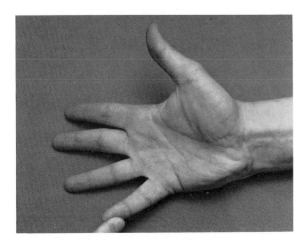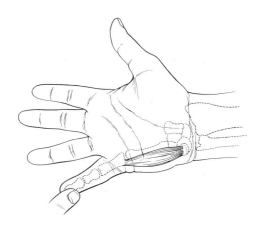

Fig. A.21

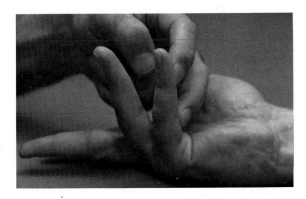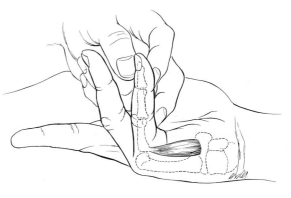

Fig. A.22

Figure No.	Muscle	Abbreviation	Action	Nerve	Cord	Root
	Interosseous		*Line of reference is axis of middle finger*			
	Dorsal		*Dorsal ABduct 'DAB'*			
A.23	1st	1st DIO	Abducts index finger	Ulnar	Medial	T1
A.24	2nd	2nd DIO	Abducts middle finger radially	Ulnar	Medial	T1
A.25	3rd	3rd DIO	Abducts middle finger ulnar-wards	Ulnar	Medial	T1
A.26	4th	4th DIO	Abducts ring finger	Ulnar	Medial	T1
	Palmar		*Palmar ADduct 'PAD'*			
A.27	1st	1st PIO	Adducts index finger	Ulnar	Medial	T1
A.28	2nd	2nd PIO	Adducts ring finger	Ulnar	Medial	T1
A.29	3rd	3rd PIO	Adducts small finger	Ulnar	Medial	T1

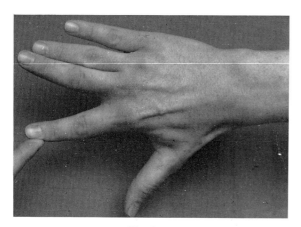

Fig. A.23

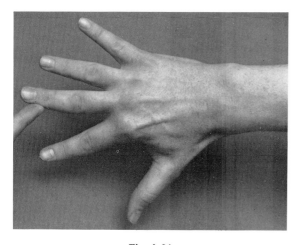

Fig. A.24

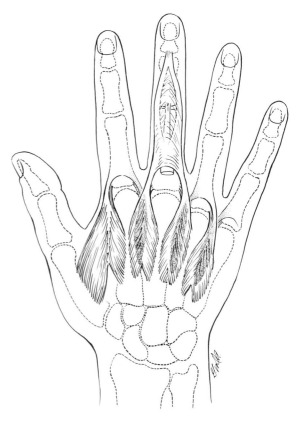

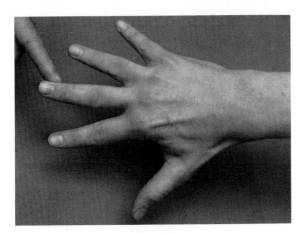

Fig. A.25

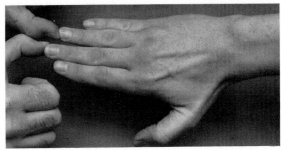

Fig. A.28

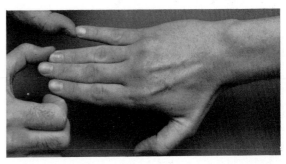

Fig. A.29

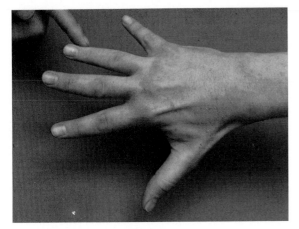

Fig. A.26

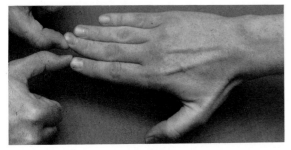

Fig. A.27

Figure No.	Muscle	Abbreviation	Action	Nerve	Cord	Root
A.30	Extensor pollicis longus	EPL	Extension of IP joint of thumb (with AP and APB)	Posterior interosseous (radial)	Posterior	C7 8
A.31	Extensor pollicis brevis	EPB	Extension of MP joint of thumb	Posterior interosseous	Posterior	C7 8
A.32	Abductor pollicis longus	APL	Extension of CM joint of thumb Radial deviation of wrist	Posterior interosseous	Posterior	C7 8
A.33	Extensor digitorum	ED	Extension of MP joints	Posterior interosseous	Posterior	C7 (8)
A.34	Extensor indicis	EI	Extension of index	Posterior interosseous	Posterior	C7 8

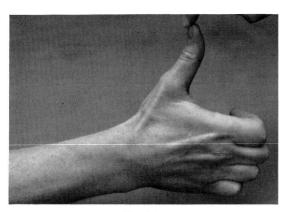 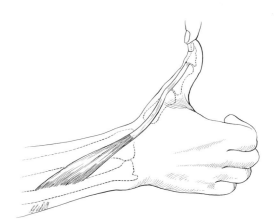

Fig. A.30

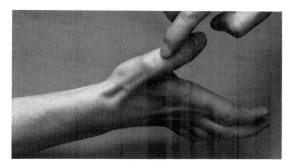 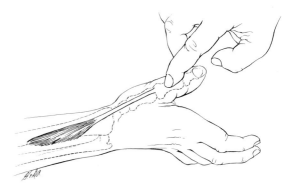

Fig. A.31

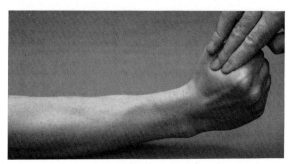 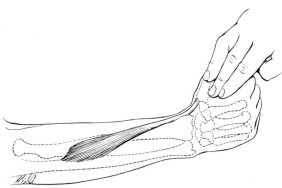

Fig. A.32

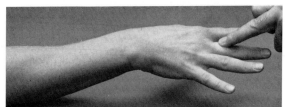 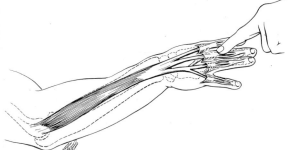

Fig. A.33

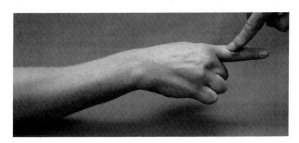 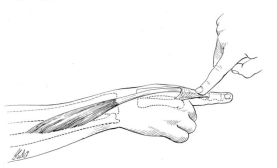

Fig. A.34

A.35	Extensor digiti minimi	EDM	Extension of small	Posterior interosseous	Posterior	C7 8
A.36	Extensor carpi ulnaris	ECU	Extension of wrist Ulnar deviation of wrist	Posterior interosseous	Posterior	C7 (8)
A.37	Extensor carpi radialis longus and brevis	ECRL ECRB	Extension of wrist Radial deviation of wrist	Radial	Posterior	C6 7

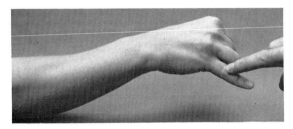

Fig. A.35

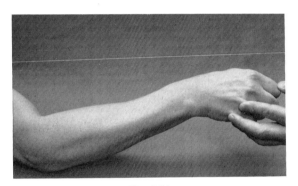

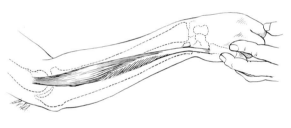

Fig. A.36

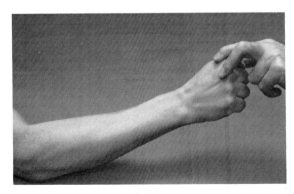

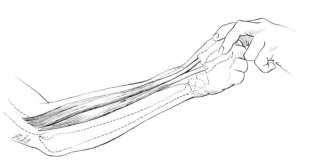

Fig. A.37

Index

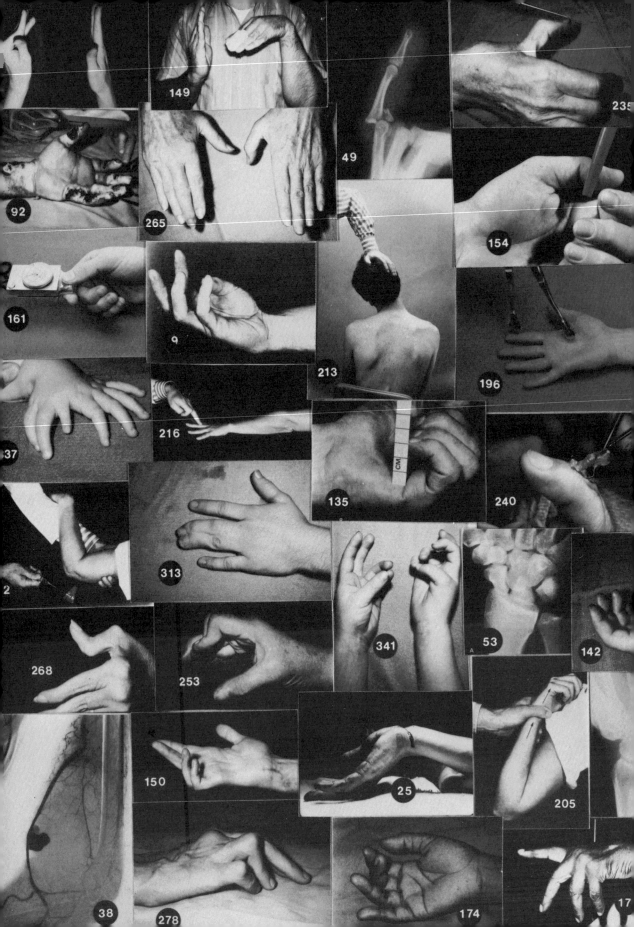